Barcelona Oct 1 2008

To Shantel Archuleta,

Best of luck in your future endeavours, and happy cooking!

Stephan Mayer

THERAPEUTIC HYPOTHERMIA

edited by

Stephan A. Mayer
Columbia University Medical Center
New York, New York, U.S.A.

Daniel I. Sessler
University of Louisville
Louisville, Kentucky, U.S.A.

MARCEL DEKKER

MARCEL DEKKER NEW YORK

Published in 2005 by
Taylor & Francis Group
6000 Broken Sound Parkway NW, Suite 300
Boca Raton, FL 33487-2742

Printed in the United States of America on acid-free paper
10 9 8 7 6 5 4 3
International Standard Book Number 0-8247-5478-6 (Hardcover)
International Standard Book Number-13: 978-0-000-00000-0 (Hardcover)

Library of Congress Cataloging-in-Publication Data

Catalog record is available from the Library of Congress

T&F informa

Taylor & Francis Group
is the Academic Division of T&F Informa plc.

Visit the Taylor & Francis Web site at
http://www.taylorandfrancis.com

Foreword

I don't know who first suggested that cooling the body might be beneficial. It's clearly an old idea. Perhaps it originated with the observation that cooling a localized injury reduced pain and swelling. Or maybe it came from the first person to watch a ground squirrel awaken from a winter's hibernation. Somewhere, sometime, someone watched an apparently dead child or sailor awaken after immersion in icy water. Or did overly aggressive efforts to reduce a patients fever have some surprising consequences. Regardless, "therapeutic hypothermia" is something that has captured the imagination of both the lay public (think "suspended animation" and a plethora of science fiction stories and movies) and the medical profession.

Medical interest in hypothermia dates to at least the mid-19th century, but its first clinical uses can be found in the 1940's. In 1942, Temple Fay, in Philadelphia reported on several patients with severe head injuries who made apparently remarkable recoveries after being cooled. In the 1950's, cooling for both cardiac surgery and neurosurgery was tried in many centers. I suspect that many readers have seen pictures of anesthetized patients immersed in bathtubs of ice prior to undergoing open cardiac procedures in the pre-bypass era. However, such interest waned rapidly—in large part due to severe complications. These were due to our limited understanding of the consequences of cooling and the relatively primative technology for monitoring and providing physiologic support.

This changed radically due to two events. The introduction of cardiopulmonary bypass allowed cardiac patients to be easily cooled and rewarmed—resulting in the near-routine use of hypothermia for many procedures, including deep hypothermia and circulatory arrest (which to this day provides incontrovertable evidence that hypothermia can protect the brain). Then, in the 1980's, several laboratories demonstrated in animals that *mild* hypothermia—which could be easily achieved with simple methods—resulted in protection of the brain during global and focal cerebral ischemia and trauma. Other studies showed that cooling instituted even AFTER an insult could improve outcome.

The genie was, thereafter, out of the proverbial bottle. Mild or moderate hypothermia was rapidly applied in many different situations: operative neurosurgery (particularly neurovascular surgery), cardiac arrest, head trauma etc. Many uncontrolled "studies" began to appear in the literature. As one example, a recent survey from Great Britain reported that hypothermia was being used in over 50% of patients undergoing intracranial aneurysm surgery. The problem, of course, was that such therapy was being applied without accompanying evidence of actual efficacy—at a time when other work was demonstrating the clear adverse events of cooling on such things as perioperative myocardial ischemia, coagulation, postoperative awakening, wound infections etc.

At the present time, the best available information regarding hypothermia is exceptionally mixed. In 2001, Clifton et al. reported that mild hypothermia instituted after severe closed head injury did not improve outcome. Other studies failed to show improved neurologic outcome in routine cardiac surgery patients cooled on bypass. Then, in 2002, two groups separately demonstrated that post-resuscitation cooling improved neurologic outcome in cardiac arrest victims. More recently, however, our group was unable to demonstrate any benefit to intraoperative cooling in patients undergoing open aneurym clippings.

There is a great deal more work to be done. This book does an outstanding job of reviewing our understanding of the physiology of body temperature alternations, of the impact of cooling on critical organs, and of updating the current status of clinical hypothermia. However, so much more information is needed. Does hypothermia improve outcome after trauma when instituted sooner than was possible in the Clifton trial? Does hypothermia improve outcome after stroke? Can hypothermia be applied successfully to a broader range of patients with cardiac arrest? Are there other conditions that might benefit? This book should provide a wonderful starting point for those interested in answering these questions.

Preface

Therapeutic hypothermia is becoming an important treatment for patients with acute brain injury, and is now under investigation for treatment of acute myocardial infarction. Although the cardiac and neuroprotective effects of hypothermia have been recognized in animals for decades, clinical interest was dormant until a resurgence of experimental studies in the early 1990's reawakened interest. These studies — many performed in the laboratory of one of our contributors, Dr. Myron Ginsberg — made it clear that even tiny variations in brain temperature powerfully modulate the extent of neuronal damage in various models of ischemic and traumatic brain injury.

Therapeutic hypothermia has attracted interest lately because pharmacologic interventions have consistently failed to improve outcome after stroke and trauma. Interest is largely predicated on evidence that hypothermia acts via a diverse array of molecular mechanisms and may thus prove to be the best method of inducing neuroprotection. This has led to an understanding that body temperature, like other physiologic parameters, should be deliberately optimized in individual patients. New technologies including circulating-water garments and endovascular heat-exchange cathethers make it relatively easy to manipulate body temperature.

The apogee of clinical work in therapeutic hypothermia to date occurred in February of 2002 with the publication of two landmark clinical trials demonstrating dramatic improvement in outcome with mild-to-moderate hypothermia for survivors of out-of-hospital cardiac arrest. It is our expectation that these are just the first of many outcomes studies that will demonstrate the benefits of therapeutic hypothermia in various patient populations.

In short, therapeutic temperature modulation and hypothermia is not only a major new field of investigation, it is a new and important development in the clinical practice of emergency medicine, neurology, neurosurgery, critical care medicine, cardiology, and neurological and cardiac anesthesiology. Our purpose in creating this book was to provide health care providers and investigators with a comprehensive reference on this new and previously under-emphasized field of medicine. Our hope is that the information within will encourage clinicians to use therapeutic hypothermia when appropriate and investigators to develop new indications for therapeutic thermal management with the ultimate goal of saving lives and improving outcomes in patients with ischemic events.

STEPHAN A. MAYER, MD
New York, NY

DANIEL A. SESSLER, MD
Louisville, KY

August 19, 2004

Contents

Section Two: Consequences of Hypothermia

Section Three: Therapeutic Temperature Modulation

Section Four: Clinical Applications of Therapeutic Hypothermia

Contributors

Ozan Akça Outcomes Research™ Institute and Department of Anesthesiology and Perioperative Medicine, University of Louisville, Louisville, Kentucky, U.S.A.

Peter J.D. Andrews Anaesthetics, Pain Medicine, and Intensive Care, Western General Hospital, Edinburgh, Scotland

Ludmila Belayev Cerebral Vascular Disease Research Center, Department of Neurology, University of Miami School of Medicine, Miami, Florida, U.S.A.

Stephen Bernard Intensive Care Unit, Dandenong Hospital, Dandenong, Australia

Jan Claassen Division of Critical Care Neurology, Department of Neurology, Columbia University College of Physicians and Surgeons, New York, New York, U.S.A.

Anupa Deogaonkar Cleveland Clinic Foundation, Cleveland, Ohio, U.S.A.

Simon R. Dixon William Beaumont Hospital, Royal Oak, Michigan, U.S.A.

Michael De Georgia Neurological Intensive Care Unit, Cleveland Clinic Foundation, Cleveland, Ohio, U.S.A.

Myron D. Ginsberg Cerebral Vascular Disease Research Center, Department of Neurology, University of Miami School of Medicine, Miami, Florida, U.S.A.

Bridget A. Harris Western General Hospital, University of Edinburgh, Edinburgh, Scotland

Bradley J. Hindman Department of Anesthesiology, Roy J. and Lucille A. Carver College of Medicine, The University of Iowa, Iowa City, Iowa, U.S.A.

Roman Hlatky Department of Neurosurgery, Baylor College of Medicine, Houston, Texas, U.S.A.

Rainer Kollmar Department of Neurology, University of Heidelberg, Im Neuenheimer Feld, Heidelberg, Germany

Rainer Lenhardt Outcomes Research™ Institute and the Department of Anesthesiology and Perioperative Medicine, University of Louisville, Louisville, Kentucky, U.S.A.

Donald W. Marion The Brain Trauma Foundation, New York, New York, U.S.A.

Stephan A. Mayer Division of Critical Care Neurology, Department of Neurology, Columbia University College of Physicians and Surgeons, New York, New York, U.S.A.

Fabian Meisel University of Heidelberg, Im Neuenheimer Feld, Heidelberg, Germany

Thomas L. Merrill Biomedical Engineering Department, Wyeth Research, Princeton, New Jersey, U.S.A.

William W. O'Neill William Beaumont Hospital, Royal Oak, Michigan, U.S.A.

Claudia S. Robertson Department of Neurosurgery, Baylor College of Medicine, Houston, Texas, U.S.A.

Stefan Schwab Department of Neurology, University of Heidelberg, Im Neuenheimer Feld, Heidelberg, Germany

Daniel I. Sessler Outcomes Research™ Institute and Department of Anesthesiology and Perioperative Medicine, University of Louisville, Louisville, Kentucky, U.S.A.

Gary K. Steinberg Stanford Stroke Center, Stanford University School of Medicine, Stanford, California, U.S.A.

Thorsten Steiner University of Heidelberg, Im Neuenheimer Feld, Heidelberg, Germany

Christine A. C. Wijman Department of Neurology and Neurological Sciences, Stanford University School of Medicine, Stanford, California, U.S.A.

Midori A. Yenari Department of Neurosurgery, Stanford University School of Medicine, Stanford, California, U.S.A.

AUTHOR DISCLOSURES

Ozan Akça, MD has no conflicts of interest to disclose.

Peter J.D. Andrews, MD has no conflicts of interest to disclose

Ludmila Belayev, MD has no conflicts of interest to disclose.

Stephen Bernard, MD has no conflicts of interest to disclose.

Jan Claassen, MD has no conflicts of interest to disclose.

Michael De Georgia, MD has received grant support from Radiant Medical, Inc.

Anupa Deogaonkar, MD has no conflicts of interest to disclose.

Simon R. Dixon, MD has no conflicts of interest to disclose.

Myron D. Ginsberg, MD has no conflicts of interest to disclose.

Bridget A. Harris, MD has no conflicts of interest to disclose.

Bradley J. Hindman, MD has no conflicts of interest to disclose.

Roman Hlatky, MD has no conflicts of interest to disclose.

Rainer Kollmar, MD has no conflicts of interest to disclose.

Rainer Lenhart, MD has no conflicts of interest to disclose.

Donald W. Marion, MD has no conflicts of interest to disclose.

Stephan A. Mayer, MD holds stock options from and is on the scientific advisory board of Radiant Medical Inc.; has received research funding, speaking honoraria, consulting fees and stock options from Medivance, Inc; and has received consulting fees from Seacoast Technologies, Inc.

Fabian Meisel, MD has no conflicts of interest to disclose.

Thomas L. Merrill, Ph.D. has no conflicts of interest to disclose.

William W. O'Neill, MD is a consultant for Radiant Medical, Inc.

Claudia S. Robertson, MD has no financial conflicts of interest to disclose.

Stefan Schwab, MD has no conflicts of interest to disclose.

Daniel I. Sessler, MD is a consultant for Radiant Medical, Inc. Kimberly Clark, Inc. and Cardinal Health, Inc. The Outcomes Research Institute is primarily funded by the National Institutes of Health but also has had research contracts with numerous corporations. Currently, the Institute has research contracts with Engineered Medical Systems, Inc. and Augustine Medical, Inc.

Gary K. Steinberg, MD is on the Scientific Advisory board and holds stock options in Innercool Therapies.

Thorsten Steiner, MD has no conflicts of interest to disclose.

Christine A.C. Wijman, MD has received consulting fees from Medivance, Inc.

Midori A. Yenari, MD has no conflicts of interest to disclose.

1

Thermoregulation and Heat Balance

DANIEL I. SESSLER
Outcomes Research™ Institute
and Department of Anesthesiology
and Perioperative Medicine,
University of Louisville,
Louisville, Kentucky, U.S.A.

INTRODUCTION

Body temperature is normally exquisitely regulated in mammals and birds through a wide range of environmental conditions. Even during hibernation, core temperature remains tightly regulated (1,2). Normal core temperature in humans averages 37°C and is remarkably similar in nearly all mammalian species. Even heterotherms ("cold-blooded" species) maintain a body temperature near 37°C when given suitable environmental choices (3).

Slight deviations from normal core temperature are associated with serious complications including morbid myocardial outcomes (4), coagulopathy (5,6), and reduced resistance to infection (7,8). However, just a few degrees reduction in temperature also provides substantial protection against ischemia in numerous animal models (9), and interestingly, heterotherms use behavioral responses to reduce core temperature in response to hypoxia (10). There is currently considerable interest in therapeutic hypothermia because, in animals at least, mild hypothermia provides better protection against tissue ischemia than any known drug. With few exceptions (11,12), the putative benefits of therapeutic hypothermia have yet to be proven in humans—although several major outcome studies are currently in progress.

The thermoregulatory system, like other physiological systems, uses positive and negative feedback to minimize body temperature perturbations. Temperatures are sensed and controlled, to some extent, throughout the body. However, the dominant controller in mammals is the hypothalamus (13). (Interestingly, the primary thermoregulatory controller in birds is the spinal cord (14).) The thermoregulatory system uses peripheral temperatures as an early-warning system to enable effective responses even before any deviation in core temperature occurs. In fact, the thermoregulatory system is based on multiple signals from nearly every type of tissue. So much redundancy is built into this critical control system that it cannot be defeated by severing any single spinal pathway. The processing of thermoregulatory information occurs in three phases: afferent thermal sensing, central regulation, and efferent responses.

A complexity of the thermoregulatory system is that peripheral tissues (the arms and legs) provide substantial insulation for the core thermal compartment (the trunk and head). This allows the body to use peripheral tissues as a buffer so that it is unnecessary to modulate thermoregulatory defenses in response to every minor environmental perturbation. Thermal buffering by peripheral tissues is usually beneficial in that it minimizes requirements for specific defenses, which may be metabolically costly or deplete scarce resources. However, insulating properties of peripheral tissues—and their sheer mass—complicate efforts to therapeutically modulate core temperature.

REVIEW

Thermoregulation

Body temperature is among the best regulated physiological parameters, rarely deviating by more than a few tenths of a degree Celsius. It is better regulated, e.g., than either heart rate or blood pressure. Core temperature deviations of even a couple of degrees Celsius in either direction are associated with complications (4–8).

However, known complications fail to explain why mammals expend considerable effort to regulate temperature to within a few tenths of a degree. For example, it is not obvious why the body would regulate core temperature to a precision of tenths of degree when the normal circadian temperature approaches 1°C (15,16). However, similarly precise control is maintained in most species. It thus seems logical to assume that core temperature is well controlled for compelling physiological reasons—even if the reasons are not yet apparent.

Afferent Input

There are temperature-sensitive cells throughout the body, including the skin surface. Cold-sensitive cells increase their firing rate as they cool, whereas warm-sensitive cell do the opposite. Both are phenomenally sensitive. Human skin, e.g., can detect temperature changes of as little as a few thousandths of a degree Celsius (17).

Cold signals travel primarily via A∂ nerve fibers and warm information by unmyelinated C fibers, although there is some overlap (18). The C fibers also detect and convey pain sensation, which is why intense heat cannot be distinguished from sharp pain. Most ascending thermal information traverses the spinothalamic tracts in the anterior spinal cord.

With the exception of the skin surface (19), relative importance of thermal input from various regions of the body is difficult or impossible to determine. However, various animal studies suggest that the hypothalamus, other parts of the brain, the spinal cord, deep abdominal and thoracic tissues, and the skin surface each contribute very roughly 20% of the total thermal input to the central regulatory system (14,19,20). Thus, although the hypothalamus is the dominant thermoregulatory controller, its temperature per se is not more important than other sites.

Central Control

Temperatures that are sensed throughout the body are integrated at various levels within the neuraxis. This hierarchical arrangement presumably developed when the evolving thermoregulatory control system co-opted previously existing mechanisms (e.g., shivering from muscles previously used for posture and locomotion) (13). A consequence is that destroying the hypothalamus does not completely obliterate thermoregulatory control because other centers compensate to some degree (14). However, these "older" systems are less precise, thus markedly degrading the quality of regulation (21,22).

Body temperature is compared to thresholds, which are defined by the core temperature triggering a specific response. Normally, the thresholds for first warm response (sweating) and first cold response (vasoconstriction) differ by only a few tenths of a degree Celsius (23). Body temperature is presumably accurately sensed even within this range, but does not trigger defenses. Temperatures between the sweating and vasoconstriction threshold define the interthreshold range. The interthreshold range also defines the limits of normal body temperature at any given time because temperatures exceeding this range trigger effective thermoregulatory responses that usually return core temperature to within these limits (Fig. 1).

Once triggered, the slope of response intensity vs. core temperature defines the gain of a thermoregulatory response. Response intensity no longer increasing with further deviation in core temperature identifies the maximum intensity. Typically, the gain of thermoregulatory responses is high. For example, vasomotion usually progresses from completely dilated to completely constricted with a deviation in body temperature of only a couple of tenths of a degree Celsius (Fig. 2) (24). Sweating (25) and shivering (26) are equally responsive.

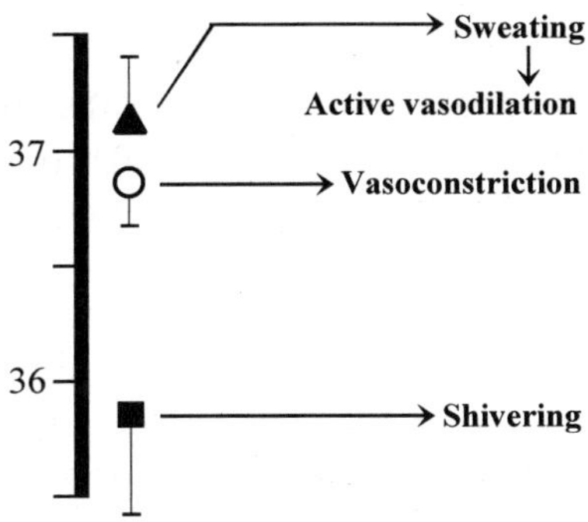

Figure 1 Normal thresholds, as a function of core temperature. The most important thermoregulatory responses in adult humans are sweating, arteriovenous shunt vasoconstriction, and shivering. Active vasodilation is triggered by an unknown factor released from sweat glands. Temperatures between the sweating and vasoconstriction thresholds do not activate thermoregulatory defenses and define the interthreshold range and normal body temperature. Results are presented as means ± SDs.

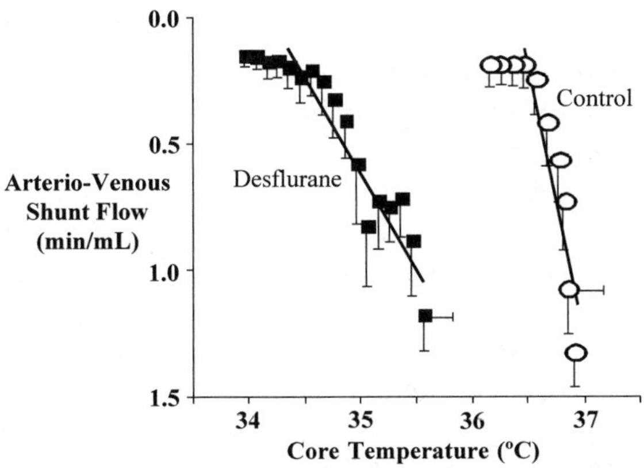

Figure 2 The gain of thermoregulatory responses is high. For example, vasomotion usually progresses from completely dilated to completely constricted with a deviation in body temperature of only a couple of tenths of a degree Celsius (right side of Figure); even during anesthesia, only about 0.5°C is required for the transition from complete dilation to complete constriction. Results are presented as means ± SDs. (From Ref. 24.)

Because the initial warm- and cold-response thresholds are so close and the gain of thermoregulatory responses so great, the system is often modeled as a setpoint. In this simplification, the system behaves like a household thermostat: temperatures exceeding the setpoint maximally trigger warm defenses, whereas lower temperatures maximally trigger cold responses. Although crude, this model reasonably approximates normal temperature control. The difficulty, though, is that it fails to explain the interthreshold range or "null zone" (27) in which no responses are activated. More importantly, the setpoint model fails seriously with some disease states and in the presence of drugs that impair thermoregulatory control (28). In these cases of unregulated hyperthermia or hypothermia, normal thermoregulatory responses are either inadequate or overwhelmed.

All thermoregulatory responses interact with other regulatory systems, as might be expected for systems that share final common pathways. For example, dehydration augments vasoconstriction (29) and reduces the intensity of sweating (30). Similarly, vasoconstriction is influenced by body position and, in turn, influences blood pressure and heart rate (31).

The precision of temperature regulation is similar in men and women, but the setpoint is a few tenths of a degree greater in women even in the luteal phase of the menstrual cycle (i.e., first 10 days) (23); it is yet a few tenths of a degree higher during the follicular phase (32,33). Infants, even premature ones, use nonshivering thermogenesis in preference to shivering (34,35). However, their setpoint and precision of regulation appears similar to that in adults. Most elderly humans also regulate temperature well. However, a subset of subjects exceeding 80 years of age have a shivering threshold that is a degree or more below normal (Fig. 3) (36).

Efferent Responses

Thermoregulatory responses consist of effectors that increase metabolic heat production or alter environmental heat loss. Because each has its own threshold, they are activated in an orderly progression according to need. When one response is

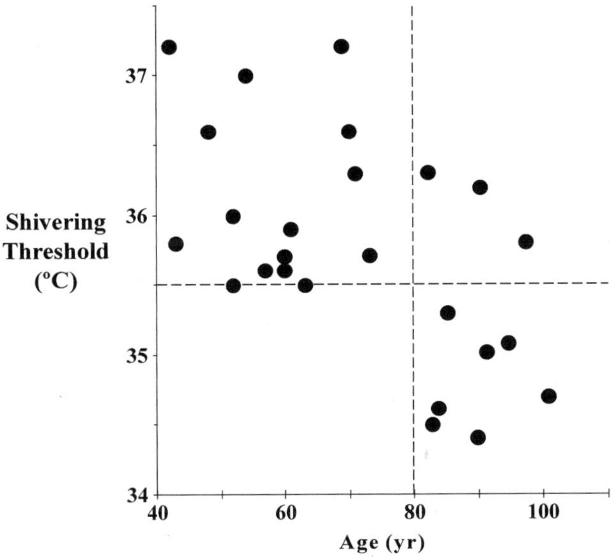

Figure 3 Most elderly humans regulate temperature well. However, a subset of subjects exceeding 80 years of age have a shivering threshold that is a degree or more below normal. (From Ref. 36.)

unavailable, others compensate. For example, decreased muscle mass, neuromuscular diseases, and muscle relaxants all inhibit shivering, which increases the minimum tolerable ambient temperature. Similarly, anticholinergic drugs inhibit sweating, which decreases the maximum tolerable temperature.

The single most important thermoregulatory defense consists of behavioral compensations, such as putting on a sweater or opening a window. In extreme forms (i.e., building shelters, using air conditioning), behavioral thermoregulation allows humans to live in virtually all regions of the earth. The major autonomic defenses, again, in adult humans are sweating, vasoconstriction, and shivering.

Cutaneous vasoconstriction is the most used autonomic thermoregulatory defense. Skin blood flow can be divided into capillary flow, which is mostly nutritional, and thermoregulatory flow through arteriovenous shunts in the fingers and toes. The arteriovenous shunts are anatomically and functionally distinct from the capillaries supplying nutritional blood to the skin (thus vasoconstriction does not compromise the needs of peripheral tissues) (37).

Shunts are typically 100 μm in diameter, which means that one shunt can convey 10,000-fold as much blood as a comparable length of capillary 10 μm in diameter (38). (Laminar flow is proportional to the fourth power of the radius.) Shunt flow is mediated by alpha-adrenergic sympathetic nerves that respond to both local temperature and central signals (39), but within the normal range of skin temperatures, control of shunt flow is mostly central. Roughly 10 % of cardiac output traverses arteriovenous shunts; consequently, shunt vasoconstriction increases mean arterial pressure by ≈15 mm Hg (31).

Nonshivering thermogenesis is the dominant mechanism for increasing metabolic heat production in small mammals (40,41). It can double or triple heat production. Human infants also use nonshivering thermogenesis in preference to shivering and can double heat production without shivering (35). However, the efficacy of this response diminishes over the initial months of life and is subsequently replaced by shivering. If adult humans can activate nonshivering thermogenesis at all, the magnitude is of questionable practical importance (42–44).

Nonshivering thermogenesis is adrenergically mediated via an uncoupling protein, sometimes called thermogenin, in brown adipose tissue (45). This specialized fat is brown because it is densely packed with mitochondria. The uncoupling protein is a proton/anion transporter that disperses the mitochondrial proton gradient by short-circuiting the ADP-phosphorylation system, thus uncoupling substrate oxygenation from ATP synthesis (46). This allows metabolic energy generated by lipid oxidation to be dissipated as heat rather than preserved in high-energy chemical species. Physiological control of brown fat thermogenesis, like most thermoregulatory responses, is largely under central control (41). Autoradiographic [^{14}C] deoxyglucose techniques further localize the control site to the anterior hypothalamus (47).

Brown fat is predominantly located around the kidneys and between the scapulae; nonshivering thermogenesis thus has the advantage of producing heat centrally where it is most needed and least likely to be dissipated to a cool environment. The thermodynamic efficiency of shivering and nonshivering thermogenesis (heat produced by metabolism of a given substrate) is identical. Nonshivering thermogenesis is nonetheless more effective because shivering generates heat peripherally where it is more easily dissipated to the environment. Furthermore, the muscular activity must be supported by augmented peripheral blood flow, which also facilitates loss of core heat to the environment. The efficacy of nonshivering thermogenesis may be one reason that most small animals activate this defense before shivering.

The threshold for shivering is a full degree below the vasoconstriction threshold. Furthermore, even vigorous shivering cannot sustain more than a twofold increase in metabolic rate, and as mentioned above, the efficacy of shivering is inherently limited because the body's largest muscles are located peripherally. Shivering might thus best be viewed as a "last resort" response that is avoided unless the environment is so extreme that behavioral responses and vasoconstriction both fail. The rapid tremor (up to 250 Hz) and unsynchronized muscular activity of thermogenic shivering suggest no central oscillator. However, superimposed on the fast activity, there usually is a slow (4–8 cycles/min), synchronous "waxing-and-waning" pattern, which presumably is centrally mediated (Fig. 4) (48,49).

Sweating is mediated by postganglionic, cholinergic nerves (50). It thus is an active process that is prevented by nerve block or atropine administration (51,52). Even untrained individuals can sweat up to 1 L/hr, and athletes can sweat at twice that rate. Sweating is the only mechanism by which the body can dissipate heat in an environment exceeding core temperature. Fortunately, the process is remarkably effective, dissipating 0.58 kcal/g of evaporated sweat. As with other thermoregulatory defenses, the gain of sweating is steep (Fig. 5).

Active vasodilation is mediated by a yet-to-be-identified factor released from sweat glands; the mediator may be a protein because it is not blocked by any standard drugs (53). (Nitric oxide was an attractive mechanism, but does not appear to be the mediator (54,55).) Because active vasodilation

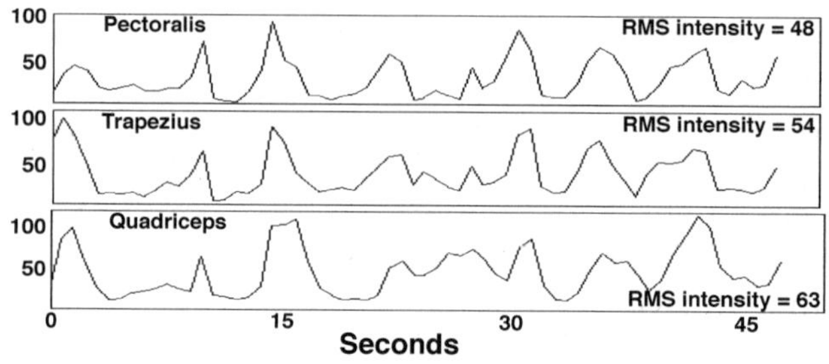

Figure 4 Electromyographic shivering signals from the pectoralis, trapezius, and quadriceps. The signals have been amplitude demodulated to remove the ≈250-Hz background signal, leaving only the 4–8 cycle/min waxing-and-waning pattern. Note that the waxing-and-waning pattern is nearly synchronous in these three widely separated muscles. This indicates that shivering has at least a degree of central control.

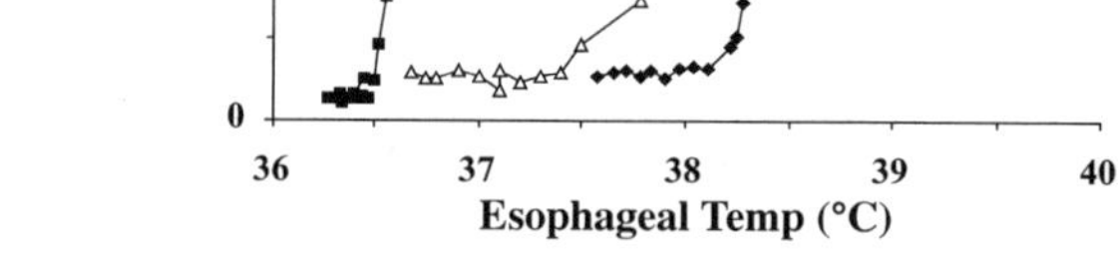

Figure 5 The gain of sweating is high. In this example, the sweating threshold without anesthesia increased to maximum intensity with an increase in core temperature of only 0.5°C. Anesthesia increased the threshold for sweating, but not the gain or maximum intensity. Sweating is the body's only mechanism for dissipating heat when ambient temperature exceeds core temperature. Fortunately, it is remarkably effective: in a dry convective environment, sweating can dissipate many times the basal metabolic rate. (From Ref. 25.)

requires intact sweat gland function, it also is largely inhibited by nerve block. During extreme heat stress, blood flow through the top millimeter of skin can reach 7.5 L/min—equaling the entire resting cardiac output (56). The threshold for active vasodilation usually is similar to the sweating threshold, but the gain may be less. Consequently, maximum cutaneous vasodilation usually is delayed until core temperature is well above that provoking maximum sweating intensity.

Heat Balance

Body temperature is normally precisely regulated throughout a wide range of environments. When deviations in core temperature occur, they are usually related to one of the three causes: (1) fever (a regulated increase in the setpoint); (2) impairment of thermoregulatory control, even in a moderate environment; or (3) metabolic heat production or environmental exposure so extreme that the thermoregulatory system fails to compensate adequately.

Fever is by far the most common thermal disturbance and is discussed in more detail in Chapter 2. General anesthesia is an example of thermoregulatory failure in a moderate environment (28). Similarly, alcoholics often present with hypothermia even in relatively warm weather because intoxication impairs behavioral thermoregulation (57). Examples of excessive heat production include heat stroke (58), malignant hyperthermia (59), and neuroleptic malignant syndrome (60).

Tissue temperature is related to heat content by the specific heat of tissue, which is ≈ 0.83 kcal kg^{-1} $°C^{-1}$ (61,62). Body temperature perturbations are thus a direct consequence of alterations in tissue heat content. How heat is generated and distributed within the body is thus of considerable interest, as is transfer of heat between peripheral tissues and the core. The principles of thermodynamics and heat transfer are discussed in greater detail in Chapter 9.

Heat Production

Metabolism is normally the only internal source of heat, although internal heating can result from drinking warm beverages, microwave radiation, magnetic resonance gradient coils, or endovascular heat-exchange catheters.

According to the First Law of Thermodynamics, energy generation by a chemical reaction is determined only by the substrates and products of the reaction. Nearly all of this energy is eventually converted to heat. The major substrates for human metabolism are glucose, protein, and fat; the major products of aerobic metabolism are generally carbon dioxide and water. Combustion of glucose and protein produces 4.1 kcal/kg, whereas fat releases 9.3 kcal/kg.

Even in the absence of nonshivering thermogenesis, the metabolic rate of body tissues is proportional to temperature; typically, the rate increases 6–9% per degree Celsius (Fig. 6) (63,64). The brain and major organs in the trunk are the most metabolically active tissues and generate more metabolic heat than muscle at rest (65,66). In contrast, heat production by skeletal muscle can, at least briefly, exceed the basal metabolic rate by a factor of 10.

Thermal Compartments

Humans are often described as having a core and peripheral thermal compartment. There is no firm anatomic or functional distinction between these putative compartments and the concept is not strictly supported physiologically. Sophisticated mathematical models thus include many more compartments to increase predictive accuracy (67). Nonetheless, the two-compartment model is remarkably useful.

The core compartment consists of the trunk and head, which contain the most metabolically active tissues. Of course the skin and most peripheral tissues of the trunk and head are not technically part of the core; however, little accuracy is lost by ignoring this mass. Truncal tissues are highly perfused and thus have a nearly homogeneous temperature. It is important to realize, though, that even within the core thermal compartment there are real temperature differences and that "core temperature" is simply an average of the tissues in this compartment. For example, liver temperature is typically a degree Celsius warmer than other core tissues.

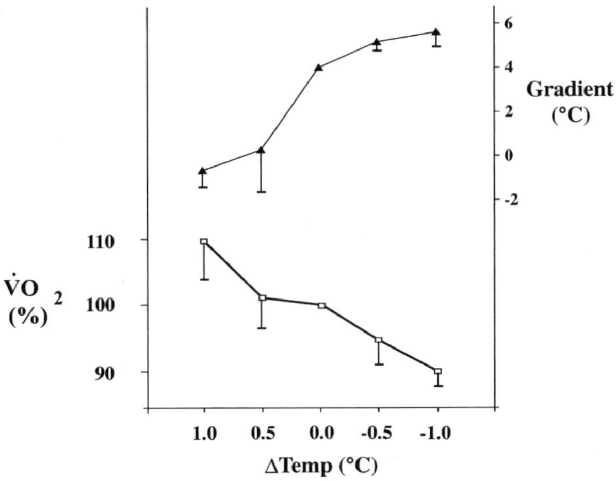

Figure 6 Because subclinical shivering could confound evaluation of nonshivering, this study was conduced in anesthetized and paralyzed volunteers. Oxygen consumption decreased in proportion to core temperature. The slopes of the lines of regression were similar before and after vasoconstriction: 9 ± 5 vs. 9 ± 3%/°C (P = NS). Change in tympanic membrane temperature (ΔTemp) in this graph was calculated relative to the individual volunteer's threshold for vasoconstriction, which averaged 35.2 ± 0.8°C. Oxygen consumption is expressed as a percentage of the oxygen consumption measured at the individual vasoconstriction threshold temperature. The onset of intense peripheral thermoregulatory vasoconstriction is indicated by a forearm minus fingertip, skin-temperature gradient = 4°C at ΔTemp = 0°C. Results are presented as means ± SDs. (From Ref. 63.)

The peripheral compartment, in contrast, consists of the arms and legs. In an adult with normal morphology, each compartment comprises roughly half the body mass (68,69). A cardinal feature of the peripheral compartment is that heat content and distribution change substantially over time and as a function of environmental exposure (56). This is in distinct contrast to the core whose temperature is usually precisely regulated.

Peripheral tissues are typically 2°C to 4°C lower than core temperature in a moderate environment (69). However, the core-to-peripheral tissue temperature gradient can become large under extreme thermal (70) or physiological (71) circumstances. During cardiopulmonary bypass, especially to low core temperatures, there can be enormous differences between core and peripheral temperatures (Fig. 7); core temperature thus poorly represents mean body temperature under this circumstance (72,73). Lower core-to-peripheral temperature gradients result when the environment is warm or when thermoregulatory vasodilation facilitates flow of metabolic heat (which is

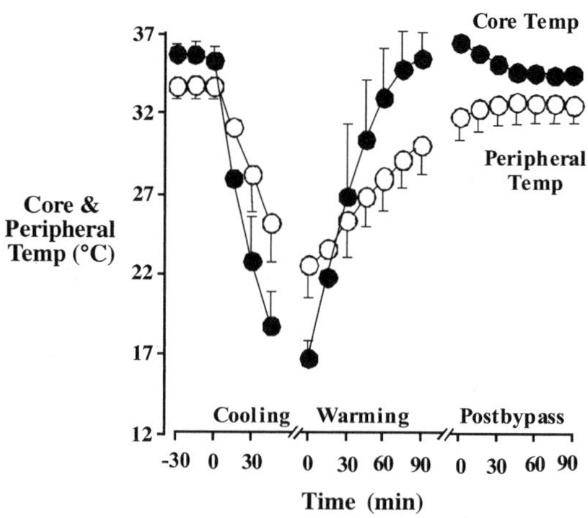

Figure 7 Core (solid circles) and peripheral (open circles) temperatures during and after cardiopulmonary bypass. The arms and legs were considered to be the peripheral compartment; peripheral tissue temperature is the volume-weighted average temperature of this compartment. The beginning of bypass cooling was designated elapsed time zero for cooling. Because the duration of cooling differed among patients, a second zero elapsed time was defined as the beginning of rewarming. Similarly, the end of rewarming identified elapsed time zero for the postbypass period. Note that peripheral temperature was initially 2–3 °C less than core temperature, but during bypass was sometimes greater than core temperature and at other times much less than core temperature. An hour or so after completion of bypass, the normal core-to-peripheral tissue-temperature gradient was restored. Results are presented as means ± SDs. (From Ref. 73.)

largely generated in the core) to the periphery (74). In contrast, vasoconstriction constrains metabolic heat to the core, increasing the core-to-peripheral temperature gradient.

There are typically substantial longitudinal tissue-temperature gradients within the extremities, with distal tissues being several degrees cooler than those positioned more proximally. There are also often substantial radial tissue-temperature gradients, which become especially large in extreme thermal environments (70,72,73). As might be expected, proximal-to-distal and radial gradients are especially severe during cardiopulmonary bypass at low temperatures (Fig. 8). However, similar gradients can probably be observed during cold-water immersion.

In a warm environment, especially in vasodilated subjects, tissue temperature in much of the peripheral compartment can equal core temperature. Some authors refer to this situation as an expansion of the core compartment. However, temperature of these tissues will decrease and again become nonuniform in a cooler environment. It is thus easier to consider physical size of the compartments to be fixed, and instead allow temperature of the peripheral compartment to vary.

Natural Internal Heat Flow

Heat distribution within core tissues is rapid. Tissue temperatures within the core compartment are thus relatively homogeneous. In contrast, heat flows relatively slowly to peripheral tissues (all thermodynamic processes are fully reversible so statements about flow of heat apply equally to cooling tissues). The major mechanism mediating flow of heat from the core to peripheral tissues, and distally within the peripheral compartment, is bloodborne convection (75). The convective component can very roughly be modeled as a large and relatively rapid longitudinal flow of heat within the big axial vessels of the extremities. The major factors influencing convective distribution of heat are peripheral blood flow, countercurrent heat exchange between adjacent arteries and veins, and the core-to-peripheral temperature gradient.

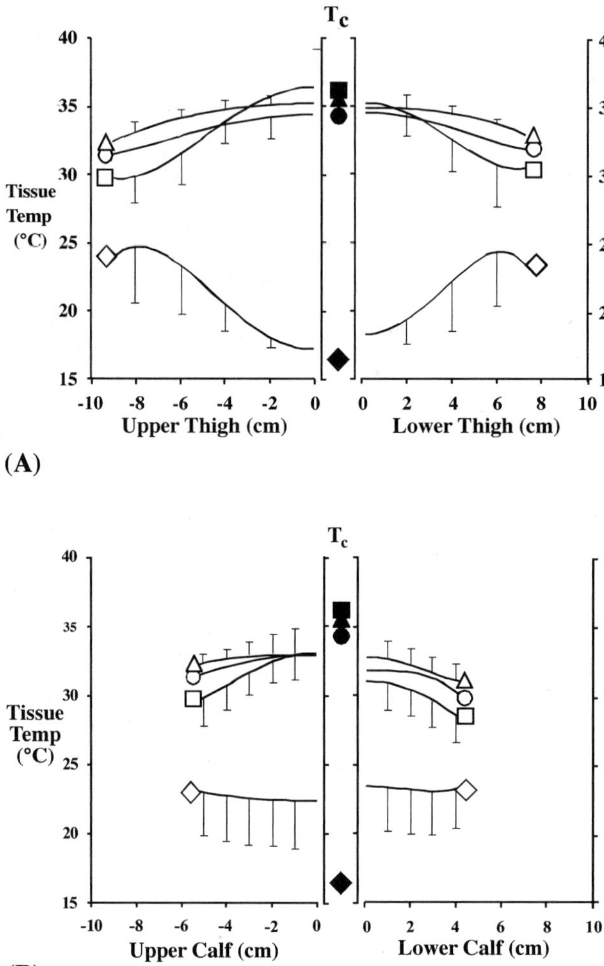

(A)

(B)

Figure 8 (A) Average radial upper- and lower thigh temperatures at the onset of cooling (open triangles), at the start of rewarming (open diamonds), at the end of rewarming (open rectangles), and 1 hr after the end of rewarming (open circles). (B) Average radial upper- and lower calf temperatures at the onset of cooling (open triangles), at the start of rewarming (open diamonds), at the end of rewarming (open rectangles), and 1 hr after the end of rewarming (open circles). Temperatures were estimated using average fourth-order regression coefficients calculated from individual calf skin and muscle temperatures. Distance zero indicates the center of each extremity segment. Solid symbols indicate the corresponding core temperatures at each time. Data are presented as means ± SDs. (From Ref. 73.)

The conductive component, in contrast, is a slower radial flow of heat from relatively warm tissue at the central axis to cooler tissues near the skin. Conductive flow is largely determined by the diffusion coefficient, which is to a great extent a function of tissue characteristics. For example, fat insulates nearly three times as well as muscle (76) and therefore provides substantial insulation (77,78). Hence, conductive heat transfer depends mostly on intrinsic tissue characteristics rather than thermoregulatory factors such as vasomotion. Of course convection and conduction each contribute to both longitudinal and radial heat flow but conduction is too slow to dissipate heat over the length of an extremity.

Deposition of heat into peripheral tissues is augmented by heat that is produced by local tissue metabolism and diminished by regional cutaneous heat loss to the environment. Regional heat transfer and local production are fully described by the bioheat equation (79). However, a precise solution to this equation requires numerous input values that cannot normally be measured. Consequently, a number of equations have been developed to quantify various aspects of tissue heat transfer and local heat production in terms of measurable quantities (80,81).

Modifications of the bioheat equation have been used to construct numerous models of tissue heat distribution. Even simple models perform reasonably well under a restricted set of circumstances such as cold-water immersion. However, they usually prove less accurate under other conditions, prompting refinements in subsequent generations of the models (82–84). Consequently, some models have become quite complicated (67).

Nonetheless, most models of tissue heat flow have been validated only to a limited extent and many do not include a sophisticated thermoregulatory component. Ignoring thermoregulatory compensations is acceptable in a situation of extreme thermal stress in which it is reasonable to assume that warm or cold defenses are maximally activated. It may also be acceptable during general anesthesia when thermoregulatory defenses are markedly impaired by drugs. However, failure to include thermoregulatory defenses can be a substantial limitation in more typical environments where active control—

rather than environmental exposure—is the major determinant of core temperature. Heat balance models have thus usually proven less helpful than initially hoped, leaving investigators largely dependent on experimental data. Fortunately, detailed measurements are now becoming available in a variety of circumstances (68,69,72,73,85,86).

All metabolic heat must eventually be dissipated to the environment to maintain a thermal steady state. About 95% of this heat traverses the skin surface, with the remaining small amount being lost through the respiratory tract (87). In the absence of sweating, only about 10% of cutaneous heat loss is evaporation in adults (although the fraction can be considerable in infants, especially premature infants) (88). Sweating, though, is remarkably effective and can dissipate 10 times the basal metabolic rate in a dry, convective environment (89,90). The upper chest and face are most sensitive to temperature. However, the common belief that half of body heat is lost through the head only applies when the rest of the body is covered by an arctic survival suit (91). Instead, with comparable levels of insulation, heat loss is roughly proportional to surface area over the entire body and is not much changed by thermoregulatory vasomotion (92–95).

Forced Internal Heat Flow

There are two major factors that limit the efficacy of active surface warming or cooling. The first is simply the mass of peripheral tissues. The peripheral compartment, roughly half the body mass, is thus about 35 kg in a typically sized adult. The specific heat of humans is $\approx$ 0.83 kcal/kg/°C (61). Nearly 100 kcal must thus be absorbed to reduce temperature of peripheral tissues by 3°C. This corresponds to a cooling rate of 83 W, which is substantial. Of course an additional comparable amount of heat must also be extracted to cool the core compartment, doubling the total heat exchange requirement.

The second factor is that the insulating property of tissues restricts flow of heat between the compartments. As above, heat flow within the body can be divided into two categories: radial conduction and longitudinal convection (80). Initial transfer of heat applied to the skin surface is conducted to tissues just under the skin. Subsequently, though, longitudinal transfer of heat between the core and peripheral thermal compartments is largely mediated by bloodborne convection. Peripheral-to-core heat transfer is thus a function of vasomotor tone which influences both the amount of blood flowing to extremities and the extent to which countercurrent mechanisms reduce heat transfer.

Thermoregulatory vasoconstriction is an effective defense against core hypothermia. However, it also limits transfer of heat from the core to peripheral tissues during induction of therapeutic hypothermia. Anesthetics inhibit thermoregulation and thus initially cause vasodilation; however, thermoregulatory vasodilation reemerges when subjects become sufficiently hypothermic (typically at core temperatures of about 34.5°C) (96,97). However, general anesthetics also induce nonthermoregulatory dilation (98); thus there is little restriction of heat flow between peripheral and core tissues during anesthesia (99,100). However, without anesthesia, vasoconstriction can be a major factor determining the rate of intercompartmental heat transfer. The rate of core warming with surface warming is thus about what would be expected based on systemic heat balance during anesthesia, but is considerably less without anesthesia (Fig. 9). Another way to express this concept is to quantify the amount of heat that is prevented from reaching the core during active surface warming (Fig. 10).

Dissipation of Heat to the Environment

There are four modes by which heat can be dissipated from the body to the environment. They are radiation, convection, conduction, and evaporation (Fig. 11). All obey the laws of thermodynamics and are thus fully reversible; that is, heat can be comparably absorbed as well as dissipated by each mechanism.

Radiation is probably the most important source of heat loss in a typical hospital environment (101). Radiation transfers heat from one surface to another via photons and is thus

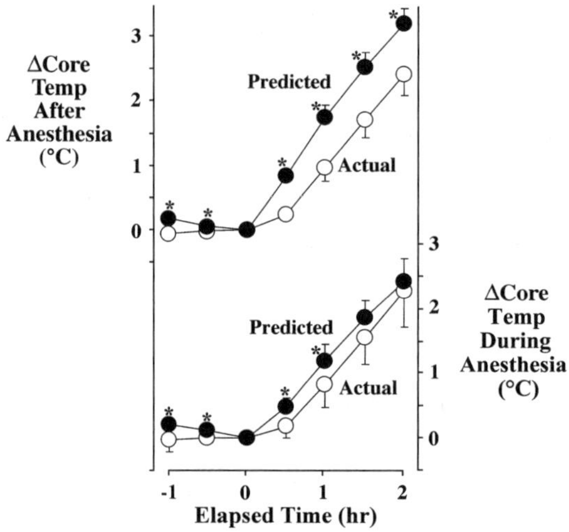

Figure 9 Predicted core temperature is the change that would be expected were applied heat evenly distributed within the body. The difference between predicted and measured increases in core heat content thus identified the extent to which vasoconstriction isolated core tissues from peripherally applied heat. These volunteers demonstrated thermoregulatory arteriovenous shunt vasoconstriction throughout the study. Consequently, postanesthetic isolation of core tissues results from direct (nonthermoregulatory) anesthetic-induced vasodilation. Time zero indicates the beginning of forced-air warming. Data are presented as means ± SDs. Asterisks (*) indicate statistically significant differences between each set of values. (From Ref. 102.)

independent of the intervening media. The amount of heat lost by radiation is a function of the emissivity of the two surfaces and the difference between the fourth power of their temperatures in degrees Kelvin. Emissivity defines an object's ability to absorb and emit heat; these two effects are always identical, otherwise objects would continue to absorb or lose heat indefinitely. Objects that absorb and emit heat perfectly are termed "black bodies" and have an emissivity of one. In contrast, perfect mirrors have an emissivity of zero. Human skin (of all

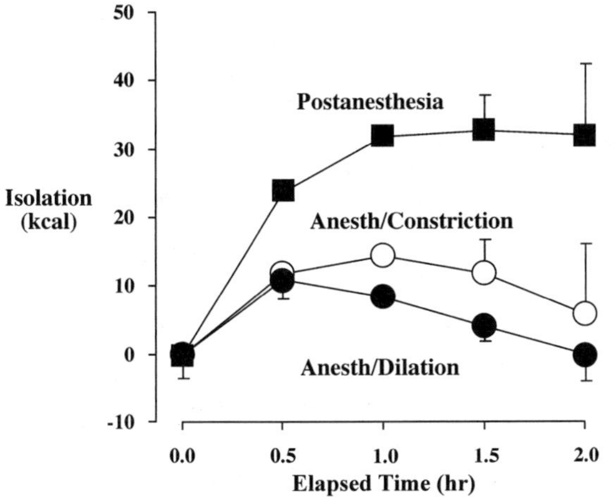

Figure 10 There was considerably more isolation of core tissues after anesthesia than during anesthesia. In contrast, thermoregulatory arteriovenous shunt vasoconstriction only minimally restricted peripheral-to-core heat transfer during anesthesia. These data indicate that direct, anesthetic-induced vasodilation influences intercompartmental heat transfer and distribution of body heat more than thermoregulatory shunt vasomotion. Time zero indicates the beginning of forced-air warming. Isolation was significantly greater postanesthesia than during anesthesia at all times after zero elapsed minutes. However, the amount of isolated heat did not differ significantly during anesthesia when the volunteers had arteriovenous shunt vasodilation ("Anesth/Dilation") than when thermoregulatory vasoconstriction had been triggered ("Anesth/Constriction"). Data are presented as means ± SDs. (From Ref. 102.)

colors) acts very much like a black body and has an emissivity near 0.95 for infrared radiation.

Conduction is the transfer of heat directly from one surface to an adjacent surface. Heat transfer is proportional to the difference in the surface temperatures and any insulation between them. This insulation might be a real barrier (such as an air gap) or effective insulation when one of the

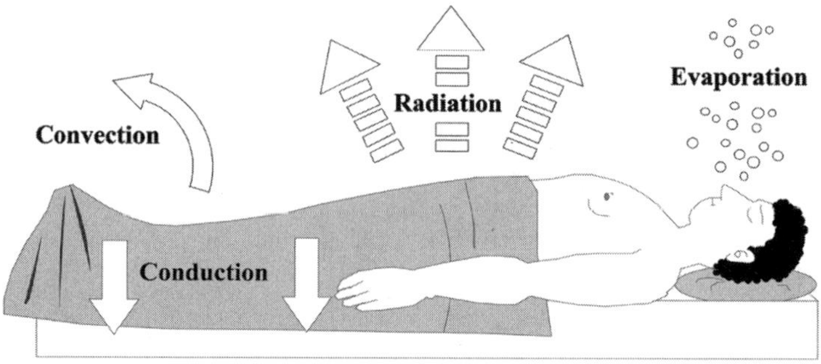

Figure 11 Cartoon illustrating the four types of heat transfer. In a typical hospital environment, radiation and convection dominate with conduction and evaporation each contributing only about 5%. Heat lost by radiation is a function of the emissivity of the two surfaces and the difference between the fourth power of their temperatures in degrees Kelvin. Conductive heat transfer is proportional to the difference in the surface temperatures and any insulation between them. Convective loss is calculated similarly, but is augmented by a factor related to the square root of air speed. Evaporative heat loss is derived from the heat of vaporization of water, which is a substantial 0.58 kcal/g. Evaporation is the only mechanism by which the body can dissipate heat when ambient temperature exceeds core temperature. (Courtesy of James Hyson, M.D.)

surfaces conducts heat poorly. For example, air is a poor conductor so relatively little heat is lost by conduction into still air—even cold air. Water, in contrast, conducts about 30 times as well as air. Water immersion is thus the fastest way to transfer heat in or out of the body from the skin surface.

Convection shares the same fundamental mechanism as conduction and is thus sometimes termed "facilitated conduction." It usually refers to transfer of heat from the skin surface into ambient air but applies equally with other fluids such as water. Conduction into air is slow because air is such a good insulator. The specific problem is that a layer of warm insulating air builds up near the skin surface, thus limiting additional heat loss. Convection solves this problem by moving the warm air away from the skin, thus again allowing heat to flow from the skin to adjacent air. The improvement in heat transfer is proportional to the square root of the air velocity. (Convection is the basis of the popular "wind-chill factor.") Even in the relatively still air of a hospital room (with a typical velocity near 20 cm/sec), convection remains the second most important source of heat loss. It becomes the dominant source of heat loss in highly convective environments such as laminar flow units or outdoors on a windy day.

Evaporative heat loss is derived from the heat of vaporization of water, which is a substantial 0.58 kcal/g. To put this in perspective, evaporation of 1 g of water at 100°C requires nearly six times as much energy as heating it from 0°C to 100°C. Adults fortunately normally lose little water through intact skin. Only about 5% of the basal metabolic rate is thus lost from evaporation of transcutaneous water under normal (nonsweating) circumstances. Respiratory evaporative losses are also small, usually less than 10% of the basal metabolic rate (87). As might thus be expected, airway heating and humidification is an ineffective way of warming patients (103).

FUTURE DIRECTIONS

The thermoregulatory system precisely defends core temperature (23), presumably because even small deviations are associated with severe consequences (104). On the other hand, there is considerable evidence that mild hypothermia provides substantial protection against tissue ischemia (12,105). The difficulty is that central thermoregulatory control is well maintained during most illnesses, including mild and moderate stroke (105). Because these responses are effective, it is usually difficult to induce therapeutic hypothermia.

Many drugs have been shown to profoundly impair thermoregulatory control and thus permit induction of therapeutic hypothermia. However, most are general anesthetics and thus unsuitable for most patients (28). A key goal is thus to discover or develop new drugs or combinations of drugs that will facilitate induction of therapeutic hypothermia. Unless relatively effective methods of defeating thermoregulatory defenses are developed, induction of deliberate hypothermia for protection of ischemic tissue is unlikely to become practical. Chapter 8 is devoted to pharmacological and nonpharmacological methods of defeating thermoregulatory responses to induced hypothermia.

A consequence of peripheral tissue mass and its insulating properties is that warming or cooling the core from the skin surface is relatively slow. However, it is distinctly faster during anesthesia. It is obviously impractical to maintain general anesthesia just to improve the efficacy of surface heat exchange. However, it may be possible to discover or develop drugs that facilitate exchange of heat between peripheral and core tissues that are safer and easier to use than anesthetics.

Systems such as endovascular catheters that directly exchange heat with core tissues (107) (Chapter 10) will change core temperature much faster for a given amount of heat exchange (108). Direct central cooling may also provoke less in the way of thermoregulatory defenses because it bypasses thermal receptors in the skin surface that normally contribute 20% to control of arteriovenous shunt vasoconstriction and to shivering (19). Experience with endovascular thermal manipulation remains limited. Additional work is needed to fully evaluate the safety and efficacy of endovascular heat exchange and other novel methods for attaining therapeutic hypothermia.

REFERENCES

1. Daan S, Barnes BM, Strijkstra AM. Warming up for sleep?—ground squirrels sleep during arousals from hibernation. Neurosci Lett 1991; 128:265–268.
2. Satinoff E. Disruption of hibernation caused by hypothalamic lesions. Science 1967; 155:1031–1033.
3. Crawshaw LI. Temperature regulation in vertebrates. Annu Rev Physiol 1980; 42:473–491.
4. Frank SM, Fleisher LA, Breslow MJ, Higgins MS, Olson KF, Kelly S, Beattie C. Perioperative maintenance of normother-

mia reduces the incidence of morbid cardiac events: a randomized clinical trial. JAMA 1997; 277:1127–1134.

5. Schmied H, Kurz A, Sessler DI, Kozek S, Reiter A. Mild intraoperative hypothermia increases blood loss and allogeneic transfusion requirements during total hip arthroplasty. Lancet 1996; 347:289–292.
6. Winkler M, Akça O, Birkenberg B, Hetz H, Scheck T, Arkilic CF, Kabon B, Marker E, Grubl A, Czepan R, Greher M, Goll V, Gottsauner-Wolf F, Kurz A, Sessler DI. Aggressive warming reduces blood loss during hip arthroplasty. Anesth Analg 2000; 91:978–984.
7. Kurz A, Sessler DI, Lenhardt RA. Study of wound infections and temperature group: perioperative normothermia to reduce the incidence of surgical-wound infection and shorten hospitalization. N Engl J Med 1996; 334:1209–1215.
8. Melling AC, Ali B, Scott EM, Leaper DJ. Effects of preoperative warming on the incidence of wound infection after clean surgery: a randomized controlled trial. Lancet 2001; 358:876–880.
9. Bickler PE, Buck LT, Hansen BM. Effects of isoflurane and hypothermia on glutamate receptor-mediated calcium influx in brain slices. Anesthesiology 1994; 81:1461–1469.
10. Rausch RN, Crawshaw LI, Wallace HL. Effects of hypoxia, anoxia, and endogenous ethanol on thermoregulation in goldfish, *Carassius auratus*. Am J Physiol Regul Integr Comp Physiol 2000; 278:R545–R555.
11. Bernard SA, Gray TW, Buist MD, Jones BM, Silvester W, Gutteridge G, Smith K. Treatment of comatose survivors of out-of-hospital cardiac arrest with induced hypothermia. N Engl J Med 2002; 346:557–563.
12. Hypothermia after Cardiac Arrest Study Group. Mild therapeutic hypothermia to improve the neurologic outcome after cardiac arrest. N Engl J Med 2002; 346:549–556.
13. Satinoff E. Neural organization and evolution of thermal regulation in mammals—several hierarchically arranged integrating systems may have evolved to achieve precise thermoregulation. Science 1978; 201:16–22.
14. Simon E. Temperature regulation: the spinal cord as a site of

extrahypothalamic thermoregulatory functions. Rev Physiol Biochem Pharmacol 1974; 71:1–76.

15. Sessler DI, Lee KA, McGuire J. Isoflurane anesthesia and circadian temperature cycles. Anesthesiology 1991; 75:985–989.
16. Tayefeh F, Plattner O, Sessler DI, Ikeda T, Marder D. Circadian changes in the sweating-to-vasoconstriction interthreshold range. Pflügers Arch 1998; 435:402–406.
17. Hardy JD, Oppel TW. The thermal response of the skin to radiation. Physics 1936; 7:466–479.
18. Poulos DA. Central processing of cutaneous temperature information. Fed Proc 1981; 40:2825–2829.
19. Cheng C, Matsukawa T, Sessler DI, Kurz A, Merrifield B, Lin H, Olofsson P. Increasing mean skin temperature linearly reduces the core-temperature thresholds for vasoconstriction and shivering in humans. Anesthesiology 1995; 82:1160–1168.
20. Jessen C, Feistkorn G. Some characteristics of core temperature signals in the conscious goat. Am J Physiol 1984; 247: R456–R464.
21. Kosaka M, Simon E, Walther O-E, Thauer R. Response of respiration to selective heating of the spinal cord below partial transection. Experientia 1969; 25:36–37.
22. Kosaka M, Simon E, Thauer R. Shivering in intact and spinal rabbits during spinal cord cooling. Experientia 1967; 23:385–387.
23. Lopez M, Sessler DI, Walter K, Emerick T, Ozaki M. Rate and gender dependence of the sweating, vasoconstriction, and shivering thresholds in humans. Anesthesiology 1994; 80:780–788.
24. Kurz A, Xiong J, Sessler DI, Dechert M, Noyes K, Belani K. Desflurane reduces the gain of thermoregulatory arteriovenous shunt vasoconstriction in humans. Anesthesiology 1995; 83:1212–1219.
25. Washington D, Sessler DI, Moayeri A, Merrifield B, Prager M, McGuire J, Belani K, Hudson S, Schroeder M. Thermoregulatory responses to hyperthermia during isoflurane anesthesia in humans. J Appl Physiol 1993; 74:82–87.

26. Ikeda T, Kim J-S, Sessler DI, Negishi C, Turakhia M, Jeffrey R. Isoflurane alters shivering patterns and reduces maximum shivering intensity. Anesthesiology 1998; 88:866–873.

27. Mekjavic IB, Sundberg CJ, Linnarsson D. Core temperature "null zone."J Appl Physiol 1991; 71:1289–1295.

28. Sessler DI. Perioperative hypothermia. N Engl J Med 1997; 336:1730–1737.

29. O'Brien C, Young AJ, Sawka MN. Hypohydration and thermoregulation in cold air. J Appl Physiol 1998; 84:185–189.

30. Montain SJ, Latzka WA, Sawka MN. Control of thermoregulatory sweating is altered by hydration level and exercise intensity. J Appl Physiol 1995; 79:1434–1439.

31. Greif R, Laciny S, Rajek A, Doufas AG, Sessler DI. Blood pressure response to thermoregulatory vasoconstriction during isoflurane and desflurane anesthesia. Acta Anaesthesiol Scand 2003; 47:847–852.

32. Tankersley CG, Nicholas WC, Deaver DR, Mikita D, Kenney WL. Estrogen replacement in middle-aged women: thermoregulatory responses to exercise in the heat. J Appl Physiol 1992; 73:1238–1245.

33. Hessemer V, Brück K. Influence of menstrual cycle on thermoregulatory, metabolic, and heart rate responses to exercise at night. J Appl Physiol 1985; 59:1911–1917.

34. Sinclair JC. Thermal control in premature infants. Annu Rev Med 1972; 23:129–148.

35. Mestyan J, Jarai I, Bata G, Fekete M. The significance of facial skin temperature in the chemical heat regulation of premature infants. Biol Neonate 1964; 7:243–254.

36. Vassilieff N, Rosencher N, Sessler DI, Conseiller C. The shivering threshold during spinal anesthesia is reduced in the elderly. Anesthesiology 1995; 83:1162–1166.

37. Rowell LB. Cardiovascular aspects of human thermoregulation. Circ Res 1983; 52:367–379.

38. Hales JRS. Skin arteriovenous anastomoses, their control and role in thermoregulation. In: Johansen K, Burggren W, eds.

Cardiovascular Shunts: Phylogenetic, Ontogenetic and Clinical Aspects. Copenhagen: Munksgaard, 1985:433–451.

39. Hales JRS, Jessen C, Fawcett AA, King RB. Skin AVA and capillary dilatation and constriction induced by local skin heating. Pflügers Arch 1985; 404:203–207.
40. Foster DO, Frydman ML. Nonshivering thermogenesis in the rat. II. Measurements of blood flow with microspheres point to brown adipose tissue as the dominant site of the calorigenesis induced by noradrenaline. Can J Physiol Pharmacol 1978; 56:110–122.
41. Fuller CA, Horwitz BA, Horowitz JM. Shivering and nonshivering thermogenic responses of cold-exposed rats to hypothalamic warming. Am J Physiol 1975; 228:1519–1524.
42. Brück K, Baum E, Schwennicke HP. Cold-adaptive modifications in man induced by repeated short-term cold-exposures and during a 10-day and -night cold-exposure. Pflügers Arch 1976; 363:125–133.
43. Jessen K. An assessment of human regulatory nonshivering thermogenesis. Acta Anaesthesiol Scand 1980; 24:138–143.
44. Jessen K, Rabøl A, Winkler K. Total body and splanchnic thermogenesis in curarized man during a short exposure to cold. Acta Anaesthesiol Scand 1980; 24:339–344.
45. Nedergaard J, Cannon B. The uncoupling protein thermogenin and mitochondrial thermogenesis. New Comp Biochem 1992; 23:385–420.
46. Ricquier R, Casteilla L, Bouillaud F. Molecular studies of the uncoupling protein. FASEB J 1991; 5:2237–2242.
47. Morimoto A, Murakami N, Nakamori T, Watanabe T. Suppression of non-shivering thermogenesis in the rat by heat-seeking behaviour during cold exposure. J Physiol 1986; 380:541–549.
48. Sessler DI, Rubinstein EH, Moayeri A. Physiological responses to mild perianesthetic hypothermia in humans. Anesthesiology 1991; 75:594–610.
49. Israel DJ, Pozos RS. Synchronized slow-amplitude modulations in the electromyograms of shivering muscles. J Appl Physiol 1989; 66:2358–2363.

50. Hemingway A, Price WM. The autonomic nervous system and regulation of body temperature. Anesthesiology 1968; 29:693–701.

51. Greif R, Laciny S, Rajek AM, Larson MD, Bjorksten AR, Doufas AG, Bakhshandeh M, Mokhtarani M, Sessler DI. Neither nalbuphine nor atropine posses special antishivering activity. Anesth Analg 2001; 93:620–627.

52. Boudet J, Qing W, Boyer-Chammard A, Del Franco G, Bergougnan JL, Rosen P, Meyer P. Dose–response effects of atropine in human volunteers. Fundam Clin Pharmacol 1991; 5:635–640.

53. Rowell LB. Active neurogenic vasodilation in man. In: Vanhoutte P, Leusen I, eds. Vasodilatation. New York: Raven Press, 1981:1–17.

54. Warren JB. Nitric oxide and human skin blood flow responses to acetylcholine and ultraviolet light. FASEB J 1994; 8:247–251.

55. Dietz NM, Rivera JM, Warner DO, Joyner MJ. Is nitric oxide involved in cutaneous vasodilation during body heating in humans? J Appl Physiol 1994; 76:2047–2053.

56. Detry J-MR, Brengelmann GL, Rowell LB, Wyss C. Skin and muscle components of forearm blood flow in directly heated resting man. J Appl Physiol 1972; 32:506–511.

57. Johnston CE, Bristow GK, Elias DA, Giesbrecht GG. Alcohol lowers the vasoconstriction threshold in humans without affecting core cooling rate during mild cold exposure. Eur J Appl Physiol Occup Physiol 1996; 74:293–295.

58. Bouchama A, Knochel JP. Heat stroke. N Engl J Med 2002; 346:1978–1988.

59. Jurkat-Rott K, McCarthy T, Lehmann-Horn F. Genetics and pathogenesis of malignant hyperthermia. Muscle Nerve 2000; 23:4–17.

60. Guze BH, Baxter LR Jr. Current concepts. Neuroleptic malignant syndrome. N Engl J Med 1985; 313:163–166.

61. Burton AC. Human calorimetry: the average temperature of the tissues of the body. J Nutr 1935; 9:261–280.

62. Cooper TE, Trezek GJ. Correlation of thermal properties of

some human tissue with water content. Aerospace Med 1971; 42:24–27.

63. Hynson JM, Sessler DI, Moayeri A, McGuire J. Absence of nonshivering thermogenesis in anesthetized humans. Anesthesiology 1993; 79:695–703.

64. Plattner O, Semsroth M, Sessler DI, Papousek A, Klasen C, Wagner O. Lack of nonshivering thermogenesis in infants anesthetized with fentanyl and propofol. Anesthesiology 1997; 86:772–777.

65. Crosby G, Crane AM, Sokoloff L. A comparison of local rates of glucose utilization in spinal cord and brain in conscious and nitrous oxide- or pentobarbital-treated rats. Anesthesiology 1984; 61:434–438.

66. Fagher B, Liedholm H, Monti M, Moritz U. Thermogenesis in human skeletal muscle as measured by direct microcalorimetry and muscle contractile performance during β-adrenoceptor blockade. Clin Sci 1986; 70:435–441.

67. Wissler EH. Comparison of computed results obtained from two mathematical models—a simple 14-node model and a complex 250-node model. J Physiol 1971; 63:455–458.

68. Matsukawa T, Sessler DI, Christensen R, Ozaki M, Schroeder M. Heat flow and distribution during epidural anesthesia. Anesthesiology 1995; 83:961–967.

69. Matsukawa T, Sessler DI, Sessler AM, Schroeder M, Ozaki M, Kurz A, Cheng C. Heat flow and distribution during induction of general anesthesia. Anesthesiology 1995; 82:662–673.

70. Bristow GK, Giesbrecht GG, Sessler DI. Leg temperature and heat content in humans during immersion hypothermia and rewarming. Aviat Space Environ Med 1994; 65:220–226.

71. Buck SH, Zaritsky AL. Occult core hyperthermia complicating cardiogenic shock. Pediatrics 1989; 83:782–784.

72. Rajek A, Lenhardt R, Sessler DI, Kurz A, Laufer G, Christensen R, Matsukawa T, Hiesmayer M. Tissue heat content and distribution during and after cardiopulmonary bypass at 31°C and 27°C. Anesthesiology 1998; 88:1511–1518.

73. Rajek A, Lenhardt R, Sessler DI, Grabenwöger M, Kastner J,

Mares P, Jantsch U, Gruber E. Tissue heat content and distribution during and after cardiopulmonary bypass at 17°C. Anesth Analg 1999; 88:1220–1225.

74. Sessler DI, Schroeder M, Merrifield B, Matsukawa T, Cheng C. Optimal duration and temperature of pre-warming. Anesthesiology 1995; 82:674–681.
75. Bazett HC, Love L, Newton M, Eisenberg L, Day R, Forster R II. Temperature changes in blood flowing in arteries and veins in man. Blood and Heat Exchange 1948; 1:3–19.
76. Andersen P, Saltin B. Maximal perfusion of skeletal muscle in man. J Physiol 1985; 366:233–249.
77. LeBlanc J. Subcutaneous fat and skin temperature. Can J Biochem Physiol 1954; 32:354–358.
78. Tikuisis P, Bell DG, Jacobs I. Shivering onset, metabolic response, and convective heat transfer during cold air exposure. J Appl Physiol 1991; 70:1996–2002.
79. Pennes HH. Analysis of tissue and arterial blood temperatures in the resting human forearm. J Appl Physiol 1948; 1:93–122.
80. Sessler DI, Sessler AM. Experimental determination of heat flow parameters during induction of anesthesia. Anesthesiology 1998; 89:657–665.
81. Wissler EH. A mathematical model of the human thermal system. Bull Math Biophys 1964; 26:147–166.
82. Ducharme MB, Tikuisis P. In vivo thermal conductivity of the human forearm tissues. J Appl Physiol 1991; 70:2682–2690.
83. Ducharme MB, VanHelder WP, Radomski MW. Tissue temperature profile in the human forearm during thermal stress at thermal stability. J Appl Physiol 1991; 71:1973–1978.
84. Ducharme MB, Tikuisis P. Forearm temperature profile during the transient phase of thermal stress. Eur J Appl Physiol Occup Physiol 1992; 64:395–401.
85. Rajek A, Greif R, Sessler DI, Baumgardner J, Laciny S, Bastanmehr H. Core cooling by central-venous infusion of 4°C and 20°C fluid: isolation of core and peripheral thermal compartments. Anesthesiology 2000; 93:629–637.

86. Lenhardt R, Negishi C, Sessler DI, Ozaki M, Tayefeh F, Kurz A. Paralysis only slightly reduces the febrile response to interleukin-2 during isoflurane anesthesia. Anesthesiology 1998; 89:648–656.

87. Bickler P, Sessler DI. Efficiency of airway heat and moisture exchangers in anesthetized humans. Anesth Analg 1990; 71:415–418.

88. Hey EN, Katz G. Evaporative water loss in the new-born baby. J Physiol 1969; 200:605–619.

89. Adams WC, Mack GW, Langhans GW, Nadel ER. Effects of varied air velocity on sweating and evaporative rates during exercise. J Appl Physiol 1992; 73:2668–2674.

90. Buono MJ, Sjoholm NT. Effect of physical training on peripheral sweat production. J Appl Physiol 1988; 65:811–814.

91. Froese G, Burton AC. Heat losses from the human head. J Appl Physiol 1957; 10:235–241.

92. Sessler DI, Moayeri A, Støen R, Glosten B, Hynson J, McGuire J. Thermoregulatory vasoconstriction decreases cutaneous heat loss. Anesthesiology 1990; 73:656–660.

93. Sessler DI, McGuire J, Moayeri A, Hynson J. Isoflurane-induced vasodilation minimally increases cutaneous heat loss. Anesthesiology 1991; 74:226–232.

94. Simbruner G, Weninge RM, Popow C, Herholdt WJ. Regional heat loss in newborn infants: Part I. Heat loss in healthy newborns at various environmental temperatures. S Afr Med J 1985; 68:940–944.

95. Simbruner G, Weninger W, Popow C, Herholdt WJ. Regional heat loss in newborn infants: Part II. Heat loss in newborns with various diseases—a method of assessing local metabolism and perfusion. S Afr Med J 1985; 68:945–948.

96. Matsukawa T, Kurz A, Sessler DI, Bjorksten AR, Merrifield B, Cheng C. Propofol linearly reduces the vasoconstriction and shivering thresholds. Anesthesiology 1995; 82:1169–1180.

97. Xiong J, Kurz A, Sessler DI, Plattner O, Christensen R, Dechert M, Ikeda T. Isoflurane produces marked and nonlinear decreases in the vasoconstriction and shivering thresholds. Anesthesiology 1996; 85:240–245.

98. Altura BM, Altura BT, Carella A, Turlapaty PDMV, Weinberg J. Vascular smooth muscle and general anesthetics. Fed Proc 1980; 39:1584–1591.

99. Plattner O, Xiong J, Sessler DI, Christensen R, Turakhia M, Dechert M, Clough D. Rapid core-to-peripheral tissue heat transfer during cutaneous cooling. Anesth Analg 1996; 82:925–930.

100. Clough D, Kurz A, Sessler DI, Christensen R, Xiong J. Thermoregulatory vasoconstriction does not impede core warming during cutaneous heating. Anesthesiology 1996; 85:281–288.

101. Hardy JD, Milhorat AT, DuBois EF. Basal metabolism and heat loss of young women at temperatures from 22 degrees C to 35 degrees C. J Nutr 1941; 21:383–403.

102. Plattner O, Ikeda T, Sessler DI, Christensen R, Turakhia M. Postanesthetic vasoconstriction slow postanesthetic peripheral-to-core transfer of cutaneous heat, thereby isolating the core thermal compartment. Anesth Analg 1997; 85:899–906.

103. Deriaz H, Fiez N, Lienhart A. Influence d'un filtre hygrophobe ou d'un humidificateur-réchauffeur sur l'hypothermie peropératoire. Ann Fr Anesth Réanim 1992; 11:145–149.

104. Sessler DI. Complications and treatment of mild hypothermia. Anesthesiology 2001; 95:531–543.

105. Alfonsi P, Coggia M, Leflon-Guibout V, Sessler DI, Goeau-Brissonniere O, Chauvin M. Mild hypothermia does not increase bacterial proliferation on implanted vascular grafts. Am J Surg 2002; 184:37–40.

106. Zweifler RM, Sessler DI, Zivin JA. Thermoregulatory vasoconstriction and shivering impede therapeutic hypothermia in acute ischemic stroke victims. J Stroke Cerebrovasc Dis 1997; 6:100–104.

107. Dae MW, Gao DW, Ursell PC, Stillson CA, Sessler DI. Safety and efficacy of endovascular cooling and rewarming for induction and reversal of hypothermia in human-sized pigs. Stroke 2003; 34:734–738.

108. Doufas AG, Akça O, Barry A, Petrusca DA, Suleman MI, Morioka N, Guarnaschelli JJ, Sessler DI. Initial experience with a novel heat-exchanging catheter in neurosurgical patients. Anesth Analg 2002; 95:1752–1756.

2

Hyperthermia and Fever

RAINER LENHARDT

Outcomes Research™ Institute and the Department of Anesthesiology and Perioperative Medicine, University of Louisville, Louisville, Kentucky, U.S.A.

INTRODUCTION

The human body has the ability to maintain core temperature within a precise range. Complex physiological mechanisms are in effect to prevent major deviations of body temperature in response to environmental conditions. These mechanisms are designed to promote heat loss or heat conservation as a response to constantly changing ambient temperatures. Control of these mechanisms resides in the hypothalamus and depends on the input of afferent neurons from various sites on the body (1,2).

Any elevation in body temperature above 38°C is considered hyperthermia (3,4). Whenever heat production exceeds heat loss, heat is stored and body temperature increases. This increase may be controlled (5) or uncontrolled (6). A controlled increase of core body temperature can be observed when exogenous or endogenous pyrogens trigger an elevated temperature setpoint in the hypothalamus (7). In this situation, the hypothalamus generates thermoregulatory responses such as vasoconstriction and shivering. These thermoregulatory mechanisms reduce heat loss and increase heat production to a predetermined temperature (setpoint). In contrast, uncontrolled hyperthermia can be generated by excessive heat exposure or by drug-related impairment of thermoregulatory response mechanisms such as active vasodilation or sweating (Table 1). Hyperthermia is metabolically stressful in both cases (8), but actively maintaining a fever can require especially large increases in metabolic heat production (9).

Increased body temperature is observed in many patients; however, it may be especially harmful in patients with brain disease or other neurological derangements. It is thus critical to obtain temperature readings on a regular basis. In case of an elevated core body temperature, it is advisable to search for the underlying cause. The distinction between controlled and uncontrolled hyperthermia is an important precondition to implementing appropriate treatment in hyperthermic patients.

This article is designed to give an overview on the various causes of hyperthermia with special emphasis on fever in general and in neurology critical care patients.

Table 1 Differences Between Hyperthermia and Fever

Hyperthermia	Fever
Uncontrolled	Controlled by the hypothalamus
Disordered central thermoregulation	Coordinated effector responses (vasoconstriction, shivering)
Excessive thermal challenge	"Setpoint" elevation
Impaired peripheral heat loss	Thermoregulatory response mechanisms intact
	Heat response mechanisms shifted to a higher value

REVIEW

Unregulated Hyperthermia

Exercise-Induced Hyperthermia

Strenuous exercise increases core body temperature considerably. An increase in core temperature during exercise was first reported in the Boston Marathon of 1903. Long distance runners can develop core temperatures of up to 41°C (10). During intense exercise, muscle activity increases internal heat production 15 to 20 times more than resting levels. Heat production by skeletal muscles exceeds heat loss, although sweating, active vasodilation, and evaporation are at their maximum. Consequently, hyperthermia remains throughout the exercise.

If strenuous exercise is performed in a warm, humid environment, heat stress can become overwhelming. Hyperthermia can be aggravated by inadequate fluid intake, which predisposes one to dehydration. A dehydrated athlete will have an impaired ability to sweat and will thus accumulate body heat. In addition, high humidity prevents heat loss, thereby causing a further imbalance between heat loss and heat production. Subsequently, heat stroke may develop.

Heat Stroke

Exercise-induced hyperthermia can result in heat illness. Another cause for heat illness is extended exposure to hot ambient temperatures coupled with high humidity. Heat illness occurs when the body produces more heat than it can dissipate. This occurs most often in conjunction with dehydration. The severity of heat illness depends on the intensity and duration of internal heat production or external heat exposure. It progresses from the mild stage of heat cramps and heat fatigue through the more serious condition of heat exhaustion and on to heat stroke, which can be fatal.

Heat cramps are often the first symptom to occur during heat illness. Heat cramps are painful contractions of muscles thought to be caused by dehydration, which creates an imbalance between fluid and electrolytes. The body's thermoregulatory responses are intact. Replacing fluid, which restores the fluid and electrolyte balance, is sufficient to treat or prevent this common syndrome. A more severe form of heat illness, which includes weakness, dizziness, nausea, and confusion, is accompanied by signs of dehydration such as tachycardia and hypotension. This phase is called heat fatigue. As symptoms continue to worsen, mental confusion develops, and an elevation of body temperature can be measured. Sweating continues at this stage. Eventually, the body loses its ability to sweat because of profound dehydration and hyperthermia becomes intense (body temperature above 41 °C). Disorientation, loss of coordination, hot, dry skin, and coma occur. Other clinical manifestations diagnosed in the hospital may be severe rhabdomyolysis, acute tubular necrosis, and disseminated intravascular coagulopathy. These symptoms are mainly seen in younger patients. This condition is known as heat stroke. At this point, immediate cooling and hospitalization are required.

Severe heat stroke requires treatment with rapid intravenous infusion of 2 to 3 L of ice-cold saline. This treatment simultaneously replenishes intravascular volume and rapidly cools the core thermal compartment. In-hospital treatment includes additional aggressive body surface cooling. Antipyretics do not have a role in the management of heat stroke.

Drug-Induced Hyperthermia

Drugs can cause hyperthermia via several mechanisms (Table 2). First, drugs can centrally inhibit sweating and vasodilation, thus allowing core temperature to increase passively in a hot environment. Second, drugs can inhibit

Table 2 Drugs Potentially Causing Increased Core Temperatures

Drugs facilitating hyperthermia	Drugs commonly triggering fever
Most anesthesia drugs	Penicillins
Atropine	Cephalosporins
Amphetamine	Phenytoin
MDMA	Amphotericin B
Cocaine	

peripheral thermoregulatory defense mechanisms. Third, drugs can produce a hypermetabolic state that increases heat production beyond the body's compensatory abilities. It is important to identify the source of drug-induced hyperthermia in order to treat it appropriately.

Most drugs used in anesthesia centrally impair thermoregulation by increasing the temperature at which the warm-response mechanisms, sweating and vasodilation, will be triggered (the thermoregulatory thresholds). If a patient is warmed actively during anesthesia, severe hyperthermia can result because sweating and active vasodilation do not function adequately (11). It is therefore prudent to measure core temperatures when patients are actively warmed during anesthesia.

Other drugs frequently used in anesthesia and intensive care can peripherally inhibit thermoregulatory effectors such as sweating. Atropine, e.g., increases the threshold for sweating by roughly 1.0°C (12) and can prevent sweating (13). The whole body sweating rate is about 45% lower in exercising humans after receiving atropine rather than saline (14). Consequently, atropine should be used with caution in a hot environment.

Some drugs can produce a hypermetabolic state that increases heat production beyond the body's compensatory abilities. Amphetamine, a frequently abused sympathomimetic drug, can cause hyperthermia. Derivatives of amphetamine have become increasingly popular. The drug 3,4-methylenedioxymethamphetamine (MDMA, Ecstasy) has numerous toxic side effects of which hyperthermia and hyponatremia are among the most serious.

Another substance commonly used as a recreational drug is cocaine. Among its other potentially lethal side effects, this drug has a propensity to cause hyperthermia. It was long believed that cocaine caused a hypermetabolic state with increased heat production. The intrinsic thermogenic property of cocaine underlies recent epidemiological data showing that mortality rates for cocaine overdose increase substantially in hot weather (15). In a recent study, however, Crandall et al. found that even small doses of cocaine are able to elevate the temperature thresholds for sweating and active vasodilation in the presence of external heat stress (16). Thus, cocaine appears to elevate core body temperature by both increasing heat production and impairing heat dissipation. This unique property is not shared by other sympathomimetic drugs, such as ephedrine or methamphetamine, which cause hyperthermia mainly by increasing skeletal muscle metabolism (17,18).

Malignant Hyperthermia and the Neuroleptic Malignant Syndrome

Malignant hyperthermia is a rare congenital disturbance of calcium regulation in skeletal muscle. This syndrome is caused by volatile anesthetics and the depolarizing paralytic agent succinylcholine (Table 3). It is characterized by a sudden excessive increase in core body temperature and is generally lethal, if untreated. The increase in body temperature during malignant hyperthermia results from an enormous escalation of metabolic heat produced by internal organs and skeletal muscles. Central thermoregulation presumably remains intact during acute crises, but efferent heat loss mechanisms may be compromised by intense peripheral vasoconstriction resulting from circulating catecholamine concentrations of up to 20 times normal.

A clinically similar syndrome, neuroleptic malignant syndrome, is expressed by hypermetabolic fever triggered by the use of psychotropic drugs, such as phenothiazines, tricyclic antidepressants, and monoamine oxidase inhibitors (Table 3).

Table 3 Drugs Causing Malignant Hyperthermia or Malignant Neuroleptic Syndrome

Drugs potentially triggering malignant hyperthermia	Drugs potentially triggering malignant neuroleptic syndrome
Volatile anesthetics: sevoflurane, desflurane, isoflurane, enflurane, halothane	Phenothiazines
	Tricyclic antidepressants
	Monoamine oxidase inhibitors
Succinylcholine	

Positive caffeine-contracture muscle biopsies in some patients with neuroleptic malignant syndrome suggest a pathophysiology similar to that of malignant hyperthermia.

Fever (Regulated Hyperthermia)

Definition of Fever

Any elevation in body temperature identifies hyperthermia. Certainly, core temperatures above 38°C are never normal. As early as 1868, Carl Reinhold August Wunderlich established 38°C as the upper limit of "subfebrile" body temperature (19). Whenever heat production exceeds heat loss, excessive heat remains in the body and core temperature increases. This increase may be unregulated hyperthermia because of conditions mentioned above or it may be fever. Clinicians have appreciated that the febrile range has an upper limit (20), in that the elevation of body temperature during fever does not exceed safe limits. In this respect, fever appears to be a tightly regulated hyperthermia.

Fever has been defined as "a state of elevated core temperature, which is often part of the defense responses of multicellular organisms (host) to the invasion of life (microorganisms) or inanimate matter recognized as pathogenic or alien by the host" (21). Thus, fever is a complex physiological response to a pathogenic trigger that is aimed at facilitating survival of the host. How fever is mediated remains controversial, although several pathways have been identified experimentally.

Pathogenesis of Fever

In the 1940s, fever was shown to be mediated by soluble "endogenous pyrogens" released by immune stimulation. Endotoxin or the lipopolysaccharide (LPS) complex in the cell wall of gram-negative bacteria readily triggers the release of these compounds by leucocytes and phagocytic macrophages.

Endogenous pyrogens are cytokines that induce fever. These cytokines are thought to either cross the blood–brain barrier by facilitated transport mechanisms (22), diffuse into areas of the brain where there is no blood–brain barrier (23), or interact with peripheral neural components of the immune system to signal the hypothalamus to increase the thermal setpoint (24).

For instance, some peripherally secreted cytokines may be transported directly from blood to brain reaching neurons in the preoptic area by facilitated transport across the blood–brain barrier in this region. In fact, some saturable transport systems for interleukin-1 and interleukin-6 have been described (25). Yet, fever caused by intravenous administration of LPS typically develops within minutes, and it is questionable whether endogenous pyrogens can enter the brain quickly enough to cause such quick onset of fever. Carrier-mediated transport of cytokines into the brain may nonetheless play a role in the later stages of fever.

It has also been suggested that circulating pyrogens might gain access to the preoptic area by crossing the capillaries at the circumventricular vascular organs [organum vasculosum laminae terminalis (OVLT)], which have been shown to lack a blood–brain barrier (23). Thus, bloodborne cytokines may diffuse into the surrounding preoptic area, causing prostaglandins (e.g., PGE_2) to be released. Prostaglandins might then mediate the passage of pyrogenic messages from blood to brain. In fact, prostaglandins produce a fever of short duration when injected into the rostral hypothalamus (26).

On the other hand, there is considerable evidence that cytokine signaling to the central nervous system is mediated primarily by stimulation of peripheral vagal afferent nerves (27). This conclusion is based on observations that (1) the vagus contains afferent fibers that communicate information from the viscera to the brain (28), (2) vagal electrical activity increases following injection of interleukin-1β into the hepatic portal vein, and (3) vagotomy prevents at least some types of fever (24,29).

Recently, a new hypothesis of peripheral cytokine signaling to the brain was suggested (30). This theory proposes that intravenous LPS rapidly triggers the release of substances such as complement fragments C3a and C5a that, in turn, bind to macrophages in the liver (Kupffer cells). In response, Kupffer cells rapidly release mediators (perhaps cytokines and PGE_2) capable of activating subdiaphragmatic vagal afferents. The vagus then sends signals to the A1/A2 noradrenergic cell groups in the brain stem, from where they are transmitted via neurons of the ventral noradrenergic bundle to the preoptic area. Consequently, noradrenergic input at the preoptic area triggers postsynaptic release of PGE_2, thus resulting in the development of fever. It has to be emphasized that this theory accounts for the rapid onset of LPS-induced fever, whereas the maintenance of fever may be caused by other mechanisms.

The regulation of fever is accomplished by two families of endogenous cytokines: some pyrogens and others cryogens (or antipyretics). The family of endogenous pyrogens includes interleukin-1 (31), interleukin-6 (32), interleukin-8, interferon-α (33), and macrophage inflammatory protein-1β (34). The other cytokines are endogenous antipyretics, which limit the magnitude and the duration of fever and include such substances as interleukin-10 (35–37), arginine vasopressin (38), α-melanocyte-stimulating hormone, and glucocorticoids (39). Other substances such as tumor necrosis factor alpha (TNF-α) have been shown to have pyrogenic and antipyretic properties, depending on the experimental conditions (40–42). To date, TNF-α is thought to be the main cytokine regulator of fever, as has been demonstrated by the use of pharmacological TNF-α neutralizing agents and gene knockout techniques (43).

The sum of the interaction between these endogenous pyrogens and antipyretics is responsible for the ultimate magnitude of fever. It has been postulated, although not proved, that pyrogens and their antagonists, the antipyretics, bind to their own specific receptors, some of which are near the preoptic region of the anterior hypothalamus (5,44). Here, receptors of the endogenous pyrogen complex activate phospholipase A_2, resulting in the liberation of plasma membrane arachidonic acid as a substrate for the cyclooxygenase pathway. Cyclooxygenase liberates prostaglandin E_2. This small lipid mediator diffuses across the blood–brain barrier, where it decreases the firing rate of preoptic warm-sensitive neurons and excites cold-sensitive neurons in the medial rostral hypothalamus. The change in neuronal signaling causes the hypothalamus to elevate the thermal setpoint. This mechanism differs from "normal" thermoregulation, which is not dependent on circulating factors, and explains why drugs like aspirin decrease fever, but have little influence on normal body temperature (45).

Course of Fever

During the first phase of fever, pyrogens decrease the firing rate in warm-sensitive neurons, and the setpoints of all thermoregulatory responses (vasoconstriction, shivering, vasodilation, and sweating) shift to higher temperatures. Once the setpoint exceeds core temperature, the usual thermoregulatory effectors are mobilized to increase core temperature. These responses include vasoconstriction to decrease heat loss, shivering to increase metabolic heat production, and behavioral responses dictated by thermal discomfort. During steady-state fever, core temperature is closely regulated around the elevated setpoint (Fig. 1).

The final phase of fever is defervescence, when body temperature returns to afebrile conditions. It occurs when the concentrations of preoptic pyrogenic substances decrease

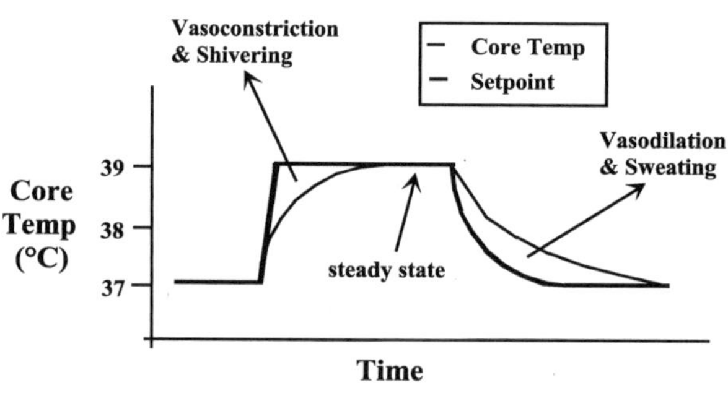

Figure 1 Typical course of a monophasic fever. As the setpoint is shifted to a higher temperature, the body increases heat retention and production by initiating vasoconstriction and shivering. When the setpoint returns to normal, the body tries to dissipate heat with vasodilation and sweating.

and warm-sensitive neurons return to their original, relatively high, firing rates, thus reducing the setpoint temperature. Consequently, heat-loss mechanisms such as active vasodilation and sweating are initiated, whereas heat-retention and heat-production mechanisms are discontinued.

The "setpoint theory" for fever is supported by a study in which fever was triggered experimentally with interleukin-2 in human volunteers (7). In this study, the sweating threshold during fever was 1.6°C higher and the vasoconstriction threshold 1.7°C higher than normal body temperature. The sweating-to-vasoconstriction interthreshold range did not change significantly, the difference being only 0.1°C, which is similar to that at normal body temperature. These data suggest that fever synchronously augments thermoregulatory thresholds without a change in interthreshold range and can thus be considered an increase in the setpoint (Fig. 2).

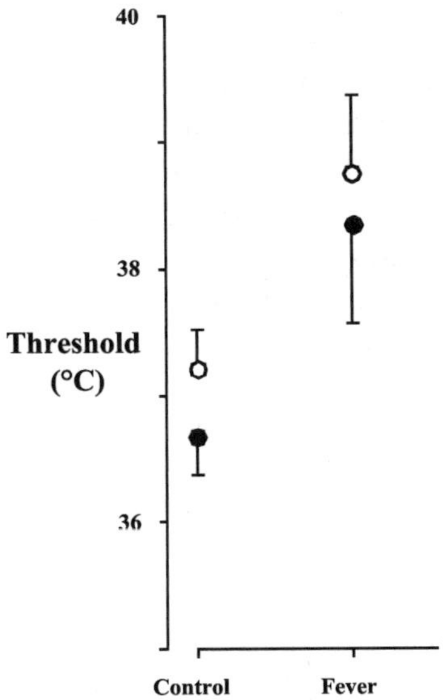

Figure 2 Threshold shifts during normothermia and during fever. Solid circles depict the threshold temperatures for vasoconstriction; open circles depict thresholds temperatures for sweating. (From Ref. 7.)

Benefits of Fever

Hyperthermia stimulates immune function (46). Both local and systemic hyperthermia have been used for the treatment of malignant disease (47,48). Cancer cells are more sensitive to hyperthermia per se, and the difference between malignant and normal cells is further enhanced when hyperthermia is combined with chemotherapy or ionizing radiation (49). Systemic hyperthermia has even been considered as a possible treatment for human immunodeficiency virus infections (50).

Studies of the phylogeny of fever have shown this response to be widespread within the animal kingdom. Mammals, birds, reptiles, and fish can all develop fever when infected (reptiles and fish, of course, use behavioral regulation to control body temperature). It is unlikely that a metabolically expensive response such as fever would have been retained in so many species for so long without providing significant benefit. This has been seen as a strong evidence for fever being an adaptive response to infection (51).

Classic studies in the 1970s demonstrated increased mortality when fever is prevented in infected lizards by denying them access to a warm environment or by administration of aspirin (52–54). Aspirin administration also increases mortality in infected mammals. The protective effects of fever result from increased immune and cytotoxic function, not from direct actions on bacterial or viral pathogens. Specifically, fever increases neutrophil and macrophage motility and activity, activates T lymphocytes, causes secretion of antibacterial chemicals, and decreases serum iron, which is required for bacterial growth (55–57).

Hemodynamic Consequences of Fever

As mentioned earlier, fever is a host defense response that may benefit some critically ill patients. Others, however, may not tolerate the cardiovascular demands caused by the increase in sympathetic tone.

In the basal state, impulses from cutaneous cold receptors tonically stimulate thermoregulatory neurons concentrated in the hypothalamus; these in turn activate sympathetic nerves in the lateral horn of the spinal cord whose postganglionic fibers terminate on cutaneous vascular bed. Tonic sympathetic arteriovenous shunt tone is thus relatively well maintained, producing a relatively high basal cutaneous vascular resistance (58).

During the rising phase of fever, increased sympathetic nervous system activity augments tone at cutaneous vessels and other organs, thus increasing systemic vascular resistance. However, the increase is modest because resistance is already high in the basal state. Consequently, thermoregulatory vasoconstriction, per se, usually has little cardiovascular effect (59). In contrast, shivering, which often accompanies the development of fever, can double or triple the metabolic rate and markedly increase heart rate and cardiac output (60).

As core temperature reaches its new (elevated) steady state, the discharge rate of thermoregulatory neurons returns to prefebrile levels. Sympathic stimulation to the cutaneous vascular bed is thus withdrawn and cutaneous blood flow returns toward basal levels. During defervescence, the thermoregulatory setpoint returns toward prefebrile levels. Sympathetic nervous activity in peripheral vascular bed is therefore reduced, permitting passive vasodilation. More importantly, however, active vasodilation via stimulation of sweat glands is initiated (58).

Active vasodilation enormously increases capillary blood flow (61) and, therefore, heat delivery from the core to the skin surface. Increased cutaneous perfusion is accompanied by a marked decrease in systemic vascular resistance. As might be expected, decreased mean arterial pressure stimulates an increase in heart rate and cardiac output (62). This is the same cardiovascular compensation observed during passive hyperthermia. It is not unusual for heart rates under these circumstances to exceed 130 beats per minute, making tachycardia the major cardiovascular issue.

Fever in the General Intensive Care Unit

Fever is common in surgical intensive care units. Routine postoperative fever is a well-recognized symptom that accompanies the inflammatory response to surgical procedures. It is generally benign and of short duration. It is most often of noninfectious origin, self-limiting, and does not need therapeutical intervention. In contrast, prolonged fever (>5 days) is usually caused by infection and is associated with a poor outcome (63).

Fever is also frequent in medical intensive care units. Fevers occur secondarily to nosocomial pneumonia, pulmonary emboli, myocardial infarction, gastrointestinal bleeding, acute pancreatitis, and adrenal insufficiency. In both medical and surgical ICUs, causes of fever are evenly divided between noninfectious and infectious etiologies (64,65). However, fever must always be considered given the potential consequences of inadequate or delayed treatment in this fragile population. Only after infectious causes have been excluded are noninfectious reasons for a fever considered.

Fever may be a striking sign of infection in ICU patients. The most common infections reported in ICU patients are pneumonia, sinusitis, bloodstream infections, and catheter-related infections (66). Less likely to be found are urinary tract infections and *Clostridium difficile* diarrhea.

Noninfectious fever can be caused by a variety of drugs (Table 2), because ICU patients are exposed to a battery of different medications. Drug-induced fevers should be considered in patients with an otherwise unexplained fever, in particular, if they were receiving betalactamase antibiotics (67) or diphenylhydantoin (68–70). Similarly, fever may be triggered secondary to blood transfusion (71) or platelet transfusion (72). Another noninfectious cause of fever is acalculous cholecystitis. In this frequently unrecognized disease, pain, vomiting, and fever may be the only symptoms. Thus, fever might be a major symptom to suspect this potentially fatal disease in ICU patients (73).

Fever in the Neurointensive Care Unit

Despite the use of antibiotic and antipyretic therapy, febrile episodes occur in more than half the patients admitted to the ICU for subarachnoid, central nervous system infection, seizure control, hemorrhagic stroke, or closed head injury (74).

The exact mechanism by which brain injury induces hyperthermia remains unknown; however, various processes are involved. Hyperthermia might increase the release of excitatory neurotransmitters (75–78), and it might trigger an abundant amount of oxygen free radicals (79–81). Hyperthermia may also aggravate blood–brain barrier disruption (82), impair cytoskeletal proteolysis (83,84), and enhance inhibition of enzymatic protein kinases (85,86), which, in turn, would impair recovery of energy metabolism.

Fever after trauma or ischemia may aggravate the damage caused by the original injury. Animal studies have shown that hyperthermia impairs the outcome after both focal and global ischemia (82,83,87) and after traumatic brain injury (88). In a canine study, successful treatment of elevated core temperatures reduced mortality and morbidity after transient global cerebral ischemia (89). Even delayed hyperthermia after ischemic or traumatic brain injury correlates with an increase in injury volume and mortality (82,88,90).

The deleterious effect of fever has also been demonstrated in patients with brain injury. For instance, each day patients with subarachnoid hemorrhage (SAH) have a fever increases the risk of poor outcome (91). If these patients suffer from symptomatic vasospasm, they have an increased risk of developing a fever. Likewise, in this population, the presence of a ventriculostomy increases the risk of becoming febrile by more than eightfold. A limitation of these studies, though, is that fever may simply be a marker for worse intracranial injury.

Several studies in stroke patients have demonstrated an association between fever and more severe symptoms, although none have demonstrated causality. In one study, fever in the first 7 days after a stroke was an independent predictor of poor outcome during the first month poststroke (92). Whereas an earlier study indicates that fever and even subfebrility carry a bad prognosis with respect to residual neurological symptoms (93), a more recent prospective trial demonstrated that in acute human stroke, an association exists between body temperature and initial stroke severity, infarct size, mortality, and outcome (94).

No study has proven that fever in patients with head injury is associated with poor outcome. However, given the body of evidence that has accumulated in recent years showing that temperature elevations exacerbate the degree of neuronal injury in both animals and humans, it seems prudent to at least prevent fever in patients with traumatic brain injuries.

A recent study of 387 patients identified risk factors for fever ($T \geq 38.3°C$) in the neurological intensive care unit (95). Fever occurred in 23% of patients; approximately one-half were due to documented infection, and one-quarter were unexplained despite a complete evaluation, and thus possibly central in origin. After controlling for ICU length of stay, coma predicted both types of fever, mechanical ventilation predicted infections fever, and placement of a ventriculostomy (usually for ventricular hemorrhage) predicted unexplained fever. Subarachnoid hemorrhage increased the risk of developing both of these types of fever even after controlling for these risk factors; over 60% developed fever at some point during their ICU stay.

FUTURE DIRECTIONS

In the sense that the brain houses the central mechanism for the regulation of body temperature, almost all illnesses that cause fever must interact with the central nervous system. Thus, some patients may suffer from neurological impairment resulting from fever itself, whereas in others fever will be the sole manifestation of a central nervous system infection. In general, in patients with intracranial disease requiring admission to an ICU, fever may play a deleterious role. It is believed that fever aggravates neuronal damage irrespective of the etiology (96). If a prospective, prophylactic fever-management study provides evidence that such management is efficacious and safe, the next step will be to determine how to keep brain and core temperatures within normal range. In two studies, intravascular cooling catheters have safely reduced core temperatures (97,98); other related studies are planned.

Many patients are heavily sedated during their stay in the ICU. Sedatives and anesthetics profoundly impair thermoregulatory responses in nonneurological and neurosurgical patients (99). However, reduction of hyperthermic temperatures remains tricky in neurointensive care patients, because therapeutic reductions in core temperature trigger aggressive thermoregulatory defenses. The most important autonomic cold defenses in humans are arteriovenous shunt vasoconstriction (100) and shivering (101). This has led to a search for drugs that impair vasoconstriction and shivering without causing excessive sedation or respiratory toxicity. Although the combination of buspirone and meperidine appears helpful (102), as does the combination of dexmedetomidine and meperidine (103), the optimal drug or drug combination has yet to be identified.

In summary, the focus of ongoing research is to determine if a reduction of fever in neurointensive care patients will decrease mortality and morbidity. At the same time, the search continues to find a tool to effectively reduce increased core body and brain temperatures without triggering thermoregulatory defense mechanisms.

REFERENCES

1. Guyton AC, Hall J. Textbook of Medical Physiology. 10th ed. Philadelphia: W.B. Saunders, 2001.
2. Schafer J. Body temperature regulation. In: LR J, ed. Essential Medical Physiology. Philadelphia: Lippincott-Raven, 1998:815–824.
3. Mackowiak PA, Wasserman SS, Levine MM. A critical appraisal of 98.6°F, the upper limit of the normal body temperature, and other legacies of Carl Reinhold August Wunderlich. JAMA 1992; 268:1578–1580.
4. Committee ASCc. Definitions for sepsis and organ failure and guidelines for the use of innovative therapies in sepsis. Chest 1992; 101:1644–1655.
5. Saper CB, Breder CD. Neurologic basis of fever. N Engl J Med 1994; 330:1880–1886.
6. Simon HB. Hyperthermia. N Engl J Med 1993; 329:483–487.

7. Lenhardt R, Negishi C, Sessler DI, Ozaki M, Ettinger K, Bastanmehr H, Lobo E. The effect of pyrogen administration on sweating and vasoconstriction thresholds during desflurane anesthesia. Anesthesiology 1999; 90:1587–1595.

8. Styrt B, Sugarman B. Antipyresis and fever. Arch Intern Med 1990; 150:1589–1597.

9. Romanovsky AA, Szekely M. Fever and hypothermia: two adaptive thermoregulatory responses to systemic inflammation. Med Hypotheses 1998; 50:219–226.

10. Armstrong LE, Crago AE, Adams R, Roberts WO, Maresh CM. Whole-body cooling of hyperthermic runners: comparison of two field therapies. Am J Emerg Med 1996; 14:355–358.

11. Washington D, Sessler DI, Moayeri A, Merrifield B, Prager M, McGuire J, Belani K, Hudson S, Schroeder M. Thermoregulatory responses to hyperthermia during isoflurane anesthesia in humans. J Appl Physiol 1993; 74:82–87.

12. Greif R, Laciny S, Rajek AM, Larson MD, Bjorksten AR, Doufas AG, Bakhshandeh M, Mokhtarani M, Sessler DI. Neither nalbuphine nor atropine posses special antishivering activity. Anesth Analg 2001; 93:620–627.

13. Boudet J, Qing W, Boyer-Chammard A, Del Franco G, Bergougnan JL, Rosen P, Meyer P. Dose–response effects of atropine in human volunteers. Fundam Clin Pharmacol 1991; 5:635–640.

14. Cadarette BS, Levine L, Rock PB, Stephenson LA, Kolka MA. Effects of atropine on thermoregulatory responses to exercise in different environments. Aviat Space Environ Med 1986; 57:1050–1055.

15. Marzuk PM, Tardiff K, Leon AC, Hirsch CS, Portera L, Iqbal MI, Nock MK, Hartwell N. Ambient temperature and mortality from unintentional cocaine overdose. JAMA 1998; 279:1795–1800.

16. Crandall CG, Vongpatanasin W, Victor RG. Mechanism of cocaine-induced hyperthermia in humans. Ann Intern Med 2002; 136:785–791.

17. Astrup A, Bulow J, Madsen J, Christensen NJ. Contribution of BAT and skeletal muscle to thermogenesis induced by ephedrine in man. Am J Physiol 1985; 248:E507–E515.

18. Makisumi T, Yoshida K, Watanabe T, Tan N, Murakami N, Morimoto A. Sympatho-adrenal involvement in methamphetamine-induced hyperthermia through skeletal muscle hypermetabolism. Eur J Pharmacol 1998; 363:107–112.

19. Wunderlich CRA. Das Verhalten von Eigenwärme in Krankheiten. Leipzig: Wigard, 1868.

20. Mackowiak PA, Boulant JA. Fever's glass ceiling. Clin Infect Dis 1996; 22:525–536.

21. IUPS Thermal Commission. Glossary of terms for thermal physiology. 2d ed. Eur J Physiol 1987; 410:567–587.

22. Banks WA, Kastin AJ, Durham DA. Bidirectional transport of interleukin-1 alpha across the blood–brain barrier. Brain Res Bull 1989; 23:433–437.

23. Blatteis C. Role of the OVLT in the febrile response to circulating pyrogens. Prog Brain Res 1992; 91:409–412.

24. Watkins LR, Goehler LE, Relton JK, Tartaglia N, Silbert L, Martin D, Maier SF. Blockade of interleukin-1 induced hyperthermia by subdiaphragmatic vagotomy: evidence for vagal mediation of immune-brain communication. Neurosci Lett 1995; 183:27–31.

25. Banks W, Plotkin S, Kastin A. Permeability of the blood–brain barrier to soluble cytokine receptors. Neuroimmunomodulation 1995; 2:161–165.

26. Sitt J. Prostaglandine E as a mediator of the febrile response. Yale J Biol Med 1986; 59:137–149.

27. Fleshner M, Goehler LE, Hermann J, Relton JK, Maier SF, Watkins LR. Interleukin-1 beta induced corticosterone elevation and hypothalamic NE depletion is vagally mediated. Brain Res Bull 1995; 37:605–610.

28. Leslie R, Reynolds J, Lawes I. Central connections of the nucleus of the vagus nerve. In: Ritter R, Ritter S, Barnes C, eds. Neuroanatomy and Physiology of the Abdominal Vagal Afferents. Ann Arbor, MI: CRC Press, 1992:81–98.

29. Niijima A. The afferent discharges from sensors from interleukin-1 beta in hepatoportal system in the anesthetized rat. J Physiol 1992; 446:236.

30. Blatteis C, Sehic E. Fever: how may circulating pyrogens signal the brain? News Physiol Sci 1997; 12:1–9.

31. Dinarello CA, Wolff SM. The role of interleukin-1 in disease. N Engl J Med 1993; 328:106–113.

32. Dinarello CA, Cannon JG, Mancilla J, Bishai I, Lees J, Coceani F. Interleukin-6 as an endogenous pyrogen: induction of prostaglandin E2 in brain but not in peripheral blood mononuclear cells. Brain Res 1991; 562:199–206.

33. Nakashima T, Hori T, Kuriyama K, Matsuda T. Effects of interferon-alpha on the activity of preoptic thermosensitive neurons in tissue slices. Brain Res 1988; 454:361–367.

34. Davatelis G, Wolpe SD, Sherry B, Dayer JM, Chicheportiche R, Cerami A. Macrophage inflammatory protein-1: a prostaglandin-independent endogenous pyrogen. Science 1989; 243:1066–1068.

35. Fiorentino DF, Zlotnik A, Vieira P, Mosmann TR, Howard M, Moore KW, O'Garra A. IL-10 acts on the antigen-presenting cell to inhibit cytokine production by Th1 cells. J Immunol 1991; 146:3444–3451.

36. Fiorentino DF, Zlotnik A, Mosmann TR, Howard M, O'Garra A. IL-10 inhibits cytokine production by activated macrophages. J Immunol 1991; 147:3815–3822.

37. Nava F, Calapai G, Facciola G, Cuzzocrea S, Marciano MC, De Sarro A, Caputi AP. Effects of interleukin-10 on water intake, locomotory activity, and rectal temperature in rat treated with endotoxin. Int J Immunopharmacol 1997; 19:31–38.

38. Pittman QJ, Wilkinson MF. Central arginine vasopressin and endogenous antipyresis. Can J Physiol Pharmacol 1992; 70:786–790.

39. Morrow LE, McClellan JL, Conn CA, Kluger MJ. Glucocorticoids alter fever and IL-6 responses to psychological stress and to lipopolysaccharide. Am J Physiol 1993; 264:R1010–1016.

40. Mier JW, Vachino G, Van Der Meer JWM, Numerof RP, Adams S, Cannon JG, Bernheim HA, Atkins MB, Parkinson DR, Dinarello CA. Induction of circulating tumor necrosis factor (TNF-alpha) as the mechanism for the febrile response

to interleukin-2 (IL-2) in cancer patients. J Clin Immunol 1988; 8:426–436.

41. Dinarello CA, Cannon JG, Wolff SM, Bernheim HA, Beutler B, Cerami A, Figari IS, Palladino JMA, O'Connor JV. Tumor necrosis factor (cachectin) is an endogenous pyrogen and induces production of interleukin 1. J Exp Med 1986; 163:1433–1450.
42. Klir JJ, McClellan JL, Kozak W, Szelenyi Z, Wong GH, Kluger MJ. Systemic but not central administration of tumor necrosis factor-alpha attenuates LPS-induced fever in rats. Am J Physiol 1995; 268:R480–486.
43. Leon LR. Invited review: cytokine regulation of fever: studies using gene knockout mice. J Appl Physiol 2002; 92:2648–2655.
44. Mackowiak PA. Concepts of fever. Arch Intern Med 1998; 158:1870–1881.
45. Satinoff E. Salicylate: action on normal body temperature in rats. Science 1972; 176:532–533.
46. Kluger MJ, Ringler DH, Anver MR. Fever and survival. Science 1975; 188:166–168.
47. Field SB. Hyperthermia in the treatment of cancer. Phys Med Biol 1987; 32:789–811.
48. Falk MH, Issels RD. Hyperthermia in oncology. Int J Hyperthermia 2001; 17:1–18.
49. Engin K, Tupchong L, Waterman FM, Komarnicky L, Mansfield CM, Hussain N, Hoh LL, McFarlane JD, Leeper DB. Multiple field hyperthermia combined with radiotherapy in advanced carcinoma of the breast. Int J Hyperthermia 1994; 10:587–603.
50. Pennypacker C, Nys N, Perelson A, Nelson G, Sessler DI. Localized or systemic in vivo heat-inactivation of human immunodeficiency virus (HIV): a mathematical analysis. J Acquir Immun Defic Syndr 1995; 8:321–329.
51. Kluger MJ. The evolution and adaptive value of fever. Am Sci 1978; 66:38–43.
52. Kluger MJ. Is fever beneficial? Yale J Biol Med 1986; 59:89–95.

53. Bernheim HA, Kluger MJ. Fever: effect of drug-induced antipyresis on survival. Science 1976; 193:237–239.

54. Bernheim HA, Bodel PT, Askenase PW, Atkins E. Effects of fever on host defence mechanisms after infection in the lizard *Dipsosaurus dorsalis*. Br J Exp Pathol 1978; 59:76–84.

55. Bennett IL Jr, Nicastri A. Fever as a mechanism of resistance. Bacteriol Rev 1960; 24:16–34.

56. Hanson DF, Murphy PA, Silicano R, Shin HS. The effect of temperature on the activation of thymocytes by interleukins I and II. J Immunol 1983; 130:216–221.

57. Duff GW, Durum SK. Fever and immunoregulation: hyperthermia, interleukins 1 and 2, and T-cell proliferation. Yale J Biol Med 1982; 55:437–442.

58. Rowell LB. Active neurogenic vasodilation in man. In: Vanhoutte P, Leusen I, eds. Vasodilatation. New York: Raven Press, 1981:1–17.

59. Rowell LB. Cardiovascular aspects of human thermoregulation. Circ Res 1983; 52:367–379.

60. Giesbrecht GG, Sessler DI, Mekjavic IB, Schroeder M, Bristow GW. Treatment of immersion hypothermia by direct body-to-body contact. J Appl Physiol 1994; 76:2373–2379.

61. Detry J-MR, Brengelmann GL, Rowell LB, Wyss C. Skin and muscle components of forearm blood flow in directly heated resting man. J Appl Physiol 1972; 32:506–511.

62. Rowell LB. Human Circulation Regulation During Physical Stress. New York: Oxford University Press, 1986.

63. Circiumaru B, Baldock G, Cohen J. A prospective study of fever in the intensive care unit. Intensive Care Med 1999; 25:668–673.

64. O'Grady NP, Barie PS, Bartlett J, Bleck T, Garvey G, Jacobi J, Linden P, Maki DG, Nam M, Pasculle W, Pasquale MD, Tribett DL, Masur H. Practice parameters for evaluating new fever in critically ill adult patients. Task Force of the American College of Critical Care Medicine of the Society of Critical Care Medicine in collaboration with the Infectious Disease Society of America. Crit Care Med 1998; 26:392–408.

65. Cunha BA, Shea KW. Fever in the intensive care unit. Infect Dis Clin North Am 1996; 10:185–209.

66. Vincent JL, Bihari DJ, Suter PM, Bruining HA, White J, Nicolas-Chanoin MH, Wolff M, Spencer RC, Hemmer M. The prevalence of nosocomial infection in intensive care units in Europe. Results of the European Prevalence of Infection in Intensive Care (EPIC) Study. EPIC International Advisory Committee. JAMA 1995; 274:639–644.

67. Huckell VF, Staniloff HM, Britt BA, Morch JE. Electrocardiographic abnormalities associated with malignant hyperthermia susceptibility. J Electrocardiol 1982; 15:137–141.

68. Carpenter J, Sander G, Newby N, Kendrick M. Phenytoin hypersensitivity presenting as postoperative fever. Neurosurgery 1980; 6:426–429.

69. Mackowiak PA. Drug fever: mechanisms, maxims and misconceptions. Am J Med Sci 1987; 294:275–286.

70. Tabor PA. Drug-induced fever. Drug Intell Clin Pharm 1986; 20:413–420.

71. Rutledge R, Sheldon GF, Collins ML. Massive transfusion. Crit Care Clin 1986; 2:791–805.

72. Heddle NM. Pathophysiology of febrile nonhemolytic transfusion reactions. Curr Opin Hematol 1999; 6:420–426.

73. Kalliafas S, Ziegler DW, Flancbaum L, Choban PS. Acute acalculous cholecystitis: incidence, risk factors, diagnosis, and outcome. Am Surg 1998; 64:471–475.

74. Kilpatrick MM, Lowry DW, Firlik AD, Yonas H, Marion DW. Hyperthermia in the neurosurgical intensive care unit. Neurosurgery 2000; 47:850–855; discussion 855–856.

75. Globus MY, Ginsberg MD, Busto R. Excitotoxic index—a biochemical marker of selective vulnerability. Neurosci Lett 1991; 127:39–42.

76. Takagi K, Ginsberg MD, Globus MY, Martinez E, Busto R. Effect of hyperthermia on glutamate release in ischemic penumbra after middle cerebral artery occlusion in rats. Am J Physiol 1994; 267:H1770–1776.

77. Suehiro E, Fujisawa H, Ito H, Ishikawa T, Maekawa T. Brain temperature modifies glutamate neurotoxicity in vivo. J Neurotrauma 1999; 16:285–297.

78. Asai S, Zhao H, Kohno T, Takahashi Y, Nagata T, Ishikawa K. Quantitative evaluation of extracellular glutamate concentration in postischemic glutamate re-uptake, dependent on brain temperature, in the rat following severe global brain ischemia. Brain Res 2000; 864:60–68.

79. Chatzipanteli K, Alonso OF, Kraydieh S, Dietrich WD. Importance of posttraumatic hypothermia and hyperthermia on the inflammatory response after fluid percussion brain injury: biochemical and immunocytochemical studies. J Cereb Blood Flow Metab 2000; 20:531–542.

80. Kil HY, Zhang J, Piantadosi CA. Brain temperature alters hydroxyl radical production during cerebral ischemia/reperfusion in rats. J Cereb Blood Flow Metab 1996; 16:100–106.

81. Lin B, Busto R, Globus MY, Martinez E, Ginsberg MD. Brain temperature modulations during global ischemia fail to influence extracellular lactate levels in rats. Stroke 1995; 26:1634–1638.

82. Dietrich WD, Busto R, Halley M, Valdes I. The importance of brain temperature in alterations of the blood–brain barrier following cerebral ischemia. J Neuropathol Exp Neurol 1990; 49:486–497.

83. Morimoto T, Ginsberg MD, Dietrich WD, Zhao W. Hyperthermia enhances spectrin breakdown in transient focal cerebral ischemia. Brain Res 1997; 746:43–51.

84. Eguchi Y, Yamashita K, Iwamoto T, Ito H. Effects of brain temperature on calmodulin and microtubule-associated protein 2 immunoreactivity in the gerbil hippocampus following transient forebrain ischemia. J Neurotrauma 1997; 14:109–118.

85. Chopp M, Knight R, Tidwell CD, Helpern JA, Brown E, Welch KM. The metabolic effects of mild hypothermia on global cerebral ischemia and recirculation in the cat: comparison to normothermia and hyperthermia. J Cereb Blood Flow Metab 1989; 9:141–148.

86. Busto R, Globus MY, Neary JT, Ginsberg MD. Regional alterations of protein kinase C activity following transient cerebral ischemia: effects of intraischemic brain temperature modulation. J Neurochem 1994; 63:1095–1103.

87. Minamisawa H, Smith ML, Siesjo BK. The effect of mild hyperthermia and hypothermia on brain damage following 5, 10, and 15 minutes of forebrain ischemia. Ann Neurol 1990; 28:26–33.

88. Dietrich WD, Alonso O, Halley M, Busto R. Delayed posttraumatic brain hyperthermia worsens outcome after fluid percussion brain injury: a light and electron microscopic study in rats. Neurosurgery 1996; 38:533–541; discussion 541.

89. Wass CT, Lanier WL, Hofer RE, Scheithauer BW, Andrews AG. Temperature changes of $\geq 1\,^{\circ}$C alter functional neurologic outcome and histopathology in a canine model of a complete cerebral ischemia. Anesthesiology 1995; 83:325–335.

90. Baena RC, Busto R, Dietrich WD, Globus MY, Ginsberg MD. Hyperthermia delayed by 24 hours aggravates neuronal damage in rat hippocampus following global ischemia. Neurology 1997; 48:768–773.

91. Oliveira-Filho J, Ezzeddine MA, Segal AZ, Buonanno FS, Chang Y, Ogilvy CS, Rordorf G, Schwamm LH, Koroshetz WJ, McDonald CT. Fever in subarachnoid hemorrhage: relationship to vasospasm and outcome. Neurology 2001; 56:1299–1304.

92. Azzimondi G, Bassein L, Nonino F, Fiorani L, Vignatelli L, Re G, D'Alessandro R. Fever in acute stroke worsens prognosis. A prospective study. Stroke 1995; 26:2040–2043.

93. Hindfelt B. The prognostic significance of subfebrility and fever in ischaemic cerebral infarction. Acta Neurol Scand 1976; 53:72–79.

94. Reith J, Jorgensen HS, Pedersen PM, Nakayama H, Raaschou HO, Jeppesen LL, Olsen TS. Body temperature in acute stroke: relation to stroke severity, infarct size, mortality, and outcome. Lancet 1996; 347:422–425.

95. Commichau C, Mayer SA, Scarmeas N. Risk factors for fever in critically-ill neurologic patients. Neurology 2003; 60:837–841.

96. Ginsberg MD, Busto R. Combating hyperthermia in acute stroke: a significant clinical concern. Stroke 1998; 29:529–534.

97. Schmutzhard E, Engelhardt K, Beer R, Brossner G, Pfausler B, Spiss H, Unterberger I, Kampfl A. Safety and efficacy of a novel intravascular cooling device to control body temperature in neurologic intensive care patients: a prospective pilot study. Crit Care Med 2002; 30:2481–2488.

98. Doufas AG, Akça O, Barry A, Petrusca DA, Suleman MI, Morioka N, Guarnaschelli JJ, Sessler DI. Initial experience with a novel heat-exchanging catheter in neurosurgical patients. Anesth Analg 2002; 95:1752–1756.

99. Sessler DI. Perioperative hypothermia. N Engl J Med 1997; 336:1730–1737.

100. Hales JRS. Skin arteriovenous anastomoses, their control and role in thermoregulation. In: Johansen K, Burggren W, eds. Cardiovascular Shunts: Phylogenetic, Ontogenetic and Clinical Aspects. Copenhagen: Munksgaard, 1985:433–451.

101. De Witte J, Sessler DI. Perioperative shivering: physiology and pharmacology. Anesthesiology 2002; 96:467–484.

102. Mokhtarani M, Mahgoub AN, Morioka N, Doufas AG, Sessler DI. Buspirone and meperidine synergistically reduce the shivering threshold. Anesth Analg 2001; 93:1233–1239.

103. Doufas AG, Lin C-M, Suleman M-I, Liem EB, Lenhardt R, Morioka N, Akça O, Shah YM, Kurz A, Sessler DI. Dexmedetomidine and meperidine additively reduce the shivering threshold in humans. Stroke 2003; 34:1218–1223.

3

Temperature Monitoring

ROMAN HLATKY and CLAUDIA S. ROBERTSON

Department of Neurosurgery,
Baylor College of Medicine,
Houston, Texas, U.S.A.

INTRODUCTION

Measurement of body temperature is among the most traditional practices in medicine. In the 5th century, Hippocrates used the distinction between heat and cold to describe certain diseases. Quantitative temperature measurements became feasible in diagnosing human illness with the development of the first thermometer by Galileo at the turn of the 15th century (1).

Brain temperature per se depends on a balance among brain metabolism, cerebral blood flow (CBF), and the external environment (radiation, conduction, and convection). Under normal conditions, three main factors determine the temperature of the brain: local heat production, cerebral blood flow, and the temperature of the blood perfusing the brain. The brain is a major consumer of energy and produces considerable heat, which is not easily dispersed because of the insulation provided by the skull. The brain uses about 20% of the oxygen and 25% of the glucose required by the body at rest, while representing only 2–3% of the total body weight. Of the total carbohydrate consumed by the brain, 95% undergoes oxidative metabolism; 43% of the energy originally held in glucose is captured by the adenosine triphosphate (ATP), and the remainder is given off as heat (2).

The primary thermoregulatory center in mammals is the anterior preoptic region in the hypothalamus; in humans, it maintains the body temperature between 36.5°C and 37.5°C (3). Abnormal temperatures are common in critically ill patients. In the surgical intensive care unit (ICU) setting, rectal temperatures on admission were normal in only 30% of patients, exceeded 37.6°C in 38%, and were below 36.8°C in 32% (4).

Temperature monitoring was identified as an essential service for critical care units by the Task Force on Guidelines of the Society of Critical Care Medicine recommendations for services and personnel for delivery of care in a critical care setting (5). Critically ill patients are at high risk for temperature disorders because of debilitation, impaired behavioral thermoregulation (voluntary control of the thermal environment), frequent use of sedative drugs, and high predisposition to infection. Consequently, critically ill patients should have core temperature measured at least every 4 hr. And because the morbidity and mortality associated with hypothermia and hyperthermia can be severe and depend on the severity and duration of the abnormality, temperature should be continuously monitored in patients having temperatures greater than 39°C or less than 36°C. Core temperature should also be continuously monitored in patients who are being therapeutically cooled or warmed to prevent excessive or inadequate treatment.

Fluctuations of brain temperature occur in physiological as well as pathological conditions, and are indications of changes in brain metabolism, cerebral blood flow, neuronal activity, and brain function. During periods of cerebral ischemia, even small changes in the temperature of the ischemic brain tissue may alter survival of neurons (6). Many experimental and clinical studies have been undertaken to devise a reliable technique for obtaining useful brain temperature measurement during patient treatment. Current literature supports a good general correlation between brain and core body temperature (7–9). However, in circumstances where the direct monitoring of brain temperature adds minimal risk to the usual monitoring, brain temperature per se can be obtained (10–13).

Continuous monitoring of brain temperature was originally performed by placing a thermocouple into an intraventricular catheter for intracranial pressure monitoring (12). Today, thermometers or thermistors are combined with other probes [for measuring intracranial pressure, oxygen, and other metabolites], so that brain temperature can be measured continuously in the lateral ventricles or in the parenchyma. These techniques have brought to light regional differences in brain temperature, with deeper zones generally being warmer than surface structures (14). Accurate measurement of temperature depends on the type of thermometer used and the site of temperature measurement.

REVIEW

Types of Thermometers

Mercury

A mercury-in-glass thermometer is the most common type in clinical use. Falsely low measurements may result from failure to leave the thermometer in place for a minimum of 3 min equilibration time. Falsely high temperatures result from failure to shake the mercury down. Because of range limitations, different models of mercury thermometers must be used when patients are especially hypothermic.

Liquid Crystal Display

Liquid crystal display (LCD) thermometers usually involve liquid crystals embedded in thin adhesive strips that are directly attached to patients' skin. The crystals may be sensitive to temperature changes as small as 0.2°C, but the displays usually limit discrimination of temperature changes to roughly 0.5°C. LCD thermometers can be applied to any area of the skin, but are most commonly applied to the forehead for ease of use and steady perfusion. Skin temperature measurements poorly reflect core body temperature when the skin is hypoperfused, as may occur with vasoconstriction or hypotension. Forehead skin temperature is typically lower than core temperatures by 2.2°C (15), and changes in LCD forehead temperature lag behind changes in core temperature by more than 12 min (16). The LCD strip may be left in place for several hours without skin irritation, but must be discarded after use (17). LCD skin thermometry is probably best used in patients with stable, normal hemodynamics, who are not anticipated to experience major temperature shifts and in whom the trend of temperature change is more important than the accuracy of the measurement (18).

Thermocouples

Thermocouples and thermistors are frequently used as probes in electric thermometers that convert the electrical temperature signal into analog or digital displays. Thermocouples consist of a tight junction of two dissimilar metals. The voltage change across the junction can be precisely related to temperature. The measuring thermocouple must be calibrated against a second constant-temperature junction for absolute temperature measurements. The measured voltage changes are of the order of 50 μV/°C, and must be amplified to generate a usable temperature display. In the range of 20–50°C, thermocouples may have a linearity error of less than 0.1 (17). Thermocouples are faster and cheaper but less sensitive than semiconductor thermistors. However, they are sufficiently accurate and precise for clinical work and thermoregulatory research.

Thermistors

Thermistors consist of semiconductor metal oxides in which the electrical resistance changes inversely with temperature.

A linearity error of up to 4°C may occur over the temperature range of 20–50°C, but this can be substantially reduced by making mathematical adjustments or placing a fixed resistance in parallel with the thermistor, which decreases its sensitivity and usable temperature range (17). Thermistors are more sensitive, faster responding, but less linear and more costly than thermocouples or semiconductors (17).

Other semiconductor thermometers measure temperature by taking advantage of the fact that the base-to-emitter voltage change of a transistor is temperature-dependent, whereas the collector current of the silicon resistor is constant. Both thermocouples and thermistors can be fashioned into thin wires and embedded in flexible probes that are suitable for placing in body cavities to measure deep temperature.

Zero Heat Flow Thermometry

Zero-heat-flow thermometry involves placing a thermistor, a heat-flow sensor, and a heater immediately adjacent to the skin. Heat loss from the skin is detected by the flow sensor and is compensated for by the heater. In this manner, the skin beneath the probe is isolated from ambient temperature changes and more directly reflects deep body temperature or core temperature (19,20). Response time to changes in core temperature is approximately 10 min (20), but may be substantially longer in obese patients (17). Inaccuracies during hypoperfusion have been reported (17). Despite its convenience, this type of thermometer remains infrequently used in the clinical setting because of its cost, 30-min warm-up time, and the inadequate data on local variation of deep body temperature at different sites.

Radiotelemetry Thermometers

Radiotelemetry thermometers have been fabricated in the form of ingestible pills. The temperature sensor in the pill is an inductor and functions in such a way that temperature-dependent changes in inductance result in changes in radiofrequency. Changes in radiofrequency can then be detected by a remote unit and electronically translated into a digital display of temperature. Temperature differences of up to 2°C may occur simply as a result of the pill's transit in the intestine (21).

Infrared Thermometers

Infrared emission detection tympanic thermometers (22) use an infrared sensor that detects infrared energy emitted by the core-temperature tissues behind the tympanic membrane. The infrared emissions through the tympanic membrane vary linearly with core temperature. The thermometer's sensor sends a signal to a microprocessor, which converts the signal into a digitally displayed temperature. Measurements of temperature by this method may be subject to errors as a result of improper positioning of the sensor (22).

Sites of Temperature Measurement

Sublingual

Sublingual temperature measurement is convenient but has numerous limitations for critically ill patients. Although open- vs. closed-mouth breathing (22) and use of nasogastric tubes do not alter temperature measurement (23), oral temperature is altered if measured during or immediately after the patient has consumed hot or cold drinks. Falsely low oral temperatures may occur because of cooling from tachypnea (24). Sixty percent of sublingual temperatures are more than 0.55°C lower than simultaneously measured rectal temperatures; 53% differ by 0.55–1.1°C; and 6% differ by more than 1.1°C. However, these results partly reflect the fact that rectal temperatures tend to exceed core temperature. Continuous sublingual measurement interferes with the patient's ability to eat and speak, and it is difficult to maintain a good probe position. Sublingual measurement is best suited for intermittent monitoring when highly accurate measurement of core temperature is unnecessary.

Axillary

Axillary temperatures have been used as an index of core temperature and may be taken with a mercury-in-glass thermometer or a flexible probe. Positioning the sensor over the axillary artery is thought to improve accuracy. The accuracy and precision of axillary temperature measurement are less than at other sites (25,26), perhaps in part because of the difficulty of maintaining a good probe position.

Rectal

Rectal temperature is conveniently measured with a mercury-in-glass thermometer or a flexible temperature sensor. It remains among the most commonly used method of measuring core temperature in clinical use. Readings are more accurate when the sensor is passed more than 10 cm (4 in.) into the rectum (26). Rectal temperature correlates well in most patients with distal esophageal, bladder, and tympanic temperatures (27,28), but tend to exceed true core values. However, it is the slowest of the central measurement sites to respond to induced changes in temperature, especially with malignant hyperthermia and heat stroke (29,30).

Tympanic

Tympanic membrane temperature must be measured with a specifically designed thermometer, which is a bit tricky to position. Contrary to rumors, these thermocouples are soft and flexible, and do not cause rupture of the tympanic membrane, even when inserted by unskilled clinicians.

Tympanic membrane temperature correlates well with rectal and distal esophageal temperature (31–34). During induced hypothermia in animals, tympanic temperature better approximates brain temperature than distal esophageal temperature (33). Recently, infrared oral canal thermometers, which are often incorrectly considered "tympanic," have become popular. They are far less accurate than true tympanic membrane measurements as determined by a properly positioned thermocouple.

Esophageal

Esophageal temperature is usually measured with an electric, flexible temperature sensor and varies with the position of the sensor in the esophagus. In the proximal esophagus, as well as in the midportion near the trachea and bronchi, temperature is influenced by that of the ambient air (31). During hypothermia, temperatures in different portions of the esophagus may differ by up to 1.5°C (31). Stable, more accurate temperatures are reached when the sensor is 45 cm from the nose in adults (31). Because of the proximity of the distal esophagus to the great vessels and heart, distal esophageal temperature responds rapidly to changes in core temperature (17,35). Some recommend placing probes where the loudest heart sounds are heard (35,36), whereas others opt for a deeper, more distal position (37,38). Complications apart from mild discomfort and epistaxis are rare. Cold cardioplegia and flooding the thorax with iced saline also alter esophageal temperatures disproportionately, although the effect is transient and usually of little clinical consequence (39). In patients who are anesthetized or sedated, distal esophageal temperatures may be the most reliable measure of core temperature.

Nasopharyngeal

Nasopharyngeal temperatures are readily monitored during anesthesia and usually correlate well with other centrally measured temperatures (35). However, temperatures may vary as a function of probe position and nasopharyngeal bleeding can occur—although this is a rare complication (39,40).

Bladder

Urinary bladder temperature can be easily measured with a specially designed temperature probe embedded in a Foley catheter (27,28,41). Bladder temperature is convenient to measure and, under steady-state conditions, is more reproducible than that taken at other relatively peripheral sites (41). However, bladder temperature sensors are influenced by urinary flow and may not provide a reliable measure of core temperature during hypothermic cardiopulmonary bypass.

Central Venous

Central venous temperature may be measured with a thermistor-equipped pulmonary artery catheter. The temperature sensor is located near the distal end of the catheter and can record accurate great vessel temperatures when the tip of the catheter is correctly positioned in the pulmonary artery (42). Central venous temperature is often considered the reference site against which other monitoring sites are compared.

Brain

Brain temperature may be directly measured with a temperature sensor, which is either incorporated in a ventriculostomy catheter or directly placed into brain tissue (Figure 1) (11,12). In patients who require monitoring of intracranial pressure for clinical management of their neurological disorder, brain temperature monitoring adds minimal risk.

Measurement of Core Temperature

Core temperature refers to the deep body temperature that is carefully regulated by the hypothalamus to be independent of transient small changes in ambient temperature. Core temperature exists more as a physiologic concept than as the temperature of an anatomic location. Ideal sites of temperature measurement would be protected from heat loss, painless, and convenient to use. The choice of site used to monitor temperature must be individualized, but certain generalizations can be made. Core temperature is best measured from the pulmonary artery, distal esophagus, tympanic membrane, or nasopharynx. Oral, axillary, rectal, and bladder temperatures approximate core temperature in most clinical circumstances, except during rapid changes in temperature.

Klein et al. (42) compared pulmonary artery with tympanic membrane temperature and rectal temperature (calibrated glass mercury) to determine consistency among these measures. Pulmonary artery and tympanic membrane tem-

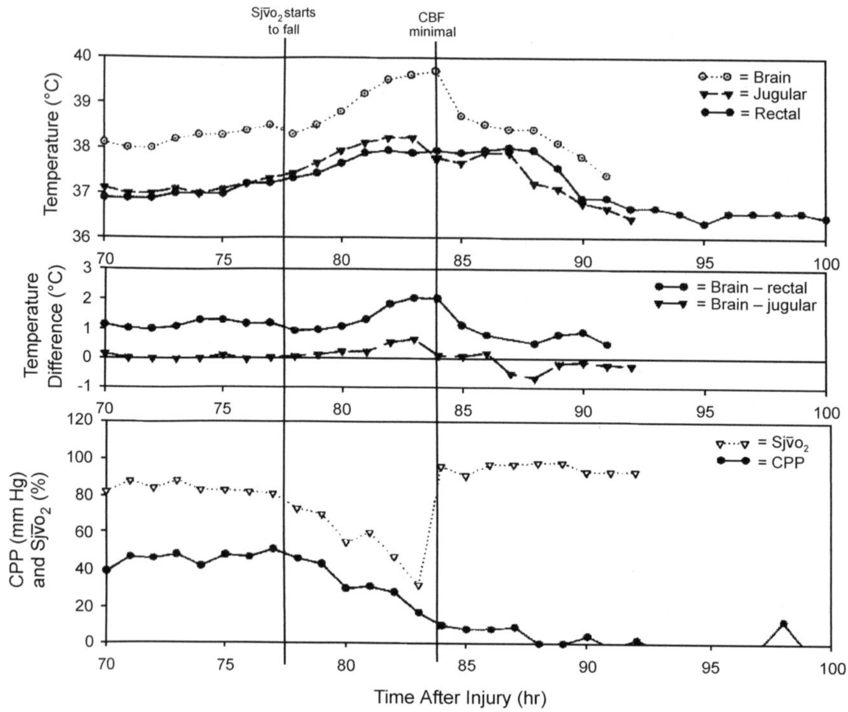

Figure 1 Example of changes in brain, rectal, and jugular bulb temperatures as cerebral blood flow (CBF) decreases due to severe intracranial hypertension. In this example, cerebral perfusion pressure and CBF fall progressively over time. As CBF initially falls, brain temperature and the brain–rectal temperature gradient increase. As CBF drops to minimal levels, brain temperature falls, the brain–rectal temperature gradient decreases, and the brain–jugular temperature gradient reverses. $SjvO_2$, jugular venous oxygen saturation; CPP, cerebral perfusion pressure. (From Ref. 54.)

peratures were highly correlated ($r = 0.909$). Mean tympanic membrane temperature was slightly higher than mean pulmonary artery temperature (mean difference = 0.42°C). Tympanic temperature measurements would be an appropriate substitute for core temperature if the pulmonary artery catheter has been removed or the pulmonary artery thermistor was nonfunctional. In addition, this study emphasizes that to effectively track temperature in any given patient, the site for temperature measurement should be consistent.

Determinants of Brain Temperature

Brain temperature is determined by a number of factors, including cerebral metabolic rate, cerebral blood flow, and arterial blood temperature. Brain temperature is also influenced by the surrounding environment (43,44). Cerebral metabolic activity generates heat and results in a small temperature gradient (less than 1°C) between deep brain temperature and that of the superficial parenchyma through which the proximal cerebral arteries course (44). CBF and the blood–brain temperature gradient determine the magnitude and direction of heat exchange in the brain (44,45).

Cerebral blood flow (CBF) and brain temperature are related in two ways. First, the blood flow to the brain supplies the nutrients that are necessary to generate heat through cerebral metabolism. If CBF is sufficiently reduced to limit metabolism in the brain, then brain temperature decreases as CBF does (Figure 1). A strong direct relationship between CBF and brain temperature was demonstrated in several models of cerebral ischemia (46,47).

Second, CBF is normally tightly coupled to cerebral metabolic rate. In normal subjects, cerebral metabolism and therefore CBF is altered by induced changes in brain temperature. In patients with brain injury, the findings have been more variable. Marion et al. (48) found a significantly lower global CBF in brain-injured patients during induced hypothermia ($p = 0.021$). CBF decreased by 5.2% per °C during the cooling period; however, the absolute blood flow increased after 23 hr compared to the first CBF measurement, which was obtained in the emergency department (48). Metz and coworkers (49) demonstrated only minor changes in CBF with hypothermia in brain-injured patients during the early hypothermia period (3.5 h) and during the late cooling period (after 24 h). In contrast, Shiozaki et al. (50) found, in brain-injured patients with mild hypothermia, a reduction in CBF of 15.2 mL/100 g/min

($p < 0.0001$) compared to brain-injured patients without cooling treatment. Soukup et al. (51) show a close relationship between brain temperature and CBF. Patients with a brain temperature exceeding 36°C had greater CBF values than patients with a brain temperature below 36°C.

Relationship Between Brain and Core Temperature

Deep brain temperature is slightly greater than core temperature measured from pulmonary artery or other great vessels during steady state conditions. That brain temperature exceeds core temperature is normal: core temperature is the average temperature of the deep, well-perfused body structures. It is not the highest temperature in the body because some organs generate more heat (and are at higher temperatures) than others. For example, the liver also exceeds core temperature.

Although these core and brain temperatures trend together, the gradient between the two temperatures tends to increase with fever and during active systemic cooling. Gradients between brain and other sites of core temperature measurements also occur. Although these temperature gradients are known to exist, they are probably not important for most clinical situations where temperature perturbations are not extreme and not changing rapidly.

Rossi et al. (52) compared pulmonary artery temperature and brain temperature measured from a sensor incorporated into a ventriculostomy catheter in 20 patients with neurological disorders. Brain and pulmonary artery temperatures were 38.4 ± 0.8 and 38.1 ± 0.8°C, respectively, with an average difference of 0.3°C between the two temperatures. The difference between brain and core temperature increased significantly as body core temperature increased (Figure 2) (52). Deep brain temperature (e.g., hypothalamus, midbrain, corpus callosum) measured in 16 monkeys were 0.4–0.6°C higher than arterial blood temperatures measured in the aortic arch (53).

Comparisons of core temperature from other sites and brain temperature have yielded results that are similar to

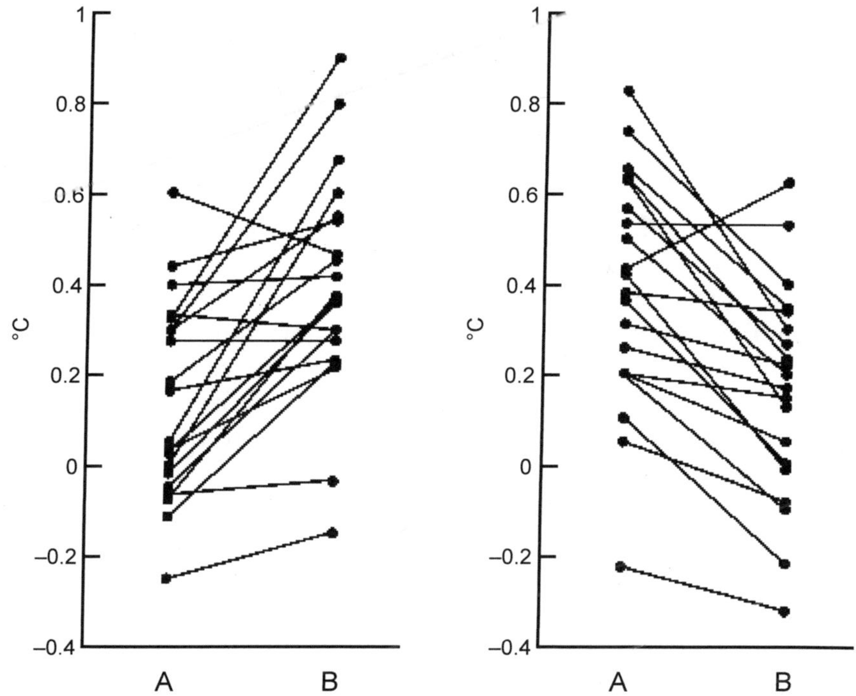

Figure 2 Left panel: Mean differences between brain (ICT) and core (T_c) temperatures before (A) and at the peak (B) of 119 febrile episodes recorded in 20 patients. One line represents one patient ($p < 0.05$). Right panel: Mean differences between ICT and T_c at the peak (A) and after (B) 121 febrile episodes ($p < 0.05$). (From Ref. 52.)

these pulmonary artery temperature findings. Rumana et al. (54) compared rectal, jugular venous, and brain temperatures in patients with traumatic brain injury. Jugular bulb temperature was similar to rectal temperature and both averaged 1.1°C less than the temperature of the brain (54). Mellergard et al. (8,11,12) found an average gradient of 0.33°C between brain temperature, measured through a ventriculostomy catheter, and rectal temperature. Verlooy et al. (55) observed an average 0.5°C difference between bladder temperature and brain temperature. Tympanic temperature has been shown to be 0.3–0.5°C lower than epidural temperature (11).

In a study comparing brain temperature with esophageal temperature in humans, thermocouples were placed 4 cm into the brain tissue and compared with esophageal temperatures at three different levels (10, 17, and 25 cm) in the esophagus (39). The mean difference between the brain temperature and esophageal temperature was 1.5±0.73°C at 10 cm, 0.6±0.63°C at 17 cm, and 0.25±0.21°C at 24 cm. Another report compared esophageal temperature to brain temperature and intraventricular temperature in a 12-year-old male patient who underwent surgery for resection of a pineal tumor (13). The intraventricular temperature was 0.5°C above the esophageal temperature, and the brain tissue temperature was 0.7°C higher than esophageal temperature (13).

It has been suggested that the temperature gradient between brain and core temperatures is a result of the phenomenon of countercurrent exchange within the brain (56). The normal arterial jugular venous differences in blood temperature, when calculated based on oxygen consumption, blood flow, and heat production in healthy individuals, should be 0.39°C (57). However, most reports have found jugular bulb temperature to be similar to core temperature, despite a higher temperature in the brain (7). Because of the extensive capillary network within brain tissue, it is likely that the brain acts as a countercurrent heat exchange. As arterial blood travels deeper into the brain tissues, heat is gained, and as blood moves to more peripheral cooler tissues in the brain, heat is lost.

During a neurosurgical procedure, the exposure of the brain to environmental temperature alters these normal relationships between temperature in the brain and other sites of core temperature measurement. In a study of 10 patients undergoing cerebellopontine angle tumor removal, Schuhmann et al. (58) monitored brain, esophageal, bladder, ipsilateral and contralateral tympanic membrane, and scalp temperatures. During monitoring, esophageal temperature increased from 35.3±0.2 to 36.0±0.3°C. After dura opening, brain temperature was −0.14±0.1°C below esophageal temperature. At the end of tumor removal, this difference increased to −0.43±0.31°C ($P < 0.05$). Contralateral tympanic temperature was −0.29±0.18°C below brain temperature at dura opening.

Contralateral tympanic temperature reflected the behavior of esophageal temperature adequately (r = 0.938), however, with a mean difference of -0.39 ± 0.04°C (72). In contrast, ipsilateral tympanic temperature readings closely followed temperature changes in the area of surgery. Bladder temperature reflected esophageal temperature, except in periods of rapid temperature changes. The authors concluded that in posterior fossa surgery, local brain temperature is most accurately reflected by esophageal temperature, and they considered bladder temperature and contralateral tympanic temperature also sufficient to assess brain surface temperature in the posterior fossa (58).

Core body temperature is the most important determinant of the temperature gradient between the brain and core temperature sites (8,11,12,54,55,59). Other factors that have been suggested to alter this temperature gradient include the absence of a bone flap (52), CBF especially when the level is very low (51,54), and level of consciousness (60).

Brain Temperature During Induction of Hypothermia

In normal subjects, brain temperature is closely reflected by nasopharyngeal, esophageal, tympanic membrane, as well as bladder and rectal temperatures. However, when rapid changes in body temperature are induced or occur from a disease process, transient temperature gradients can develop between these sites of measurement. In general, the more profound the change in temperature the greater is the disparity between temperature measurements in the different sites. A number of studies have compared measurements at different sites during both hyperthermia and hypothermia.

Experimental Studies

In an experimental study using dogs and pigtail monkeys, Eshel and Safar (61) monitored brain (epidural), esophageal, rectal, and nasopharyngeal temperatures during hyperthermia induced by immersion into water at 45°C. While normothermic, brain, rectal, esophageal, and nasopharyngeal temperatures correlated well in both species. In dogs, brain, esophageal, nasopharyngeal, and rectal temperatures correlated well during heating, until vigorous panting lowered nasopharyngeal and brain temperatures. In monkeys, brain, esophageal, and rectal temperatures correlated well during heating until blood pressure began to fall. When cerebral perfusion pressure decreased below 50 mm Hg, brain and nasopharyngeal temperatures declined significantly compared with rectal temperature, which remained high despite severe arterial hypotension (61). Esophageal temperature remained at levels between brain and rectal temperatures.

In another experimental study, Ao et al. (62) measured brain, jugular vein, cisterna magna, pulmonary artery, and rectal temperatures in dogs during induced hypothermia. Jugular, cisterna magna and pulmonary arterial, but not rectal temperature, were close to brain temperature during stable hypothermia.

Human Studies

Stone et al. (63) sought to determine which of the standard temperature monitoring sites best approximates brain temperature when deep hypothermia is rapidly induced and reversed during cardiopulmonary bypass. Twenty-seven patients underwent cardiopulmonary bypass and deep hypothermic circulatory arrest in order for each to have a giant cerebral aneurysm surgically clipped. Brain temperatures were directly measured with a thermocouple embedded in the cerebral cortex. Eight other body temperatures were simultaneously monitored with less invasive sensors at standard sites (63).

In this study, brain temperature decreased from 32.6 ± 1.4 to 16.7 ± 1.7°C in 28 ± 7 min, and none of the monitored sites tracked cerebral temperature well throughout the entire hypothermic period. During rapid temperature change, nasopharyngeal, esophageal, and pulmonary artery temperatures corresponded to brain temperature with smaller mean differences than did those of the tympanic membrane, bladder, rectum, axilla, and sole of the foot. At circulatory arrest, nasopharyngeal, esophageal, and pulmonary artery mean temperatures were within 1 °C of brain temperature, even though individual patients frequently exhibited disparate values at those sites (63).

Stone et al. (63) concluded that when profound hypothermia is rapidly induced and reversed, temperature measurements made at standard monitoring sites may not reflect cerebral temperature. Measurements from the nasopharynx, esophagus, and pulmonary artery tend to match brain temperature best, but an array of data give a better overall picture.

In summary, direct measurement of brain temperature is the only absolutely reliable way to measure the temperature in the brain during conditions of profound or rapidly changing temperature, but nasopharyngeal or tympanic membrane temperatures are probably the best indirect estimation of brain temperature in such circumstances. In normal clinical conditions, including routine neurosurgery, any of the standard core-temperature monitoring sites give a reasonable approximation of brain temperature.

Temperature Monitoring During Pathological Conditions

Hyperthermia and fever are common in patients with neurological and neurosurgical disorders. Even in normal subjects, the temperature gradient between the brain and core temperature sites increases as core temperature increases. In most circumstances, these small differences between temperature monitoring sites are not clinically important. In the patient with a neurological disorder, however, an accurate measurement of brain temperature might be important, because experimental studies suggest that even small changes in brain temperature can determine survival of neurons during a period of cerebral ischemia (6).

Albrecht et al. (64) studied the incidence and timing of fever in patients with brain injury resulting from ischemia or trauma. During the initial 72 hr of hospitalization, temperature increases to 38 °C or more were observed in 83% of patients with cardiac arrest, 70% of those with subarachnoid hemorrhage, and 68% of those with closed-head injury. In another study of 428 patients admitted to an ICU during a 6-month period because of neurological disease, nearly one-half of the patients developed fever (65). In patients with acute intracerebral hemorrhage, the duration of fever was strongly related to a poor neurological outcome. The risk of a poor outcome was increased by 8.33 for 24–48 hr with fever (95% CI, 1.75–39.67) and by 13.52 for more than 48 hr with fever (95% CI, 2.22–82.23) (66). Similar relationships between fever and poor neurological outcome have been observed with ischemic stroke (67,68) and with traumatic brain injury (51,69,70).

However, it is important to realize that these correlations—impressive as they are—do not necessarily indicate causality. The observed association between fever and neurological outcome may simply indicate that fever is a manifestation of a more severe neurological injury. No clinical studies to date have clearly implicated fever as causing a worse neurological outcome. The need for direct monitoring of brain temperature in the patient with a neurological disorder will have to balance the risk of the monitoring against the potential benefit of having this brain-specific information.

FUTURE DIRECTIONS

Further technological development of brain temperature monitors will largely depend on the clinical importance of precise brain temperature measurements. Fortunately, measurement of core temperature at routine sites is nearly always sufficient for clinical purposes. If more precise measurement of brain temperature is desired, then currently invasive monitors are required. Noninvasive and regional measurements of tissue temperature using imaging techniques, such as magnetic resonance imaging, already exist and may someday be clinically practical.

REFERENCES

1. Frank SM. Body temperature monitoring. Anesth Clin North Am 1994; 12:387–407.

2. Fitch W. Brain metabolism. In: Cottrell JE, Smith DS, eds. Anesthesia and Neurosurgery. St. Louis: Mosby, 1994:1–16.

3. Sessler DI. Temperature monitoring. In: Miller RD, ed. Anesthesia. 4th ed. New York: Churchill Livingstone, 1994:1363–1382.

4. Kholoussy AM, Sufian S, Pavlides C. Central peripheral temperature gradient: its value and limitations in the management of critically ill surgical patients. Am J Surg 1980; 140:609–615.

5. Task Force on Guidelines. Recommendations for services and personnel for delivery of care in a critical care setting. Crit Care Med 1988; 16:809–815.

6. Busto R, Dietrich WD, Globus MYT. Small differences in intraischemic brain temperature critically determine the extent of ischemic neuronal injury. J Cereb Blood Flow Metab 1987; 7:729–738.

7. Crowder CM, Tempelhoff R, Theard A, Cheng MA, Todorov A, Dacey RG. Jugular bulb temperature: comparison with brain surface and core temperature in neurosurgical patients during mild hypothermia. J Neurosurg 1996; 85:98–103.

8. Mellegard P, Nordstrom CH. Intracerebral temperature in neurosurgical patients. Neurosurgery 1991; 28:709–713.

9. Mellegard P. Changes in human intracerebral temperature in response to different methods of brain cooling. Neurosurgery 1992; 31:671–677.

10. Horrow JC, Rosenberg H. Does urinary catheter temperature reflect core temperature during cardiac surgery? Anesthesiology 1988; 69:686–689.

11. Mellegard P, Nordstrom CH. Epidural temperature and possible intracerebral temperature gradients in man. Br J Neurosurg 1990; 4:31–38.

12. Mellergard P, Nordstrom CH, Christensson M. A method for monitoring intracerebral temperature in neurosurgical patients. Neurosurgery 1990; 27:654–657.

13. Shiraki K, Sagawa S, Tajima F, Yokota A, Hashimoto M, Brengelmann GL. Independence of brain and tympanic

temperatures in an unanesthetized human. J Appl Physiol 1988; 65:482–486.

14. Hirashima Y, Takaba M, Endo S. Intracerebral temperature in patients with hydrocephalus of varying aetiology. J Neurol Neurosurg Psychiatry 1998; 64:792–794.
15. Burgess GE III, Cooper JR, Marino RJ. Continuous monitoring of skin temperature using a liquid-crystal thermometer during anesthesia. South Med J 1978; 71:516–521.
16. Roberts NH. The comparison of surface and core temperature devices. Am Assoc Nurse Anesth 1980; 48:53–67.
17. Silverman RW, Lomax F. The measurement of temperature for thermoregulatory studies. Pharmacol Ther 1985; 27:233–239.
18. Ikeda T, Sessler DI, Marder D, Xiong J. The influence of thermoregulatory vasomotion and ambient temperature variation on the accuracy of core-temperature estimates by cutaneous liquid-crystal thermometers. Anesthesia 1997; 86:603–612.
19. Fukuoka M, Yamori Y, Toyoshima T. Twenty-four hour monitoring of deep body temperature with a novel flexible probe. J Biomed Eng 1987; 9:173–185.
20. Lees DE, Kim YD, MacNamara TE. Noninvasive determination of core temperature during anesthesia. South Med J 1980; 73:1322–1334.
21. Watson BW. Clinical uses of radio pills. Br J Hosp Med 1981; 25:618–627.
22. Erickson R. Thermometer placement for oral temperature measurement in febrile adults. Int J Nurs Stud 1976; 13:199–205.
23. Heinz J. Validation of sublingual temperatures in patients with nasogastric tubes. Heart Lung 1985; 14:128–137.
24. Tandberg D, Sklar D. Effect of tachypnea on the estimation of body temperature by an oral thermometer. N Engl J Med 1985; 313:945–956.
25. Cork RC, Vaughan RW, Humphrey LS. Precision and accuracy of intraoperative temperature monitoring. Anesth Analg 1983; 62:211–223.

26. Ramsay JG, Ralley FE, Whalley DG. Site of temperature monitoring and prediction of afterdrop after open heart surgery. Can Anaesth Soc J 1985; 32:607–615.

27. Bone ME, Feneck RO. Bladder temperature as an estimate of body temperature during cardiopulmonary bypass. Anaesthesia 1988; 43:181–192.

28. Moorthy SS, Winn BA, Jallard MS. Monitoring urinary bladder temperature. Heart Lung 1985; 14:90–99.

29. Iaizzo PA, Kehler CH, Zink RS, Belani KG, Sessler DI. Thermal response in acute porcine malignant hyperthermia. Anesth Analg 1996; 82:803–809.

30. Ash CJ, Cook JR, McMurray TA, Anner CR. The use of rectal temperature to monitor heat stroke. MOMed 1992; 89:283–288.

31. Crocker BD, Okumura F, McCuaig DI, Denborough MA. Temperature monitoring during general anaesthesia. Br J Anaesth 1980; 52:1223–1232.

32. Davis FM, Barnes PK, Bailey JS. Aural thermometry during profound hypothermia. Anaesth Intensive Care 1981; 9:124–129.

33. Benzinger M. Tympanic thermometry in surgery and anesthesia. JAMA 1969; 209:1207–1219.

34. Childs C, Harrison R, Hodkinson C. Tympanic membrane temperature as a measure of core temperature. Arch Dis Child 1999; 80:262–266.

35. Cork RC, Vaughan RW, Humphrey LS. Precision and accuracy of intraoperative temperature monitoring. Anesth Analg 1983; 62:211–214.

36. Horrow JC, Rosenberg H. Does urinary catheter temperature reflect core temperature during cardiac surgery. Anesthesiology 1988; 69:986–989.

37. Whitby JD, Dunkin LJ. Temperature differences in the oesophagus. Br J Anaesth 1968; 40:991–995.

38. Kaufman RD. Relationship between esophageal temperature gradient and heart and lung sounds heard by esophageal stethoscope. Anesth Analg 1987; 66:104–108.

39. Muravchick S. Deep body thermometry during general anesthesia. Anesthesiology 1983; 58:271–275.

40. Whitby JD, Dunkin LJ. Cerebral, oesophageal and nasopharyngeal temperatures. Br J Anaesth 1971; 43:673–676.

41. Lilly JK, Boland JP, Zekan S. Urinary bladder temperature monitoring. Crit Care Med 1980; 8:742–744.

42. Klein DG, Mitchell C, Petrinec A, Monroe MK, Oblak M, Ross B, Youngblut JM. A comparison of pulmonary artery, rectal, and tympanic membrane temperature measurement in the ICU. Heart Lung 1993; 22:435–441.

43. Whitby JD, Dunkin LJ. Cerebral, oesophageal and nasopharyngeal temperatures. Br J Anaesth 1971; 43:673–676.

44. Baker MA, Stocking RA, Meehan JP. Thermal relationship between tympanic membrane and hypothalamus in conscious cat and monkey. J Appl Physiol 1972; 32:739–742.

45. Hayward JN, Baker MA. Role of arterial blood in the regulation of brain temperature in the monkey. Am J Physiol 1968; 215:389–403.

46. Chen H, Chopp M, Welch KMA. Effect of mild hyperthermia on the ischemic infarct volume after middle cerebral artery occlusion in the rat. Neurology 1991; 41:1133–1135.

47. Minamisawa H, Mellegard P, Smith M. Preservation of brain temperature during ischemia in rats. Stroke 1990; 21:87–91.

48. Marion DW, Obrist WD, Carlier PM. The use of moderate therapeutic hypothermia for patients with severe head injuries: a preliminary report. J Neurosurg 1993; 79:354–362.

49. Metz C, Holzschuh M, Bein T. Moderate hypothermia in patients with severe head injury: cerebral and extracerebral effects. J Neurosurg 1996; 85:533–541.

50. Shiozaki T, Sugimoto H, Taneda M. Effect of mild hypothermia on uncontrollable intracranial hypertension after severe head injury. J Neurosurg 1993; 79:363–368.

51. Soukup J, Zauner A, Doppenberg EM, Menzel M, Gilman C, Young HF, Bullock R. The importance of brain temperature in patients after severe head injury: relationship to intracranial

pressure, cerebral perfusion pressure, cerebral blood flow, and outcome. J Neurotrauma 2002; 19:559–571.

52. Rossi S, Zanier ER, Mauri I, Columbo A, Stocchetti N. Brain temperature, body core temperature, and intracranial pressure in acute cerebral damage. J Neurol Neurosurg Psychiatry 2001; 71:448–454.

53. Hayward JN, Baker MA. Role of cerebral arterial blood in the regulation of brain temperature in the monkey. Am J Physiol 1968; 215:389–403.

54. Rumana CS, Gopinath SP, Uzura M, Valadka AB, Robertson CS. Brain temperature exceeds systemic temperature in head-injured patients. Crit Care Med 1998; 26:562–565.

55. Verlooy J, Heytens L, Veeckmans S. Intracerebral temperature monitoring in severely head injured patients. Acta Neurochir (Wien) 1995; 134:76–78.

56. Hayward JN, Baker MA. A comparative study of the role of the cerebral arterial blood in the regulation of brain temperature in five mammals. Brain Res 1969; 16:417–440.

57. Brengelmann GL. Body temperature regulation. In: Patton HD, Fuchs AF, Hille B, Scher AM, Steiner R, eds. Textbook of Physiology. Philadelphia: W.B. Saunders, 1989:1584–1596.

58. Schuhmann MU, Suhr DF, v Gosseln HH, Brauer A, Jantzen JP, Samii M. Local brain surface temperature compared to temperatures measured at standard extracranial monitoring sites during posterior fossa surgery. J Neurosurg Anesthesiol 1999; 11:90–95.

59. Henker RA, Brown SD, Marion DW. Comparison of brain temperature with bladder and rectal temperatures in adults with severe head injury. Neurosurgery 1998; 42:1071–1075.

60. Mellergard P. Intracerebral temperature in neurosurgical patients: intracerebral temperature gradients and relationships to consciousness level. Surg Neurol 1995; 43:91– 95.

61. Eshel GM, Safar P. Do standard monitoring sites affect true brain temperature when hyperthermia is rapidly induced and reversed. Aviat Space Environ Med 1999; 70:1193–1196.

62. Ao H, Moon JK, Tanimoto H, Sakanashi Y, Terasaki H. Jugular vein temperature reflects brain temperature during hypothermia. Resuscitation 2000; 45:111–118.

63. Stone JG, Young WL, Smith CR, Solomon RA, Wald A, Ostapkovich N, Shrebnick DB. Do standard monitoring sites reflect true brain temperature when profound hypothermia is rapidly induced and reversed? Anesthesiology 1995; 82:344–351.

64. Albrecht RF, Wass CT, Lanier WL. Occurrence of potentially detrimental temperature alterations in hospitalized patients at risk for brain injury. Mayo Clin Proc 1998; 73:629–635.

65. Kilpatrick MM, Lowry DW, Firlik AD. Hyperthermia in neurosurgical intensive care unit. Neurosurgery 2000; 47:850–856.

66. Schwarz S, Hafner K, Aschoff A. Incidence and prognostic significance of fever following intracerebral hemorrhage. Neurology 2000; 94:354–361.

67. Azzimondi G, Bassein L, Nonino F. Fever in acute stroke worsens prognosis: a prospective study. Stroke 1995; 26:2040–2043.

68. Reith J, Jorgensen HS, Pedersen PM, Nakayama H, Raaschou HO, Jeppesen LL, Olsen TS. Body temperature in acute stroke: relationship to stroke severity, infarct size, mortality and outcome. Lancet 1996; 347:422–425.

69. Albrecht RF, Wass CT, Lanier WL. Occurrence of potentially detrimental temperature alterations in hospitalized patients at risk of brain injury. Mayo Clin Proc 1998; 73:629–635.

70. Natale JE, Joseph JG, Helfaer MA. Early hyperthermia after traumatic brain injury in children: risk factors, influence on length of stay, and effect on short-term neurologic status. Crit Care Med 2000; 28:2608–2615.

4

Biological and Molecular Mechanisms of Hypothermic Neuroprotection

MYRON D. GINSBERG and LUDMILA BELAYEV

Cerebral Vascular Disease Research Center,
Department of Neurology,
University of Miami School of Medicine,
Miami, Florida, U.S.A.

INTRODUCTION

Any discussion of the role of therapeutic hypothermia in medical practice must distinguish among three historical epochs: the initial historical period; the subsequent application of profound degrees of hypothermia for medical and surgical procedures; and the "modern" period of therapeutic hypothermia, which was ushered in by observations that mild-to-moderate temperature decreases were also therapeutic.

As reviewed elsewhere (1,2), the first documented applications of therapeutic hypothermia were use as a local anesthetic during surgical procedures, and, early in the 20th century, use of local or generalized cooling to treat head injury, tumors, and other conditions (3,4). These procedures were commonly complicated by sudden heart failure, possibly attributable to ventricular fibrillation (5).

The second historical milestone was the use of profound hypothermia, often with extracorporeal circulation, to protect the brain during cardiac surgical procedures that required interruption of the circulation (6) and during neurosurgical procedures to clip cerebral aneurysms or resect arteriovenous malformations (7,8). This approach employed levels of systemic hypothermia as low as 4–15°C, which resulted in severe medical complications including ventricular fibrillation and other cardiac arrhythmias, hypotension, acidosis, coagulopathies, and suppression of immune function (2,9). In an effort to minimize systemic complications, methods for selective brain cooling were attempted (10) and feasibility was demonstrated in animal studies (11). In the clinic, it was also appreciated that the expected hypoxic–ischemic sequelae of drowning were substantially diminished in cases of *cold water* immersion (12).

The modern era of therapeutic hypothermia was heralded by studies in the 1960s, which demonstrated that the duration of cerebral ischemia compatible with complete functional and histological recovery increased continuously as temperature declined and could be extended fivefold by reducing temperature from 37°C to 25°C (13). Other studies showed that brain energy metabolite depletion and acidosis during hypoxia–ischemia could be lessened by temperature decrements of only 1–3°C (14). These observations reinforced the need for stringent control of body temperature in animal experimentation. In contrast, animal studies conducted prior to the mid-1980s failed to monitor or regulate brain temperature.

Serendipitous laboratory observations led to the realization that unmonitored variability in brain temperature declines during ischemia studies led to variable neuropathological outcomes (15) and that, therefore, the temperature of the brain or cranium needed to be directly monitored and regulated to achieve interpretable outcomes in ischemia experiments (16). These observations stimulated experimentation using mild-to-moderate degrees of hypothermia to achieve neuroprotection in cerebral ischemia, leading in turn to a burgeoning mechanistic literature, which will be reviewed below.

REVIEW

Hypothermic Neuroprotection: Experimental Evidence and Proof-of-Principle

Global Ischemia

In the seminal paper of Busto et al. (16), anesthesized rats received a 20-min global forebrain ischemic insult, with brain temperature monitoring via a thermocouple stereotaxically inserted into the striatum. Brain temperature was regulated by a warming lamp over the head and was held during the ischemic insult at fixed levels ranging from 33°C to 39°C. Following normothermic ischemia and 3-day survival, there was marked loss of CA1 hippocampal pyramidal neurons and ischemic neuronal pathology in the striatum. These changes were markedly reduced in animals with intraischemic brain cooling to 33–34°C and were further diminished in uncontrolled animals with ischemic brain temperature declines to 30°C (Fig. 1). This study thus provided proof-of-principle that hypothermic neuroprotection could be achieved by brain temperature reductions as small as 2°C.

Other laboratories using small animal (rat, gerbil) ischemia models offered compelling confirmatory evidence of high-grade neuroprotection of vulnerable neuronal populations, and of improved neurobehavioral performance with small (e.g., 2–3°C) temperature decrements (17–24). Moderate hypothermia also proved to be neuroprotective in large animal models of cardiac arrest and cardiopulmonary bypass (9,25,26).

Focal Ischemia

Hypothermia is also clearly neuroprotective in focal cerebral ischemia. Thus, infarct volume was reduced when hypothermia was instituted near the end of middle cerebral artery (MCA) occlusion, or during the early reperfusion period (27–29). In

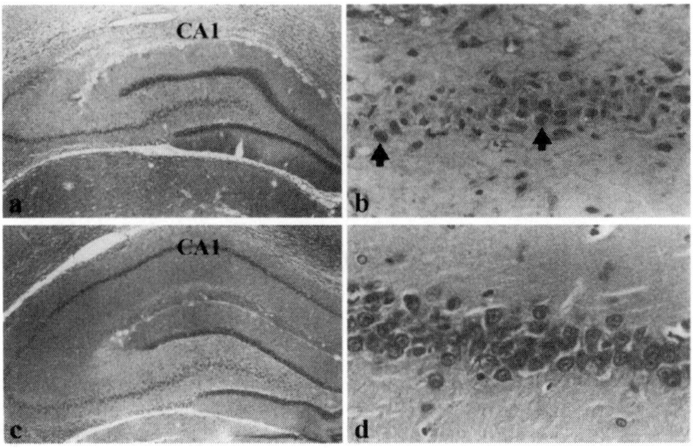

Figure 1 Paraffin-embedded coronal rat brain sections stained with hematoxylin and eosin from normothermic (a and b) and hypothermic (c and d) ischemic rats. (a) Two months after 12.5 min of normothermic (37°C) global ischemia, severe necrosis of CA1 hippocampus was apparent. (b) Higher magnification of injured CA1 sector showed only two viable neurons (arrowheads) among reactive astrocytes and microglia. (c) In contrast to normothermic results, a relatively intact CA1 sector was present after hypothermic (30°C) global ischemia. (d) Higher magnification of CA1 showed many viable neurons containing a distinct nucleus and nucleolus. (From Ref. 21.)

one study (30), mild hypothermia (33°C) during a 1-hr ischemia period and first hour of reperfusion reduced infarct volume by 48% compared to normothermic–ischemic animals. The most pronounced therapeutic effects of hypothermia, amounting to reductions of over 90% in infarct size, were observed in temporary 3-hr MCA occlusion in which cooling to 32°C was started at the onset of ischemia and was maintained for several hours (31).

Importantly, significant protection was observed even when hypothermia was delayed by 3 hr (31). Hypothermia imposed during either the first or second 90-min epoch of a 3-hr ischemic insult reduced infarct volume by 45–50% compared to normothermic animals (37°C) (31). Other studies supported the therapeutic efficacy of moderate intraischemic cooling in focal ischemia (Fig. 2) (32–34). In spontaneously hypertensive rats (SHRs)—a strain more resistant to neuroprotection—cooling by 3°C during temporary MCA occlusion markedly reduced brain infarction, and cooling to 29°C conferred complete neuroprotection (35).

Intraischemic Vs. Postischemic Cooling: The Problem of Enduring Neuroprotection

The multiple variations of experimental design in hypothermic neuroprotection studies conducted by numerous laboratories have afforded insights into how the severity of the ischemic insult and the depth, duration, and delay in initiation of moderate hypothermia interact to affect therapeutic efficacy. Thus, when postischemic hypothermia (30°C for 3 hr) was initiated 3 min after a 10-min normothermic global forebrain ischemic insult in rats, CA1 pyramidal neurons showed high-grade protection when examined histopathologically after only a 3-day survival; however, in animals surviving for 7 days, the degree of protection was diminished, and in animals allowed to survive for 2 months, no protection was evident (36). This finding was in contrast to *intraischemic* cooling of the same degree, which conferred permanent protection at 2 months. These results showed that postischemic hypothermia might retard the evolution of histopathological alterations while not permanently protecting against them.

In another study, prolonging a normothermic global ischemic insult in gerbils from 3 to 5 min tended to override the protective effect of postischemic cooling (32°C for 12 hr beginning 1 hr after ischemia), whereas by increasing the duration of postischemic hypothermia from 12 to 24 hr, near-total preservation of CA1 neurons was achieved at 30 days following the 5-min insult (37). Extending the survival period to 6 months revealed 70% neuroprotection of CA1 neurons, indicating that although some CA1 neurons continued to die over a prolonged period, substantial enduring protection (both histological and behavioral) was nonetheless achieved (38). In a model of severe 10-min normothermic forebrain ischemia in rats, a 48-hr period of induced mild hypothermia (32–34°C) starting at

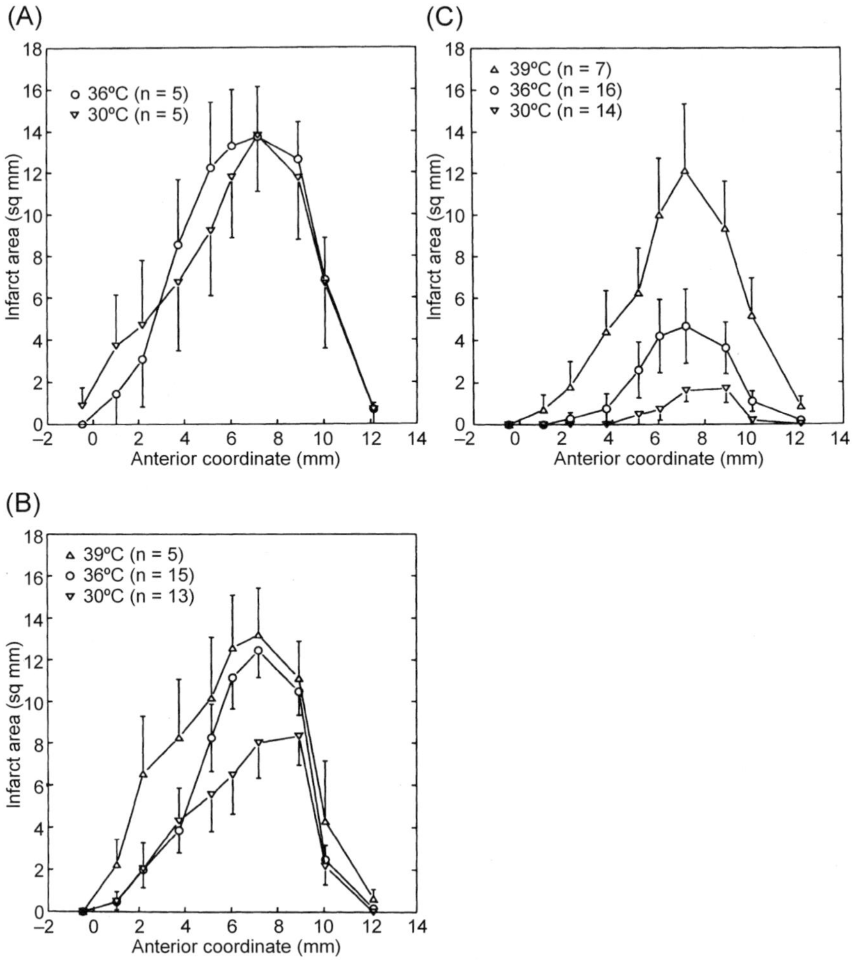

Figure 2 Cortical infarct areas in rats with MCA occlusion and 3-day survival, plotted as a function of the anteroposterior stereotactic coordinate, in animals with different intraischemic brain temperatures (30°C, 36°C, or 39°C). (A) Permanent MCA occlusion by proximal electrocoagulation combined with hypotension to 50 mm Hg for 30 min. (B) Permanent proximal MCA occlusion without hypotension. (C) Reversible 2-hr proximal MCA clip occlusion. Values are mean ± SEM. Intraischemic hypothermia was highly neuroprotective (and hyperthermia was highly injurious) in the reversible MCA occlusion paradigm (C). (From Ref. 32.)

6-hr postischemia resulted in only 14% CA1 neuronal loss at 28-day survival, contrasting with 99% cell loss in untreated rats, establishing that indefatigable neuroprotection was possible with very prolonged postischemic cooling (39). Other workers have also shown substantial protection in global ischemia even when the onset of hypothermia (32.5–33.5°C) was delayed by 6 hr (40).

Remarkable confirmation of enduring neuroprotection was provided by electrophysiological studies performed in hippocampal slices taken from gerbils 5 weeks after being subjected to 5-min forebrain ischemia, either untreated or given 48 hr of hypothermia (32–34°C). In slices from treated animals, resting membrane potential, action potential amplitude and duration, and synaptic currents evoked by Schaffer collateral stimulation resembled those of sham animals without ischemia (41)—a definitive proof of functional integrity. In hippocampal slices studied in vitro, the CA1 pyramidal cells recovered their postsynaptic population spike after 7 min of hypoxia at 34°C, but failed to do so after hypoxia at 37°C (42).

Postischemic cooling is also neuroprotective in focal ischemia. In our laboratory, for example, a 5-hr cooling paradigm was assessed in rats with 2-hr MCA occlusion by the intraluminal suture method. Cooling to a target cranial temperature of 32°C improved neurobehavioral score and reduced cortical infarction by ~90%, showing equal efficacy whether initiated during ischemia or at the onset of the recirculation period; lowering temperature further (to 27°C), in fact, tended to be less efficacious (43) (Fig. 3). A similarly designed study showed that delaying the induction of mild hypothermia by 2 hr after the onset of temporary (2-hr) MCA occlusion still afforded sustained protection following 2-month survival (22). In another focal ischemia study in rats, cooling to 34°C for 48 hr starting 30 min following the onset of reperfusion substantially reduced cortical and striatal injury following 2-month survival, supporting enduring neuroprotection (44). Other studies have abundantly confirmed the protective efficacy of postischemic hypothermia (45–47).

Taken together, these studies highlight the subtle interplay between depth, duration, and delay of cooling, and suggest

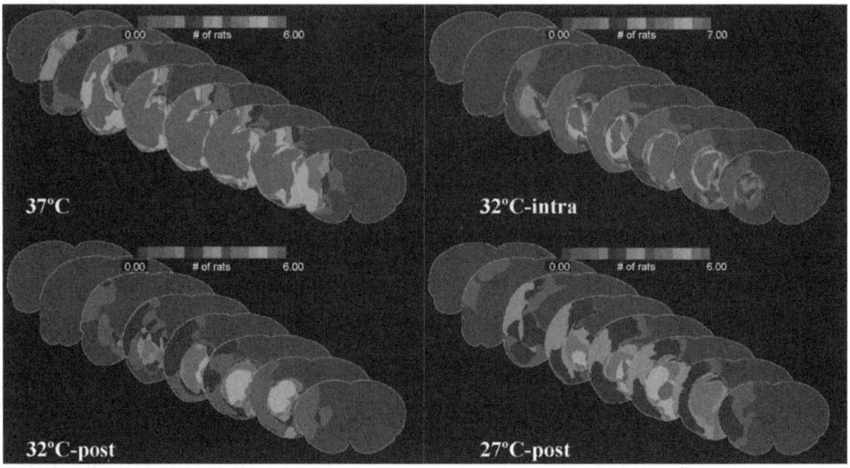

Figure 3 Histopathological infarct frequency maps constructed by computerized image mapping at eight coronal brain levels in rats with 2-hr MCA occlusion and 3-day survival, treated with various hypothermic regimens: "37°C," cranial normothermia; "32°C–intra," 5-hr cranial cooling to target temperature of 32°C, begun at the onset of MCA occlusion; "32°C–post" and "27°C–post," 5-hr cranial cooling to target temperatures of 32°C or 27°C, respectively, begun at the time of recirculation following 2-hr MCA occlusion. Colors depict numbers of rats with histological evidence of infarction at each pixel location. Both intraischemic and postischemic cooling to 32°C led to marked reductions in the frequency of cortical infarction compared to normothermic animals; postischemic cooling to 27°C conferred no additional benefit. (From Ref. 43.)

that these differences might, in turn, reflect a multifaceted complexity in the pathophysiology of hypothermic neuroprotection (48).

Mechanistic Effects of Hypothermia

Hemodynamic Effects

Both increases and decreases of cerebral blood flow (CBF) have been reported with hypothermia. Autoradiographic studies conducted in a 20-min global forebrain ischemia model in rats revealed that the severe CBF decrement produced *during* the insult was not influenced by intraischemic temperatures ranging from 30 °C to 36 °C (49). More profound hypothermia (25 °C, without ischemia) reduced CBF in dogs (50). In contrast, a recent study found that mild selective brain cooling (31 °C, with maintenance of normal core body temperature) more than doubled cortical CBF (51). Temperature influences on CBF are considered in greater detail in Chapter 5 ("Brain Metabolism") (52).

General Metabolic Influences

It has long been recognized that hypothermia reduces cerebral oxygen consumption (cerebral metabolic rate for oxygen, or $CMRO_2$). This is expressed by the temperature coefficient Q_{10} defined as:

$$\frac{\mathrm{CMRO_2 \ at\ } x\,^\circ\mathrm{C}}{\mathrm{CMRO_2 \ at\ } [x - 10]\,^\circ\mathrm{C}}$$

Thus, the Q_{10} measured in dogs cooled from 37 °C to 27 °C was 2.23 (53)—identical to the value (2.3) obtained in human subjects (54). In pediatric patients undergoing hypothermic cardiopulmonary bypass, an exponential relationship was found between temperature and metabolic rate, with an average temperature coefficient of 3.65 (55). Although this temperature dependence of $CMRO_2$ probably helps to account for the cerebroprotection conferred by profound hypothermia, such as during cardiopulmonary bypass procedures, it does little by itself to explain why mild or moderate hypothermia is also neuroprotective. Although hypothermia tends to increase hemoglobin oxygen-binding affinity (thus decreasing the arterial pO_2 at which hemoglobin is 50% oxygen-saturated), this effect appeared not to be relevant to its protective effect in focal cerebral ischemia (56).

Bioenergetics and Intermediary Metabolism

Early evidence suggesting that mild-to-moderate hypothermia might modulate metabolic function emerged from studies in the rabbit retina preparation—an exquisitely controllable and sensitively monitored in vitro model (57). Here, large reductions in oxygen and glucose consumption and in electrophysiological function were produced by temperature decrements of only 3–6°C. In other studies in gerbils subjected to brief ischemia, reduction of head temperature by 3°C (a decrement sufficient to diminish hippocampal injury) delayed the rate of hippocampal adenosine triphosphate (ATP) decline during ischemia but did not prevent its eventual depletion (58). Similarly, following 20 min of global ischemia, brain ATP and phosphocreatine were nearly depleted and brain glucose substrate was exhausted, irrespective of intraischemic brain temperature (30°C, 33°C, or 39°C) (59).

Magnetic resonance spectroscopy has permitted a more detailed analysis of the metabolic effects of hypothermia. In neonatal rats with hypoxia–ischemia, temperature decreases to 34°C or 31°C suppressed the decline of brain ATP and phosphocreatine concentrations (60). In severe forebrain ischemia in rats, brain pH declined to ~6.5–6.6 irrespective of temperature (34°C, 36°C, or 38°C); however, in the postischemic period, pH recovered at a somewhat faster rate in the 34°C group (61). Other magnetic resonance spectroscopy studies have reported that hypothermia attenuates the development of cerebral acidosis during prolonged ischemia (62) and decreases the rate of decline of high-energy phosphates by ≈5% per 1°C (63). Multiparametric probe measurements during profound hypothermic circulatory arrest (18°C) in a human subject during aneurysm surgery revealed a rate of hydrogen ion increase one-third that seen at 35°C, and a more rapid rate of recovery of tissue acidosis (64). However, in brain microdialysis studies performed during experimental global ischemia, *extracellular* lactate rose by sevenfold to eightfold irrespective of brain temperature (30°C, 37°C, or 39°C), but early postischemic lactate clearance was more rapid in the 30°C group (65). Lactate accumulation during complete cerebral ischemia in dogs was also unaffected by selective brain cooling to 33°C (66).

Magnetic resonance spectroscopy studies employing carbon-13 to trace the glycolytic and tricarboxylic acid pathways of normal rats revealed that hypothermia to 31°C (without ischemia) led to a 30–40% depression of both neocortical and hippocampal metabolism, together with a 20–25% decrease in the steady-state fractional enrichment of metabolites, suggesting that hypothermia caused an increased fraction of glucose metabolism to be shunted through the pentose phosphate pathway (67).

Postischemic Metabolic Recovery

Autoradiographic studies of local cerebral glucose utilization and local cerebral blood flow following global ischemia have shown significantly greater recovery of local cerebral glucose utilization throughout cortical and subcortical structures of rats with intraischemic hypothermia compared to normothermic animals (68), as well as improved postischemic metabolic activation in response to peripheral stimuli following global ischemia conducted under hypothermic compared to normothermic conditions (69).

Ionic Alterations and Ischemic Depolarizations

Cellular ionic dyshomeostasis is a pivotal event in triggering ischemic brain damage. Ischemia-induced depletion of cellular high-energy metabolites (ATP and phosphocreatine) results in the failure of membrane ATPases and leads quickly to stereotypic perturbations of the brain's ionic gradients (70,71). There is egress of intracellular potassium and calcium ions into the extracellular compartment and a reciprocal movement of extracellular sodium ion and water into cells, leading to intracellular swelling. Extracellular potassium ion concentrations may increase to ~60–70 mmol/L due to rapidly developing increases in the permeability of both voltage-operated and receptor-operated ion channels. In the core of the focal ischemic lesion, where CBF is markedly reduced, terminal anoxic depolarization soon occurs. The surrounding ischemic penumbra, by contrast, initially undergoes fluctuating ionic disturbances, signaled by a negative shift of the direct current (DC) potential and termed "ischemic depolarizations." These events impose a metabolic demand on the energetically compromised penumbral tissue and hasten its irreversible deterioration (72–75).

Hypothermia has beneficial influences on ionic alterations in ischemia. Direct measurements of brain surface potassium concentration during total ischemia in dogs revealed that hypothermia (28°C) reduced ischemic potassium efflux rate by about 50% (76). In a study of focal cerebral ischemia, extracellular potassium ion concentration ($[K^+]_e$) was measured in the ischemic core and penumbra of normothermic and hypothermic rats (77). During the 1-hr MCA occlusion period, $[K^+]_e$ rose to a similar extent in normothermic and hypothermic (32°C) animals, but at 1 hr of reperfusion, $[K^+]_e$ in the ischemic core of normothermic animals showed incomplete recovery and was refractory to direct cortical stimulation, whereas $[K^+]_e$ in hypothermic rats had returned to preischemic levels and was responsive to cortical stimulation. Correspondingly, there proved to be marked diminution in infarct size in the hypothermic group (77).

Ischemic depolarizations are highly sensitive to mild-to-moderate hypothermia. In rats studied during 90-min MCA occlusion, continuous cortical DC potential measurements revealed only a single depolarization event in hypothermic (30°C) animals, contrasting with multiple depolarizations in normothermic rats (78). *Hyperthermia* (40°C) further increased these depolarizations; a number of depolarizations were highly correlated to the volumes of the resulting infarcts.

Studies of global ischemia have yielded consonant findings. Thus, in rats subjected to cardiac arrest at various pericranial temperatures, decreasing the temperature from 39°C to 25°C increased the time to cortical depolarization from 76 to 326 sec. This temporal prolongation paralleled the hypothermia-associated decrease in glucose metabolic rate and, hence, was thought to reflect the rate of energy store depletion (79,80). Similarly, hypothermia to 31°C increased the time to onset of depolarization by ≈4 min after near-complete forebrain ischemia in rats, but did not affect repolarization time after the insult (81). Hypothermic ischemia thus produced a duration of depolarization equivalent to that produced by shorter periods of ischemia at higher temperature. However, when the 37°C–10-min and 31°C–14-min ischemia groups were matched for equivalent durations of depolarization, the hypothermic group showed markedly improved histological outcome in hippocampal CA1 neurons. This observation suggested that mechanisms other than the delay to depolarization are involved in hypothermic neuroprotection (81).

In another study of global ischemia in rats, cortical hypoperfusion to ~9% of control CBF levels triggered anoxic depolarization in normothermic animals, whereas hypothermia (31–33 °C) delayed the appearance of anoxic depolarization and raised the blood flow threshold for its emergence to 4–5% of control CBF values (82). Intracellular measurements from single CA1 pyramidal neurons exposed to an ischemic medium showed a failure of membrane potential restoration after a 35 °C or 37 °C insult, but a return of membrane potential to control levels in 75% of neurons after an insult carried out at 27 °C or 33 °C (83); these workers concluded that 33 °C was the critical temperature for neuroprotection in this system.

In an important recent study of transient global ischemia in gerbils, the time of onset of ischemic depolarization lengthened from 1.3 min at 37°C to 2.4 min at 31°C, and logistic regression analysis demonstrated a close relationship between the duration of ischemic depolarization and neuronal damage (84). The durations of ischemic depolarization causing 50% neuronal damage at 37°C, 34°C, and 31°C were 8, 14, and 26 min, respectively; neurons were thus capable of withstanding almost threefold longer ischemia times at 31 °C than at 37 °C.

Neurotransmitters

Neurotransmitters play an important role in the pathogenesis of ischemic brain injury. The ischemia-induced release and extracellular accumulation of excitatory amino acids result in the activation of postsynaptic glutamate receptors, leading to increases in intracellular free calcium ion concentration and a cascade of deleterious events, eventuating in cell death (85–87). Multiple neurotransmitters and neuromodulators are massively released in ischemia, including glutamate, glycine, GABA, dopamine, norepinephrine, serotonin, adenosine, and others (88–90). Hypothermic temperatures tend to inhibit the biosynthesis, release, and/or reuptake of these various neurotransmitters (91,92).

Global Ischemia

In our laboratory, extracellular neurotransmitter levels were measured by microdialysis in the striatum of rats subjected to 20 min of global forebrain ischemic insults at various intra-ischemic brain temperatures. At 36°C, extracellular glutamate and dopamine levels increased significantly during ischemia and the early recirculation period (by 500-fold and 7-fold, respectively). In contrast, animals with brain temperatures maintained at 33°C or 30°C during ischemia showed complete inhibition of glutamate release (Fig. 4) and attenuation of dopamine release by 60% (49,88,89).

Microdialysis studies in other laboratories have confirmed these findings by showing marked attenuations of glutamate, aspartate, and glycine release from the hypothermic–ischemic brain (93–98). In one such investigation (95)—a study of global ischemia in rabbits—hypothermia of 32°C sufficed to reduce hippocampal glutamate release to less than one-tenth of the values typically observed after normothermic ischemia. In another rabbit global-ischemia study, hypothermia to 29°C strikingly attenuated glutamate, aspartate, and glycine elevations and abolished the prolonged postischemic elevation of glycine levels observed in normothermic–ischemic animals (94). The latter finding is of importance in that glycine potentiates *N*-methyl-D-aspartate (NMDA) receptor-mediated responses to glutamate (99,100). The hypothermic inhibition of glutamate release has been described, as well, under ischemic conditions complicated by hyperglycemia (101).

Our laboratory proposed the concept of the excitotoxic index as a composite descriptor of excitatory/inhibitory amino acid neurotransmitter balance based on microdialysis measurements in the brain's extracellular space (102,103). This index is defined as:

$$\text{Excitotoxic index} = [\text{glutamate}] \times [\text{glycine}]/[\text{GABA}]$$

Normothermic global ischemia for 12.5 min in rats led to significant 7-fold to 12-fold increases in the excitotoxic index

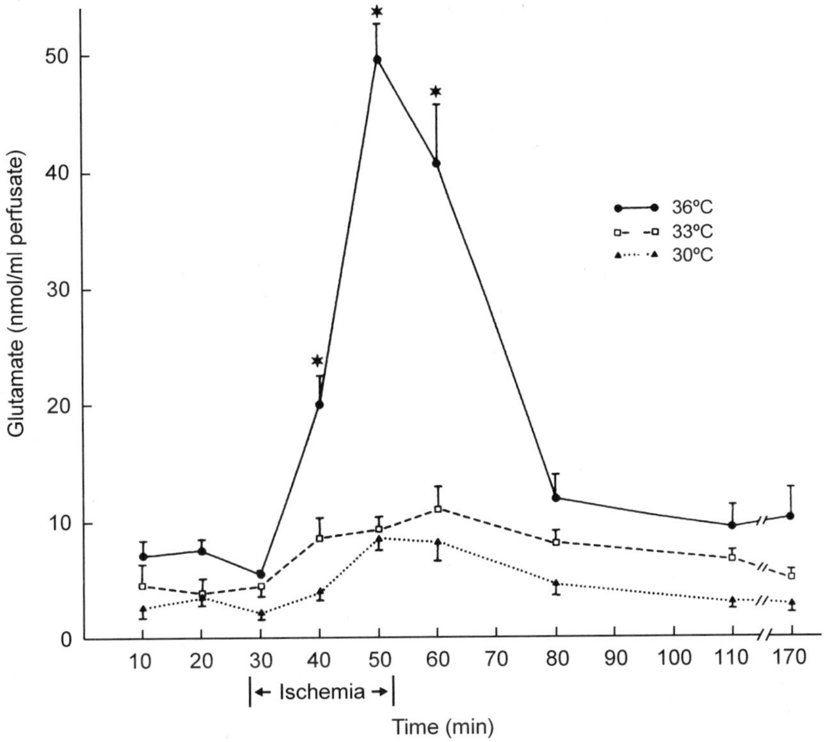

Figure 4 Time course of changes in striatal microdialysis perfusate levels of glutamate in rats subjected to 20-min global forebrain ischemia by four-vessel occlusion at intraischemic brain temperatures of 30°C, 33°C, or 36°C. In normothermic rats, a massive extracellular release of glutamate was triggered by the ischemic insult, whereas in animals with hypothermic brain temperatures (33°C or 30°C), glutamate release was almost entirely suppressed. (From Ref. 49.)

that persisted for 3–4 hr, whereas animals with postischemic hypothermia (30°C for 3 hr) showed no elevations of the excitotoxic index during the recirculation period (104).

Adenosine is also released into the brain in ischemia, but evidence suggests that this neuromodulator plays a neuroprotective—rather than a deleterious—role. In rats with 20-min global ischemia, striatal levels of adenosine were significantly greater in animals with intraischemic hypothermia than in normothermic animals, and postischemic hypoperfusion was less pronounced (105). Theophylline, an adenosine receptor antagonist, abolished the latter effect but did not affect histopathological outcome, suggesting that adenosine-mediated effects are not crucial to the protective action of intraischemic hypothermia (105).

Interestingly, hypothermia also modulates neurotransmitter release in the context of experimental traumatic brain injury. Thus, the elevated cerebrospinal fluid acetylcholine concentrations produced by normothermic trauma were not observed when hypothermic conditions (30°C) were imposed (106). In our laboratory, posttraumatic hypothermia (30°C for 3 hr) suppressed glutamate release adjacent to the impact site (107).

Focal Ischemia

Neurotransmitter release also occurs in focal cerebral ischemia and is sensitive to temperature modulations. For example, mild hypothermia attenuated cortical glutamate and glycine release produced by MCA occlusion, and these decreases paralleled the degree of histological infarct reduction (108). In our laboratory, we simultaneously measured neurotransmitter amino acids by microdialysis and CBF by laser Doppler flowmetry in the ischemic penumbral cortex of rats subjected to a 2-hr normothermic MCA occlusion (109). Extracellular glutamate increased by approximately 25-fold in the first 20–30 min, with the threshold CBF level for moderate glutamate release being 48% of control. In individual animals, the magnitude of glutamate release during ischemia was positively correlated with infarct volume. The decline in glutamate levels with ongoing ischemia suggested that neurotransmitter amino acid reuptake systems might remain functional in the penumbra during transient ischemia (109). Importantly, although hypothermia was not tested in that study, mildly *hyperthermic* ischemia (39°C) elevated peak levels of glutamate ≈7-fold above normothermic–ischemic levels and permitted glutamate release to occur at substantially lesser CBF decrements (110).

In a rabbit model of permanent focal ischemia, mild hypothermia (33°C)—a therapy that did not protect—led to glutamate efflux only in central tissue regions, suggesting that the hypothermic reduction of excitotoxic neurotransmitter release (when observed) might play a more significant role in the ischemic periphery than in core regions (111). In rats with permanent focal ischemia, a fourfold release of extracellular glutamate occurred within the first 30 min, but levels decreased over the subsequent 90 min; peak glutamate release was attenuated by one-half by hypothermia (112).

Mechanistic Studies, Transporters, and Receptor Subtypes

In mechanistic studies, the human glial glutamate transporter, hGLT-1, was transfected into hamster ovary cells, and temperature effects on transporter activity were assessed (113). Hypothermia attenuated the uptake of extracellular glutamate via hGLT-1, suggesting, paradoxically, that glutamate toxicity might initially be propagated by hypothermia because of a relative failure of glutamate uptake. In agreement with the above, a study using simulated "ischemia" (anoxia and substrate deprivation) in astrocyte cultures noted less glutamate uptake at 32°C than at normothermia (114). In cultured hippocampal neurons, hypothermia (30°C) could not prevent the massive neuronal death induced by directly applying high glutamate concentrations; the implication is that, in ischemia, hypothermia might be unable to protect once glutamate had been released (115). In another study, hypothermia (30°C or 20°C) protected cultured cortical neurons from brief excitotoxic challenges, whereas prolonged (60 min) exposures to glutamate unmasked a temperature-insensitive component of NMDA-mediated glutamate neurotoxicity (116).

The complexity of neuroprotective mechanisms is highlighted by a careful study of oxygen and/or glucose deprivation in organotypic hippocampal cultures (117). In this setting, NMDA receptor blockade was very effective in reducing the damage caused by complete oxygen-plus-glucose deprivation, whereas, by contrast, neither NMDA nor α-amino-3-hydroxy-5-methyl-4-isoxazolepropionic acid (AMPA)/kainate receptor blockade diminished the CA1 neuronal injury caused by oxygen deprivation alone. Hypothermia, however, protected against the latter type of injury, emphasizing the importance of nonglutamatergic mechanisms in hypothermic neuroprotection (117).

The influence of intraischemic hypothermia (30 °C) on the expression of glutamate receptor subtypes was examined by in situ hybridization following a 10-min global ischemic insult in rats (118). At 1-day survival, normothermic ischemia markedly suppressed the expression of AMPA receptor GluR1A, GluR2B, and GluR3C mRNAs to a similar degree in the hippocampal CA1 sector. NR1 mRNA expression in CA1 was reduced but to a lesser extent than AMPA receptor mRNA. At 7 days after normothermic ischemia, all three AMPA transcripts were nearly absent in CA1, whereas a percentage of NR1 remained. Intraischemic hypothermia fully blocked CA1 damage as well as the nonselective mRNA downregulations at 1 and 7 days. By contrast, *postischemic* hypothermia postponed neurodegeneration but only partially rescued the expression of AMPA and NR1 mRNAs at 7 days, and not at 1 day after the insult. These results suggest that intraischemic hypothermic neuroprotection occurred independently of altered subunit composition of AMPA receptors (118). A very recent publication has also reported that postischemic hypothermia (32 °C for 24 hr) in gerbils with 5-min forebrain ischemia attenuated the ischemia-induced downregulation of mRNA encoding the AMPA receptor subunit GluR2 (119).

Reactive Oxygen Species

Free radicals are chemically unstable molecules that are highly reactive because they contain an unpaired electron in one or more of their valance electron orbitals. These partially reduced species are mainly responsible for oxygen's toxicity (120). Among these reactive oxygen species are the superoxide anion radical and the highly reactive hydroxyl radical, which efficiently extracts hydrogen ions from unsaturated fatty acids to form lipid peroxides. Ensuing chain reactions in lipids facilitated by the presence of oxygen lead to the formation of new radicals that propagate the process of lipid peroxidation (121). Free radicals are also capable of inflicting damage to proteins and nucleic acids.

Our laboratory has studied hydroxyl radical production in the course of cerebral ischemia under different intraischemic temperatures. The method used was based on the chemical trapping of hydroxyl radical in the form of the stable adducts, 2,3-dihydroxybenzoic acid (2,3-DHBA) and 2,5-dihydroxybenzoic acid (2,5-DHBA), following administration of salicylate (122). In these studies, global ischemia for 20 min in normothermic rats was followed, during early recirculation, by increased DHBA levels, denoting hydroxyl radical production. By contrast, the same duration of ischemia at 30°C led to no significant hydroxyl radical signal during recirculation (122) (Fig. 5). Similar results were demonstrated in another laboratory, also using the DHBA method in the setting of 15-min global ischemia in rats; although normothermic animals showed increased levels of the hydroxylation product during reperfusion, attaining approximately 250% of control at 60 min, hypothermic ischemia (30°C) attenuated this increase to only 160% of control (123). In another study, extracellular concentrations of hydrogen peroxide were measured in gerbil hippocampus during transient forebrain ischemia and reperfusion. Hypothermia at 30°C or 34°C inhibited the increase in hydrogen peroxide concentration observed after normothermic ischemia (124). Moderate hypothermia (28°C) has also been reported to inhibit the increase in thiobarbituric acid-reactive substances produced after hemorrhage shock, which signals oxidative stress (125). Hypothermia (30°C) also suppressed evidence of hydroxyl radical formation following traumatic brain injury (107).

Inflammatory Mediators

Inflammatory processes, mediated by both humoral components (including cytokines) and cellular components (including leukocytes and microglia), contribute to ischemic brain injury (for recent reviews, see Refs. 126–128). Polymorphonuclear leukocytes (PMNLs; neutrophils) normally infiltrate into the

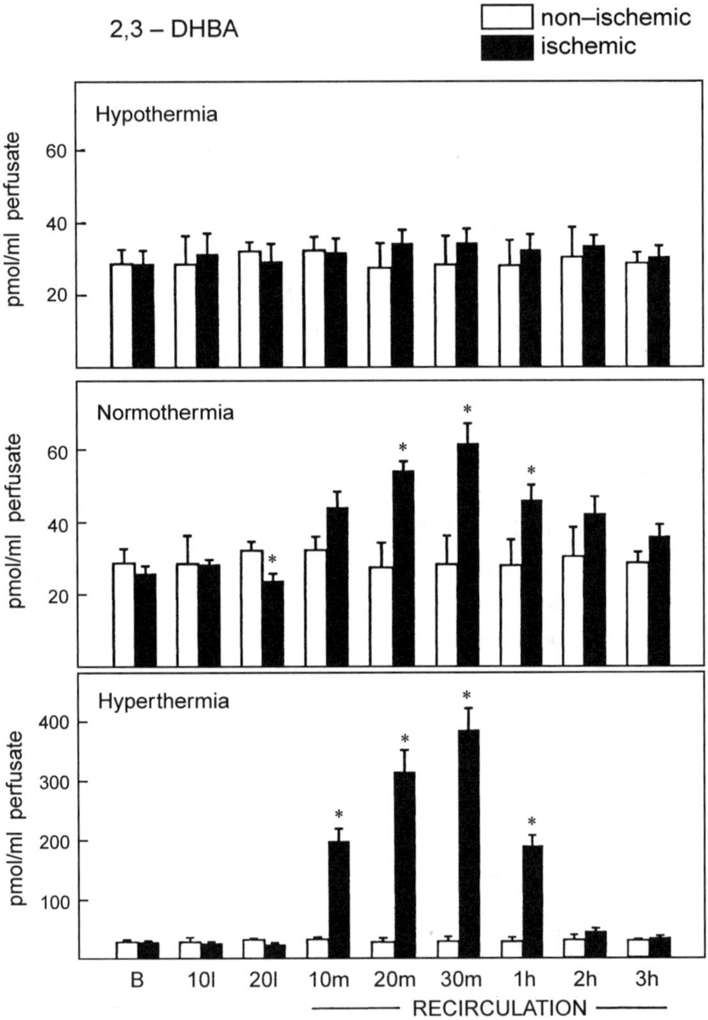

Figure 5 Levels of 2,3-DHBA—a stable adduct formed by the chemical trapping of hydroxyl radicals after salicylate administration—in the striatal microdialysis perfusate of rats with 20-min of global forebrain ischemia by bilateral carotid artery occlusions plus systemic hypotension at different levels of intraischemic brain temperatures, followed by 2 hr of normothermic recirculation. Values in nonischemic controls are also shown. Hypothermia = 30–30.5°C; normothermia = 36.5–37°C; hyperthermia = 38.5–39°C. Data are mean±SEM. $*P < 0.05$ vs. nonischemic values. Evidence of

postischemic brain. Several studies have shown that this process is attenuated by hypothermia. In a 3-hr MCA occlusion model in rats, intraischemic hypothermia (30°C) attenuated PMNL accumulation in the pericore region (i.e., the region histologically spared from infarction under hypothermic conditions) (129). In rats with 2-hr MCA occlusions treated with hypothermia (33°C for 2 hr), neutrophil accumulation decreased by over one-half (130). In a third report, rats with a 2-hr MCA occlusion treated with postischemic hypothermia (33°C for 4 hr followed by housing at cold temperature for 18 hr) showed significantly reduced neutrophil accumulation, as well as suppression of intracellular adhesion molecule-1 (ICAM-1) mRNA, which is normally overexpressed after ischemia (131). In a recent report using a rat model of 2-hr transient focal ischemia, hypothermia also reduced the number of neutrophils migrating into ischemic tissues as well as the number of microvessels expressing ICAM-1 (132).

Activation of the brain's resting microglia by an ischemic insult is attenuated by hypothermia. In gerbils with 10 min of normothermic global ischemia, microglial activation occurred at 1 day and became intense at 3 days; by contrast, hypothermic ischemia at 30°C, which conferred neuroprotection, failed to activate microglia (133). In microglial culture studies, hypothermia to 30°C markedly inhibited microglial proliferation and reduced their production of nitric oxide and superoxide radical—potential mediators of ischemic injury (134). A confirmatory study in cultured microglia reported that hypothermia (30°C or 33°C) markedly diminished lipopolysaccharide-stimulated nitric oxide and interleukin-6 (IL-6) production (135).

Immunohistochemical methods have been used recently to detect endothelial ICAM-1 expression, as well as infiltrating neutrophils, monocytes, and microglia after 2-hr MCA occlu-

---

increased hydroxyl radical activity was present during early recirculation following normothermic ischemia; this was markedly suppressed by moderate intraischemic hypothermia and greatly exaggerated by intraischemic hyperthermia. (From Ref. 122.)

sion produced by intraluminal suture in rats (136). Mild hypothermia (30°C during ischemia) reduced neutrophil infiltration by 97% on day 1 and by three quarters on day 3 postischemia, and also decreased ICAM-1-positive vessels during the first 7 days. Decreases in monocytes and activated microglia were observed in hypothermia-treated animals at 3 and 7 days (136). The latter observation is consonant with evidence that hypothermia (30°C) results in a remarkable inhibition of microglial proliferation in cell culture (134).

In a related study, hypothermic modulation of inflammatory responses elicited by the systemic injection of interleukin-1β (IL-1β)—a cytokine responsible for initiating inflammatory cascades—was examined in mice by intravital microscopy (137). Moderate hypothermia (32°C for 4 hr) caused a reduction in both leukocyte rolling and adhesion elicited by IL-1β injection (Fig. 6). In cultured cerebral endothelial cells, hypothermia attenuated nuclear factor-κB (NFκB) activation and reduced the expression of IL-8 and IL-1β (137). These results suggest that hypothermia acts, in part, by suppressing inflammatory gene transcription in cerebral endothelium. Relevant to the above, studies in experimental traumatic brain injury have also shown that trauma-induced IL-1β elevations are attenuated by hypothermia (32°C) applied immediately after the insult (138).

Figure 6 Effect of moderate hypothermia on mouse brain's inflammatory response elicited by systemic injection of IL-1β. (A) Average number of adhering leukocytes in pial venules determined over a 30-sec period 4 hr after injection of saline (sham) or IL-1β (5 mg/kg, i.p.). Hypothermia (32°C) was applied for 1 or 4 hr. (B and C) Intravital microscopic recordings of leukocyte rolling and adhesion in pial venules obtained via an open cranial window after systemic injection of acridine orange. (B) IL-1β-injected animal maintained at 37°C for 4 hr; arrows indicate numerous leukocytes adhering to intraluminal endothelium. (C) IL-1β-injected animal maintained at 32°C for 4 hr showing diminished leukocyte adhesion. (From Ref. 137.)

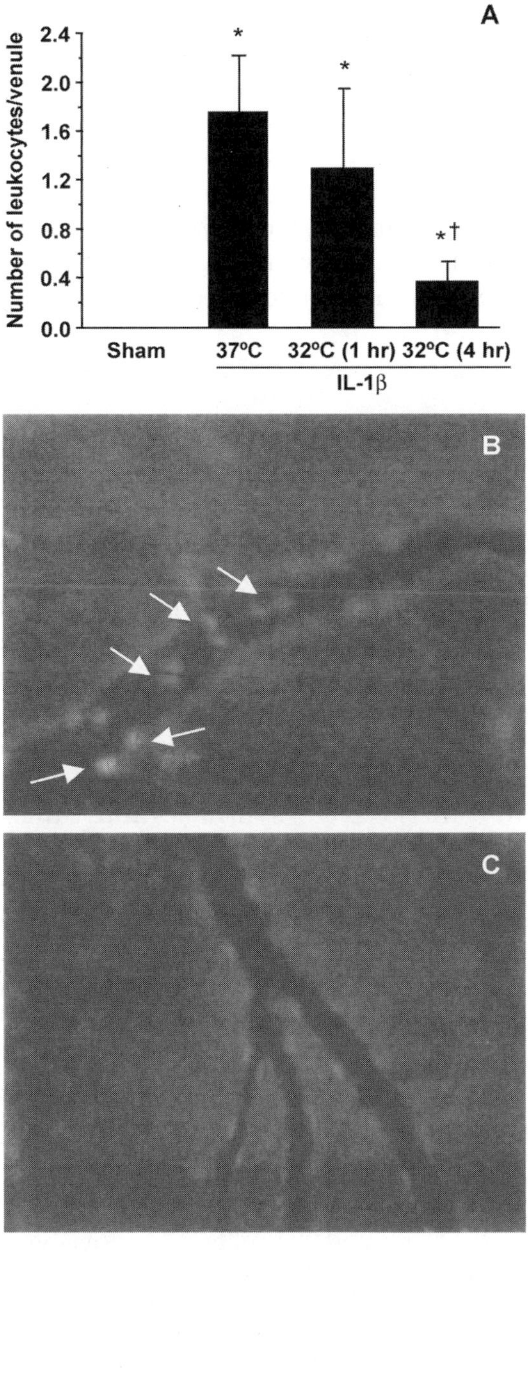
A
Number of leukocytes/venule
2.4
2.0
1.6
1.2
0.8
0.4
0.0
*
*
*†
Sham
37°C
32°C (1 hr)
32°C (4 hr)
IL-1β
B
C

The combination of therapeutic hypothermia with various anti-inflammatory strategies has also proven neuroprotective. For example, in rats with 10-min global forebrain ischemia, postischemic hypothermia (33°C for 7 hr) provided long-lasting high-grade neuroprotection when followed by repeated administration of dipyrone, an anti-inflammatory/antipyretic agent (139). In another report in rats with transient global ischemia, hypothermia combined with interleukin-10 (IL-10) therapy resulted in a degree of protection exceeding that seen with hypothermia alone (140).

NFκB

NFκB is an important transcription factor activated after ischemia, which leads to the expression of many inflammatory genes. In rats with 2-hr transient MCA occlusion maintained normothermic, NFκB cytoplasmic expression, nuclear translocation, and binding activity were observed as early as 2 hr and persisted at 24 hr (141). Hypothermia (33°C for 2 hr) decreased NFκB translocation and binding activity but did not alter its overall expression. Hypothermia also suppressed the phosphorylation of NFκB's inhibitory protein (IκB-α) and the activity of IκB kinase (IKK), as well as gene expression of two target genes of NFκB—inducible nitric oxide synthase and tumor necrosis factor-α (TNF-α) (141). Previous work had also established that mild hypothermia decreases a number of NFκB-regulated proteins such as inducible nitric oxide synthase (142), ICAM-1 (132,136), and inflammatory cytokines (138). Taken together, these data relate the protective effect of hypothermia, in part, to NFκB inhibition via decreased activity of IKK.

In a recent report (141), *delayed* hypothermia was more effective than intraischemic hypothermia in suppressing IκB phosphorylation, IKK expression, and target gene expression, despite the fact that these two cooling paradigms conferred similar degrees of neuroprotection (142). The authors attribute this to the fact that NFκB is activated by reactive oxygen species, which become more prominent during the reperfusion phase of an ischemic insult. This hypothesis highlights the important point that the mechanisms of hypothermia-mediated neuroprotection in all likelihood differ, depending on the timing of cooling.

Kinases

The previous section discussed the sensitivity of IKK activity to hypothermia. Other kinases are also hypothermia-sensitive. Thus, calcium/calmodulin-dependent protein kinase II (CaM kinase II) activity decreased significantly within seconds of recirculation following 5-min forebrain ischemia in normothermic gerbils, and this depression persisted at 1 week (143). Reductions of intracerebral temperature to 32°C prevented this decrease. Conversely, hyperthermia (39°C) markedly accentuated ischemia-induced decreases of CaM kinase II activity and led to severe neuronal loss (143). A more recent study (144), also conducted in the 5-min gerbil global ischemia model, demonstrated that CaM kinase II activity in the hippocampal cytosolic fraction decreased by about one-half of control in normothermic animals but remained close to normal under hypothermic conditions; this preservation of CaM kinase activity after ischemia paralleled the neuroprotective effect. It was recently shown in a 30-min global forebrain ischemia model in rats that CaM kinase II and protein kinase C (PKC) α, β, and γ isoforms are translocated to the synaptosomal fraction, and that mild hypothermia inhibits this translocation (145). Hypothermia also inhibited fodrin proteolysis caused by ischemia–reperfusion, implying that calpain activation had been inhibited (145).

Protein kinase C has been implicated in neurotransmitter release and glutamate receptor-mediated events. In our laboratory, we explored PKC activity in various brain regions in the course of 20 min of forebrain ischemia in rats at 30°C, 37°C, or 39°C (146). For both membrane-bound and cytosolic PKC, there was a distinct temperature effect, and for membrane-bound PKC, there was a differential effect according to brain region. In normothermic ischemic rats, extensive depressions of PKC activity were noted in the vulnerable hippocampus and striatum throughout 24 hr of postischemic recirculation, whereas the less vulnerable cortex and thalamus showed more transient and inconsistent patterns; these patterns were highly susceptible to the influence of intraischemic hypothermia (30°C) (146).

Ubiquitin

Ubiquitin is a small protein that binds to abnormal proteins produced by neural injury and facilitates their digestion by proteases (147). In gerbils exposed to 5 min of global ischemia, loss of ubiquitin was seen at 6 hr in both normothermic and hypothermic animals, whereas the hypothermic group showed subsequent restitution at 24–48 hr. Enhanced resynthesis of ubiquitin may thus contribute to hypothermic protection (148).

Cerebral Edema and Blood–Brain Barrier Disruption

Both cytotoxic edema and vasogenic edema associated with increased blood–brain barrier (BBB) permeability are components of ischemic stroke (149). Moderate hypothermia has long been recognized as a means of reducing cerebral edema and diminishing BBB permeability in focal ischemic stroke (150, 151). In rats with 2-hr MCA occlusion, tracer studies were used to demonstrate a marked biphasic opening of the cortical BBB, the second phase of which led to vasogenic edema (152); hypothermia (28–29°C for 6 hr) reduced the late-phase BBB opening. The success of hypothermia as an antiedema measure in focal ischemia has led to the use of cooling (33°C for 48–72 hr) in patients with massive hemispheral ischemic stroke as a means of controlling elevated intracranial pressure; however, rewarming of some patients was complicated by a rebound of intracranial pressure with cerebral herniation (153).

Antiedema and BBB effects of hypothermia have also been noted in the setting of global ischemia. Thus, in one study, hypothermia protected against early cytotoxic edema formation after global ischemia (154). In rats exposed to 20 min of global forebrain ischemia at temperatures of 30°C, 33°C, 36°C, or 39°C, normothermic ischemic rats showed cortical protein extravasation—denoting BBB disruption—as early as 45 min after ischemia (155). Hypothermia of 30°C or 33°C markedly suppressed this leakage, whereas ischemia at 39°C dramatically accentuated BBB disruption. Moderate hypothermia also attenuated increased BBB permeability and brain edema after experimental intracerebral hematoma (156).

Apoptotic Mechanisms

Although it is widely accepted that apoptotic mechanisms contribute, at least in part, to ischemic cell death, controversies persist as to the precise extent, anatomic sites, physiological settings, time course, and molecular mechanisms (157–160). A careful electron microscopic analysis was conducted in gerbils subjected to 5 min of global ischemia—an insult that leads to 96% death of CA1 neurons by day 4 under normothermic conditions and protection by hypothermia (161). Regardless of temperature conditions, dying neurons failed to exhibit apoptotic morphology but rather showed necrotic features or signs of selective mitochondrial injury (161). In contrast, other workers found evidence of cells meeting the electron microscopic criteria for apoptosis in a rat model of transient global ischemia following normothermic ischemia, and their diminution by hypothermia (33°C) (Fig. 7), which also resulted in increased expression of the antiapoptotic protein Bcl-2 (162).

Other global ischemia studies have found evidence of temperature-sensitive DNA fragmentation—a hallmark of apoptosis. In a gerbil study, DNA fragmentation was demonstrated in hippocampal CA1 neurons after transient forebrain ischemia, and inhibition of DNA fragmentation was proportional to the magnitude of hypothermia, with temperatures at or below 35°C being critical for the prevention of apoptosis (163). Other studies have provided supportive evidence of DNA fragmentation (164).

A careful study in transient forebrain ischemia in the rat explored molecular indices of DNA fragmentation under normothermic or hypothermic (33°C) conditions (165). At 48 hr of recovery after normothermic ischemia, in situ labeling of DNA breaks was widespread, and high-molecular weight DNA

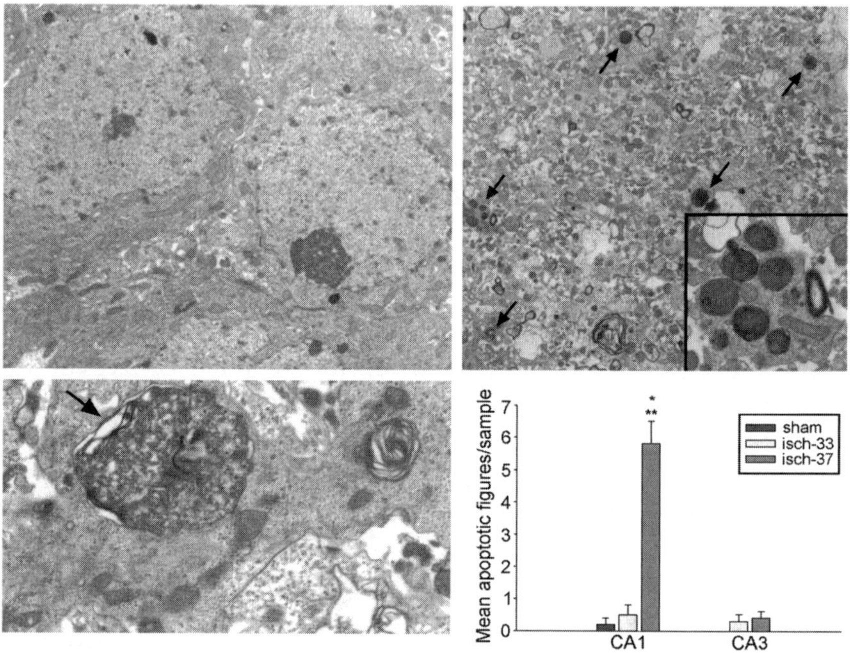

Figure 7 Rats with 10 min of forebrain ischemia produced by bilateral carotid artery occlusions plus hypotension under conditions of normothermia (brain temperature 36.5–37.5°C) or mild hypothermia (32.5–33.5°C), which was maintained for 3 hr; the survival period was 72 hr. Electron micrograph from hippocampal CA1 region of hypothermic–ischemic rat (upper left panel) shows normal neuronal morphology (original magnification, ×2900). By contrast, normothermic–ischemic brain contains numerous apoptotic neurons (upper right panel: arrows; original magnification, ×2900); inset (×10,000) shows numerous condensed homogeneous apoptotic bodies and intact mitochondrion. Lower left panel: Hypothermic–ischemic brain, showing apoptotic neuron with condensed nucleus and blebbing of nuclear membrane (arrow); note numerous intact mitochondria and relatively normal-appearing cytoplasm. Lower right panel: Numbers of apoptotic cells in CA1 were decreased in the 33°C ischemia group compared to the 37°C ischemia group (*$P < 0.001$). (From Ref. 162.)

cleavage was seen in the medial hippocampal CA1 sector; at 72-hr recovery, major oligonucleosomal DNA fragmentation was observed. In contrast, after hypothermic ischemia, DNA fragmentation was absent in CA1 (165). In rats with 1-hr transient forebrain ischemia, prolonged hypothermia (34.5°C for 16 hr) was studied (166). By the transferase dUTP nick-end labeling (TUNEL) method, TUNEL-positive cells peaked at 2 days after ischemia in normothermic animals, but their numbers were reduced by hypothermia. Correspondingly, Bax immunostaining was attenuated in the hypothermic group (166). A related study of transient forebrain ischemia in gerbils showed that a 1° temperature decrease (from 39°C to 38°C) increased the migration of fragmented DNA from nuclei into apical dendrites of CA1 pyramidal cells (167).

In focal cerebral ischemia (2-hr MCA occlusion model in rats), mild intraischemic hypothermia (33°C) needed to be maintained for 1–2 hr to obtain optimal neuroprotection against ischemic cell death, which was partially apoptotic as reflected by the TUNEL method—a technique not fully specific for apoptosis. One or 2 hr of mild hypothermia decreased TUNEL staining by 80% or more (130). In a study of 1-hr MCA occlusion in rats, immunohistochemical expression of Fas and caspase-3 could be demonstrated as early as 5 hr after reperfusion, and the expression pattern maximized at 24 hr (168). This expression was decreased in hypothermic (33°C) animals. Correspondingly, DNA fragmentation by the TUNEL method increased over the first 24 hr in normothermic animals, but was significantly decreased by hypothermia (168).

The mitochondrial release of cytochrome *c* is thought to trigger caspase activation and apoptosis. These mechanisms were studied in a rat transient focal cerebral ischemia model (169). Mild hypothermia decreased cytochrome *c* release at 5 hr after the onset of ischemia, but mitochondrial translocation of Bax was not observed until 24 hr; hypothermia did not alter Bcl-2 or Bax expression, and caspase activation was not observed. The authors conclude that the maintenance of mitochondrial integrity contributed to the protective effect of mild hypothermia, but that it was unlikely that this therapy altered the intrinsic apoptotic pathway (169). In a related study of 1-hr

MCA occlusion, immunohistochemistry revealed Bcl-2 induction in many neurons in rats treated with hypothermia (33°C), whereas Bax and cytochrome *c* were induced in only a few neurons; there was a corresponding decrease in TUNEL labeling in the hypothermic group (170).

Apoptotic cell death mechanisms appear to play a prominent role in perinatal hypoxia–ischemia but decline in importance with neuronal maturation. Thus, in the brains of 7-day-old rat pups with hypoxia–ischemia, more than 90% of damaged striatal and neocortical neurons were caspase-3-positive, but this fraction declined dramatically by postnatal day 26 (171). In newborn piglets with hypoxia–ischemia, brain cooling during resuscitation reduced the fraction of apoptotic but not necrotic cells; the fraction of apoptotic cells was thought to be related to the degree of energy depletion during the insult (172).

Caspases are thought to play a key role in cell death after neonatal hypoxia–ischemia. In a model of this condition in 7-day postnatal rat pups, hypothermia (29°C) and the intraventricular administration of a pan-caspase inhibitor were studied singly and in combination; caspase-3 activity peaked after the normothermic insult and this was reduced by either therapy alone or in combination (173). In another study, hypothermia was found to suppress caspase-3 activation in the newborn rat brain after hypoxia–ischemia (174).

Gene Expression

A number of studies have explored the expression of various genes and gene products after global and focal ischemia, as influenced by hypothermia. The heat shock proteins have been most investigated in this regard. In a study of piglets subjected to circulatory arrest at temperatures ranging from profoundly to moderately hypothermic, ischemia at 29°C failed to induce substantial expression of heat shock protein 72 (HSP72) mRNA in the cerebral cortex, whereas ischemia at more severe temperature reductions triggered HSP72 expression (175). In gerbil global ischemia, HSP72 immunoreactivity could be demonstrated in hippocampus and neocortex following normothermic ischemia, but this was absent in hypothermic–ischemic

(30°C) brains (176). These observations suggested that the neuroprotection afforded by intraischemic hypothermia could not be explained by HSP72 protein induction.

Immediate early genes have also been explored in hypothermic ischemia. In rat transient forebrain ischemia, in situ hybridization was used to examine the expression of the fos and jun families of transcription factors. A biphasic expression was seen after normothermic ischemia, with the second phase (maximal at 12–36 hr) particularly evident in vulnerable hippocampal regions (177). Induction of immediate early genes occurred more rapidly following hypothermic ischemia and was thought to reflect the faster resumption of normal intracellular signaling, possibly leading to enhanced neuronal recovery (177).

In a related study in gerbil transient forebrain ischemia, intraischemic hypothermia, which protects CA1 neurons, resulted in a prolonged elevation of activator protein-1 binding, which persisted up to 9 hr after reperfusion and was mediated, in part, via the expression of c-Fos protein (178). These results suggested that the prolonged elevation of DNA-binding activity of activator protein-1 might contribute to modulating the vulnerability or resistance of neuronal populations to ischemia.

Expression of the mRNAs for nerve growth factor, brain-derived neurotrophic factor, neurotrophin 3, and TrkB receptor was studied by in situ hybridization in normothermic and hypothermic (33°C) transient ischemia in rats (179). The expression of nerve growth factor, brain-derived neurotrophic factor, neurotrophin 3, and the neurotrophin receptor, TrkB, mRNA in ischemia-sensitive hippocampal subregions was not increased by protective levels of hypothermia. By contrast, neurotrophin mRNA alterations were induced in the ischemia-resistant dentate gyrus; the latter was speculated to confer protection to that region.

Proliferating cell nuclear antigen (PCNA) is required for DNA replication and nucleotide excision repair of damaged DNA. The PCNA mRNA levels were upregulated in the hippocampal CA1 sector at 36 hr following normothermic global forebrain ischemia, whereas protective levels of hypothermic ischemia accelerated this induction by 18 hr (180). In normothermic ischemia, nuclear PCNA immunoreactivity was largely abolished in vulnerable CA1 neurons prior to cell death, whereas after hypothermic ischemia, PCNA protein levels did not decrease. These findings implicate DNA repair processes in ischemia-sensitive neurons after ischemia (180).

Expression of the glucose-regulated protein-78 (GRP78) was explored at the mRNA and protein levels in gerbils with 15-min normothermic forebrain ischemia, reperfused either under normothermic or mildly hypothermic conditions (34°C, for 3 hr) (181). The GRP78 mRNA was reduced in the vulnerable hippocampal CA region under normothermic conditions but was not reduced under hypothermic conditions. The GRP78 protein decreased in the CA1 region under normothermia but not hypothermia. The authors concluded that hypothermia-mediated restoration of GRP78 expression may contribute to enhancement of neuronal survival (181).

FUTURE DIRECTIONS

Studies over the past decade and a half have established beyond doubt that mild-to-moderate degrees of hypothermia are neuroprotective in cerebral ischemia and, in all likelihood, in the related disorder of traumatic brain injury (the results of a recent imperfect multicenter trial notwithstanding) (182,183). Experimental studies have proven that focal cerebral ischemia (resembling clinical thromboembolic stroke), as well as transient global near-complete ischemia with recirculation (resembling cardiac arrest with resuscitation), are both amenable to hypothermic neuroprotection. Indeed, the broad therapeutic applicability of moderate hypothermia is epitomized by the recently reported randomized clinical trials of hypothermia as a successful therapy for ameliorating the neurological sequelae of cardiac arrest (184,185). Moderate hypothermia is also viewed as having strong potential as a neuroprotective strategy for perinatal hypoxic–ischemic brain injury (186,187).

As hypoxic–ischemic brain injury is engendered by a highly complex interaction of multiple biochemical and molecular mechanisms, it seems reasonable to hypothesize that the ideal neuroprotective strategy would be one that targets *multiple* injury mechanisms. It is apparent from this chapter that mild-to-moderate hypothermia is such a neuroprotectant in that it impacts a multitude of possible injury pathways. Indeed, we consider it highly probable that the ability of hypothermia to affect multiple processes is essential to its broad therapeutic efficacy.

Although the evidence presented here supports a large number of potential biological effects of moderate hypothermia, the precise weighting (i.e., relative importance) attached to these various effects is probably highly context-dependent. This point is clearly illustrated, for example, by comparing intraischemic with postischemic cooling. Intraischemic hypothermia has been clearly documented to suppress the extracellular release of excitotoxic neurotransmitters (49). Postischemic cooling, if sufficiently prolonged, also confers high-grade enduring ischemic neuroprotection (e.g., Ref. 39) despite the fact that the intraischemic release of excitatory neurotransmitters has already occurred prior to its initiation.

Viewed therapeutically, variations in the specifics of how hypothermia is administered may influence outcome. These include: (a) the delay from onset of the ischemic insult to institution of hypothermia; (b) the depth of cooling; (c) the duration of cooling; (d) the rate of rewarming; and (e) the presence or absence of pharmacological agents or other therapies. Therapeutic efficacy surely also depends on the nature of the ischemic insult itself, including whether it is focal or global; the duration of ischemia; body temperature during the insult; age of the subject; coexistence of systemic disease; and, if focal ischemia, whether or not reperfusion has occurred. It is obviously impossible to investigate these combinations comprehensively, so that intelligent decision making in designing a specific therapeutic strategy must be made based on the best synthesis of available data.

It can be recommended with confidence that therapeutic hypothermia should be instituted as rapidly as possible; there is no evidence that delaying the initiation of therapy ever provides superior results. Secondly, it is important that the target organ—the brain—be the object of cooling, i.e., that the target temperature of the brain itself be reduced sufficiently to provide a protective effect. It is likely that there is a reciprocal interaction between depth and duration of cooling: as a generalization, brain temperatures of 32–33°C tend to be highly neuroprotective if maintained for sufficient lengths of time.

Inducing hypothermia to 32–33°C in the setting of clinical stroke inevitably requires heavy sedation or anesthesia; often, it also requires ventilatory assistance and intensive care management. This therapy may predispose patients to infectious complications and other sequelae of hospitalization that are presumably worsened at lower temperatures. In this regard, the commercial development of intravascular cooling catheters over the past several years (e.g., Ref. 188) now makes it possible to attain target levels of core temperature more rapidly and to achieve more rigorous temperature control than is possible with surface-cooling methods; internal cooling, especially when accompanied by surface warming, also reduces thermal discomfort of the patient and thereby reduces the need for adjunctive antishivering therapies. It is likely that these devices will be incorporated into the design of controlled clinical trials for acute ischemic stroke and related disorders during the next decade.

It is important to recall that hypothermia has also been shown to be protective when combined with other therapeutic measures such as anti-inflammatory strategies (139), NMDA receptor blockade (189–191), and radical scavengers (192). Hypothermia may be useful as a therapeutic adjunct by slowing the process of cell death, thereby broadening the therapeutic window for neuroprotection with a coadministered pharmacological agent, or by conferring synergistic protection. As hypothermia tends to be more effective in reperfusible focal ischemia than in permanent vascular occlusion (e.g., Ref. 32), it might prove to be a valuable adjunct to thrombolytic therapy (193).

Finally, although not explicitly reviewed in this chapter, it is now apparent that the obverse of hypothermia—namely, *hyperthermia* (temperature elevation, fever)—accentuates many of the injury mechanisms reviewed above so as to worsen ischemic and traumatic brain injury. This has been abundantly substantiated in experimental studies (for reviews, see Refs. 194 and 195). In addition, numerous clinical studies have shown that even mild temperature elevations are deleterious in patients with acute stroke (196–202). The prevention of fever in patients with acute ischemic or traumatic brain injury should now be considered an obligatory part of good medical practice. Conventional antipyretics confer moderate benefit in this setting (203–205). Early-phase clinical trials using intravascular cooling catheters suggest that this approach may offer a more effective means of preventing fever in patients with acute stroke, subarachnoid hemorrhage, and traumatic brain injury (206).

ACKNOWLEDGMENTS

Our studies are supported by grants NS05820 and NS40406 of the National Institutes of Health.

REFERENCES

1. Ginsberg MD, Sternau LL, Globus MY, Dietrich WD, Busto R. Therapeutic modulation of brain temperature: relevance to ischemic brain injury. Cerebrovasc Brain Metab Rev 1992; 4:189–225.
2. Busto R, Ginsberg MD. The influence of altered brain temperature in cerebral ischemia. In: Ginsberg MD, Bogousslavsky J, eds. Cerebrovascular Disease: Pathophysiology, Diagnosis, and Management. Malden, MA: Blackwell Science, 1998:287–307.
3. Smith LW, Fay T. Observations on human beings with cancer, maintained at reduced temperatures of 75°–90° Fahrenheit. Am J Physiol 1940; 10:1–10.
4. Fay T. Observations on generalized refrigeration in cases of severe cerebral trauma. Assoc Res Nerv Ment Dis Proc 1943; 24:611–619.
5. Fay T, Smith GW. Observations on reflex responses during prolonged periods of human refrigeration. Arch Neurol Psychiatry 1941; 45:215–222.
6. Sealy WC, Brown IJ, Young WJ. A report on the use of both

extracorporeal circulation and hypothermia for open heart surgery. Ann Surg 1958; 147:603–613.

7. Botterell EH, Lougheed WM, Scott JW, Vandewater SL. Hypothermia, and interruption of carotid, or carotid and vertebral circulation, in the surgical management of intracranial aneurysms. J Neurosurg 1956; 13:1–42.

8. Spetzler RF, Hadley MN, Rigamonti D, Carter LP, Raudzens PA, Shedd SA, Wilkinson E. Aneurysms of the basilar artery treated with circulatory arrest, hypothermia, and barbiturate cerebral protection. J Neurosurg 1988; 68:868–879.

9. Weinrauch V, Safar P, Tisherman S, Kuboyama K, Radovsky A. Beneficial effect of mild hypothermia and detrimental effect of deep hypothermia after cardiac arrest in dogs. Stroke 1992; 23:1454–1462.

10. Connolly JE, Boyd RJ, Calvin JW. The protective effect of hypothermia in cerebral ischemia: experimental and clinical application by selective brain cooling in the human. Surgery 1962; 52:15–24.

11. White RJ, Massopust LJ, Wolin LR, Taslitz N, Yashon D. Profound selective cooling and ischemia of primate brain without pump or oxygenator. Surgery 1969; 66:224–232.

12. Young RS, Zalneraitis EL, Dooling EC. Neurological outcome in cold water drowning. JAMA 1980; 244:1233–1235.

13. Hirsch H, Müller HA. Funktionelle und histologische Veränderungen des Kaninchengehirns nach kompletter Gehirnischämie. Pflugers Arch 1962; 275:277–291.

14. Berntman L, Welsh FA, Harp JR. Cerebral protective effect of low-grade hypothermia. Anesthesiology 1981; 55:495–498.

15. Vibulsresth S, Dietrich WD, Busto R, Ginsberg MD. Failure of nimodipine to prevent ischemic neuronal damage in rats. Stroke 1987; 18:210–216.

16. Busto R, Dietrich WD, Globus MY, Valdes I, Scheinberg P, Ginsberg MD. Small differences in intraischemic brain temperature critically determine the extent of ischemic neuronal injury. J Cereb Blood Flow Metab 1987; 7:729–738.

17. Clifton GL, Taft WC, Blair RE, Choi SC, DeLorenzo RJ.

Conditions for pharmacologic evaluation in the gerbil model of forebrain ischemia. Stroke 1989; 20:1545–1552.

18. Minamisawa H, Nordstrom CH, Smith ML, Siesjo BK. The influence of mild body and brain hypothermia on ischemic brain damage. J Cereb Blood Flow Metab 1990; 10:365–374.
19. Minamisawa H, Smith ML, Siesjo BK. The effect of mild hyperthermia and hypothermia on brain damage following 5, 10, and 15 minutes of forebrain ischemia. Ann Neurol 1990; 28:26–33.
20. Chopp M, Chen H, Dereski MO, Garcia JH. Mild hypothermic intervention after graded ischemic stress in rats. Stroke 1991; 22:37–43.
21. Green EJ, Dietrich WD, van Dijk F, Busto R, Markgraf CG, McCabe PM, Ginsberg MD, Schneiderman N. Protective effects of brain hypothermia on behavior and histopathology following global cerebral ischemia in rats. Brain Res 1992; 580:197–204.
22. Maier CM, Sun GH, Kunis D, Yenari MA, Steinberg GK. Delayed induction and long-term effects of mild hypothermia in a focal model of transient cerebral ischemia: neurological outcome and infarct size. J Neurosurg 2001; 94:90–96.
23. Kuluz JW, Gregory GA, Yu AH, Chang Y. Selective brain cooling during and after prolonged global ischemia reduces cortical damage in rats. Stroke 1992; 23:1792–1797.
24. Nurse S, Corbett D. Direct measurement of brain temperature during and after intraischemic hypothermia: correlation with behavioral, physiological, and histological endpoints. J Neurosci 1994; 14:7726–7734.
25. Leonov Y, Sterz F, Safar P, Radovsky A, Oku K, Tisherman S, Stezoski SW. Mild cerebral hypothermia during and after cardiac arrest improves neurologic outcome in dogs. J Cereb Blood Flow Metab 1990; 10:57–70.
26. Wass CT, Lanier WL, Hofer RE, Scheithauer BW, Andrews AG. Temperature changes of $\geq 1\,^{\circ}C$ alter functional neurologic outcome and histopathology in a canine model of complete cerebral ischemia. Anesthesiology 1995; 83:325–335.
27. Lauritzen M, Hansen AJ. The effect of glutamate receptor

blockade on anoxic depolarization and cortical spreading depression. J Cereb Blood Flow Metab 1992; 12:223–229.

28. Zhang ZG, Chopp M, Chen H. Duration dependent post-ischemic hypothermia alleviates cortical damage after transient middle cerebral artery occlusion in the rat. J Neurol Sci 1993; 117:240–244.
29. Markarian GZ, Lee JH, Stein DJ, Hong SC. Mild hypothermia: therapeutic window after experimental cerebral ischemia. Neurosurgery 1996; 38:542–550.
30. Ridenour TR, Warner DS, Todd MM, McAllister AC. Mild hypothermia reduces infarct size resulting from temporary but not permanent focal ischemia in rats. Stroke 1992; 23: 733–738.
31. Xue D, Huang ZG, Smith KE, Buchan AM. Immediate or delayed mild hypothermia prevents focal cerebral infarction. Brain Res 1992; 587:66–72.
32. Morikawa E, Ginsberg MD, Dietrich WD, Duncan RC, Kraydieh S, Globus MY, Busto R. The significance of brain temperature in focal cerebral ischemia: histopathological consequences of middle cerebral artery occlusion in the rat. J Cereb Blood Flow Metab 1992; 12:380–389.
33. Chen H, Chopp M, Zhang ZG, Garcia JH. The effect of hypothermia on transient middle cerebral artery occlusion in the rat. J Cereb Blood Flow Metab 1992; 12:621–628.
34. Goto Y, Kassell NF, Hiramatsu K, Soleau SW, Lee KS. Effects of intraischemic hypothermia on cerebral damage in a model of reversible focal ischemia. Neurosurgery 1993; 32:980–985.
35. Barone FC, Feuerstein GZ, White RF. Brain cooling during transient focal ischemia provides complete neuroprotection. Neurosci Biobehav Rev 1997; 21:31–44.
36. Dietrich WD, Busto R, Alonso O, Globus MY, Ginsberg MD. Intraischemic but not postischemic brain hypothermia protects chronically following global forebrain ischemia in rats. J Cereb Blood Flow Metab 1993; 13:541–549.
37. Colbourne F, Corbett D. Delayed and prolonged post-ischemic hypothermia is neuroprotective in the gerbil. Brain Res 1994; 654:265–272.

38. Colbourne F, Corbett D. Delayed postischemic hypothermia: a six month survival study using behavioral and histological assessments of neuroprotection. J Neurosci 1995; 15: 7250–7260.

39. Colbourne F, Li H, Buchan AM. Indefatigable CA1 sector neuroprotection with mild hypothermia induced 6 hours after severe forebrain ischemia in rats. J Cereb Blood Flow Metab 1999; 19:742–749.

40. Coimbra C, Wieloch T. Moderate hypothermia mitigates neuronal damage in the rat brain when initiated several hours following transient cerebral ischemia. Acta Neuropathol (Berl) 1994; 87:325–331.

41. Dong H, Moody-Corbett F, Colbourne F, Pittman Q, Corbett D. Electrophysiological properties of CA1 neurons protected by postischemic hypothermia in gerbils. Stroke 2001; 32: 788–795.

42. Amorim P, Cottrell JE, Kass IS. Effect of small changes in temperature on CA1 pyramidal cells from rat hippocampal slices during hypoxia: implications about the mechanism of hypothermic protection against neuronal damage. Brain Res 1999; 844:143–149.

43. Huh PW, Belayev L, Zhao W, Koch S, Busto R, Ginsberg MD. Comparative neuroprotective efficacy of prolonged moderate intraischemic and postischemic hypothermia in focal cerebral ischemia. J Neurosurg 2000; 92:91–99.

44. Corbett D, Hamilton M, Colbourne F. Persistent neuroprotection with prolonged postischemic hypothermia in adult rats subjected to transient middle cerebral artery occlusion. Exp Neurol 2000; 163:200–206.

45. Colbourne F, Sutherland G, Corbett D. Postischemic hypothermia. A critical appraisal with implications for clinical treatment. Mol Neurobiol 1997; 14:171–201.

46. Yanamoto H, Nagata I, Nakahara I, Tohnai N, Zhang Z, Kikuchi H. Combination of intraischemic and postischemic hypothermia provides potent and persistent neuroprotection against temporary focal ischemia in rats. Stroke 1999; 30:2720–2726.

47. Colbourne F, Corbett D, Zhao Z, Yang J, Buchan AM.

Prolonged but delayed postischemic hypothermia: a long-term outcome study in the rat middle cerebral artery occlusion model. J Cereb Blood Flow Metab 2000; 20:1702–1708.

48. Corbett D, Nurse S. The problem of assessing effective neuroprotection in experimental cerebral ischemia. Prog Neurobiol 1998; 54:531–548.

49. Busto R, Globus MY, Dietrich WD, Martinez E, Valdes I, Ginsberg MD. Effect of mild hypothermia on ischemia-induced release of neurotransmitters and free fatty acids in rat brain. Stroke 1989; 20:904–910.

50. Rosomoff HL, Holaday DA. Cerebral blood flow and cerebral oxygen consumption during hypothermia. Am J Physiol 1954; 179:85–88.

51. Kuluz JW, Prado R, Chang J, Ginsberg MD, Schleien CL, Busto R. Selective brain cooling increases cortical cerebral blood flow in rats. Am J Physiol 1993; 265:H824–H827.

52. Steinberg G. Effects of hypothermia on cerebral metabolism, blood flow, and autoregulation. In: Mayer SA, Sessler DI, eds. Hypothermia in Neurocritical Care. New York: Marcel Dekker, Inc., 2004. In press.

53. Michenfelder JD, Milde JH. The relationship among canine brain temperature, metabolism, and function during hypothermia. Anesthesiology 1991; 75:130–136.

54. McCullough JN, Zhang N, Reich DL, Juvonen TS, Klein JJ, Spielvogel D, Ergin MA, Griepp RB. Cerebral metabolic suppression during hypothermic circulatory arrest in humans. Ann Thorac Surg 1999; 67:1895–1899.

55. Greeley WJ, Kern FH, Ungerleider RM, Boyd JL III, Quill T, Smith LR, Baldwin B, Reves JG. The effect of hypothermic cardiopulmonary bypass and total circulatory arrest on cerebral metabolism in neonates, infants, and children. J Thorac Cardiovasc Surg 1991; 101:783–794.

56. Wainwright MS, Sheng H, Sato Y, Burkhard MG, Steffen RP, Pearlstein RD, Warner DS. Pharmacological correction of hypothermic P(50) shift does not alter outcome from focal cerebral ischemia in rats. Am J Physiol Heart Circ Physiol 2002; 282:H1863–H1870.

57. Zager EL, Ames A III. Reduction of cellular energy requirements. Screening for agents that may protect against CNS ischemia. J Neurosurg 1988; 69:568–579.

58. Welsh FA, Sims RE, Harris VA. Mild hypothermia prevents ischemic injury in gerbil hippocampus. J Cereb Blood Flow Metab 1990; 10:557–563.

59. Ginsberg MD, Busto R, Martinez E, Globus MT, Valdes I, Loor JY. The effects of cerebral ischemia on energy metabolism. In: Schousboe A, Diemer NH, Kofod H, eds. Drug Research Related to Neuroactive Amino Acids—Alfred Benzon Symposium 32. Copenhagen: Munksgaard, 1992:207–224.

60. Williams GD, Dardzinski BJ, Buckalew AR, Smith MB. Modest hypothermia preserves cerebral energy metabolism during hypoxia–ischemia and correlates with brain damage: a ^{31}P nuclear magnetic resonance study in unanesthetized neonatal rats. Pediatr Res 1997; 42:700–708.

61. Haraldseth O, Gronas T, Southon T, Thommessen L, Borchgrevink G, Jynge P, Grisvold SE, Unsgard G. The effects of brain temperature on temporary global ischaemia in rat brain. A 31-phosphorous NMR spectroscopy study. Acta Anaesthesiol Scand 1992; 36:393–399.

62. Laptook AR, Corbett RJ, Burns D, Sterett R. Neonatal ischemic neuroprotection by modest hypothermia is associated with attenuated brain acidosis. Stroke 1995; 26:1240–1246.

63. Laptook AR, Corbett RJ, Sterett R, Garcia D, Tollefsbol G. Quantitative relationship between brain temperature and energy utilization rate measured in vivo using ^{31}P and ^{1}H magnetic resonance spectroscopy. Pediatr Res 1995; 38: 919–925.

64. Hoffman WE, Charbel FT, Munoz L, Ausman JI. Comparison of brain tissue metabolic changes during ischemia at 35 degrees and 18 degrees C. Surg Neurol 1998; 49:85–88.

65. Lin B, Busto R, Globus MY, Martinez E, Ginsberg MD. Brain temperature modulations during global ischemia fail to influence extracellular lactate levels in rats. Stroke 1995; 26:1634–1638.

66. Natale JA, D'Alecy LG. Protection from cerebral ischemia by

brain cooling without reduced lactate accumulation in dogs. Stroke 1989; 20:770–777.

67. Kaibara T, Sutherland GR, Colbourne F, Tyson RL. Hypothermia: depression of tricarboxylic acid cycle flux and evidence for pentose phosphate shunt upregulation. J Neurosurg 1999; 90:339–347.

68. Ginsberg MD, Busto R, Castella Y, Valdes I, Loor J. The protective effect of moderate intra-ischemic brain hypothermia is associated with improved postischemic glucose utilization and blood flow. J Cereb Blood Flow Metab 1989; 9:S380.

69. Dietrich WD, Busto R, Alonso O, Pita-Loor Y, Globus MT, Ginsberg MD. Intraischemic brain hypothermia promotes postischemic metabolic recovery and somatosensory circuit activation. J Cereb Blood Flow Metab 1991; 11:S846.

70. Hansen A, Lundbaek J, Sager T. Ionic alterations in ischemia. In: Ginsberg MD, Bogousslavsky J, eds. Cerebrovascular Disease: Pathophysiology, Diagnosis, and Management. Malden, MA: Blackwell Science, 1998:205–216.

71. Katsura K, Minamisawa H, Ekholm A, Folbergrova J, Siesjo BK. Changes of labile metabolites during anoxia in moderately hypo- and hyperthermic rats: correlation to membrane fluxes of K^+. Brain Res 1992; 590:6–12.

72. Back T, Ginsberg MD, Dietrich WD, Watson BD. Induction of spreading depression in the ischemic hemisphere following experimental middle cerebral artery occlusion: effect on infarct morphology. J Cereb Blood Flow Metab 1996; 16:202–213.

73. Belayev L, Zhao W, Busto R, Ginsberg MD. Transient middle cerebral artery occlusion by intraluminal suture: I. Three-dimensional autoradiographic image-analysis of local cerebral glucose metabolism–blood flow interrelationships during ischemia and early recirculation. J Cereb Blood Flow Metab 1997; 17:1266–1280.

74. Zhao W, Belayev L, Ginsberg MD. Transient middle cerebral artery occlusion by intraluminal suture: II. Neurological deficits, and pixel-based correlation of histopathology with local blood flow and glucose utilization. J Cereb Blood Flow Metab 1997; 17:1281–1290.

75. Back T, Nedergaard M, Ginsberg MD. The ischemic penumbra. Pathophysiology and relevance of spreading depression-like phenomena. In: Ginsberg MD, Bogousslavsky J, eds. Cerebrovascular Disease: Pathophysiology, Diagnosis, and Management. Malden, MA: Blackwell Science, 1998:276–286.

76. Astrup J, Skovsted P, Gjerris F, Sorensen HR. Increase in extracellular potassium in the brain during circulatory arrest: effects of hypothermia, lidocaine, and thiopental. Anesthesiology 1981; 55:256–262.

77. Sick TJ, Xu G, Perez-Pinzon MA. Mild hypothermia improves recovery of cortical extracellular potassium ion activity and excitability after middle cerebral artery occlusion in the rat. Stroke 1999; 30:2416–2421.

78. Chen Q, Chopp M, Bodzin G, Chen H. Temperature modulation of cerebral depolarization during focal cerebral ischemia in rats: correlation with ischemic injury. J Cereb Blood Flow Metab 1993; 13:389–394.

79. Nakashima K, Todd MM, Warner DS. The relation between cerebral metabolic rate and ischemic depolarization. A comparison of the effects of hypothermia, pentobarbital, and isoflurane. Anesthesiology 1995; 82:1199–1208.

80. Verhaegen M, Iaizzo PA, Todd MM. A comparison of the effects of hypothermia, pentobarbital, and isoflurane on cerebral energy stores at the time of ischemic depolarization. Anesthesiology 1995; 82:1209–1215.

81. Bart RD, Takaoka S, Pearlstein RD, Dexter F, Warner DS. Interactions between hypothermia and the latency to ischemic depolarization: implications for neuroprotection. Anesthesiology 1998; 88:1266–1273.

82. Kaminogo M, Ichikura A, Onizuka M, Takahata H, Matsuo Y, Kitagawa N, Shibata S. Mild hypothermia on anoxic depolarization and subsequent cortical injury following transient ischemia. Neurol Res 1999; 21:670–676.

83. Onitsuka M, Mihara S, Inokuchi H, Shigemori M, Higashi H. Mild hypothermia protects rat hippocampal CA1 neurons from irreversible membrane dysfunction induced by experimental ischemia. Neurosci Res 1998; 30:1–6.

84. Takeda Y, Namba K, Higuchi T, Hagioka S, Takata K, Hirakawa M, Morita K. Quantitative evaluation of the neuroprotective effects of hypothermia ranging from 34 degrees C to 31 degrees C on brain ischemia in gerbils and determination of the mechanism of neuroprotection. Crit Care Med 2003; 31:255–260.

85. Rothman SM, Olney JW. Glutamate and the pathophysiology of hypoxic–ischemic brain damage. Ann Neurol 1986; 19: 105–111.

86. Choi DW, Rothman SM. The role of glutamate neurotoxicity in hypoxic–ischemic neuronal death. Annu Rev Neurosci 1990; 13:171–182.

87. Benveniste H. The excitotoxin hypothesis in relation to cerebral ischemia. Cerebrovasc Brain Metab Rev 1991; 3:213–245.

88. Globus MY, Busto R, Dietrich WD, Martinez E, Valdes I, Ginsberg MD. Effect of ischemia on the in vivo release of striatal dopamine, glutamate, and gamma-aminobutyric acid studied by intracerebral microdialysis. J Neurochem 1988; 51:1455–1464.

89. Globus MY, Busto R, Dietrich WD, Martinez E, Valdes I, Ginsberg MD. Direct evidence for acute and massive norepinephrine release in the hippocampus during transient ischemia. J Cereb Blood Flow Metab 1989; 9:892–896.

90. Globus MT, Wester P, Busto R, Dietrich WD. Ischemia-induced extracellular release of serotonin plays a role in CA1 neuronal cell death in rats. Stroke 1992; 23:1595–1601.

91. Okuda C, Saito A, Miyazaki M, Kuriyama K. Alteration of the turnover of dopamine and 5-hydroxytryptamine in rat brain associated with hypothermia. Pharmacol Biochem Behav 1986; 25:79–83.

92. Graf R, Matsumoto K, Risse F, Rosner G, Heiss WD. Effect of mild hypothermia on glutamate accumulation in cat focal ischemia. Stroke 1992; 23:150.

93. Mitani A, Kataoka K. Critical levels of extracellular glutamate mediating gerbil hippocampal delayed neuronal death during hypothermia: brain microdialysis study. Neuroscience 1991; 42:661–670.

94. Baker AJ, Zornow MH, Grafe MR, Scheller MS, Skilling SR, Smullin DH, Larson AA. Hypothermia prevents ischemia-induced increases in hippocampal glycine concentrations in rabbits. Stroke 1991; 22:666–673.
95. Illievich UM, Zornow MH, Choi KT, Scheller MS, Strnat MA. Effects of hypothermic metabolic suppression on hippocampal glutamate concentrations after transient global cerebral ischemia. Anesth Analg 1994; 78:905–911.
96. Illievich UM, Zornow MH, Choi KT, Strnat MA, Scheller MS. Effects of hypothermia or anesthetics on hippocampal glutamate and glycine concentrations after repeated transient global cerebral ischemia. Anesthesiology 1994; 80:177–186.
97. Thoresen M, Satas S, Puka-Sundvall M, Whitelaw A, Hallstrom A, Loberg EM, Ungerstedt U, Steen PA. Post-hypoxic hypothermia reduces cerebrocortical release of NO and excitotoxins. Neuroreport 1997; 8:3359–3362.
98. Koinig H, Vornik V, Rueda C, Zornow MH. Lubeluzole inhibits accumulation of extracellular glutamate in the hippocampus during transient global cerebral ischemia. Brain Res 2001; 898:297–302.
99. Monaghan DT, Olverman HJ, Nguyen L, Watkins JC, Cotman CW. Two classes of *N*-methyl-D-aspartate recognition sites: differential distribution and differential regulation by glycine. Proc Natl Acad Sci USA 1988; 85:9836–9840.
100. Kvrivishvili G. Glycine and neuroprotective effect of hypothermia in hypoxic–ischemic brain damage. Neuroreport 2002; 13:1995–2000.
101. Li PA, He QP, Miyashita H, Howllet W, Siesjo BK, Shuaib A. Hypothermia ameliorates ischemic brain damage and suppresses the release of extracellular amino acids in both normo- and hyperglycemic subjects. Exp Neurol 1999; 158:242–253.
102. Globus MY, Busto R, Martinez E, Valdes I, Dietrich WD, Ginsberg MD. Comparative effect of transient global ischemia on extracellular levels of glutamate, glycine, and gamma-aminobutyric acid in vulnerable and nonvulnerable brain regions in the rat. J Neurochem 1991; 57:470–478.

103. Globus MY, Ginsberg MD, Busto R. Excitotoxic index—a biochemical marker of selective vulnerability. Neurosci Lett 1991; 127:39–42.

104. Globus MT, Busto R, Martinez E, Valdes I, Dietrich WD, Ginsberg MD. Early moderate postischemic hypothermia attenuates the rise in excitotoxic index in the hippocampus—a possible mechanism for the beneficial effects of early postischemic moderate cooling. J Cereb Blood Flow Metab 1991; 11:S10.

105. Horiguchi T, Shimizu K, Ogino M, Yamaguchi N, Suga S, Inamasu J, Kawase T. Neuroprotection role of adenosine under hypothermia in the rat global ischemia involves inhibition of not dopamine release but delayed postischemic hypoperfusion. Brain Res 2002; 952:222–231.

106. Lyeth BG, Jiang JY, Robinson SE, Guo H, Jenkins LW. Hypothermia blunts acetylcholine increase in CSF of traumatically brain injured rats. Mol Chem Neuropathol 1993; 18:247–256.

107. Globus MY, Alonso O, Dietrich WD, Busto R, Ginsberg MD. Glutamate release and free radical production following brain injury: effects of posttraumatic hypothermia. J Neurochem 1995; 65:1704–1711.

108. Huang FP, Zhou LF, Yang GY. Effects of mild hypothermia on the release of regional glutamate and glycine during extended transient focal cerebral ischemia in rats. Neurochem Res 1998; 23:991–996.

109. Takagi K, Ginsberg MD, Globus MY, Dietrich WD, Martinez E, Kraydieh S, Busto R. Changes in amino acid neurotransmitters and cerebral blood flow in the ischemic penumbral region following middle cerebral artery occlusion in the rat: correlation with histopathology. J Cereb Blood Flow Metab 1993; 13:575–585.

110. Takagi K, Ginsberg MD, Globus MY, Martinez E, Busto R. Effect of hyperthermia on glutamate release in ischemic penumbra after middle cerebral artery occlusion in rats. Am J Physiol 1994; 267:H1770–H1776.

111. Lo EH, Steinberg GK, Panahian N, Maidment NT, Newcomb R. Profiles of extracellular amino acid changes in focal

cerebral ischaemia: effects of mild hypothermia. Neurol Res 1993; 15:281–287.

112. Baker CJ, Fiore AJ, Frazzini VI, Choudhri TF, Zubay GP, Solomon RA. Intraischemic hypothermia decreases the release of glutamate in the cores of permanent focal cerebral infarcts. Neurosurgery 1995; 36:994–1001.

113. Sakai F, Amaha K. The effects of hypothermia on a cloned human brain glutamate transporter (hGLT-1) expressed in Chinese hamster ovary cells: [^{3}H]L-glutamate uptake study. Anesth Analg 1999; 89:1546–1550.

114. Huang R, Shuaib A, Hertz L. Glutamate uptake and glutamate content in primary cultures of mouse astrocytes during anoxia, substrate deprivation and simulated ischemia under normothermic and hypothermic conditions. Brain Res 1993; 618:346–351.

115. Arai H, Uto A, Ogawa Y, Sato K. Effect of low temperature on glutamate-induced intracellular calcium accumulation and cell death in cultured hippocampal neurons. Neurosci Lett 1993; 163:132–134.

116. Tymianski M, Sattler R, Zabramski JM, Spetzler RF. Characterization of neuroprotection from excitotoxicity by moderate and profound hypothermia in cultured cortical neurons unmasks a temperature-insensitive component of glutamate neurotoxicity. J Cereb Blood Flow Metab 1998; 18:848–867.

117. Newell DW, Barth A, Papermaster V, Malouf AT. Glutamate and non-glutamate receptor mediated toxicity caused by oxygen and glucose deprivation in organotypic hippocampal cultures. J Neurosci 1995; 15:7702–7711.

118. Friedman LK, Ginsberg MD, Belayev L, Busto R, Alonso OF, Lin B, Globus MY. Intraischemic but not postischemic hypothermia prevents non-selective hippocampal downregulation of AMPA and NMDA receptor gene expression after global ischemia. Mol Brain Res 2001; 86:34–47.

119. Colbourne F, Grooms SY, Zukin RS, Buchan AM, Bennett MV. Hypothermia rescues hippocampal CA1 neurons and attenuates down-regulation of the AMPA receptor GluR2 subunit after forebrain ischemia. Proc Natl Acad Sci USA 2003; 100:2906–2910.

120. Beckman JS. Interactions of oxidants, nitric oxide, and antioxidant defenses in cerebral ischemia and injury. In: Ginsberg MD, Bogousslavsky J, eds. Cerebrovascular Disease: Pathophysiology, Diagnosis, and Management. Malden, MA: Blackwell Science, 1998:455–470.

121. Watson BD, Ginsberg MD. Ischemic injury in the brain. Role of oxygen radical-mediated processes. Ann NY Acad Sci 1989; 559:269–281.

122. Globus MY, Busto R, Lin B, Schnippering H, Ginsberg MD. Detection of free radical activity during transient global ischemia and recirculation: effects of intraischemic brain temperature modulation. J Neurochem 1995; 65:1250–1256.

123. Kil HY, Zhang J, Piantadosi CA. Brain temperature alters hydroxyl radical production during cerebral ischemia/reperfusion in rats. J Cereb Blood Flow Metab 1996; 16:100–106.

124. Lei B, Adachi N, Arai T. The effect of hypothermia on H_2O_2 production during ischemia and reperfusion: a microdialysis study in the gerbil hippocampus. Neurosci Lett 1997; 222: 91–94.

125. Guven H, Amanvermez R, Malazgirt Z, Kaya E, Doganay Z, Celik C, Ozkan K. Moderate hypothermia prevents brain stem oxidative stress injury after hemorrhagic shock. J Trauma 2002; 53:66–72.

126. Barone FC, Feuerstein GZ. Inflammatory mediators and stroke: new opportunities for novel therapeutics. J Cereb Blood Flow Metab 1999; 19:819–834.

127. Emsley HC, Tyrrell PJ. Inflammation and infection in clinical stroke. J Cereb Blood Flow Metab 2002; 22:1399–1419.

128. Danton GH, Dietrich WD. Inflammatory mechanisms after ischemia and stroke. J Neuropathol Exp Neurol 2003; 62:127–136.

129. Toyoda T, Suzuki S, Kassell NF, Lee KS. Intraischemic hypothermia attenuates neutrophil infiltration in the rat neocortex after focal ischemia–reperfusion injury. Neurosurgery 1996; 39:1200–1205.

130. Maier CM, Ahern K, Cheng ML, Lee JE, Yenari MA, Steinberg GK. Optimal depth and duration of mild hypo-

thermia in a focal model of transient cerebral ischemia: effects on neurologic outcome, infarct size, apoptosis, and inflammation. Stroke 1998; 29:2171–2180.

131. Kawai N, Okauchi M, Morisaki K, Nagao S. Effects of delayed intraischemic and postischemic hypothermia on a focal model of transient cerebral ischemia in rats. Stroke 2000; 31:1982–1989.

132. Inamasu J, Suga S, Sato S, Horiguchi T, Akaji K, Mayanagi K, Kawase T. Intra-ischemic hypothermia attenuates intercellular adhesion molecule-1 (ICAM-1) and migration of neutrophil. Neurol Res 2001; 23:105–111.

133. Kumar K, Evans AT. Effect of hypothermia on microglial reaction in ischemic brain. Neuroreport 1997; 8:947–950.

134. Si QS, Nakamura Y, Kataoka K. Hypothermic suppression of microglial activation in culture: inhibition of cell proliferation and production of nitric oxide and superoxide. Neuroscience 1997; 81:223–229.

135. Maekawa S, Aibiki M, Si QS, Nakamura Y, Shirakawa Y, Kataoka K. Differential effects of lowering culture temperature on mediator release from lipopolysaccharide-stimulated neonatal rat microglia. Crit Care Med 2002; 30:2700–2704.

136. Wang GJ, Deng HY, Maier CM, Sun GH, Yenari MA. Mild hypothermia reduces ICAM-1 expression, neutrophil infiltration and microglia/monocyte accumulation following experimental stroke. Neuroscience 2002; 114:1081–1090.

137. Sutcliffe IT, Smith HA, Stanimirovic D, Hutchison JS. Effects of moderate hypothermia on IL-1 beta-induced leukocyte rolling and adhesion in pial microcirculation of mice and on proinflammatory gene expression in human cerebral endothelial cells. J Cereb Blood Flow Metab 2001; 21:1310–1319.

138. Goss JR, Styren SD, Miller PD, Kochanek PM, Palmer AM, Marion DW, DeKosky ST. Hypothermia attenuates the normal increase in interleukin 1 beta RNA and nerve growth factor following traumatic brain injury in the rat. J Neurotrauma 1995; 12:159–167.

139. Coimbra C, Drake M, Boris-Moller F, Wieloch T. Long-lasting neuroprotective effect of postischemic hypothermia and treat-

ment with an anti-inflammatory/antipyretic drug. Evidence for chronic encephalopathic processes following ischemia. Stroke 1996; 27:1578–1585.

140. Dietrich WD, Busto R, Bethea JR. Postischemic hypothermia and IL-10 treatment provide long-lasting neuroprotection of CA1 hippocampus following transient global ischemia in rats. Exp Neurol 1999; 158:444–450.

141. Han HS, Karabiyikoglu M, Kelly S, Sobel R, Yenari MA. Mild hypothermia inhibits nuclear factor-kB translocation in experimental stroke. J Cereb Blood Flow Metab 2003; 23:589–598.

142. Han HS, Qiao Y, Karabiyikoglu M, Giffard RG, Yenari MA. Influence of mild hypothermia on inducible nitric oxide synthase expression and reactive nitrogen production in experimental stroke and inflammation. J Neurosci 2002; 22:3921–3928.

143. Churn SB, Taft WC, DeLorenzo RJ. Effects of ischemia on multifunctional calcium/calmodulin-dependent protein kinase type II in the gerbil. Stroke 1990; 21:III112–III116.

144. Uno H, Kobayashi H, Handa Y, Kabuto M, Kubota T. Alterations of calcium/calmodulin-dependent protein kinase II activity in ischaemia-induced neuronal death and neuronal protection against ischaemia in the gerbil hippocampus. Acta Neurochir (Wien) 1999; 141:287–294.

145. Harada K, Maekawa T, Tsuruta R, Kaneko T, Sadamitsu D, Yamashima T, Yoshida KK. Hypothermia inhibits translocation of CaM kinase II and PKC-alpha, beta, gamma isoforms and fodrin proteolysis in rat brain synaptosome during ischemia–reperfusion. J Neurosci Res 2002; 67:664–669.

146. Busto R, Globus MY, Neary JT, Ginsberg MD. Regional alterations of protein kinase C activity following transient cerebral ischemia: effects of intraischemic brain temperature modulation. J Neurochem 1994; 63:1095–1103.

147. Rechsteiner M. Ubiquitin-mediated pathways for intracellular proteolysis. Annu Rev Cell Biol 1987; 3:1–30.

148. Yamashita K, Eguchi Y, Kajiwara K, Ito H. Mild hypothermia ameliorates ubiquitin synthesis and prevents delayed neuronal death in the gerbil hippocampus. Stroke 1991; 22:1574–1581.

149. Rosenberg GA. Ischemic brain edema. Prog Cardiovasc Dis 1999; 42:209–216.

150. Simeone FA, Frazer G, Lawner P. Ischemic brain edema: comparative effects of barbiturates and hypothermia. Stroke 1979; 10:8–12.

151. Karibe H, Zarow GJ, Graham SH, Weinstein PR. Mild intraischemic hypothermia reduces postischemic hyperperfusion, delayed postischemic hypoperfusion, blood–brain barrier disruption, brain edema, and neuronal damage volume after temporary focal cerebral ischemia in rats. J Cereb Blood Flow Metab 1994; 14:620–627.

152. Huang ZG, Xue D, Preston E, Karbalai H, Buchan AM. Biphasic opening of the blood–brain barrier following transient focal ischemia: effects of hypothermia. Can J Neurol Sci 1999; 26:298–304.

153. Schwab S, Schwarz S, Spranger M, Keller E, Bertram M, Hacke W. Moderate hypothermia in the treatment of patients with severe middle cerebral artery infarction. Stroke 1998; 29:2461–2466.

154. Schwab M, Bauer R, Zwiener U. Mild hypothermia prevents the occurrence of cytotoxic brain edema in rats. Acta Neurobiol Exp (Warsz) 1998; 58:29–35.

155. Dietrich WD, Busto R, Halley M, Valdes I. The importance of brain temperature in alterations of the blood–brain barrier following cerebral ischemia. J Neuropathol Exp Neurol 1990; 49:486–497.

156. Kawai N, Nakamura T, Nagao S. Effects of brain hypothermia on brain edema formation after intracerebral hemorrhage in rats. Acta Neurochir Suppl 2002; 81:233–235.

157. Snider BJ, Gottron FJ, Choi DW. Apoptosis and necrosis in cerebrovascular disease. Ann NY Acad Sci 1999; 893:243–253.

158. Mattson MP, Culmsee C, Yu ZF. Apoptotic and antiapoptotic mechanisms in stroke. Cell Tissue Res 2000; 301:173–187.

159. MacManus JP, Buchan AM. Apoptosis after experimental stroke: fact or fashion? J Neurotrauma 2000; 17:899–914.

160. Graham SH, Chen J. Programmed cell death in cerebral ischemia. J Cereb Blood Flow Metab 2001; 21:99–109.

161. Colbourne F, Sutherland GR, Auer RN. Electron microscopic evidence against apoptosis as the mechanism of neuronal death in global ischemia. J Neurosci 1999; 19:4200–4210.

162. Zhang Z, Sobel RA, Cheng D, Steinberg GK, Yenari MA. Mild hypothermia increases Bcl-2 protein expression following global cerebral ischemia. Mol Brain Res 2001; 95:75–85.

163. Niwa M, Hara A, Iwai T, Nakashima M, Yano H, Yoshimi N, Mori H, Uematsu T. Relationship between magnitude of hypothermia during ischemia and preventive effect against post-ischemic DNA fragmentation in the gerbil hippocampus. Brain Res 1998; 794:338–342.

164. Nakamura T, Miyamoto O, Yamagami S, Toyoshima T, Negi T, Itano T, Nagao S. The chronic cell death with DNA fragmentation after post-ischaemic hypothermia in the gerbil hippocampus. Acta Neurochir (Wien) 1999; 141:407–412.

165. Ferrand-Drake M, Wieloch T. The time-course of DNA fragmentation in the choroid plexus and the CA1 region following transient global ischemia in the rat brain. The effect of intra-ischemic hypothermia. Neuroscience 1999; 93:537–549.

166. Inamasu J, Suga S, Sato S, Horiguchi T, Akaji K, Mayanagi K, Kawase T. Postischemic hypothermia attenuates apoptotic cell death in transient focal ischemia in rats. Acta Neurochir Suppl 2000; 76:525–527.

167. Hara A, Niwa M, Iwai T, Yano H, Bunai Y, Uematsu T, Yoshimi N, Mori H. Increase of fragmented DNA transport in apical dendrites of gerbil CA1 pyramidal neurons following transient forebrain ischemia by mild hypothermia. Neurosci Lett 2000; 280:73–77.

168. Phanithi PB, Yoshida Y, Santana A, Su M, Kawamura S, Yasui N. Mild hypothermia mitigates post-ischemic neuronal death following focal cerebral ischemia in rat brain: immunohistochemical study of Fas, caspase-3 and TUNEL. Neuropathology 2000; 20:273–282.

169. Yenari MA, Iwayama S, Cheng D, Sun GH, Fujimura M, Morita-Fujimura Y, Chan PH, Steinberg GK. Mild hypothermia attenuates cytochrome *c* release but does not alter Bcl-2 expression or caspase activation after experimental stroke. J Cereb Blood Flow Metab 2002; 22:29–38.

170. Prakasa BP, Yoshida Y, Su M, Segura M, Kawamura S, Yasui N. Immunohistochemical expression of Bcl-2, Bax and cytochrome *c* following focal cerebral ischemia and effect of hypothermia in rat. Neurosci Lett 2000; 291:196–200.

171. Hu BR, Liu CL, Ouyang Y, Blomgren K, Siesjo BK. Involvement of caspase-3 in cell death after hypoxia–ischemia declines during brain maturation. J Cereb Blood Flow Metab 2000; 20:1294–1300.

172. Edwards AD, Mehmet H. Apoptosis in perinatal hypoxic–ischaemic cerebral damage. Neuropathol Appl Neurobiol 1996; 22:494–498.

173. Adachi M, Sohma O, Tsuneishi S, Takada S, Nakamura H. Combination effect of systemic hypothermia and caspase inhibitor administration against hypoxic–ischemic brain damage in neonatal rats. Pediatr Res 2001; 50:590–595.

174. Fukuda H, Tomimatsu T, Watanabe N, Mu JW, Kohzuki M, Endo M, Fujii E, Kanazaki T, Murata Y. Post-ischemic hypothermia blocks caspase-3 activation in the newborn rat brain after hypoxia–ischemia. Brain Res 2001; 910:187–191.

175. Shaver EG, Welsh FA, Sutton LN, Mora G, Gennarelli LM, Norwood CR. Deep hypothermia diminishes the ischemic induction of heat-shock protein-72 mRNA in piglet brain. Stroke 1995; 26:1273–1277.

176. Kumar K, Wu X, Evans AT, Marcoux F. The effect of hypothermia on induction of heat shock protein (HSP)-72 in ischemic brain. Metab Brain Dis 1995; 10:283–291.

177. Kamme F, Campbell K, Wieloch T. Biphasic expression of the fos and jun families of transcription factors following transient forebrain ischaemia in the rat. Effect of hypothermia. Eur J Neurosci 1995; 7:2007–2016.

178. Yoneda Y, Azuma Y, Inoue K, Ogita K, Mitani A, Zhang L, Masuda S, Higashihara M, Kataoka K. Positive correlation between prolonged potentiation of binding of double-stranded oligonucleotide probe for the transcription factor AP1 and resistance to transient forebrain ischemia in gerbil hippocampus. Neuroscience 1997; 79:1023–1037.

179. Boris-Moller F, Kamme F, Wieloch T. The effect of hypo-

thermia on the expression of neurotrophin mRNA in the hippocampus following transient cerebral ischemia in the rat. Mol Brain Res 1998; 63:163–173.

180. Tomasevic G, Kamme F, Wieloch T. Changes in proliferating cell nuclear antigen, a protein involved in DNA repair, in vulnerable hippocampal neurons following global cerebral ischemia. Mol Brain Res 1998; 60:168–176.

181. Aoki M, Tamatani M, Taniguchi M, Yamaguchi A, Bando Y, Kasai K, Miyoshi Y, Nakamura Y, Vitek MP, Tohyama M, Tanaka H, Sugimoto H. Hypothermic treatment restores glucose-regulated protein 78 (GRP78) expression in ischemic brain. Mol Brain Res 2001; 95:117–128.

182. Clifton GL, Miller ER, Choi SC, Levin HS, McCauley S, Smith KR Jr, Muizelaar JP, Wagner FC Jr, Marion DW, Luerssen TG, Chesnut RM, Schwartz M. Lack of effect of induction of hypothermia after acute brain injury. N Engl J Med 2001; 344:556–563.

183. Ginsberg MD. Therapeutic trials for traumatic brain injury—a journey in progress. Crit Care Med 2002; 30:935–936.

184. Hypothermia after Cardiac Arrest Group. Mild therapeutic hypothermia to improve the neurologic outcome after cardiac arrest. N Engl J Med 2002; 346:549–556.

185. Bernard SA, Gray TW, Buist MD, Jones BM, Silvester W, Gutteridge G, Smith K. Treatment of comatose survivors of out-of-hospital cardiac arrest with induced hypothermia. N Engl J Med 2002; 346:557–563.

186. Volpe JJ. Perinatal brain injury: from pathogenesis to neuroprotection. Ment Retard Dev Disabil Res Rev 2001; 7:56–64.

187. Tooley JR, Satas S, Porter H, Silver IA, Thoresen M. Head cooling with mild systemic hypothermia in anesthetized piglets is neuroprotective. Ann Neurol 2003; 53:65–72.

188. Inderbitzen B, Yon S, Lasheras J, Dobak J, Perl J, Steinberg GK. Safety and performance of a novel intravascular catheter for induction and reversal of hypothermia in a porcine model. Neurosurgery 2002; 50:364–370.

189. Shuaib A, Ijaz S, Mazagri R, Senthilsevlvan A. CGS-19755 is neuroprotective during repetitive ischemia: this effect is

significantly enhanced when combined with hypothermia. Neuroscience 1993; 56:915–920.

190. Green EJ, Pazos AJ, Dietrich WD, McCabe PM, Schneiderman N, Lin B, Busto R, Globus MY, Ginsberg MD. Combined postischemic hypothermia and delayed MK-801 treatment attenuates neurobehavioral deficits associated with transient global ischemia in rats. Brain Res 1995; 702:145–152.

191. Dietrich WD, Lin B, Globus MY, Green EJ, Ginsberg MD, Busto R. Effect of delayed MK-801 (dizocilpine) treatment with or without immediate postischemic hypothermia on chronic neuronal survival after global forebrain ischemia in rats. J Cereb Blood Flow Metab 1995; 15:960–968.

192. Pazos AJ, Green EJ, Busto R, McCabe PM, Baena RC, Ginsberg MD, Globus MY, Schneiderman N, Dietrich WD. Effects of combined postischemic hypothermia and delayed *N-tert*-butyl-alpha-phenylnitrone (PBN) administration on histopathological and behavioral deficits associated with transient global ischemia in rats. Brain Res 1999; 846:186–195.

193. National Institute of Neurological Disorders and Stroke rt-PA Stroke Study Group. Tissue plasminogen activator for acute ischemic stroke. N Engl J Med 1995; 333:1581–1587.

194. Ginsberg MD, Busto R. Combating hyperthermia in acute stroke: a significant clinical concern. Stroke 1998; 29:529–534.

195. Corbett D, Thornhill J. Temperature modulation (hypothermic and hyperthermic conditions) and its influence on histological and behavioral outcomes following cerebral ischemia. Brain Pathol 2000; 10:145–152.

196. Azzimondi G, Bassein L, Nonino F, Fiorani L, Vignatelli L, Re G, D'Allesandro R. Fever in acute stroke worsens prognosis. A prospective study. Stroke 1995; 26:2040–2043.

197. Reith J, Jorgensen HS, Pedersen PM, Nakayama H, Raaschou HO, Jeppesen LL, Olsen TS. Body temperature in acute stroke: relation to stroke severity, infarct size, mortality, and outcome. Lancet 1996; 347:422–425.

198. Castillo J, Davalos A, Marrugat J, Noya M. Timing for fever-related brain damage in acute ischemic stroke. Stroke 1998; 29:2455–2460.

199. Castillo J, Davalos A, Noya M. Aggravation of acute ischemic stroke by hyperthermia is related to an excitotoxic mechanism. Cerebrovasc Dis 1999; 9:22–27.

200. Grau AJ, Buggle F, Schnitzler P, Spiel M, Lichy C, Hacke W. Fever and infection early after ischemic stroke. J Neurol Sci 1999; 171:115–120.

201. Kammersgaard LP, Jorgensen HS, Rungby JA, Reith J, Nakayama H, Weber UJ, Houth J, Olsen TS. Admission body temperature predicts long-term mortality after acute stroke: the Copenhagen Stroke Study. Stroke 2002; 33:1759–1762.

202. Hajat C, Hajat S, Sharma P. Effects of poststroke pyrexia on stroke outcome: a meta-analysis of studies in patients. Stroke 2000; 31:410–414.

203. Koennecke HC, Leistner S. Prophylactic antipyretic treatment with acetaminophen in acute ischemic stroke: a pilot study. Neurology 2001; 57:2301–2303.

204. Dippel DW, van Breda EJ, van Gemert HM, van der Worp HB, Meijer RJ, Kappelle LJ, Koudstaal PJ. Effect of paracetamol (acetaminophen) on body temperature in acute ischemic stroke: a double-blind, randomized phase II clinical trial. Stroke 2001; 32:1607–1612.

205. Kasner SE, Wein T, Piriyawat P, Villar-Cordova CE, Chalela JA, Krieger DW, Morgenstern LB, Kimmel SE, Grotta JC. Acetaminophen for altering body temperature in acute stroke: a randomized clinical trial. Stroke 2002; 33:130–134.

206. Marion DW. Therapeutic moderate hypothermia and fever. Curr Pharm Des 2001; 7:1533–1536.

5

Effects of Hypothermia on Cerebral Metabolism, Blood Flow, and Autoregulation

MIDORI A. YENARI, CHRISTINE A. C. WIJMAN, and GARY K. STEINBERG

Department of Neurosurgery, Stanford University School of Medicine, Stanford, California, U.S.A.

Department of Neurology and Neurological Sciences, Stanford University School of Medicine, Stanford, California, U.S.A.

Stanford Stroke Center, Stanford University School of Medicine, Stanford, California, U.S.A.

INTRODUCTION

Deep hypothermia, achieved by lowering body temperature to the range of 20–25 °C, has been used for decades to improve the outcome from high-risk surgical procedures. At the laboratory level, hypothermia is one of the most robust neuroprotectants studied to date. Experimentally, decreases in body and brain temperature have consistently produced marked reductions in brain injury and improvement in a variety of behavioral parameters. Unfortunately, the benefits of hypothermia can be offset by undesirable side effects such as cardiac arrhythmias, shivering, coagulopathies, and reduced resistance to infection (see Chapter 6)—all of which become more serious as the depth of cooling increases.

In recent years, though, there has been increasing recognition that even small reductions in temperature are neuroprotective (1–3), leading several investigators to speculate that mild (33–36°C) to moderate (29–32°C) hypothermia may be a reasonable approach to treating a broad range of patients suffering from stroke, brain trauma, or cardiac arrest. Although it remains unclear whether mild hypothermia is beneficial in patients suffering brain trauma (4), two small randomized studies in patients suffering from cerebral ischemic injury secondary to cardiac arrest suggest that mild hypothermia improves neurological outcome (5,6).

As a result of these recent studies, there has been a remarkable resurgence of interest in this phenomenon both at the laboratory level and clinical level. Although clinical trials are in progress to determine whether hypothermia is beneficial to stroke, neonatal hypoxia, and other brain disorders, the mechanisms by which brain cooling protects tissues against ischemic injury continue to be the subject of laboratory investigations (see Chapter 4).

Although hypothermia likely interferes with a variety of damaging processes leading to ischemic brain death, it is well-known that lower temperatures reduce metabolic rate. In fact, work by several investigators indicates that hypothermia does indeed decrease metabolism and, as a consequence, modulates cerebral blood flow (CBF), although not always consistently under injury conditions. Furthermore, the effect of temperature on brain metabolism and blood flow correlates poorly with the remarkable extent of neuroprotection (7). This review focuses on the influence of temperature on cerebral metabolism and blood flow both at the laboratory and clinical levels.

REVIEW

Cerebral Metabolism

Influence of Temperature on Cerebral Metabolism in Uninjured States

A traditional view has been that hypothermia's protective effect can be attributed to a reduction of metabolic rate. The primary source of energy in the brain is glucose. To generate sufficient energy to maintain normal cerebral metabolism, the central nervous system relies on glycolysis to generate adenosine triphosphate (ATP) (8). To meet its relatively high energy demand requiring glucose and oxygen, the brain uses approximately one-fifth of all cardiac output. Normal glucose consumption is approximately 70–150 μmol/100 g/min within the grey matter and approximately 20–50 μmol/100 g/min within the white matter (9).

Experimental Studies

Cerebral metabolism, reflected in estimates of oxygen consumption, glucose utilization, and lactate concentration, is temperature-dependent, and hypothermia has been associated with decreases in each of these parameters. Hypothermia decreases the cerebral metabolic rate of glucose (CMR_{glu}) and the cerebral metabolic rate of oxygen ($CMRO_2$), and slows ATP breakdown (reviewed in Ref. 10). On average, hypothermia reduces brain oxygen consumption by approximately 5–6% per degree Celsius decrease in body temperature in the range from 22°C to 37°C (11); in anesthesized animals, $CMRO_2$ decreases linearly between 8°C and 37°C (12,13). The Q_{10} or the ratio of metabolism at 10°C intervals, for $CMRO_2$, has been estimated at 2.5 (12,13). Q_{10} is remarkably consistent between various laboratory reports, appears to be independent of age and species, and is not influenced by alpha-stat management (10,14). However, one earlier report indicated that the relative reduction in Q_{10} for temperatures less than 27°C is approximately 4 (13), although the reasons for this discrepancy are unclear. Consistent with the observations that oxygen utilization decreases as temperature is reduced, cerebral oxygen extraction, or the cerebral arteriovenous oxygen difference (typically estimated by differences in oxygen concentration in blood sampled from the carotid artery and sagittal sinus), is also temperature-dependent and decreases by approximately 50% at 28°C compared to normothermia (15).

Cerebral glucose metabolism, like $CMRO_2$, is temperature-sensitive. Perhaps unsurprisingly, the decrease in CMR_{glu} is similar to the decrease in $CMRO_2$, and the Q_{10} is nearly identical (16,17). Using autoradiography and 2-deoxyglucose (2-DG) as a tracer, regional glucose utilization can be estimated as a function of temperature. In anesthesized animals, hypothermia decreased glucose utilization, with the reductions being somewhat greater in grey matter (4.8%) than in white matter (3.5%) (14,18,19). Anesthesia itself can confound estimates of metabolism by decreasing CMR_{glu} (14,18); it is thus comforting that the cerebral metabolic rate for glucose was similar in awake, uninjured, lightly restrained rats at normothermia and body temperatures of 32°C (mild hypothermia) and 39°C (hyperthermia) (9). In the majority of brain regions analyzed, glucose utilization decreased with temperature, with a 6.5% and 9.8% change per degree Celsius in grey and white matter, respectively. Interestingly, glucose utilization changed the least within the anterior hypothalamus and the most within the posterior hypothalamus, both being brain regions critical to normal control of body temperature.

Studies have also shown that hypothermia decreases the generation of intermediates of glycolytic pathways, consistent with the notion that hypothermia preserves brain glucose metabolism (10,20). Using magnetic resonance spectroscopy (MRS), Kaibara et al. (20) showed that moderate hypothermia (31°C) reduced several metabolites of the tricarboxylic acid pathway by ~30–40% and may have actually increased metabolism through the pentose phosphate pathway (PPP). The authors proposed that shunting of glucose metabolism to the

PPP leads to increases in nicotinamide adenine dinucleotide phosphate (NADPH), which is involved in potentially protective functions such as peroxide detoxification and maintenance of membrane potentials.

Hypothermia leads to preservation of high-energy phosphate compounds as well. Early studies suggested that hypothermia reduced the hydrolysis of ATP, as estimated by the ratio of phosphocreatine (PCr) to creatine (Cr) (21); this finding has been replicated more recently using phosphorus-31 MRS (22,23). In a study by Laptook et al. (23), brain temperature was inversely correlated with PCr. Measurements of brain utilization rates of PCr, nucleoside triphosphate, and lactate to estimate ATP hydrolysis showed a 5.3% decline per degree Celsius.

Tissue pH is inversely related to temperature. Although this has been demonstrated by several laboratories (10,22,23), the precise reasons are not entirely clear. Under noninjury conditions, this may be related to inhibiting the generation of hydrogen ions through ATP hydrolysis (10).

Clinical Studies

Data are relatively sparse in humans, and most data in humans evaluating the effects of hypothermia on cerebral metabolism are derived from measurements of $CMRO_2$ during cardiopulmonary bypass. Total body hypothermia in anesthesized and paralyzed patients typically reduces $CMRO_2$, on average, between twofold to fourfold, with a 10°C reduction in temperature between 37°C and 27°C (10,24–28). Acid–base strategy (see "Influence of Temperature on Cerebral Metabolism Under Injury Conditions") does not seem to affect the hypothermic decrease in $CMRO_2$ (25,28), although shivering appears to increase it, which emphasizes the need to control shivering in such settings (24). There are some reports of metabolic changes documented in humans undergoing surgical procedures who receive intraoperative hypothermia. In one report of a patient who underwent clipping of a large carotid artery aneurysm, tissue acidosis developed more slowly and recovered more rapidly with a brain temperature at 18°C than at 35°C (29).

Influence of Temperature on Cerebral Metabolism Under Injury Conditions

Experimental Studies

Hypoxia and ischemia cause decreases in brain oxygenation and glucose concentration. With cessation of blood flow (ischemia) or critical reductions in oxygen partial pressure (hypoxia), a series of events occurs, ultimately leading to cell death. High-energy organic phosphates are quickly depleted, with substantial decreases in PCr and ATP within a minute or two of ischemia onset (8). In an attempt to maintain ATP concentration, glycolysis increases, but proceeds from aerobic to anaerobic pathways, leading to further ATP decreases and accumulation of lactic acid and tissue acidosis. Although most of these processes are potentially reversible provided energy sources are replaced in time, persistent deprivation of energy stores leads to irreversible injury, ultimately culminating in cell death. Hypothermia slows many of these processes, allowing the brain to withstand longer periods of hypoxia and ischemia, and putting it in a state of so-called "suspended animation" until blood flow can be restored. This concept was demonstrated in a paper by Sutton et al. (30), who showed that the time to total ATP depletion in piglets exposed to cardiac arrest was much slower at a brain temperature of 15°C compared to 37°C, even though the entire ATP pool was eventually depleted in both cases. In a hippocampal slice model, in which tissue slices maintained in artificial cerebrospinal fluid are exposed to hypoxia, hypothermia attenuated depletion of ATP whereas hyperthermia accelerated its loss (31). Under conditions of hypoxia–ischemia, several studies have now shown that hypothermia slows the rates of metabolite consumption and lactic acid accumulation, and reduces $CMRO_2$ (10,31–33). It must be remembered, however, that reduction of metabolic demand is only one of many mechanisms by which hypothermia confers neuroprotection in ischemia (see Chapter 4).

Hypothermia also improves glucose utilization following ischemia. Following 20 min of forebrain ischemia, CMR_{glu} was measured 2 hr later using autoradiography (2). Animals cooled to 30°C had significantly lower CMR_{glu} rates (3.3 mg/100 g/min) than animals maintained at 36°C (4.8 mg/100 g/min). Using autoradiography, Tohyama et al. (34) measured local glucose utilization in rats subjected to focal cerebral ischemia. Although ischemia suppressed glycolysis in the ischemic core regardless of brain temperature, glycolysis was increased within regions that extended to the infarct periphery. Interestingly, in rats cooled to 30°C, such increases were not observed, suggesting that moderate hypothermia mainly influences glucose metabolism in the lesion periphery or "penumbra."

By using noninvasive methods to estimate energy stores in the brain, it is possible to examine the time course of metabolite depletion and recovery within the same experimental subject. A few groups have now utilized phosphorus-32 MRS in various ischemia models. In gerbils subjected to global cerebral ischemia, mild hypothermia (34°C applied for 1 hr preinsult and 3 hr postinsult) did not alter amounts of high-energy phosphates during the ischemic period (35). However, during reperfusion, mild hypothermia was associated with faster and better ATP and PCr recovery for up to 7 days (Fig. 1). Furthermore, mild hypothermia attenuated a secondary ATP decline observed among normothermic animals at 1–7 days. Similar findings were reported earlier by Chopp et al. (33) using a feline global cerebral ischemia model. In this latter study, hypothermia to temperatures of 27°C, 32°C, and 35°C also improved metabolite recovery only during reperfusion. One might conclude from these findings that hypothermia need only be applied during the reperfusion phase. However, Dietrich et al. (36) showed that while cooling applied during both the ischemic period and shortly into the reperfusion period produces long-lasting neuroprotection, neuroprotection from cooling initiated only during reperfusion is transient. Furthermore, the extent of metabolite recovery (10–20%) was not proportional to the extent of neuroprotection (35–45%) by cooling. Therefore, the mechanism of hypothermic protection probably involves factors other than hypothermia's influence on brain metabolism.

Measurement of metabolites in young animals suggests a correlation between hypothermia and preservation of meta-

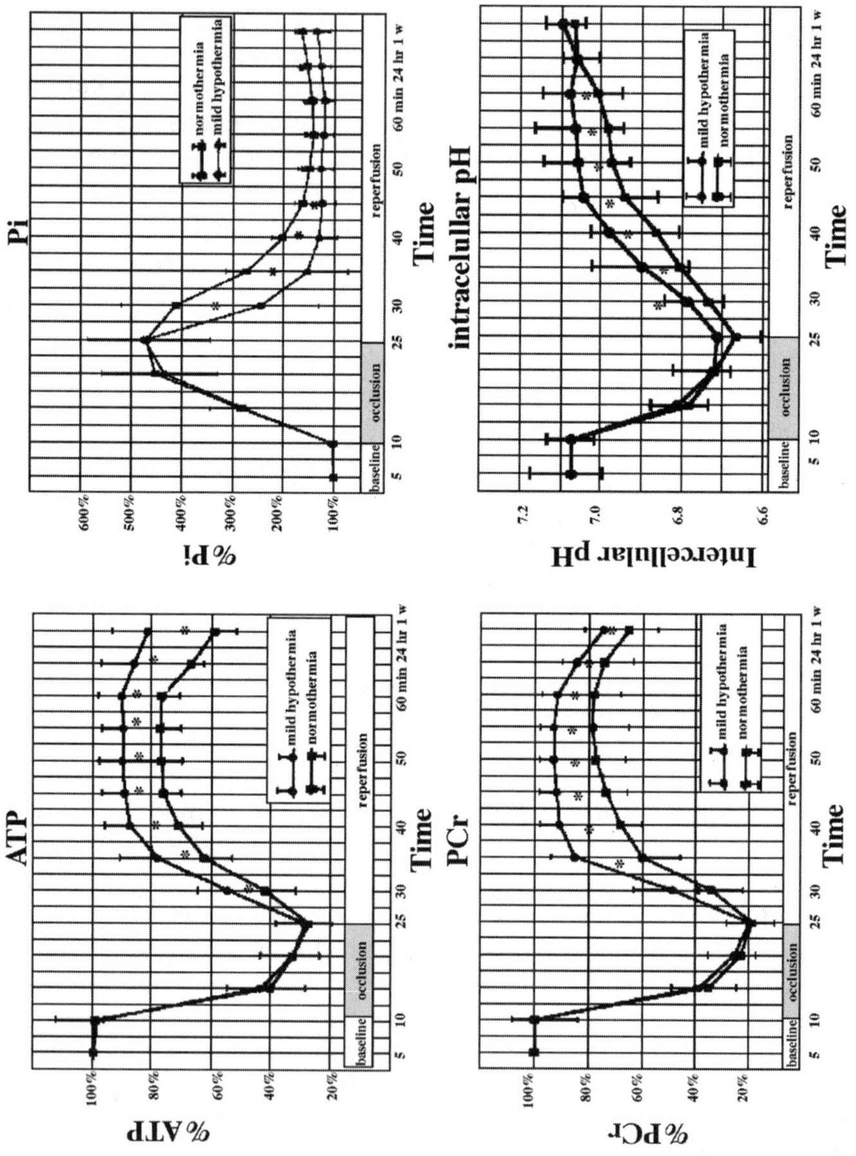
ATP
%ATP
100%
80%
60%
40%
20%
mild hypothermia
normothermia
baseline
occlusion
reperfusion
5 10 25 30 40 50 60 min 24 hr 1 w
Time
Pi
%Pi
600%
500%
400%
300%
200%
100%
normothermia
mild hypothermia
PCr
%PCr
intracelullar pH
Intercellular pH
7.2
7.0
6.8
6.6

bolic stores. Piglets subjected to circulatory arrest in a model that depletes ATP stores had slower loss and better recovery of brain energy metabolites when cooled to 15°C, compared to normothermia. For example, ATP and PCr, measured both with MRS and biochemically, were better preserved at 15°C than at normothermia (30). Seven-day-old rats subjected to hypoxia plus unilateral carotid artery occlusion showed less ischemic damage and no loss of tissue ATP when cooled to 29°C or 21°C compared to normothermic rats (37).

Whether hypothermia influences tissue lactate levels is unclear. Although most studies indicate that hypothermia decreases lactate levels after ischemia (15,38), a few studies have found that hypothermia did not significantly alter brain lactate levels (39,40). The discrepancies may depend on the time lactate levels were measured. In a model of global cerebral ischemia, lactate levels did not differ by temperature during the ischemic period; but in rats cooled to 30°C, hypothermia eventually did reduce levels 30 min into recirculation, suggesting that this may, in part, explain its protective effects (Fig. 2) (41). However, hyperthermia to temperatures of 39°C, which is known to exacerbate ischemic damage (42), did not appear to influence lactate levels (41). Because lactate accumulation is thought to contribute to tissue acidosis under ischemic conditions, the observation that hypothermia reduces lactate accumulation may, in part, explain why hypothermia also increases tissue pH in this setting (33).

Whether the mechanism of protection by mild hypothermia against cerebral ischemic insults is necessarily the preservation of metabolic stores is far from clear. Barbiturates

---

Figure 1 Mild hypothermia (34°C) preserves high-energy metabolites and intracellular pH during reperfusion, but not during ischemia. Changes in energy metabolites and intracellular pH as assessed by MRS prior to, during, and 7 days after 15 min of forebrain ischemia followed by 1 week of reperfusion in gerbils. Animals were maintained at body temperatures of 37°C (normothermia) or 34°C (mild hypothermia) from 1 hr before and 3 hr after ischemia onset. ($^*P < 0.05$) (ATP, adenosine triphosphate; Pi, inorganic phosphate; PCr, phosphocreatine). (From Ref. 35.)

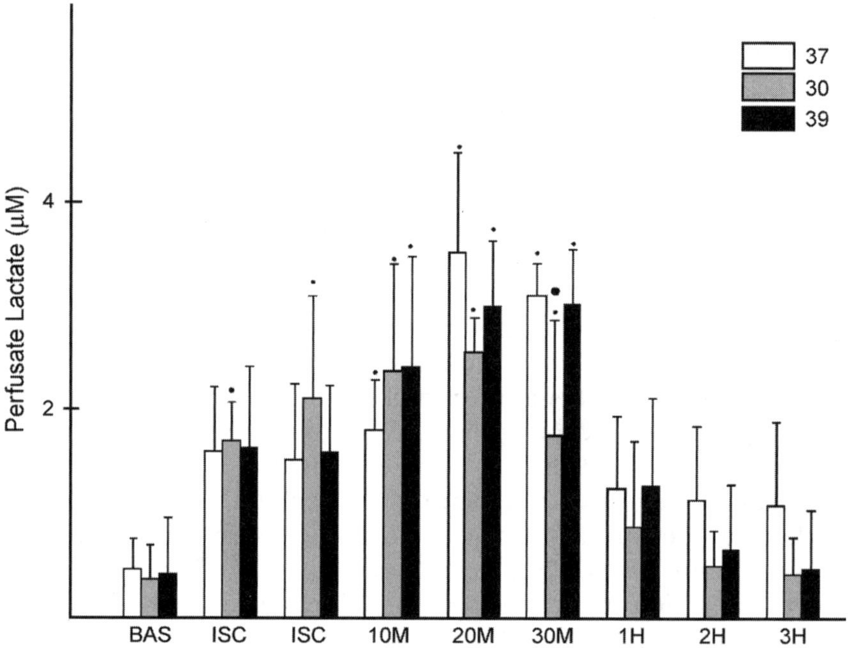

Figure 2 Influence of temperature on brain lactate levels after global cerebral ischemia. Lactate levels were measured in microdialysis perfusate from brains of rats subjected to 20 min of global cerebral ischemia. Intraischemic brain temperature was held at either 37°C, 30°C, or 39°C. Hypothermia decreased lactate levels 30 min into recirculation, whereas hyperthermia did not alter levels at all. (small circle: significant increases in lactate above corresponding control level; large circle: significantly lower lactate level in the hypothermic group compared with the other temperature groups; BAS: baseline.) (From Ref. 41.)

suppress cerebral metabolism to a similar or even greater degree than hypothermia (43), yet there is little conclusive evidence that barbiturates are truly neuroprotective (44). Hypothermia is also known to reduce the extent of focal cerebral ischemic injury in some models of permanent cerebral artery disruption (45–47). These observations (that hypothermia protects even in settings where ATP is depleted) suggest that lower temperatures may exert a protective effect by interfering with other pathological processes.

Several other studies suggest that metabolism is not significantly altered in the face of remarkable neuroprotection. In studies by Busto et al. (40,48), rodents were subjected to 20 min of forebrain ischemia, and brain levels of ATP, lactate, PCr, and glucose were measured. Although remarkable neuroprotection was observed with brain temperatures of 30–33°C, they found no difference in the levels of these various metabolites from the normothermic (36°C brain temperature) controls. They therefore concluded that the cytoprotective effect of hypothermia in this model was independent of the metabolic state of the brain. In another study of gerbils subjected to forebrain ischemia, cooling to 32.5°C initially prevented ATP depletion throughout the hippocampus, but did not do so at later time points despite improved neuronal survival (32). In a model of traumatic brain injury, similar patterns emerged. Rodents were subjected to fluid percussion injury, and CMR_{glu} was measured at the end of a 3-hr period of mild hypothermia (brain temperature of 30°C) using autoradiography and a computer-assisted mapping program. This study showed that CMR_{glu} was largely unaffected by temperature manipulation in either the injury or control groups. However, the ratio of CMR_{glu} to CBF was nearly doubled in the hypothermic group, indicating that mild hypothermia induced a moderate decline in cerebral perfusion but did not improve cerebral glucose utilization (49).

Clinical Studies

The effect of hypothermia on cerebral metabolism in humans under cerebral injury states is similar to that reported in laboratory studies. The clinical condition in which changes in cerebral metabolism due to hypothermia are most widely studied is severe traumatic brain injury. Most studies report a substantial decrease in $CMRO_2$ during mild-to-moderate (32–34°C) hypothermia compared to normothermia, albeit to varying degrees (50–52). In one study of 10 patients suffering from severe closed-head injury, therapeutic hypothermia (32–33°C) was instituted with a median delay between injury and induction time of 16 hr. Cooling initially decreased $CMRO_2$ by about 45% and further decreased it to 27% after 24 hr (51). In the same study, six patients had elevated lactate levels prior to cooling; the levels were normalized by hypothermia in all patients.

Energy Balance and Ion Fluxes

Although cerebral metabolism in both injured and non-injured brains is affected by temperature changes, its pattern is not consistently correlated with the temporal patterns of neuroprotection. Therefore, it is possible that hypothermia may have significant influences on other cellular processes that are highly energy-dependent. Many ion pumps throughout the brain are dependent on ATP to maintain highly regulated gradients. With ischemia and ATP loss, many ions will flow down their concentration gradients, leading to a variety of damaging processes such as depolarization, cellular swelling, efflux of potassium, and influx of sodium and calcium. It is well-known that sodium influxes can lead to cytotoxic edema and calcium influxes lead to direct toxicity as well as extracellular accumulation of glutamate, which in itself is damaging. In a study of cardiac arrest in rats, hypothermia to 34°C attenuated the initial rise of extracellular potassium (K_e) and delayed terminal depolarization (53). These changes were not proportionate to decreases in ATP levels, although the time courses of both events were similar (i.e., the rapid potassium efflux occurred when ATP levels dropped). This, in turn, suggests the temperature dependence of calcium influx as a consequence of potassium efflux, and raises the link between hypothermia and suppression of intracellular calcium accumulation and associated cell death pathways. Hypothermia also delayed a secondary K_e elevation during reperfusion in a model of focal cerebral ischemia (54). In a hippocampal slice model, exposure to hypoxia leads to total tissue increases in sodium and decreases in potassium. However, hypothermia to 34°C attenuated tissue sodium increases and accelerated potassium decreases, whereas hyperthermia (40°C) did the opposite (31). Although it was not clear whether the measured sodium or potassium levels reflected intracellular or extracellular concentrations, they likely reflect the movement of these ions down their concentration gradients due to loss of sodium–potassium pump function, which is highly ATP-dependent.

A clinically relevant method of estimating fluid shifts is diffusion-weighted magnetic resonance imaging (DWI). This takes advantages of micromolecular changes in fluid movement to delineate regions of ischemia and is based on the notion that cytotoxic edema effectively reduces overall tissue water diffusion (reviewed in Ref. 55). During ischemia, increases in apparent diffusion coefficient (ADC) (and increased signal intensity on DWI) are thought to reflect increased intracellular fluid, which parallels increases in intracellular sodium. A few studies have shown that ADC changes with temperature (56–58). Based on the known physical properties of water, this would predict a 2.4% change in ADC per degree Celsius (59). In fact, in nonischemic brain, ADC changes by $0.013–0.016 \times 10^{-5}$ cm^2/sec (or ca. 1.5%) per degree Celsius change in temperature (56,58). These temperature-dependent differences are relatively small compared to the extent of ADC changes seen with ischemia (>25%), but even with corrections for temperature, two groups have shown that ADC returns to control values earlier in animals exposed to mild hypothermia than in normothermic animals in models of experimental stroke (57,58). This would be consistent with the idea that hypothermia restores ion pump function; thus cytotoxic edema is reversed more effectively than under normothermic conditions.

It is unlikely, however, that hypothermia's influence on cerebral metabolism fully explains its protective effect. Cerebral metabolic rate should be reduced by $\approx$20–25% at a brain temperature of 33°C (60), but the extent of protection as documented by several laboratories (on the order of 50–80%) greatly exceeds this. Therefore, it is likely that hypothermia influences other factors such as excitatory amino acid accumulation, oxidative stress, inflammation, and apoptosis in such a way as to lead to neuroprotection.

Cerebral Blood Flow

Influence of Temperature on Cerebral Blood Flow in Uninjured States

Cerebral blood flow is normally in the range of 55 mL/100 g/min. As CBF decreases, cerebral function and viability also decrease in a graded fashion. With decreases below 40% of normal ($\approx$20 mL/100 g/min), oxygen delivery becomes sufficiently compromised, resulting in loss of synaptic firing. With reductions below 10 mL/100 g/min, ATP-dependent membrane pumps fail and ions flow down their concentration gradients, leading to collapse of membrane potentials. Cooling the brain can also lead to decreases in CBF (19). In juvenile pigs cooled to 8°C on cardiopulmonary bypass, CBF decreased linearly between temperatures of 18°C and 37°C (12). CBF reduction at 18°C was 62% of normal, but did not decrease further at temperatures below this level. Cerebral vascular resistance increased as body temperature decreased to 18°C, but then decreased further at 8°C, suggesting a loss of autoregulation.

In uninjured brain, coupling between CBF and brain metabolism appears, for the most part, preserved at different temperatures (11,19,61). Oxygen consumption decreases with temperature—a 40–50% drop at 28°C compared to normothermia—with nearly parallel decreases in CBF. However, several reports suggest that such coupling is not always maintained below ≈28–33°C. Mori et al. (62) measured CBF, arteriovenous oxygen differences, and cerebral venous oxygen saturation to calculate $CMRO_2$ in anesthesized cats. Hypothermia proportionately decreased CBF from 48 mL/100 g/min in normothermic animals to 21 and 11 mL/100 g/min at 33°C and 29°C, respectively. Cooling to 33°C led to a proportionate decrease in CBF and $CMRO_2$, indicating that hypothermia maintained coupling between blood flow and metabolism. However, at 29°C, CBF decreased more than $CMRO_2$, leading to a lower CBF/$CMRO_2$ ratio, consistent with a state of relative ischemia. Ehrlich et al. (12) also found that coupling of blood flow and metabolism (ratio of CBF/$CMRO_2$) was preserved at 28°C, but was slightly increased at 18°C and variable at 8°C, suggesting a loss of autoregulation below 28°C and possibly a state of luxury perfusion where CBF exceeds oxygen consumption.

Because of these observations, it is reasonable to assume that therapeutic hypothermia in the range of 33–35°C may be optimal to maintain normal coupling. Between 28°C and 33°C, coupling is inconsistently observed, whereas below 28°C, the majority of studies indicate that coupling is disrupted, with larger decreases in metabolism than in CBF (10,11,19,22).

However, one study in newborn piglets found the opposite result, where CBF decreased to a greater extent than $CMRO_2$ and CMR_{glu} at temperatures below 35°C (63). The reasons for this disparity are not obvious. These differences cannot merely be ascribed to differences in adult vs. developing brain because studies in other newborn animals showed patterns like those of older animals (19).

Influence of Temperature on Cerebral Blood Flow Under Injury Conditions

Experimental Studies

During various injury paradigms, CBF is altered in different ways depending on the time after the insult and the nature of the insult. Focal and global ischemias initially decrease CBF, but hyperemia is often observed upon reperfusion (64). This hyperemia is typically followed by gradual decreases in CBF during the reperfusion phase. Data regarding the influence of hypothermia on CBF are conflicting. Under noninjury conditions (as described earlier), CBF clearly decreases with temperature. However, reports examining CBF during ischemia vary. Some studies indicate that hypothermia actually increases CBF during the period of ischemia (2,65), whereas other reports note reduced CBF (66) or no effect (34,57,58,67). Mild hypothermia to 33°C also appears to blunt the early postreperfusion hyperemia and to prevent the gradual decrease in CBF during reperfusion (Fig. 3) (67). Similar patterns have been documented in experimental head injury models (62), although reports involving other experimental models indicate that hypothermia does not significantly influence CBF (68).

Like DWI, other noninvasive methods are available to estimate cerebral perfusion or blood flow, and these could potentially be applied in clinical trials of hypothermia. Using a spin-tagging perfusion-weighted magnetic resonance imaging (PWI), Jiang et al. (57) showed that hypothermia to 30°C decreased CBF by 46% in nonischemic animals. In ischemic animals, CBF decreased during the ischemic period, but hypothermia did not affect this. Hypothermia did improve CBF

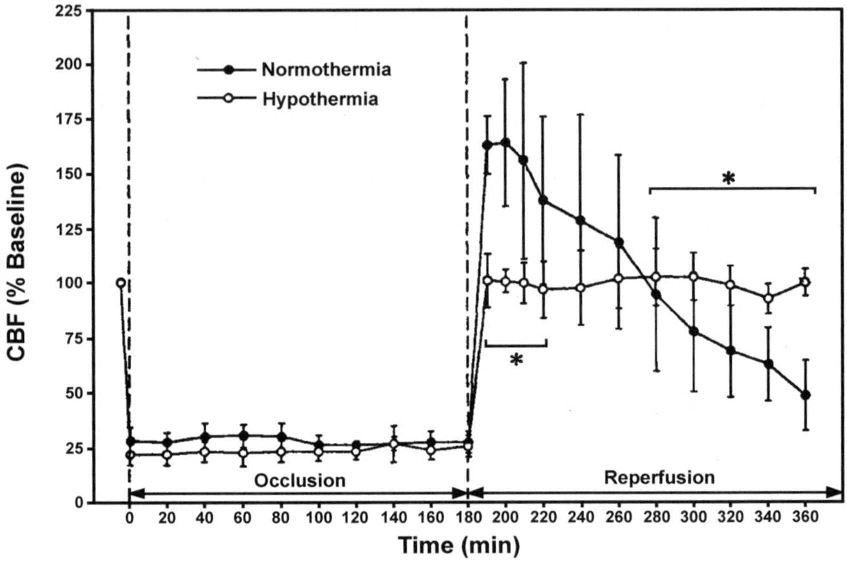

Figure 3 Influence of mild hypothermia on CBF following focal cerebral ischemia. Rats were subjected to middle cerebral artery occlusion for 3 hr followed by 3 hr of reperfusion. Brain temperature was maintained at 37°C (normothermia) or reduced to 32–33°C within 10 min of occlusion and maintained during the ischemic period (hypothermia). CBF, as measured by laser Doppler flowmetry, did not differ by hypothermia during occlusion. However, upon reperfusion, CBF increased, then gradually deteriorated in normothermic animals. In contrast, hypothermia blunted the initial reperfusion hyperemia and maintained CBF at preocclusion levels. (*$P < 0.01$). (From Ref. 67.)

recovery during reperfusion. Using a bolus contrast-tracking PWI method to measure cerebral perfusion, our laboratory showed that hypothermia, in spite of marked lesion reduction, did not alter the area of perfusion deficit either before, during, or after focal cerebral ischemia (58). The reasons for these differences are not entirely clear, but may be due to experimental variables, such as the type of anesthesia used, and inherent difficulties in detecting very small differences using PWI in small rodent brains.

Because selective brain cooling (rather than whole body cooling) may be a desirable clinical approach to applying therapeutic hypothermia (see Chapter 11), it is worth understanding how CBF and metabolism are affected by selected cooling. Under noninjury conditions, nitrous oxide-anesthesized rats cooled to a brain temperature of 30°C with body temperature maintained at 37°C showed a doubling of cortical blood flow as estimated by laser Doppler flowmetry compared to 37°C (69). This unlikely result contrasts with other studies in which whole body cooling was applied and CBF was reduced. The authors suggested that the reason for their observations may be a relative lack of vasoconstriction in the cerebrovascular bed relative to increased vascular resistance in other organs that did not receive cooling.

Using a metal plate to selectively regulate brain temperature to prespecified levels (33°C, 36°C, and 37°C), Ibayashi et al. (70) showed that brain cooling in this range linearly decreased blood flow in the cortex without altering blood pressure and arterial blood gases. However, surface cooling did not appear to decrease temperature and CBF as effectively in deeper structures including the thalamus. When forebrain ischemia was applied in their model, hypothermia to 30°C did not alter cortical or thalamic blood flow, tissue lactate, or pyruvate, but ATP levels were higher. Hypothermia lowered arterial pH into the normal range—from 7.58 in normothermic ischemic animals to 7.45 in hypothermic ones. Unfortunately, ischemic brain injury was not assessed in this model; therefore, it is unclear whether such a cooling strategy is necessarily neuroprotective. However, in a similar study by Kuluz et al. (71), selective brain cooling using ice packs did result in better hippocampal neuron survival, although CBF and metabolism were not measured.

Clinical Studies

Like the data reported in experimental studies, reports of hypothermia on CBF at the clinical level have also been inconsistent. In patients on cardiopulmonary bypass, most reports show a decline in CBF as temperature is lowered (24,26,27), whereas others have reported increases (28,72,73).

These conflicting results may be explained, in part, by differences in acid–base management and depth of hypothermia in various studies.

In patients with severe traumatic brain injury, mild-to-moderate (32–34°C) hypothermia has been shown to decrease CBF in most studies (52,74), although some studies have reported no change (51). Such differences may be explained, in part, by the impact of severe traumatic brain injury itself on CBF, as CBF is typically decreased within the first few hours after injury, followed by a relative increase. With the renewed interest in therapeutic hypothermia, it is likely that more clinical data will become available in the near future.

Cerebral Autoregulation and Acid–Base Management

Influence of Hypothermia on Acid–Base Changes

When body temperature is lowered, blood becomes more viscous, the solubility of gases in the blood increases, and important acid–base changes occur. pH increases approximately 0.016 points for every degree Celsius lowering of body temperature (75). There are currently two types of blood gas management strategies that are used in clinical practice during hypothermia: pH-stat and alpha-stat methods.

During the pH-stat method, arterial pH and pCO_2 are maintained at 7.40 and 40 mm Hg, respectively, after correction for the patient's body temperature. The blood gas analyzer measures the blood gas at 37°C and corrects the obtained values for the reported body temperature of the patient. This strategy typically requires increasing CO_2 to maintain pH and pCO_2 at normal levels. This strategy can result in relative hypoventilation, leading to vasodilatation and an increase in CBF (25,76). In the alpha-stat method, pH is maintained at 7.40 and pCO_2 at 40 mm Hg without correcting for body temperature, resulting in an increase in pH and a decrease in pCO_2 during hypothermia. This strategy leads to relative hyperventilation and a decrease in CBF. Each of these acid–base strategies has theoretical advantages and disadvantages, and there is currently no consensus on which strategy is optimal in terms of cerebral protection or perfusion during therapeutic hypothermia (76,77).

Both laboratory and clinical studies have shown that pH-stat management results in higher CBF compared to alpha-stat management, and that cerebral autoregulation is more likely to be maintained during alpha-stat (25,28,72,78–80). In a study examining rat pial arteriole reactivity using a closed cranial window, baseline vessel diameter measured during moderate hypothermia (30°C) was reduced using the alpha-stat method, but not the pH-stat method (80). Vasodilation induced by hypotension was significantly reduced under hypothermic conditions in both circumstances, but more so during pH-stat management than during alpha-stat management. Vasodilation by hypercapnia, however, was preserved in both groups. Verhaegen et al. (78) found that CBF responses to controlled hemorrhagic hypotension in rats at 30.5°C were preserved during alpha-stat management, but were abolished during pH-stat management.

Murkin et al. (25) published a landmark study in 1987 on 38 patients undergoing cardiopulmonary bypass at approximately 26°C by comparing pH-stat and alpha-stat management. Cerebral oxygen consumption decreased in both groups during hypothermia regardless of pH management strategy (Fig. 4). CBF decreased in the alpha-stat group, but increased in the pH-stat group, during hypothermic bypass (Fig. 5). Furthermore, during pH-stat management, CBF was independent of cerebral oxygen consumption but dependent on cerebral perfusion pressure (CPP), suggesting a loss of cerebral autoregulation. In contrast, in the alpha-stat group, CBF was correlated with cerebral oxygen consumption and not with CPP, suggesting the preservation of cerebral autoregulation (25). Stephan et al. (28) studied 35 patients undergoing hypothermic cardiopulmonary bypass at 26°C. Patients were randomized to pH-stat and alpha-stat management. Overall, hypothermia was associated with an 18% reduction in CBF in the alpha-stat group, but with a 191% increase in CBF in the pH-stat group compared to postinduction values. Cerebral oxygen and glucose uptake were decreased by 60–74% in both

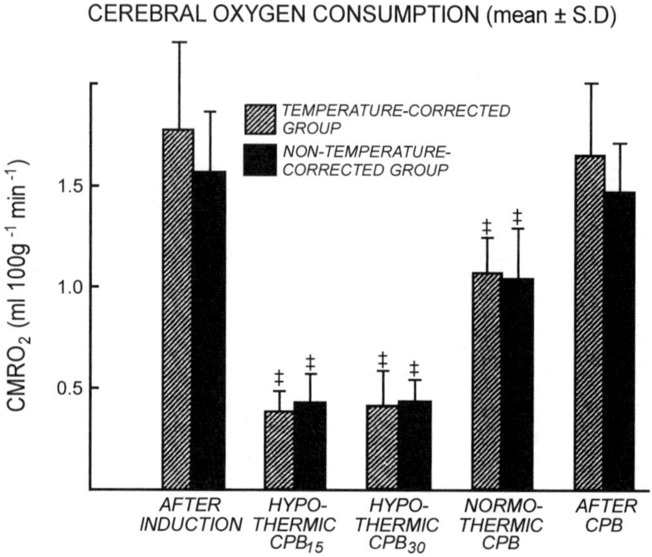

Figure 4 Influence of maintaining temperature-corrected (pH-stat) or non-temperature-corrected (alpha-stat) pCO_2 at 40 mm Hg on cerebral oxygen consumption in patients undergoing cardiopulmonary bypass at 26°C. No significant differences in cerebral metabolic rate for oxygen ($CMRO_2$) occur between the two groups at any point in time. (From Ref. 25.)

groups, indicating that coupling of flow and metabolism was lost in the pH-stat group. In another study of 70 patients undergoing coronary artery bypass graft surgery on cardiopulmonary bypass, CBF was significantly greater in the pH-stat group than in the alpha-stat group (79). Cerebral autoregulation as measured by the cerebral extraction ratio for oxygen was disturbed in both groups, but more so during pH-stat management than alpha-stat management.

Thus, during moderate and deep hypothermia, pH-stat management appears to result in luxury perfusion with vasodilation and loss of autoregulatory function, a state similar to normothermia with severe hypercapnia and/or hypoxia. It is unclear to what depth of hypothermia this phenomenon persists, or to what extent it affects various cerebral injury states.

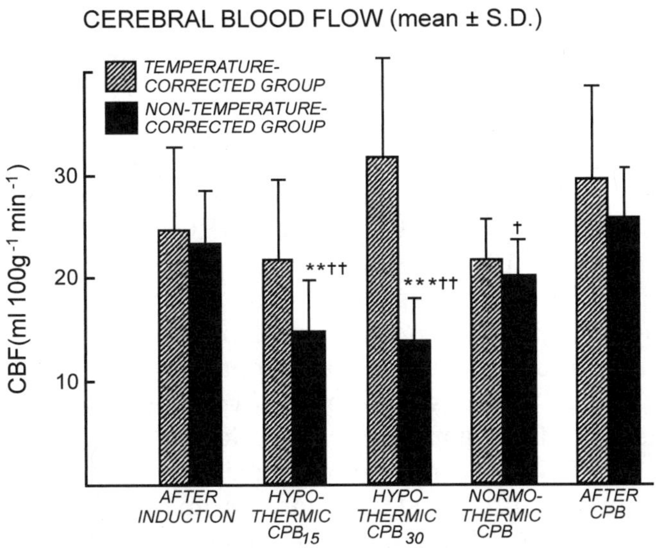

Figure 5 Influence of maintaining temperature-corrected (pH-stat) and non-temperature-corrected (alpha-stat) pCO_2 at 40 mm Hg on CBF in patients undergoing cardiopulmonary bypass at 26°C. In the temperature-corrected (pH-stat) group, CBF is significantly increased during hypothermic cardiopulmonary bypass compared to the non-temperature-corrected (alpha-stat) group (***P* < 0.005, ****P* < 0.001). (From Ref. 25.)

Several randomized clinical studies on the effect of acid–base management strategy on neurological outcome in adult patients maintained on hypothermic cardiopulmonary bypass during coronary artery bypass surgery have shown a significantly higher incidence of postoperative cognitive decline in patients managed on pH-stat strategy as compared to alpha-stat strategy (72,81). This observation has been attributed to a higher load of gaseous and particulate microemboli to the brain during higher blood flow states (82,83). Cerebral microemboli have been associated with cerebral dysfunction following cardiopulmonary bypass surgery, and pathological studies have demonstrated thousands of microemboli in the brain after surgery (83). Moreover, an increasing duration of cardiopulmonary bypass increases emboli load.

In contrast to the findings of cardiopulmonary bypass in adult patients, neurological outcome in infants and young animals undergoing deep hypothermic circulatory arrest (DHCA) is better with the pH-stat strategy (22,84–86). Kirshbom et al. (87) compared alpha-stat and pH-stat in a porcine model of cardiac arrest with aortopulmonary collaterals, which showed improved CBF and $CMRO_2$ and better cerebroprotection with pH-stat management. Furthermore, several retrospective and prospective clinical studies have found better neurological outcomes during pH-stat management in neonates undergoing cardiopulmonary bypass with DHCA (85–88). These findings have been attributed to differences in the nature of intraoperative neurological injury between adults and infants undergoing cardiac surgery. In infants, brain injury results most commonly from global hypoperfusion during periods of decreased or arrested CBF. Furthermore, infant cardiac surgery is typically performed at deeper levels of hypothermia with a potentially more pronounced divergence between the two pH management strategies. The proposed mechanisms by which pH-stat management may be beneficial in this setting are by an increase in the rate of brain cooling and by a slower rate of brain oxygen depletion during DHCA (82,89). Kurth et al. (89) studied 16 piglets who were cooled with pH-stat or alpha-stat cardiopulmonary bypass to 19°C and subjected to 1 hr of circulatory arrest. The authors found greater CBF and an increased cortical oxygen saturation during pH-stat management. Furthermore, cortical deoxygenation during arrest was slower in the pH-stat group than in the alpha-stat managed group.

Little is known about acid–base management strategy under cerebral injury conditions. But in a 2-hr middle cerebral artery occlusion model in rats during normothermia, followed by 5 hr of reperfusion during hypothermia (33°C), pH-stat management decreased cerebral infarct volume and edema and increased CBF compared to alpha-stat management, presumably by increasing CBF (90).

In patients with severe traumatic brain injury under mild hypothermia, one study evaluated the effects of hypothermia (34°C) and two different acid–base strategies (52). Twenty patients with severe traumatic brain injury were consecutively subjected to normocapnia–normothermia, hypocapnia–normothermia, hypocapnia–hypothermia, or normocapnia–hypothermia. The study showed a significant correlation of decrease in CBF with decrease of pCO_2 during hypocapnia, but not with body temperature. The authors felt that these CBF changes were directly related to changes in pCO_2 during different acid–base strategies under hypothermic conditions, rather than hypothermia itself.

In summary, there are two distinct protocols for acid–base management during hypothermia that significantly affect CBF especially at lower body temperatures. Most data on the effects of these strategies on neurological outcome are derived from laboratory and clinical studies during cardiopulmonary bypass and circulatory arrest under deep hypothermia of relatively short duration. These data cannot be directly translated to other disease states. The balance between advantages and disadvantages of each of the two acid–base strategies may vary under different cerebral injury conditions and different depths of hypothermia.

Influence of Hypothermia on Cerebral Autoregulation

Autoregulation of blood flow is the capacity of an organ to regulate its blood supply according to its underlying functional or metabolic needs. In the brain, autoregulation is often characterized as its ability to maintain constant CBF over a wide range of CPP, generally between 50 and 150 mm Hg. The limits of this autoregulation curve vary in individuals and are influenced by numerous factors, including longstanding hypertension, CBF itself, sympathetic nerve activity, arterial CO_2 partial pressure, pharmacological agents, and cerebral injury (91). If CPP exceeds the limits of the autoregulation curve, cerebral hypoperfusion or hyperperfusion may develop, which may result in cerebral ischemia and edema, respectively.

Cerebral autoregulation is thought to be localized in small arteries and arterioles ranging between 25 and >400 μm in diameter. The precise mechanisms that underlie cerebral autoregulation are not entirely understood. Several hypotheses have been proposed, including: (a) contraction and relaxation of smooth muscle cells in the vascular wall in response to variations in intravascular pressure and circumferential wall strain; (b) production of vasoactive substances by cells in the brain in response to a decrease in CBF; and (c) release of endothelial-derived relaxing and contracting factors in response to alterations in sheer stress or intravascular pressure (92).

Experimental Studies

In most studies of CBF in noninjured animals under hypothermic conditions, CBF declines almost in parallel with $CMRO_2$ (24,25,93) or CMR_{glu} (14,94) between 38°C and 28°C, suggesting that autoregulation is largely maintained. Below 28°C, metabolic rate seems to decrease more than CBF, resulting in a state of excess blood flow (10,87,95). This uncoupling of CBF and metabolism occurs with both acid–base management strategies, but more so with pH-stat management.

The result is a state of hypothermic hyperemia that may lead to an increase in oxygen tension and free radical production, including nitric oxide, which may further increase CBF through vasodilation (10). In a study of pigs undergoing progressive cooling to 28°C, 18°C, and 8°C with alpha-stat management during cardiopulmonary bypass, CBF decreased steadily to 18°C, but not subsequently. Cerebral vascular resistance steadily increased as animals were cooled, but then decreased between 18°C and 8°C, suggesting that autoregulation was lost at temperatures below 18°C (12). In rats, hypothermia (30°C) reduced CBF, but had no effect on cerebral autoregulation during alpha-stat management (78). In a study of juvenile swine under mild hypothermia (32°C) using pH-stat blood gas management, hypothermia improved brain tolerance for decreases in CPP in that CBF decreased less than $CMRO_2$ during hypothermia—a finding that may be explained by hypercarbia during hypothermia (96).

Clinical Studies

Studies of cerebral autoregulation under hypothermic conditions in humans are somewhat less consistent. In a study of healthy volunteers, dynamic autoregulation was measured by the response of CBF velocity to a transient decrease of the mean arterial pressure, induced by rapid deflation of a thigh cuff. Cerebral autoregulation decreased with only a slight decrease (0.3 °C) in body temperature and increased with slight increases in body temperature (0.4 °C) (97).

Several studies report preserved autoregulation during hypothermia in patients on cardiopulmonary bypass (10,98). Other studies, however, report uncoupling of CBF and cerebral metabolic rate under hypothermic conditions, to a greater extent during pH-stat management than during alpha-stat management (see previous section) (25,28,79). The uncoupling appears to be typically in the direction of excessive CBF for the metabolic requirements rather than insufficient CBF potentially leading to cerebral ischemia. Grubhofer et al. (99) observed increased jugular venous bulb oxygen saturation in response to increased CPP among patients on cardiopulmonary bypass under moderate hypothermia (29C) during alpha-stat management, suggesting impaired autoregulation in these patients.

Data are scarce on the effects of hypothermia on cerebral autoregulation under injury conditions in humans. Most studies are derived from patients with severe traumatic brain injury under mild-to-moderate hypothermia, and report a decrease in CBF and cerebral metabolic rate during mild hypothermia. It is unclear whether the two remain coupled under these circumstances. In a study of 14 stroke patients with large infarcts of the middle cerebral artery territory, static cerebral autoregulation in the nonaffected hemisphere was intact under alpha-stat management and a target body temperature of 33 °C (100). In a small study of patients with acute liver failure and raised intracranial pressure, moderate hypothermia (32 °C) restored autoregulation and reactivity to carbon dioxide (101).

Summary

In summary, cerebral autoregulation is generally preserved, at least to some extent, in uninjured brain during mild-to-moderate hypothermia and alpha-stat acid–base management; however, there are several studies in humans that have demonstrated impaired autoregulation under these circumstances. Some of the inconsistencies in the results of these studies may be explained by differences in study design, including depth of hypothermia, techniques for measuring cerebral autoregulation, acid–base management strategy, and disease state (102).

Most of the knowledge of the effects of hypothermia on cerebral metabolism, blood flow, pH management, and autoregulation is derived from laboratory models, under relatively short durations of moderate-to-deep hypothermia. In humans, most data are derived from patients with uninjured brains during cardiopulmonary bypass, under deep hypothermia. Little is thus known about these parameters during mild, resuscitative (postinjury), and prolonged hypothermia, particularly in the presence of various types of brain injury. Currently available data should therefore be applied to critically ill neurological patients only with considerable caution.

FUTURE DIRECTIONS

Cerebral blood flow and metabolism are sensitive to changes in temperature. Hypothermia decreases both parameters under normal and ischemic conditions, but the extent of neuroprotection, especially that provided by mild hypothermia, exceeds that predicted simply by lowered oxygen consumption and reduced CBF.

Although blood flow and metabolism in uninjured brain and metabolism in injured brain bear direct correlations to temperature, the extent of protection is not predicted by these changes. As mentioned above, the Q_{10} values for both oxygen and glucose metabolism are both approximately 2–4. Mild and moderate hypothermia (30–35°C) has been shown to be equally protective with reduced tissue damage on the order of 50% or greater (reviewed in Ref. 2). However, based on a Q_{10} of 2, this would predict a decrease in cerebral metabolic rate by only 15–20% (7). Therefore, the mechanisms of neuroprotection are likely to extend beyond the parameters of altered metabolism or blood flow. Other factors, such as the influence of temperature on excitotoxin release, inflammation, gene expression, and oxidative stress, may also contribute significantly to the underlying mechanism of protection, and are the subject of investigation in several laboratories.

Changes in CBF during hypothermia may be more affected by acid–base changes than hypothermia itself. Regardless, CBF appears to remain adequate for metabolic demands under most circumstances. But because the effects of acid–base management on CBF are substantial, further studies are required under various injury paradigms, both in the laboratory and clinic. Hypothermia nonetheless remains one of the most robust neuroprotectants studied to date in the laboratory and holds substantial potential as a clinical tool.

ACKNOWLEDGMENTS

Preparation of this chapter was supported by NINDS grants RO1 NS40516 (M.A.Y.) and RO1 NS027292 (G.K.S.). The authors wish to thank Beth Hoyte, Suzun Lamaina, and Dave Schaal for assistance in preparing this chapter.

REFERENCES

1. Busto R, Dietrich WD, Globus MY, Ginsberg MD. The importance of brain temperature in cerebral ischemic injury. Stroke 1989; 20:1113–1114.
2. Ginsberg MD, Sternau LL, Globus MY-T, Dietrich WD, Busto R. Therapeutic modulation of brain temperature: relevance to ischemic brain injury. Cerebrovasc Brain Metab Rev 1992; 4:189–225.
3. Maier CM, Ahern K, Cheng ML, Lee JE, Yenari MA, Steinberg GK. Optimal depth and duration of mild hypothermia in a focal model of transient cerebral ischemia: effects on neurologic outcome, infarct size, apoptosis, and inflammation. Stroke 1998; 29:2171–2180.
4. Clifton GL, Miller ER, Choi SC, Levin HS, McCauley S, Smith

KR Jr, Muizelaar JP, Wagner FC Jr, Marion DW, Luerssen TG, Chesnut RM, Schwartz M, Penrod LE, Kelsey SF, Obrist WD, Kochanek PM, Palmer AM, Wisniewski SR, DeKosky ST. Lack of effect of induction of hypothermia after acute brain injury. N Engl J Med 2001; 344:556–563.

5. The Hypothermia after Cardiac Arrest Study Group. Mild therapeutic hypothermia to improve the neurologic outcome after cardiac arrest. N Engl J Med 2002; 346:549–556.
6. Bernard SA, Gray TW, Buist MD, Jones BM, Silvester W, Gutteridge G, Smith K. Treatment of comatose survivors of out-of-hospital cardiac arrest with induced hypothermia. N Engl J Med 346:557–563.
7. Hartung J, Cottrell JE. Mild hypothermia and cerebral metabolism. J Neurosurg Anesthesiol 1994; 6:1–3.
8. Plum F, Pulsinelli WA. Cerebral metabolism and hypoxic–ischemic brain injury. In: Asbury AK, McKhann GM, McDonald WI, eds. Diseases of the Nervous System/Clinical Neurobiology. Vol. 2. Philadelphia: W. B. Saunders Co., 1992:1002–1015.
9. McCulloch J, Savaki HE, Jehle J, Sokoloff L. Local cerebral glucose utilization in hypothermic and hyperthermic rats. J Neurochem 1982; 39:255–258.
10. Erecinska M, Thoresen M, Silver IA. Effects of hypothermia on energy metabolism in mammalian central nervous system. J Cereb Blood Flow Metab 2003; 23:513–530.
11. Hagerdal M, Harp J, Nilsson L, Siesjo BK. The effect of induced hypothermia upon oxygen consumption in the rat brain. J Neurochem 1975; 24:311–316.
12. Ehrlich MP, McCullough JN, Zhang N, Weisz DJ, Juvonen T, Bodian CA, Griepp RB. Effect of hypothermia on cerebral blood flow and metabolism in the pig. Ann Thorac Surg 2002; 73:191–197.
13. Michenfelder JD, Milde JH. The relationship among canine brain temperature, metabolism, and function during hypothermia. Anesthesiology 1991; 75:130–136.
14. Krafft P, Frietsch T, Lenz C, Piepgras A, Kuschinsky W, Waschke KF. Mild and moderate hypothermia (alpha-stat) do

not impair the coupling between local cerebral blood flow and metabolism in rats. Stroke 2000; 31:1393–1400.

15. Conroy BP, Lin CY, Jenkins LW, DeWitt DS, Zornow MH, Uchida T, Johnston WE. Hypothermic modulation of cerebral ischemic injury during cardiopulmonary bypass in pigs. Anesthesiology 1998; 88:390–402.
16. Nakashima K, Todd MM, Warner DS. The relation between cerebral metabolic rate and ischemic depolarization. A comparison of the effects of hypothermia, pentobarbital, and isoflurane. Anesthesiology 1995; 82:1199–1208.
17. Astrup J, Sorensen PM, Sorensen HR. Inhibition of cerebral oxygen and glucose consumption in the dog by hypothermia, pentobarbital, and lidocaine. Anesthesiology 1981; 55:263–268.
18. Frietsch T, Krafft P, Piepgras A, Lenz C, Kuschinsky W, Waschke KF. Relationship between local cerebral blood flow and metabolism during mild and moderate hypothermia in rats. Anesthesiology 2000; 92:754–763.
19. Palmer C, Vannucci RC, Christensen MA, Brucklacher RM. Regional cerebral blood flow and glucose utilization during hypothermia in newborn dogs. Anesthesiology 1989; 71:730–737.
20. Kaibara T, Sutherland GR, Colbourne F, Tyson RL. Hypothermia: depression of tricarboxylic acid cycle flux and evidence for pentose phosphate shunt upregulation. J Neurosurg 1999; 90:339–347.
21. Hagerdal M, Harp J, Siesjo BK. Effect of hypothermia upon organic phosphates, glycolytic metabolites, citric acid cycle intermediates and associated amino acids in rat cerebral cortex. J Neurochem 1975; 24:743–748.
22. Aoki M, Nomura F, Stromski ME, Tsuji MK, Fackler JC, Hickey PR, Holtzman DH, Jonas RA. Effects of pH on brain energetics after hypothermic circulatory arrest. Ann Thorac Surg 1993; 55:1093–1103.
23. Laptook AR, Corbett RJ, Sterett R, Garcia D, Tollefsbol G. Quantitative relationship between brain temperature and energy utilization rate measured in vivo using ^{31}P and ^{1}H magnetic resonance spectroscopy. Pediatr Res 1995; 38:919–925.

24. Stone HH, Donnelly C, Frobese AS. The effect of lowered body temperature on the cerebral hemodynamics and metabolism of man. Surg Gynecol Obstet 1956; 102:313–317.

25. Murkin JM, Farrar JK, Tweed WA, McKenzie FN, Guiraudon G. Cerebral autoregulation and flow/metabolism coupling during cardiopulmonary bypass: the influence of p_aCO_2. Anesth Analg 1987; 66:825–832.

26. Croughwell N, Smith LR, Quill T, Newman M, Greeley W, Kern F, Lu J, Reves JG. The effect of temperature on cerebral metabolism and blood flow in adults during cardiopulmonary bypass. J Thorac Cardiovasc Surg 1992; 103:549–554.

27. Greeley WJ, Kern FH, Ungerleider RM, Boyd JL III, Quill T, Smith LR, Baldwin B, Reves JG. The effect of hypothermic cardiopulmonary bypass and total circulatory arrest on cerebral metabolism in neonates, infants, and children. J Thorac Cardiovasc Surg 1991; 101:783–794.

28. Stephan H, Weyland A, Kazmaier S, Henze T, Menck S, Sonntag H. Acid–base management during hypothermic cardiopulmonary bypass does not affect cerebral metabolism but does affect blood flow and neurological outcome. Br J Anaesth 1992; 69:51–57.

29. Hoffman WE, Charbel FT, Munoz L, Ausman JI. Comparison of brain tissue metabolic changes during ischemia at 35 degrees and 18 degrees C. Surg Neurol 1998; 49:85–88; discussion, 88–89.

30. Sutton LN, Clark BJ, Norwood CR, Woodford EJ, Welsh FA. Global cerebral ischemia in piglets under conditions of mild and deep hypothermia. Stroke 1991; 22:1567–1573.

31. Amorim P, Cottrell JE, Kass IS. Effect of small changes in temperature on CA1 pyramidal cells from rat hippocampal slices during hypoxia: implications about the mechanism of hypothermic protection against neuronal damage. Brain Res 1999; 844:143–149.

32. Welsh FA, Sims RE, Harris VA. Mild hypothermia prevents ischemic injury in gerbil hippocampus. J Cereb Blood Flow Metab 1990; 10:557–563.

33. Chopp M, Knight R, Tidwell CD, Helpern JA, Brown E, Welch KM. The metabolic effects of mild hypothermia on global

cerebral ischemia and recirculation in the cat: comparison to normothermia and hyperthermia. J Cereb Blood Flow Metab 1989; 9:141–148.

34. Tohyama Y, Sako K, Yonemasu Y. Hypothermia attenuates hyperglycolysis in the periphery of ischemic core in rat brain. Exp Brain Res 1998; 122:333–338.

35. Kimura T, Sako K, Tanaka K, Kusakabe M, Tanaka T, Nakada T. Effect of mild hypothermia on energy state recovery following transient forebrain ischemia in the gerbil. Exp Brain Res 2002; 145:83–90.

36. Dietrich WD, Busto R, Alonso O, Globus MY, Ginsberg MD. Intraischemic but not postischemic brain hypothermia protects chronically following global forebrain ischemia in rats. J Cereb Blood Flow Metab 1993; 13:541–549.

37. Young RS, Olenginski TP, Yagel SK, Towfighi J. The effect of graded hypothermia on hypoxic–ischemic brain damage: a neuropathologic study in the neonatal rat. Stroke 1983; 14:929–934.

38. Mori K, Maeda M, Miyazaki M, Iwase H. Effects of mild (33 degrees C) and moderate (29 degrees C) hypothermia on cerebral blood flow and metabolism, lactate, and extracellular glutamate in experimental head injury. Neurol Res 1998; 20:719–726.

39. Natale JA, D'Alecy LG. Protection from cerebral ischemia by brain cooling without reduced lactate accumulation in dogs. Stroke 1989; 20:770–777.

40. Busto R, Globus MY, Dietrich WD, Martinez E, Valdes I, Ginsberg MD. Effect of mild hypothermia on ischemia-induced release of neurotransmitters and free fatty acids in rat brain. Stroke 1989; 20:904–910.

41. Lin B, Busto R, Globus MY, Martinez E, Ginsberg MD. Brain temperature modulations during global ischemia fail to influence extracellular lactate levels in rats. Stroke 1995; 26:1634–1638.

42. Kim Y, Busto R, Dietrich WD, Kraydieh S, Ginsberg MD. Delayed postischemic hyperthermia in awake rats worsens the histopathological outcome of transient focal cerebral ischemia. Stroke 1996; 27:2274–2280.

43. Nemoto EM, Klementavicius R, Melick JA, Yonas H. Suppression of cerebral metabolic rate for oxygen ($CMRO_2$) by mild hypothermia compared with thiopental. J Neurosurg Anesthesiol 1996; 8:52–59.

44. Yenari MA, Steinberg GK. Pharmacological advances in cerebrovascular protection. In: Awad I, ed. Cerebrovascular Neurosurgery. Current Techniques in Neurosurgery. 3rd ed. Philadelphia: Current Medicine, 1998:98–116.

45. Yanamoto H, Nagata I, Niitsu Y, Zhang Z, Xue JH, Sakai N, Kikuchi H. Prolonged mild hypothermia therapy protects the brain against permanent focal ischemia. Stroke 2001; 32:232–239.

46. Kader A, Brisman MH, Maraire N, Huh JT, Solomon RA. The effect of mild hypothermia on permanent focal ischemia in the rat. Neurosurgery 1992; 31:1056–1060; discussion, 1051–1060.

47. Baker CJ, Onesti ST, Barth KN, Prestigiacomo CJ, Solomon RA. Hypothermic protection following middle cerebral artery occlusion in the rat. Surg Neurol 1991; 36:175–180.

48. Busto R, Dietrich WD, Globus MY, Valdes I, Scheinberg P, Ginsberg MD. Small differences in intraischemic brain temperature critically determine the extent of ischemic neuronal injury. J Cereb Blood Flow Metab 1987; 7:729–738.

49. Zhao W, Alonso OF, Loor JY, Busto R, Ginsberg MD. Influence of early posttraumatic hypothermia therapy on local cerebral blood flow and glucose metabolism after fluid-percussion brain injury. J Neurosurg 1999; 90:510–519.

50. Marion DW, Obrist WD, Carlier PM, Penrod LE, Darby JM. The use of moderate therapeutic hypothermia for patients with severe head injuries: a preliminary report. J Neurosurg 1993; 79:354–362.

51. Metz C, Holzschuh M, Bein T, Woertgen C, Frey A, Frey I, Taeger K, Brawanski A. Moderate hypothermia in patients with severe head injury: cerebral and extracerebral effects. J Neurosurg 1996; 85:533–541.

52. Vigue B, Ract C, Zlotine N, Leblanc PE, Samii K, Bissonnette B. Relationship between intracranial pressure, mild hypo-

thermia and temperature-corrected p_aCO_2 in patients with traumatic brain injury. Intensive Care Med 2000; 26:722–728.

53. Katsura K, Minamisawa H, Ekholm A, Folbergrova J, Siesjo BK. Changes of labile metabolites during anoxia in moderately hypo- and hyperthermic rats: correlation to membrane fluxes of K^+. Brain Res 1992; 590:6–12.
54. Sick TJ, Tang R, Perez-Pinzon MA. Cerebral blood flow does not mediate the effect of brain temperature on recovery of extracellular potassium ion activity after transient focal ischemia in the rat. Brain Res 1999; 821:400–406.
55. Moseley ME, Wendland MF, Kucharczyk J. Magnetic resonance imaging of diffusion and perfusion. Top Magn Reson Imaging 1991; 3:50–67.
56. Hasegawa Y, Latour LL, Sotak CH, Dardzinski BJ, Fisher M. Temperature dependent change of apparent diffusion coefficient of water in normal and ischemic brain of rats. J Cereb Blood Flow Metab 1994; 14:383–390.
57. Jiang Q, Chopp M, Zhang ZG, Helpern JA, Ordidge RJ, Ewing J, Jiang P, Marchese BA. The effect of hypothermia on transient focal ischemia in rat brain evaluated by diffusion- and perfusion-weighted NMR imaging. J Cereb Blood Flow Metab 1994; 14:732–741.
58. Yenari MA, Onley D, Hedehus M, deCrespigny A, Sun GH, Moseley ME, Steinberg GK. Diffusion- and perfusion-weighted magnetic resonance imaging of focal cerebral ischemia and cortical spreading depression under conditions of mild hypothermia. Brain Res 2000; 885:208–219.
59. Le Bihan D, Delannoy J, Levin RL. Temperature mapping with MR imaging of molecular diffusion: application to hyperthermia. Radiology 1989; 171:853–857.
60. Todd MM, Warner DS. A comfortable hypothesis reevaluated. Cerebral metabolic depression and brain protection during ischemia. Anesthesiology 1992; 76:161–164.
61. Busija DW, Leffler CW. Hypothermia reduces cerebral metabolic rate and cerebral blood flow in newborn pigs. Am J Physiol 1987; 253:H869–873.

62. Mori K, Maeda M, Miyazaki M, Iwase H. Effects of mild and moderate hypothermia on cerebral metabolism and glutamate in an experimental head injury. Acta Neurochir Suppl 1998; 71:222–224.

63. Okubo K, Itoh S, Isobe K, Kusaka T, Nagano K, Kondo M, Onishi S. Cerebral metabolism and regional cerebral blood flow during moderate systemic cooling in newborn piglets. Pediatr Int 2001; 43:496–501.

64. Olsen TS. Regional cerebral blood flow after occlusion of the middle cerebral artery. Acta Neurol Scand 1986; 73:321–337.

65. Jenkins LW, DeWitt DS, Johnston WE, Davis KL, Prough DS. Intraischemic mild hypothermia increases hippocampal CA1 blood during forebrain ischemia. Brain Res 2001; 890:1–10.

66. Lo EH, Steinberg GK. Effects of hypothermia on evoked potentials, magnetic resonance imaging, and blood flow in focal ischemia in rabbits. Stroke 1992; 23:889–893.

67. Karibe H, Zarow GJ, Graham SH, Weinstein PR. Mild intraischemic hypothermia reduces postischemic hyperperfusion, delayed postischemic hypoperfusion, blood–brain barrier disruption, brain edema, and neuronal damage volume after temporary focal cerebral ischemia in rats. J Cereb Blood Flow Metab 1994; 14:620–627.

68. Koizumi H, Fujisawa H, Ito H, Maekawa T, Di X, Bullock R. Effects of mild hypothermia on cerebral blood flow-independent changes in cortical extracellular levels of amino acids following contusion trauma in the rat. Brain Res 1997; 747:304–312.

69. Kuluz JW, Prado R, Chang J, Ginsberg MD, Schleien CL, Busto R. Selective brain cooling increases cortical cerebral blood flow in rats. Am J Physiol 1993; 265:H824–H827.

70. Ibayashi S, Takano K, Ooboshi H, Kitazono T, Sadoshima S, Fujishima M. Effect of selective brain hypothermia on regional cerebral blood flow and tissue metabolism using brain thermo-regulator in spontaneously hypertensive rats. Neurochem Res 2000; 25:369–375.

71. Kuluz JW, Gregory GA, Yu AC, Chang Y. Selective brain cooling during and after prolonged global ischemia reduces cortical damage in rats. Stroke 1992; 23:1792–1796.

72. Venn GE, Patel RL, Chambers DJ. Cardiopulmonary bypass: perioperative cerebral blood flow and postoperative cognitive deficit. Ann Thorac Surg 1995; 59:1331–1335.

73. Henriksen L. Brain luxury perfusion during cardiopulmonary bypass in humans. A study of the cerebral blood flow response to changes in CO_2, O_2, and blood pressure. J Cereb Blood Flow Metab 1986; 6:366–378.

74. Marion DW, Penrod LE, Kelsey SF, Obrist WD, Kochanek PM, Palmer AM, Wisniewski SR, DeKosky ST. Treatment of traumatic brain injury with moderate hypothermia. N Engl J Med 1997; 336:540–546.

75. Swain JA, McDonald TJ Jr, Robbins RC, Balaban RS. Relationship of cerebral and myocardial intracellular pH to blood pH during hypothermia. Am J Physiol 1991; 260:H1640–1644.

76. Kofstad J. Blood gases and hypothermia: some theoretical and practical considerations. Scand J Clin Lab Invest Suppl 1996; 224:21–26.

77. Tallman RD Jr. Acid–base regulation, alpha-stat, and the emperor's new clothes. J Cardiothorac Vasc Anesth 1997; 11:282–288.

78. Verhaegen MJ, Todd MM, Hindman BJ, Warner DS. Cerebral autoregulation during moderate hypothermia in rats. Stroke 1993; 24:407–414.

79. Patel RL, Turtle MR, Chambers DJ, Newman S, Venn GE. Hyperperfusion and cerebral dysfunction. Effect of differing acid–base management during cardiopulmonary bypass. Eur J Cardiothorac Surg 1993; 7:457–463; discussion, 464.

80. Irikura K, Miyasaka Y, Nagai S, Yuzawa I, Morii S, Fujii K. Moderate hypothermia reduces hypotensive, but not hypercapnic vasodilation of pial arterioles in rats. J Cereb Blood Flow Metab 1998; 18:1294–1297.

81. Murkin JM, Martzke JS, Buchan AM, Bentley C, Wong CJ. A randomized study of the influence of perfusion technique and pH management strategy in 316 patients undergoing coronary artery bypass surgery: II. Neurologic and cognitive outcomes. J Thorac Cardiovasc Surg 1995; 110:349–362.

82. Hindman BJ. Choice of alpha-stat or pH-stat management

and neurologic outcomes after cardiac surgery: it depends. Anesthesiology 1998; 89:5–7.

83. Brown WR, Moody DM, Challa VR, Stump DA, Hammon JW. Longer duration of cardiopulmonary bypass is associated with greater numbers of cerebral microemboli. Stroke 2000; 31:707–713.

84. Hiramatsu T, Miura T, Forbess JM, Du Plessis A, Aoki M, Nomura F, Holtzman D, Jonas RA. pH strategies and cerebral energetics before and after circulatory arrest. J Thorac Cardiovasc Surg 1995; 109:948–957; discussion, 948–957.

85. Jonas RA, Bellinger DC, Rappaport LA, Wernovsky G, Hickey PR, Farrell DM, Newburger JW. Relation of pH strategy and developmental outcome after hypothermic circulatory arrest. J Thorac Cardiovasc Surg 1993; 106:362–368.

86. du Plessis AJ, Jonas RA, Wypij D, Hickey PR, Riviello J, Wessel DL, Roth SJ, Burrows FA, Walter G, Farrell DM, Walsh AZ, Plumb CA, del Nido P, Burke RP, Castaneda AR, Mayer JE Jr, Newburger JW. Perioperative effects of alpha-stat versus pH-stat strategies for deep hypothermic cardiopulmonary bypass in infants. J Thorac Cardiovasc Surg 1997; 114:991–1000; discussion, 1000–1001.

87. Kirshbom PM, Skaryak LR, DiBernardo LR, Kern FH, Greeley WJ, Gaynor JW, Ungerleider RM. pH-stat cooling improves cerebral metabolic recovery after circulatory arrest in a piglet model of aortopulmonary collaterals. J Thorac Cardiovasc Surg 1996; 111:147–155.

88. Hickey PR. Neurologic sequelae associated with deep hypothermic circulatory arrest. Ann Thorac Surg 1998; 65:S65–S69; discussion, S69–S70, S66–S74.

89. Kurth CD, O'Rourke MM, O'Hara IB. Comparison of pH-stat and alpha-stat cardiopulmonary bypass on cerebral oxygenation and blood flow in relation to hypothermic circulatory arrest in piglets. Anesthesiology 1998; 89:110–118.

90. Kollmar R, Frietsch T, Georgiadis D, Schabitz WR, Waschke KF, Kuschinsky W, Schwab S. Early effects of acid–base management during hypothermia on cerebral infarct volume, edema, and cerebral blood flow in acute focal cerebral ischemia in rats. Anesthesiology 2002; 97:868–874.

91. Drummond JC. The lower limit of autoregulation: time to revise our thinking? Anesthesiology 1997; 86:1431–1433.

92. Chillon J-M, Baumbach G. Autoregulation: arterial and intracranial pressure. In: Edvinsson KDL, ed. Cerebral Bloodflow and Metabolism. 2nd ed. Philadelphia: Lippincott, Williams, and Wilkins, 2002:395–412.

93. Michenfelder JD, Theye RA. Hypothermia: effect on canine brain and whole-body metabolism. Anesthesiology 1968; 29: 1107–1112.

94. Frietsch T, Piepgras A, Krafft P, Schwab S, Kuschinsky W, Waschke KF. Acid–base management—is it relevant for the study design of hypothermic neuroprotection? Eur J Anaesthesiol 2002; 19:389–394.

95. Skaryak LA, Chai PJ, Kern FH, Greeley WJ, Ungerleider RM. Blood gas management and degree of cooling: effects on cerebral metabolism before and after circulatory arrest. J Thorac Cardiovasc Surg 1995; 110:1649–1657.

96. Bauer R, Fritz H, Walter B, Schlonski O, Jochum T, Hoyer D, Zwiener U, Reinhart K. Effect of mild hypothermia on cerebral oxygen uptake during gradual cerebral perfusion pressure decrease in piglets. Crit Care Med 2000; 28:1128–1135.

97. Doering TJ, Aaslid R, Steuernagel B, Brix J, Niederstadt C, Breull A, Schneider B, Fischer GC. Cerebral autoregulation during whole-body hypothermia and hyperthermia stimulus. Am J Phys Med Rehabil 1999; 78:33–38.

98. Johnsson P, Messeter K, Ryding E, Nordstrom L, Stahl E. Cerebral blood flow and autoregulation during hypothermic cardiopulmonary bypass. Ann Thorac Surg 1987; 43:386–390.

99. Grubhofer G, Lassnigg AM, Schneider B, Rajek MA, Pernerstorfer T, Hiesmayr MJ. Jugular venous bulb oxygen saturation depends on blood pressure during cardiopulmonary bypass. Ann Thorac Surg 1998; 65:653–657; discussion, 658.

100. Georgiadis D, Schwarz S, Evans DH, Schwab S, Baumgartner RW. Cerebral autoregulation under moderate hypothermia in patients with acute stroke. Stroke 2002; 33:3026–3029.

101. Jalan R, Olde Damink SW, Deutz NE, Hayes PC, Lee A.

Restoration of cerebral blood flow autoregulation and reactivity to carbon dioxide in acute liver failure by moderate hypothermia. Hepatology 2001; 34:50–54.

102. Prough DS, Bedell EA. Is reduced cerebral perfusion pressure better tolerated during hypothermia? Crit Care Med 2000; 28:1243–1244.

6

Complications of Hypothermia

OZAN AKÇA
Outcomes Research™ Institute
and Department of Anesthesiology
and Perioperative Medicine,
University of Louisville,
Louisville, Kentucky, U.S.A.

INTRODUCTION

In the last decade, a series of randomized clinical trials have demonstrated several hypothermia-induced complications. Most of the work was done in the perioperative setting, but there is little reason for believing that patients undergoing therapeutic hypothermia in the intensive care unit (ICU) will be any less susceptible to the major complications of thermal perturbations.

Although hypothermia is generally classified into four distinct qualitative groups—mild (33–36°C), moderate (26–33°C), deep (20–26°C), and profound (<20°C)—there is no widely accepted definition of these groups. Generally, a core temperature lower than 36°C is defined as hypothermia. Important adverse effects of mild hypothermia are listed in Table 1. Only evidence-based complications will be discussed in this chapter. The focus will be on the effects of hypothermia on the cardiovascular system, coagulation, immunological function, and metabolism, including specific complications such as shivering, insulin resistance, and altered drug kinetics.

REVIEW

Cardiovascular Consequences

Background

Myocardial infarction is a leading cause of morbidity and mortality, and perioperative hypothermia increases the risk of myocardial infarction. Severe cardiovascular effects of moderate-to-deep hypothermia include morbid myocardial outcomes such as ventricular arrhythmias, myocardial ischemia, and hypotension. The circulatory effects of hypothermia begin with increased systemic vascular resistance and increased afterload, which is the result of generalized vasoconstriction as the body attempts to conserve heat (1). Although mild hypertension can occur during initiation of cooling, at deeper levels hypothermia tends to reduce heart rate, blood pressure, and cardiac output. As cooling proceeds, fluid leaves the intravascular space, resulting in mild hemoconcentration by approximately 5% per °C reduction in temperature (2) which can impede microcirculatory flow. Cold-induced diuresis caused by suppression of antidiuretic hormone release and shunting of the peripheral blood volume centrally further depletes intravascular volume (3). After a prolonged period of hypothermia, cooled patients may be at risk for hypovolemia and hypotension, particularly after rewarming (with accompanying vasodilation) has started.

Why hypothermia increases myocardial risk remains unknown, but shivering has been suggested as a possible culprit. Shivering, which increases oxygen consumption substantially (4), could cause hypoxemia, myocardial ischemia, and myocardial infarction in high-risk patients by increasing myocardial

Table 1 Major Complications of Hypothermia

	Author	N	ΔT_{core} (°C)	Normothermic group	Hypothermic group	P
Morbid cardiac events (%)	Frank et al. (17)	300	1.3	1	6	<0.05
Postoperative ventricular tachycardia (%)	Frank et al. (17)	300	1.3	2	8	<0.05
Surgical wound infection (%)	Kurz et al. (41)	200	1.9	6	19	<0.01
	Melling et al. (63)	238	0.35	6	14	0.026
Thermal comfort at first postoperative hour (mm VAS[a])	Kurz et al. (88)	74	2.5	≈50	~25	<0.01
Decrease in muscle glutamine concentration (%)	Carli et al. (62)	12		18	50	<0.05
Duration of hospitalization (days)	Kurz et al. (41)	200	1.9	12.1 ± 4.4	14.7 ± 6.5	<0.01
Duration of postanesthetic recovery (min)	Lenhardt et al. (85)	150	1.9	53 ± 36	94 ± 65	<0.001

Above table includes only some of the important prospective, randomized human trials. N = total number of subjects. ΔT_{core} = difference in core temperature between the treatment groups.

[a] VAS = visual analogue scale, 0–100 mm represents cold to warm extremes (Fig. 6).

demand (5). However, it is difficult to credit increased myocardial problems associated with hypothermia to shivering alone. For instance, the increase in oxygen consumption during shivering is less than might be expected. Although cold-induced shivering in young, healthy volunteers typically doubles oxygen consumption (6), postoperative shivering usually increases oxygen consumption only slightly (7,8). The second problem is that elderly patients rarely shiver because advanced age per se impairs thermoregulatory responses (9). Shivering appears to be especially rare in frail patients, who are at the highest risk for cardiac complications (10,11,2). The third issue is that shivering does not appear to be an important cause of postoperative hypoxemia. Instead, hypoxemia itself inhibits shivering (12–15). Finally, several studies indicate that myocardial ischemia is unrelated to shivering (16,17). Available evidence thus suggests that shivering, while uncomfortable for patients and disturbing for caregivers, does not directly trigger myocardial ischemia or infarction.

Induction of therapeutic hypothermia is likely to provoke responses similar to those of normal volunteers rather than of postoperative patients in whom thermoregulation remains blunted by residual anesthesia. Hypothermia-induced cardiac complications seem most likely to result from a threefold increase in plasma norepinephrine concentrations (18) and consequent hypertension (19), especially in the elderly (20) (Fig. 1). Each factor might augment cardiac irritability and facilitate development of ventricular arrhythmias.

Hypothermia can affect the myocardial conduction system, resulting in arrhythmias and ventricular ectopy. These complications are uncommon with mild hypothermia, but tend to occur predictably as temperature descends from moderate to deep levels of hypothermia. At temperatures below 32°C there is a tendency to develop atrial fibrillation (21), and below 30°C spontaneous ventricular fibrillation can occur (1). For this reason, 32–33°C is widely considered the lowest safe level of therapeutic hypothermia in the ICU setting. Hypothermia may cause conduction disturbances and ventricular irritability through direct effects on the myocardium, by potentiating the effects of various drugs that can irritate the heart (such as bupivacaine), or by provoking hypokalemia (22,23). Nonuni-

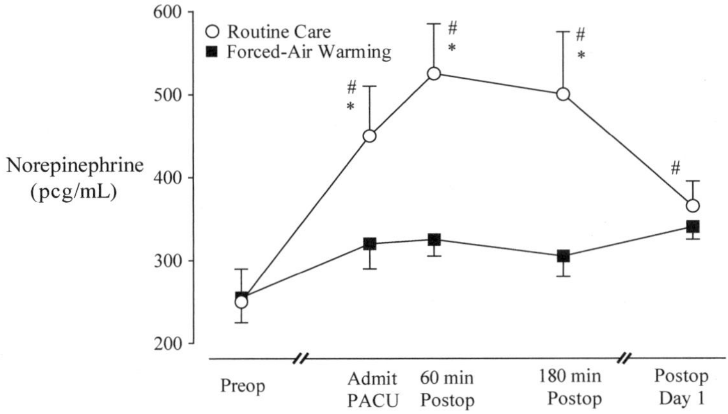

Figure 1 Plasma norepinephrine levels measured in arterial blood in routine care (hypothermic, $N = 37$) and forced-air warming (normothermic, $N = 37$) groups. Norepinephrine levels were significantly greater than the preoperative baseline in the routine care group on admission to the PACU, at 60 and 180 min, and 1 day postoperatively. Between-group comparisons showed NE levels were significantly greater in the routine-care group on admission to the PCU and at 60 and 180 min postoperatively. Data presented as mean ± SEM. $*P < 0.01$ vs. forced-air warming. $\#P < 0.05$ vs. preoperative. (Figure modified from Ref. 18; used by permission.)

form cooling or rewarming of the heart may cause regional heterogeneity of conduction, action potential duration, and refractory periods (24). This in turn favors the occurrence of unidirectional conduction block, reentrant dysrhythmias, and other conduction disturbances.

Clinical Outcomes

Frank et al. retrospectively analyzed the effects of perioperative hypothermia on myocardial morbidity (16). In this multivariate analysis, there was a significantly higher incidence of postoperative myocardial ischemia on ECG in vascular surgery patients who arrived in the ICU with temperatures <35°C compared to those who were normothermic (36% vs. 13%) (4). In addition, hypothermia was associated with an increased frequency of postoperative angina (18% vs. 2%). Because of the retrospective analysis technique, it was hard to avoid the possibility that older, sicker patients and those having the largest and longest procedures were the patients who became the most hypothermic. But in a follow-up prospective, randomized study, Frank et al. demonstrated that high-risk patients who were only 1.3°C hypothermic were three times more likely to experience adverse myocardial outcomes (17).

More recently, Nesher et al. showed that during coronary artery bypass graft surgery, patients kept normothermic had significantly lower concentrations of cardiac-specific troponin I (25), a cardiac protein marker that correlates with the extent of myocardial injury (Fig. 2). In this study, the aggressive temperature management group was kept normothermic for most of the intraoperative period and always ≈1°C warmer than the routine temperature management group. Available evidence thus suggests that even mild hypothermia substantially increases the risk of morbid myocardial events in high-risk patients.

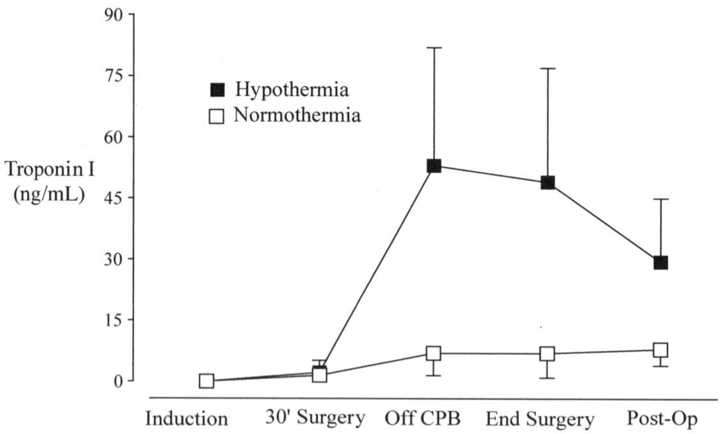

Figure 2 Perioperative levels of specific cardiac troponin I (ng/mL). Groups were significantly different in samples taken when the patients came off CPB, at the end of surgery, and 2 hr postoperatively ($P < 0.01$). There were 30 patients per group; levels for both groups were 0 ng/mL at induction. (Figure modified from Ref. 25; used by permission.)

In contrast to this theory, a recent therapeutic hypothermia study for cardiac arrest evaluated the cardiovascular effects of reducing core temperature to $\approx 33\,^{\circ}\mathrm{C}$. The investigators showed that heart rate decreased 20–30 beats per minute and systemic vascular resistance increased by $\approx 50\%$. However, there was no effect on blood pressure (26). Additionally, in the cooled patients, there were no clinically important arrhythmias or significant changes in creatinine kinase myocardial band (CK-MB), an enzyme that is elevated after myocardial infarctions. However, this clinical outcome study did not report plasma catecholamine concentrations to explore possible mechanisms.

Effects on Coagulation

Background

The effects of hypothermia on platelet functions have been studied in detail in the last two decades. Three general mechanisms contribute to temperature-related coagulation disorders: platelet function, clotting factor enzyme function, and fibrinolytic activity.

The number of platelets remains normal during mild hypothermia. However, in the late 1980s, Valeri et al. demonstrated that mild hypothermia seriously impairs platelet function (27). This impairment is strictly a local phenomenon: bleeding time is comparably increased by systemic or local hypothermia. However, wound temperature is largely determined by core temperature and, therefore, higher in normothermic patients than in the hypothermic ones. Subsequent work indicated that the defect resulted from reduced release of thromboxane A_2 (28–30).

Standard coagulation tests, including the prothrombin time (PT) and the partial thromboplastin time (PTT), remain normal in blood taken from hypothermic patients (31). A possible reason for this finding is that the tests are normally performed at $37\,^{\circ}\mathrm{C}$ regardless of the patient's actual body temperature. However, coagulation time is prolonged when these tests are performed at hypothermic temperatures (32,33).

The fibrinolytic system normally regulates the balance between formation of hemostatic plugs and restoration of blood flow after clot formation. Fibrin is a major structural element in formed clots, but is subject to degradation by plasmin. Plasmin is the activated enzymatic form of plasminogen. The conversion of plasminogen to plasmin is the major fibrinolytic mechanism. This reaction is enhanced by two types of plasminogen activators, with tissue-type plasminogen activator the most important. Inadequate fibrinolysis predisposes patients to thrombosis, whereas excessive fibrinolysis predisposes them to hemorrhage. Preliminary data indicate that fibrinolysis remains normal during mild hypothermia, suggesting that hypothermia-induced coagulopathy does not result from excessive clot lysis. The corresponding effects of thermal disturbances on plasminogen activator have yet to be determined, but thromboelastogram data suggest that hypothermia impairs clot formation, rather than facilitating clot degeneration (34).

Clinical Outcomes

Schmied et al. first demonstrated that mild hypothermia increases blood loss (35). They found that an intraoperative core temperature decrease of 1.6°C increased blood loss by 500 mL (30%) and significantly increased allogeneic transfusion requirement. The same group subsequently confirmed the hemostatic benefits of maintaining intraoperative normothermia in a retrospective analysis (36). In a follow-up study, Winkler et al. showed that even very mild hypothermia (≈0.5°C) increases perioperative (mostly intraoperative) blood loss (37). This observation was confirmed in another study, again with hip arthroplasty patients, in which Widman et al. (38) showed a 200-mL increase in intraoperative blood loss with a core temperature reduction of only 0.5°C. In another study of blood loss during hip arthroplasty, though, Johansson et al. failed to identify any relationship between body temperature and blood loss (39). There were differences in surgical techniques and in the populations evaluated in these study, although most patients were undergoing hip arthroplasties.

The reason for the discrepancy between the abovementioned well-designed and conducted studies remains unclear.

In a different surgical setting, Persson and Lundberg showed that very mild hypothermia (0.5 to 1°C) increased blood loss ≈70% during subtotal hysterectomy (40). A concern about this study, however, was that the way intraoperative blood loss was measured was not noted in detail, possibly because it was not initially one of the major outcomes for the study. Kurz et al. similarly showed a slight increase in transfusion requirements necessary to reach target hemoglobin concentrations in colorectal surgery patients who were ≈2°C hypothermic, but again blood loss was not a major a priori outcome (41). Recently, The Hypothermia after Cardiac Arrest Study Group found a slight increase in bleeding in the hypothermic patients, but this difference was not statistically significant (42). Slight elevations of the PT and PTT within the normal range (measured at normal body temperature) were found during and after rewarming in traumatic brain injury (TBI) patients (43). However, platelet counts did not decrease and bleeding complications were no more frequent in the hypothermic patients, despite preexisting intracranial hemorrhage in many patients. Careful analysis of CT scans in another trial of hypothermia for TBI showed no effect on the incidence of delayed traumatic intracerebral hemorrhage (44). Prospective randomized studies of hypothermia and coagulation are shown in Table 2.

Available data are most consistent with the conclusion that mild hypothermia causes a clinically important coagulopathy that increases intraoperative blood loss and transfusion requirement. However, the extent to which reduced platelet function and impaired coagulation enzyme function contributes to hypothermia-induced coagulopathy remains unknown. The effect of hypothermia on coagulation remains inadequately evaluated outside the operative setting. Although there is no reason to believe that therapeutic hypothermia will not produce a similar coagulopathy in the ICU, preliminary observations have not found that intracranial bleeding is an important risk of therapeutic hypothermia for traumatic brain injury.

Table 2 The Effects of Hyperthermia on Coagulation

	Author	Surgery	N	ΔT_{core} (°C)	Normothermic group	Hypothermic group	P
Intraoperative blood loss (mL)	Schmied et al. (35)	Arthroplasty	60	1.6	1700 ± 300	2200 ± 500	<0.001
	Persson and Lundberg (40)	Hysterectomy	59	1.0	186 ± 27	308 ± 47	<0.05
	Widman et al. (38)	Arthroplasty	46	0.5	516 ± 272	702 ± 344	<0.05
	Winkler et al. (37)	Arthroplasty	150	0.5	488 (368–721)	618 (480–864)	0.002
	Johansson et al. (39)	Arthroplasty	50	0.9	698 ± 314	665 ± 292	N.S.
	Kurz et al. (41)	Colorectal	200	1.9	0.4 ± 1.0	0.8 ± 1.2	0.01
Allogeneic transfusion requirement (units)	Schmied et al. (35)	Arthroplasty	60	1.6	1	8	<0.05

Data presented as means ± SD or medians (interquartile ranges).

Resistance to Infection

Background

In vitro evidence shows that bacterial growth decreases during hypothermia (45). Hypothermia nonetheless increases infection risk by reducing host resistance to infection, especially oxidative killing of bacteria by neutrophils. Perioperative hypothermia may increase the risk of infection by decreasing subcutaneous oxygen tension. This reduction results in part because hypothermia triggers thermoregulatory vasoconstriction (46). As a consequence, hypothermia significantly decreases subcutaneous oxygen tension (47), and the incidence of wound infections correlates well with subcutaneous oxygen tension (48,49) (Fig. 3).

Another serious consequence of hypothermia is that mild core hypothermia directly impairs immune function, including T-cell-mediated antibody production (50,51) and oxidative bacterial killing by neutrophils (52) (Fig. 4). Bacterial killing by neutrophils is reduced as temperature decreases from

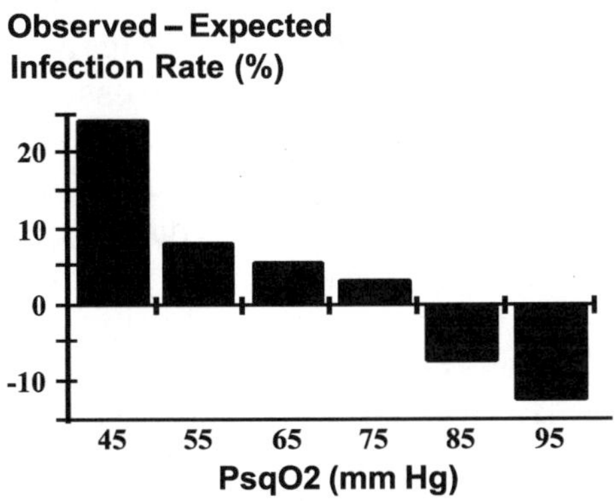

Figure 3 Surgical wound infection rates among 130 patients, stratified by maximum subcutaneous wound oxygen tension ($PsqO_2$ max). The bars represent the difference between observed rates and those expected based on the Study on the Effect of Nosocomial Infection Control (SENIC) multivariate risk index. These differences are statistically significant ($P = 0.002$; $r^2 = 0.93$, linear regression). (Figure modified from Ref. 48; used by permission.)

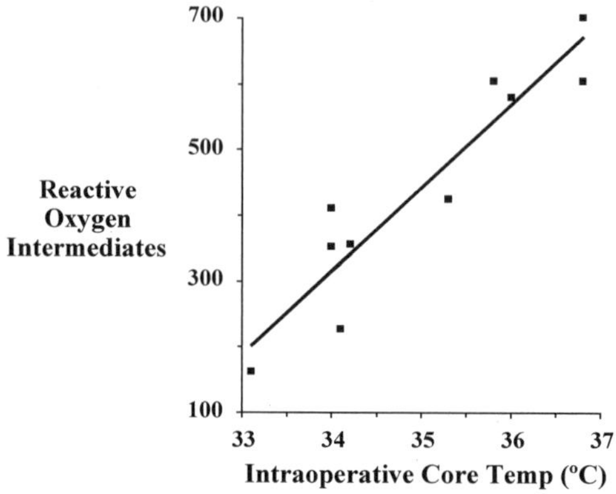

Figure 4 Intraoperative polymorphonuclear leukocyte production of reactive oxygen species (mean fluorescence units) was linearly related to intraoperative core temperature in patients undergoing colorectal surgery: reactive oxygen = $130(T_{\text{Core}}) - 4000$, $r^2 = 0.88$. (From Ref. 54; used by permission.)

hyperthermic values to severe hypothermic temperatures such as 26°C (53,54). Decreased killing results mostly because production of oxygen radicals and nitroso free radicals is oxygen-dependent in the range of oxygen partial pressures found in wounds (55,56).

Hypothermia decreases the number and function of circulating neutrophils. Although this effect of hypothermia increases the sensitivity to infections, it may also simultaneously reduce the severity of endotoxin-associated injury. In rats, hypothermia to 27°C decreases the neutrophil count, myeloperoxidase activity, and IL-1β level, and increases concentrations of the anti-inflammatory cytokine IL-10 in bronchoalveolar lavage fluid (57,58).

There are thus several routes by which hypothermia may reduce resistance to infection. Most importantly, hypothermia directly impairs neutrophil function and indirectly impairs function by triggering subcutaneous vasoconstriction, thereby reducing tissue oxygenation and oxidative killing by neutrophils. Hypothermia also decreases circulating neutrophil number and reduces concentrations of proinflammatory cytokines.

The first few hours following bacterial contamination constitute a decisive period during which infections are established (59). The effects of antibiotic administration or hypoperfusion are especially important during this period. Specifically, antibiotics limit infection when given within a couple of hours of bacterial inoculation, but are virtually worthless when given subsequently (59,60). Similarly, wound hypoperfusion achieved by epinephrine infiltration or "dehydration shock" aggravates test infections when induced up to 2.5 hr after the inoculation, but subsequently has no effect (59).

Clinical Outcomes

Consistent with the above observations, mild hypothermia reduces resistance to test infections in animals (61). In a multicenter, randomized study, a decrease of intraoperative core body temperature of only 1.9°C increased the incidence of surgical wound infections following colon resection by a factor of three (41). These were clinically important infections as indicated by the fact that the infected patients remained 1 week longer in the hospital. Interestingly, hypothermia also increased the duration of hospitalization by 20% even when infected patients were excluded from the analysis (41). This result might suggest that hypothermia per se interferes with the healing process and is consistent with the observation that collagen deposition (i.e., scar formation) was significantly reduced in the hypothermic patients. It is also consistent with studies by Carli et al. showing that mild hypothermia provokes postoperative protein wasting (62).

The deleterious effect of hypothermia on postoperative wound infections was confirmed by Melling et al. (63). In this randomized, blinded study, 421 patients undergoing clean surgery of short duration were assigned to routine care, preoperative whole body (systemic) warming, or preoperative warming of the surgical site. Prewarming reduced the infection rate from 14% in unwarmed patients to only 5% in all warmed patients (systemic or local; $P = 0.001$). The difference was still significant when unwarmed patients were compared to only the systemically warmed patients (14% vs. 6% infection rate,

$P = 0.026$). Although wound scores were also lower in the warmed group, the development of other wound complications, such as hematoma, seroma, and wounds requiring aspiration, did not differ between the groups. Curiously, the authors failed to report intraoperative core temperatures so the degree of hypothermia is difficult to estimate.

Despite the strong evidence showing the correlation between hypothermia and wound infections, respiratory infections have always been of greater interest during therapeutic hypothermia. Because the potential patient population receiving therapeutic hypothermia is generally critically ill, concerns about pneumonia are justified. A recent review article from the Cochrane Database reported that in moderate-to-severe head injury patients, mild hypothermia nearly doubled the incidence of pneumonia (OR: 1.95, 95% CI: 1.18–3.23) (64). An increased rate of pneumonia in severely head-injured patients subjected to mild hypothermia was also reported in an earlier retrospective study (65). Bernard et al. also reported a high rate of nosocomial pneumonia (45%) in their prospective cohort study (66). Although the findings from these studies are alarming, there are problems with the study designs. The first study (64) consisted only of a meta-analysis, whereas the second study (65) was retrospective. Finally, the cohort study did not include a control group (66). A recent outcome study from the Hypothermia after Cardiac Arrest Study Group showed only a nonsignificant difference in the pneumonia incidence in the hypothermic and normothermic groups (42). However, if the pneumonia and sepsis data are combined in this study, there is a statistically significant difference between the groups. Available data thus suggest that mild hypothermia is likely to promote pneumonia; however, the magnitude of the risk remains unclear and additional study is thus warranted.

Pharmacokinetics and Pharmacodynamics

Pharmacokinetics refers to the distribution and clearance of drugs; in contrast, pharmacodynamics refers to the physiologic effect of a given plasma concentration. Drug metabolism is a highly temperature-dependent function. It is therefore unsurprising that hypothermia alters the pharmacokinetics of many drugs (Table 3).

Background

Volatile Anesthetics

The solubility of volatile anesthetics increases in hypothermic patients (67). Interestingly, this does not alter anesthetic potency, which depends on partial pressure rather than tissue concentration; however, it may slow recovery from anesthesia as more anesthetic needs to be exhaled. But for a practical matter, volatile anesthetic washout rates appear to be similar in normothermic and hypothermic individuals (68). The minimum alveolar concentrations (MAC) of halothane and isoflurane in rats both decrease roughly 5% per °C reduction in core body temperature (69). Minimum alveolar concentration also varies with the circadian rhythm (70), which likely results from diurnal temperature fluctuations (71).

Muscle Relaxants and Neostigmine

Skeletal muscle shows a slight temperature sensitivity during drug-free conditions (72,73). However, the direct effects of hypothermia on muscle activity are probably of limited clinical importance. On the other hand, hypothermia extensively alters kinetics of numerous drugs, including muscle relaxants.

Vecuronium's duration of action is more than doubled in patients with a core body temperature of 34.5°C compared to those maintained at 36.5°C (74) (Fig. 5). In a subsequent study, it was shown that the first twitch amplitude and train-of-four ratio each decreased ≈20% for a °C reduction in adductor pollicis temperature (75). This reduction is clinically important. Hypothermic prolongation of vecuronium action results, by and large, via a pharmacokinetic effect, with only limited contribution from pharmacodynamic variation (76,77).

For example, hypothermia prolongs the duration of action of vecuronium by reducing clearance and the rate of effect-site equilibration. Plasma clearance of vecuronium decreased 11% per °C, and the rate constant for drug equilibration between

Table 3 Kinetic Effects of Hypothermia

Drug	N	ΔT_{core} (°C)[a]	Onset of effect	Duration of action	Recovery	Clearance	[Plasma]	Equilibration rate[b]	C–R slope[c]
Vecuronium (77)	12	3.0				Decreased		Decreased	Increased
Vecuronium (74)	20	2.0		Increased	Increased				
Vecuronium (76)	10	2.2	No change					No change	No change
Neostigmine (81)	7	2.0	Increased	No change		No change			
Morphine (83)	18 dogs	7.0				Decreased	Increased		
Fentanyl (82)	7 pigs	6.0					Increased		
Propofol (78)	6	3.0				Decreased	Increased		
Atracurium (78)	6	3.0		Increased					
Isoflurane, N_2O and fentanyl (85)	150	1.9			Increased				
Halothane and N_2O (86)	84[d]	3 max			No change				

[a] Difference in core body temperature between normothermic and hypothermic groups.
[b] Drug equilibration between plasma and effect site.
[c] Concentration–response relationship.
[d] Infants and children weighing <50 kg.

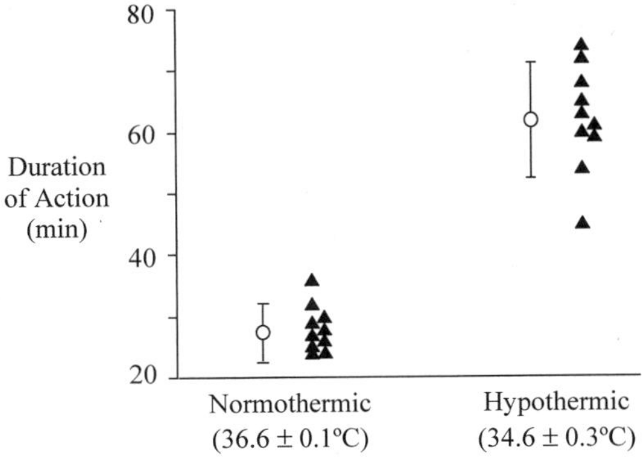

Figure 5 Duration of action of vecuronium in 10 normothermic (35.5 ± 0.1°C) and 10 mildly hypothermic (34.6 ± 0.4°C) patients. Duration of action was significantly prolonged during hypothermia. Data presented as mean ± SD. (Figure modified from Ref. 74; used by permission.)

plasma and the effect site was decreased about 0.023 min per °C (77). The decrease in plasma clearance (pharmacokinetics) with hypothermia results both from the decreased specific hepatic clearance of vecuronium and from an overall decrease in renal blood flow, which decreases clearance of all metabolites nonspecifically. However, as mentioned above, there was a slight decrease in pharmacodynamics resulting in slightly delayed equilibration of vecuronium between the circulation and the neuromuscular junction.

Atracurium duration depends less on core temperature than vecuronium: a 3°C reduction in core temperature increases the duration of muscle relaxation only by 60% (78). This reduced dependence on temperature most likely results because atracurium is partially degraded in plasma by an enzyme-independent mechanism that is presumably less temperature-dependent than enzymatic pathways. With both atracurium and vecuronium, the recovery index (time for 25–75% twitch recovery) remains normal during hypothermia. Rocuronium, a close pharmacological relative of vecuronium, has also decreased plasma clearance with hypothermia (79).

Additionally, its duration of action is prolonged during cardiac bypass surgery in hypothermic patients (80).

The efficacy of the neuromuscular blocking agents does not appear to be altered by hypothermia. Recently, it was shown in healthy human volunteers that the efficacy of neostigmine was not influenced by hypothermia to 34.5°C (81). Although the central volume of distribution decreased by 38% and the onset time for maximum effect was delayed for an additional minute compared to normothermia (36.5°C), neither the clearance nor the duration of action was altered.

Intravenous Sedatives

During a constant infusion, the plasma concentration of propofol is approximately 30% greater in volunteers maintained at 34°C than in those kept normothermic. This difference most likely results from reduced intercompartmental clearance between the deep and shallow compartments as mild hypothermia does not significantly alter hepatic blood flow (78). Hypothermia also increases steady-state plasma concentrations of fentanyl by about 5% per °C (82). The findings with muscle relaxants, propofol, and fentanyl suggest that hypothermia has substantial effects on the kinetics of many drugs. Data from animal studies are generally consistent with available human results and similarly demonstrate reduced drug clearance during hypothermia (83).

Clinical Outcomes

As hypothermia reduces the clearance rate of anesthetics, it is reasonable to expect prolonged sedation in the recovery phase of anesthesia in hypothermic patients. However, most of the studies that targeted recovery duration as an outcome suffer from major methodological flaws that preclude accurate interpretation of the results (84). Among the flaws were failures to randomize patients to normothermia or hypothermia, using inappropriate temperature monitoring sites (e.g., axilla), and allowing unblinded investigators to evaluate outcomes.

On the other hand, some prospective, randomized trials have explored the effects of mild perioperative hypothermia on operating room discharge criteria of adult and pediatric patients. Lenhardt et al. found that the recovery duration was prolonged in patients assigned to hypothermia even when core normothermia was not a discharge criterion in an adult patient population (85). Interestingly, similar prolongation of recovery duration was not observed in infants and children (86).

The clinical importance of temperature-induced pharmacokinetic and pharmacodynamic variation remains to be explored. However, it is likely that the substantial pharmacokinetic variations that have been identified apply equally in patients undergoing therapeutic hypothermia. Failure to adjust drug doses in hypothermic patients is thus likely to result in excessive plasma concentrations and toxicity. Considerably more work is required to identify the specific effects of temperature on the kinetics and action of drugs commonly used during therapeutic hypothermia.

Other Effects of Hypothermia

Shivering and Patient Comfort

Shivering is an involuntary, oscillatory muscular activity that augments metabolic heat production (see Chapter 1 for more background on the physiology of shivering). Shivering causes significant discomfort and metabolic stress. It also increases intraocular and intracranial pressures (87). Shivering can double oxygen consumption and carbon dioxide production; however, the increases are typically much smaller. It is frequently stated that these large increases in metabolic requirement might provoke clinical decompensation in patients with existing intrapulmonary shunts, fixed cardiac output, or limited respiratory reserve. However, there is little evidence to support these claims. Furthermore, shivering intensity is markedly reduced in elderly and frail patients (10); it thus seems unlikely that shivering itself provokes serious adverse outcomes in these patients. A variety of drugs can be used to suppress shivering, and, of course, muscle relaxants obliterate this response (see Chapter 8).

Even in the absence of shivering, mild hypothermia produces marked postoperative thermal discomfort (68). For example, Kurz et al. showed that mildly hypothermic patients felt unpleasantly cold, a sensation that persisted for more than 2 hr (88) (Table 1 and Fig. 6). Without adequate treatment to suppress thermoregulatory responses to shivering, surface cooling may thus be poorly tolerated. Maher and Hachinski induced mild hypothermia (34–36°C) with cooling blankets in 16 unanesthetized stroke patients; in five (31%), the treatment was stopped prematurely because of patient discomfort (89). Similarly, Zweifler and Sessler found that mild hypothermia induced by surface cooling in eight unsedated stroke patients was impractical because of shivering and vasoconstriction which were triggered at temperatures just below 37°C (90). Feeling cold in the immediate postoperative period is one of the most frequent complaints from unwarmed surgical patients and one that they remember vividly often for many years.

Pulmonary Complications

Mild hypothermia may contribute to pulmonary edema formation in postoperative patients (91). In a study of patients with peripheral vascular disease, those who arrived in the ICU with temperatures <35°C were more likely to have marginal oxy-

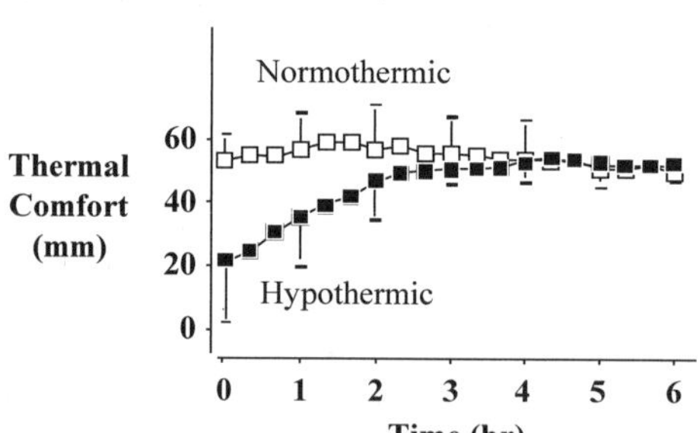

Figure 6 Hypothermic patients ($N = 35$, core temperature of 34.4 ± 0.4°C) reported feeling unpleasantly colder than the normothermic patients did ($N = 39$, core temperature of 37.0 ± 0.3°C); the sensation persisted for more than 2 hr. Data presented as mean ± SD. (Figure modified from Ref. 88; used by permission.)

genation (P_aO_2 <80% mm Hg) (16). Pulmonary edema has also been described as a complication of accidental hypothermia (92). Recently, it was shown that when oxygen, carbon dioxide, and water vapor pressures were corrected to body temperature, the alveolar–arterial oxygen tension difference increases during hypothermia (32.0°C) (93). The mechanism for hypothermia-associated pulmonary edema is unknown, but has been attributed to centrally mediated increases in pulmonary vascular permeability (3).

Metabolic Derangements

Decreasing body temperature lowers the basal metabolic rate by approximately 5% to 7% per °C (3). Hypothermia also shifts the hemoglobin–oxygen dissociation curve to the left, thus reducing oxygen availability. This may contribute to an uncompensated mild metabolic acidosis, which is commonly observed with hypothermia (23). A lower metabolic rate is associated with reduced CO_2 production, which leads to a respiratory alkalosis in vivo when patients are cooled and minute ventilation is unchanged, despite the fact that arterial blood gases measured at room temperature and not corrected for body temperature will show a normal pH (alpha-stat management, see Chapter 5). Mild intraoperative hypothermia also promotes protein catabolism and nitrogen loss after major surgical procedures (62).

Hypothermia shifts potassium intracellularly and predisposes patients to mild hypokalemia that is probable of marginal clinical importance (23,94). This shift is fully reversible with rewarming. Consequently, aggressive potassium replacement during hypothermia can lead to rebound hyperkalemia when patients are rewarmed (95). Hypophosphatemia and hypomagnesemia can also develop in hypothermic patients and may be the result of increased urinary output (96). Possibly, these electrolyte disturbances contribute to the propensity for cardiac arrhythmias during hypothermia (97). Hypothermia can also result in gastric ileus, elevated serum amylase and lipase concentrations, and hyperglycemia related to peripheral insulin resistance (3).

Clinical Monitoring

Reductions of core body temperature can alter somatosensory-evoked potentials (98) and slow conduction velocity measurements in patients undergoing neurophysiological studies. However, it would be unusual for either effect to interfere with interpretation of the results.

Pulse oximeter function is usually well maintained even in intensely vasoconstricted patients. Levinsohn et al. thus observed that the pulse oximeter cannot be used as an indicator of extremity flow, because it shows stable values until very low blood-flow rates (99). In rare cases where vasoconstriction resulting from the combination of hypothermia and vascular volume depletion obliterates the saturation signal, it can be restored by local warming or by a digital nerve block (100). Interestingly, thermoregulatory vasoconstriction per se slightly increases SaO_2, but the increase is too small to be clinically important (101).

FUTURE DIRECTIONS

Mild intraoperative hypothermia triples the risk of adverse myocardial outcomes, most of which are detected a day or two after surgery. It increases blood loss and augments allogeneic transfusion requirement by clinically important amounts. Less than a 2°C decrease in core body temperature triples the incidence of surgical wound infections following colon resection, prolongs recovery, and increases duration of hospitalization significantly. Hypothermia also increases blood loss and transfusion requirement. And finally, it markedly reduces drug metabolism. Available data further suggest that hypothermia increases the risk of pneumonia.

It is apparent from these studies that hypothermia causes numerous serious complications. To the extent that therapeutic hypothermia proves beneficial, those benefits will need to be balanced against hypothermia-induced complications. The potential adverse effects of hypothermia presumably can be minimized with meticulous critical care management with special attention to the systems at risk. Additional research is needed to develop and evaluate improved ICU management strategies for therapeutic hypothermia; areas of particular interest include antishivering medications, adequate sedation, good electrolyte management, and suitable prophylactic antibiotic protocols.

REFERENCES

1. Reuler JB. Hypothermia: pathophysiology, clinical settings, and management. Ann Int Med 1978; 89:519–527.
2. Chen RYZ, Chien S. Hemodynamic functions and blood viscosity in surface hypothermia. Am J Physiol 1978; 235:H136–H143.
3. Schubert A. Side effects of mild hypothermia. J Neurosurg Anesthiol 1995; 7:139–147.
4. Bay J, Nunn JF, Prys-Roberts C. Factors influencing arterial PO_2 during recovery from anaesthesia. Br J Anaesth 1968; 40:398–406.
5. Flacke JW, Flacke WE. Inadvertent hypothermia: frequent, insidious, and often serious. Semin Anesth 1983; 2:183–196.
6. Horvath SM, Spurr GB, Hutt BK, Hamilton LH. Metabolic cost of shivering. J Appl Physiol 1956; 8:595–602.
7. Guffin A, Girard D, Kaplan JA. Shivering following cardiac surgery: hemodynamic changes and reversal. J Cardiothorac Vasc Anesth 1987; 1:24–28.
8. Just B, Delva E, Camus Y, Lienhart A. Oxygen uptake during recovery following naloxone. Anesthesiology 1992; 76:60–64.
9. Kurz A, Plattner O, Sessler DI, Huemer G, Redl G, Lackner F. The threshold for thermoregulatory vasoconstriction during nitrous oxide/isoflurane anesthesia is lower in elderly than young patients. Anesthesiology 1993; 79:465–469.
10. Frank SM, Fleisher LA, Olson KF, Gorman RB, Higgins MS, Breslow MJ, Sitzmann JV, Beattie C. Multivariate determinants of early postoperative oxygen consumption in elderly patients. Anesthesiology 1995; 83:241–249.
11. Wagner JA, Robinson S, Marino RP. Age and temperature

regulation of humans in neutral and cold environments. J Appl Physiol 1974; 37:562–565.

12. Gautier H, Bonora M, Remmers JE. Effects of hypoxia on metabolic rate of conscious adult cats during cold exposure. J Appl Physiol 1989; 67:32–38.

13. Gautier H, Bonora M, Ben M'Barek S, Sinclair JD. Effects of hypoxia and cold acclimation on thermoregulation in the rat. J Appl Physiol 1991; 71:1355–1363.

14. Robinson KA, Haymes EM. Metabolic effects of exposure to hypoxia plus cold at rest and during exercise in humans. J Appl Physiol 1990; 68:720–725.

15. Iwashita H, Matsukawa T, Ozaki M, Sessler DI, Imamura M, Kumazawa T. Hypoxemia decreases the shivering threshold in rabbits anesthetized with 0.2 MAC isoflurane. Anesth Analg 1998; 87:1408–1411.

16. Frank SM, Beattie C, Christopherson R, Norris EJ, Perler BA, Williams GM, Gottlieb SO. Unintentional hypothermia is associated with postoperative myocardial ischemia. Anesthesiology 1993; 78:468–476.

17. Frank SM, Fleisher LA, Breslow MJ, Higgins MS, Olson KF, Kelly S, Beattie C. Perioperative maintenance of normothermia reduces the incidence of morbid cardiac events: a randomized clinical trial. JAMA 1997; 277:1127–1134.

18. Frank SM, Higgins MS, Breslow MJ, Fleisher LA, Gorman RB, Sitzmann JV, Raff H, Beattie C. The catecholamine, cortisol, and hemodynamic responses to mild perioperative hypothermia. Anesthesiology 1995; 82:83–93.

19. Greif R, Laciny S, Rajek A, Doufas AG, Sessler DI. Blood pressure response to thermoregulatory vasoconstriction during isoflurane and desflurane anesthesia. Acta Anaesthesiol Scand, 2003; 47:847–852.

20. Frank SM, El-Gamal N, Raja SN, Wu PK. Alpha-adrenoceptor mechanisms of thermoregulation during cold challenge in humans. Clin Sci 1996; 91:627–631.

21. Okada M. The cardiac rhythm in accidental hypothermia. J Electrocardiol 1984; 17:123–128.

22. Freysz M, Timour Q, Mazze R, Bertrix L, Cohen S, Samii K, Faucon G. Potentiation by mild hypothermia of ventricular conduction disturbances and reentrant arrhythmias induced by bupivicaine in dogs. Anesthesiology 1989; 70:799–804.

23. Boelhouwer RU, Bruining HA, Ong GL. Correlations of serum potassium fluctuations with body temperature after major surgery. Crit Care Med 1987; 15:310–312.

24. Bjornstad H, Tande PM, Refsum H. Cardiac electrophysiology during hypothermia. Implications for medical treatment. Arctic Med Res 1991; 50(suppl 6):71–75.

25. Nesher N, Zisman E, Wolf T, Sharony R, Bolotin G, David M, Uretzky G, Pizov R. Strict thermoregulation attenuates myocardial injury during coronary artery bypass graft surgery as reflected by reduced levels of cardiac-specific troponin I. Anesth Analg 2003; 96:328–335.

26. Bernard SA, Gray TW, Buist MD, Jones BM, Silvester W, Gutteridge G, Smith K. Treatment of comatose survivors of out-of-hospital cardiac arrest with induced hypothermia. N Engl J Med 2002; 346:557–563.

27. Valeri RC, Cassidy G, Khuri S, Feingold H, Ragno G, Altschule MD. Hypothermia-induced reversible platelet dysfunction. Ann Surg 1987; 205:175–181.

28. Michelson AD, MacGregor H, Barnard MR, Kestin AS, Rohrer MJ, Valeri RC. Reversible inhibition of human platelet activation by hypothermia in vivo and in vitro. Thromb Haemost 1994; 71:633–640.

29. Valeri CR, Khabbaz K, Khuri SF, Marquardt C, Ragno G, Feinhold H, Gray AD, Axford T. Effect of skin temperature on platelet function in patients undergoing extracorporeal bypass. J Thorac Cardiovasc Surg 1992; 104:108–116.

30. Khuri S, Wolfe JA, Josa M, Axford TC, Szymanski I, Assousa S, Ragno G, Patel M, Silverman A, Park M, Valeri CR. Hematologic changes during and after cardiopulmonary bypass and their relationship to the bleeding time and nonsurgical blood loss. J Thorac Cardiovasc Surg 1992; 104:94–107.

31. Bunker JP, Goldstein R. Coagulation during hypothermia in man. Proc Soc Exp Biol Med 1958; 97:199–202.

32. Rohrer M, Natale A. Effect of hypothermia on the coagulation cascade. Crit Care Med 1992; 20:1402–1405.

33. Reed L, Johnston TD, Hudson JD, Fischer RP. The disparity between hypothermic coagulopathy and clotting studies. J Trauma 1992; 33:465–470.

34. Kettner SC, Kozek SA, Groetzner JP, Gonano C, Schellongowski A, Kucera M, Zimpfer M. Effects of hypothermia on thrombelastography in patients undergoing cardiopulmonary bypass. Br J Anaesth 1998; 80:313–317.

35. Schmied H, Kurz A, Sessler DI, Kozek S, Reiter A. Mild intraoperative hypothermia increases blood loss and allogeneic transfusion requirements during total hip arthroplasty. Lancet 1996; 347:289–292.

36. Schmied H, Schiferer A, Sessler DI, Maznik C. The effects of red-cell scavenging, hemodilution, and active warming on allogeneic blood requirement in patients undergoing hip or knee arthroplasty. Anesth Analg 1998; 86:387–391.

37. Winkler M, Akça O, Birkenberg B, Hetz H, Scheck T, Arkilic CF, Kabon B, Marker E, Grubl A, Czepan R, Greher M, Goll V, Gottsauner-Wolf F, Kurz A, Sessler DI. Aggressive warming reduces blood loss during hip arthroplasty. Anesth Analg 2000; 91:978–984.

38. Widman J, Hammarqvist F, Sellden E. Amino acid infusion induces thermogenesis and reduces blood loss during hip arthroplasty under spinal anesthesia. Anesth Analg 2002; 95:1757–1762.

39. Johansson T, Lisander B, Ivarsson I. Mild hypothermia does not increase blood loss during total hip arthroplasty. Acta Anaesthesiol Scand 1999; 43:1005–1010.

40. Persson K, Lundberg J. Perioperative hypothermia and postoperative opioid requirements. Eur J Anaesthesiol 2001; 18:679–686.

41. Kurz A, Sessler DI, Lenhardt RA and Study of wound infections and temperature group. Perioperative normothermia to reduce the incidence of surgical-wound infection and shorten hospitalization. N Engl J Med 1996; 334:1209–1215.

42. The Hypothermia after Cardiac Arrest Study Group. Mild

therapeutic hypothermia to improve the neurologic outcome after cardiac arrest. N Engl J Med 2002; 346:549–556.

43. Clifton GL, Allen S, Barrodale P, Plenger P, Berry J, Koch S, Fletcher J, Hayes RL, Choi SC. A phase II study of moderate hypothermia in severe brain injury. J Neurotrauma 1993; 10:263–271.

44. Resnick DK, Marion DW, Darby JM. The effect of hypothermia on the incidence of delayed traumatic intracerebral hemorrhage. Neurosurgery 1994; 34:252–256.

45. Mackowiak PA. Direct effects of hyperthermia on pathogenic microorganisms: teleologic implications with regard to fever. Rev Infect Dis 1981; 3:508–520.

46. Sessler DI, Olofsson CI, Rubinstein EH. The thermoregulatory threshold in humans during nitrous oxide-fentanyl anesthesia. Anesthesiology 1988; 69:357–364.

47. Sheffield CW, Sessler DI, Hopf HW, Schroeder M, Moayeri A, Hunt TK, West JM. Centrally and locally mediated thermoregulatory responses alter subcutaneous oxygen tension. Wound Rep Reg 1997; 4:339–345.

48. Hopf HW, Hunt TK, West JM. Wound tissue oxygen tension predicts the risk of wound infection in surgical patients. Arch Surg 1997; 132:997–1005.

49. Greif R, Akça O, Horn E-P, Kurz A, Sessler DI. Outcomes Research™ Group. Supplemental perioperative oxygen to reduce the incidence of surgical wound infection. N Engl J Med 2000; 342:161–167.

50. Farkas LG, Bannantyne RM, James JS, Umamaheswaran B. Effect of two different climates on severely burned rats infected with *Pseudomonas aeruginosa*. Eur Surg Res 1974; 6:295–300.

51. Saririan K, Nickerson DA. Enhancement of murine in vitro antibody formation by hyperthermia. Cell Immunol 1982; 74:306–312.

52. Van Oss CJ, Absolam DR, Moore LL, Park BH, Humbert JR. Effect of temperature on the chemotaxis, phagocytic engulfment, digestion and O_2 consumption of human polymorphonuclear leukocytes. J Reticuloendothel Soc 1980; 27:561–565.

53. Leijh CJ, Van den Barselaar MT, Van Zwet TL, Dubbelde-

man-Rempt I, Van Furth R. Kinetics of phagocytosis of *Staphylococcus aureus* and *Escherichia coli* by human granulocytes. Immunology 1979; 37:453–465.

54. Wenisch C, Narzt E, Sessler DI, Parschalk B, Lenhardt R, Kurz A, Graninger W. Mild intraoperative hypothermia reduces production of reactive oxygen intermediates by polymorphonuclear leukocytes. Anesth Analg 1996; 82:810–816.

55. Hohn DC, MacKay RD, Halliday B, Hunt TK. The effect of oxygen tension on the microbicidal function of leukocytes in wound and in vitro. Surg Forum 1976; 27:18–20.

56. Mader JT. Phagocytic killing and hyperbaric oxygen: antibacterial mechanisms. HBO Rev 1982; 2:37–49.

57. Sarcia PJ, Scumpia PO, Moldawer LL, DeMarco VG, Skimming JW. Hypothermia induces interleukin-10 and attenuates injury in the lungs of endotoxemic rats. Shock 2003; 20:41–45.

58. Lim CM, Sun Kim M, Ahn JJ, Kim MJ, Kwon Y, Lee I, Koh Y, Kim DS, Kim WD. Hypothermia protects against endotoxin-induced acute lung injury in rats. Intensive Care Med 2003; 29:453–459.

59. Burke JF. The effective period of preventive antibiotic action in experimental incisions and dermal lesions. Surgery 1961; 50:161–168.

60. Classen DC, Evans RS, Pestotnik R, Horn SD, Menlove RL, Burke JP. The timing of prophylactic administration of antibiotics and the risk of surgical wound infection. N Engl J Med 1992; 326:281–286.

61. Sheffield CW, Sessler DI, Hunt TK. Mild hypothermia during isoflurane anesthesia decreases resistance to *E. coli* dermal infection in guinea pigs. Acta Anaesthesiol Scand 1994; 38:201–205.

62. Carli F, Emery PW, Freemantle CAJ. Effect of preoperative normothermia on postoperative protein metabolism in elderly patients undergoing hip arthroplasty. Br J Anaesth 1989; 63:276–282.

63. Melling AC, Ali B, Scott EM, Leaper DJ. Effects of preoperative warming on the incidence of wound infection after

clean surgery: a randomized controlled trial. Lancet 2001; 358:876–880.

64. Gadkary CS, Alderson P, Signorini DF. Therapeutic hypothermia for head injury. Cochrane Database Syst Rev, 2002; 1:CD001048.

65. Ishikawa K, Tanaka H, Shiozaki T, Takaoka M, Ogura H, Kishi M, Shimazu T, Sugimoto H. Characteristics of infection and leukocyte count in severely head-injured patients treated with mild hypothermia. J Trauma 2000; 49:912–922.

66. Bernard SA, Mac CJB, Buist M. Experience with prolonged induced hypothermia in severe head injury. Crit Care (Lond) 1999; 3:167–172.

67. Zhou JX, Liu J. The effect of temperature on solubility of volatile anesthetics in human tissues. Anesth Analg 2001; 93:234–238.

68. Sessler DI, Rubinstein EH, Moayeri A. Physiological responses to mild perianesthetic hypothermia in humans. Anesthesiology 1991; 75:594–610.

69. Eger EI II, Johnson BH. MAC of I-653 in rats, including a test of the effect of body temperature and anesthetic duration. Anesth Analg 1987; 66:974–976.

70. Halberg J, Halberg E, Halberg F, Munson E. Chronobiologic monitoring and analysis for anesthesiologists: another look at a chronoanesthetic index. In: Puly JE, Scheving LE, eds. Advances in Chronobiology, Part B. New York: Alan R. Liss, Inc., 1985:315–322.

71. Sessler DI, Lee KA, McGuire J. Isoflurane anesthesia and circadian temperature cycles. Anesthesiology 1991; 75:985–989.

72. Heier T, Caldwell JE, Sessler DI, Kitts JB, Miller RD. The relationship between adductor pollicis twitch tension and core, skin and muscle temperature during nitrous oxide-isoflurane anesthesia in humans. Anesthesiology 1989; 71:381–384.

73. Heier T, Caldwell JE, Sessler DI, Miller RD. The effect of local surface and central cooling on adductor pollicis twitch tension

during nitrous oxide/isoflurane and nitrous oxide/fentanyl anesthesia in humans. Anesthesiology 1990; 72:807–811.

74. Heier T, Caldwell JE, Sessler DI, Miller RD. Mild intraoperative hypothermia increases duration of action and spontaneous recovery of vecuronium blockade during nitrous oxide-isoflurane anesthesia in humans. Anesthesiology 1991; 74:815–819.

75. Heier T, Caldwell JE, Eriksson LI, Sessler DI, Miller RD. The effect of hypothermia on adductor pollicis twitch tension during continuous infusion of vecuronium in isoflurane-anesthetized humans. Anesth Analg 1994; 788:312–317.

76. Heier T, Caldwell JE, Sharma ML, Gruenke LD, Miller RD. Mild intraoperative hypothermia does not change the pharmacodynamics (concentration–effect relationship) of vecuronium in humans. Anesth Analg 1994; 78:973–977.

77. Caldwell JE, Heier T, Wright PMC, Lin S, McCarthy G, Szenohradzky J, Sharma ML, Hing JP, Schroeder M, Sessler DI. Temperature-dependent pharmacokinetics and pharmacodynamics of vecuronium. Anesthesiology 2000; 92:84–93.

78. Leslie K, Sessler DI, Bjorksten AR, Moayeri A. Mild hypothermia alters propofol pharmacokinetics and increases the duration of action of atracurium. Anesth Analg 1995; 80:1007–1014.

79. Beaufort AM, Wierda JM, Belopavlovic M, Nederveen PJ, Kleef UW, Agoston S. The influence of hypothermia (surface cooling) on the time–course of action and on the pharmacokinetics of rocuronium in humans. Eur J Anaesthesiol Suppl 1995; 11:95–106.

80. Smeulers NJ, Wierda JM, van den Broek L, Gallandat Huett RC, Hennis PJ. Effects of hypothermic cardiopulmonary bypass on the pharmacodynamics and pharmacokinetics of rocuronium. J Cardiothorac Vasc Anesth 1995; 9:700–705.

81. Heier T, Clough D, Wright PM, Sharma ML, Sessler DI, Caldwell JE. The influence of mild hypothermia on the pharmacokinetics and time course of action of neostigmine in anesthetized volunteers. Anesthesiology 2002; 97:90–95.

82. Fritz HG, Bauer R, Walter B, Moeritz K-U, Reinhart K. Effects of hypothermia (32°C) on plasma concentration of fentanyl in piglets (abstract). Anesthesiology 1999; 91:A444.

83. Bansinath M, Turndord H, Puig M. Influence of hypo and hyperthermia on disposition of morphine. J Clin Pharmacol 1988; 28:860–864.

84. Hines R, Barash PG, Watrous G, O'Connor T. Complications occurring in the postanesthesia care unit: a survey. Anesth Analg 1992; 74:503–509.

85. Lenhardt R, Marker E, Goll V, Tschernich H, Kurz A, Sessler DI, Narzt E, Lackner F. Mild intraoperative hypothermia prolongs postoperative recovery. Anesthesiology 1997; 87:1318–1323.

86. Bissonnette B, Sessler DI. Mild hypothermia does not impair postanesthetic recovery in infants and children. Anesth Analg 1993; 76:168–172.

87. Rosa G, Pinto G, Orsi P, De Blasi RA, Conti G, Sanita R, La Rosa I, Gasparetto A. Control of post anaesthetic shivering with nefopam hydrochloride in mildly hypothermic patients after neurosurgery. Acta Anaesthesiol Scand 1995; 39:90–95.

88. Kurz A, Sessler DI, Narzt E, Bakar A, Lenhardt R, Huemer G. Postoperative hemodynamic and thermoregulatory consequences of intraoperative core hypothermia. J Clin Anesth 1995; 7:359–366.

89. Maher J, Hachinski VC. Mild hypothermia in acute cerebral ischemia: a feasibility study [abstr]. Can J Neurol Sci 1993; 20(suppl 4):549.

90. Zweifler RM, Sessler DI. Thermoregulatory vasoconstriction and shivering impede therapeutic hypothermia following acute ischemic stroke. J Stroke Cerebrovasc Dis 1997; 6:152.

91. Bloch M. Cerebral effects of rewarming following prolonged hypothermia: significance for the management of severe cranio-cerebral injury and acute pyrexia. Brain 1967;90769–784.

92. Moralews CF. Noncardiogenic pulmonary edema associated with accidental hypothermia. Chest 1993; 103:971–973.

93. Hansen D, Syben R, Vargas O, Spies C, Welte M. The alveolar–arterial difference in oxygen tension increases with temperature-corrected determination during moderate hypothermia. Anesth Analg 1999; 88:538–541.

94. Bruining HA, Boelhouwer RU. Acute transient hypokalaemia and body temperature. Lancet 1982; 2:1283–1284.

95. Koht A, Cane R, Cerullo LJ. Serum potassium levels during prolonged hypothermia. Intensive Care Med 1983; 9:275–277.

96. Polderman KH, Peerdeman SM, Girbes AR. Hypophosphatemia and hypomagnesemia induced by cooling in patients with severe head injury. J Neurosurg 2001; 94:697–705.

97. Polderman KH, Girbes AR. Therapeutic hypothermia after cardiac arrest. N Engl J Med 2002; 347:63–65.

98. Reynolds PC, Antoine JA, Bettencourt J, Starck TW. Regional hypothermia affects somatosensory evoked potentials. Anesth Analg 1991; 73:653–656.

99. Levinsohn DG, Gordon L, Sessler DI. The Allen's test: analysis of four methods. J Hand Surg [Am] 1991; 16A:279–282.

100. Paulus DA, Monroe MC. Cool fingers and pulse oximetry (letter). Anesthesiology 1989; 71:168–169.

101. Hynson JM, Sessler DI, Belani K, Washington D, McGuire J, Merrifield B, Schroeder M, Moayeri A, Crankshaw D, Hudson S. Thermoregulatory vasoconstriction during propofol/nitrous oxide anesthesia in humans: threshold and SpO_2. Anesth Analg 1992; 75:947–952.

7

Complications of Rewarming

THORSTEN STEINER, FABIAN MEISEL, and STEPHAN A. MAYER

University of Heidelberg, Im Neuenheimer Feld, Heidelberg, Germany

BACKGROUND

The rewarming process may well constitute the most critical period of risk related to therapeutic hypothermia (1). Studies on the use of hypothermia in patients with brain injury or stroke have reported a high frequency of side effects related not only to cooling, but also to rewarming. Indeed, beginning with Fay's pioneering studies of hypothermia for metastatic carcinoma conducted in the 1940s and 1950s, it was noted that the majority of fatalities occurred either during or within 24 hr of the completion of rewarming (17 of 19 fatalities among 124 treated patients) (2).

As discussed later in this chapter, the most common problem during rewarming is that vasodilation reduces blood pressure. Additional data suggest that in patients who are rewarmed too rapidly, a syndrome compatible with systemic inflammatory response syndrome (SIRS) can develop. Although warming-related hypotension may be well tolerated in patients who lack intracranial pathology and have intact cerebral autoregulation, fatal "rebound" brain edema and increased intracranial pressure (ICP) have been described in stroke and trauma patients treated with hypothermia. This represents the most serious complication related to rewarming after therapeutic hypothermia.

Many other complications have been observed during rewarming. However, it remains unclear if they simply reflect a delayed effect of the initial cooling period, or whether they result from the core temperature increase per se. Another major problem in understanding complications of rewarming is the relative lack of reliable human data: most of our knowledge about physiological changes during hypothermia and rewarming is based on animal research. Finally, because hypothermia in a clinical setting cannot easily be administered locally to the brain (see Chapter 11, "Direct Brain Cooling"), most of our understanding of the physiology of rewarming is based on systemic hypothermia, which involves an interplay of both cerebral and extracerebral side effects.

REVIEW

Methods of Rewarming

Therapeutic hypothermic can be divided into three phases (Fig. 1): phase 1 (induction) is followed by phase 2 (sustaining of the target temperature). After withdrawal of the device used to actively cool the body, phase 3 (rewarming) ensues. This process is finished when a normal body temperature of 37.0°C is reached.

Depending on the clinical scenario and the depth of hypothermia, different rewarming procedures may be employed. In general, rewarming is understood as being pas-

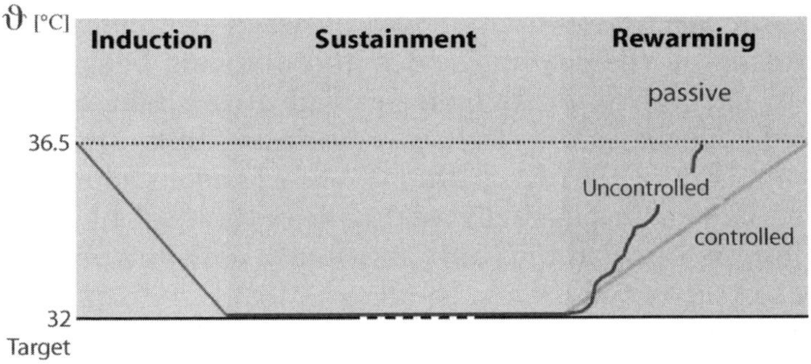

Figure 1 Different phases during hypothermia.

sive or active. Active rewarming refers to the practice of directly applying heat to normalize body temperature after induced hypothermia. Active rewarming is commonly used in the operating room to reduce postoperative shivering. Postoperative shivering is related to reductions in body temperature that can occur with general anesthesia; it can lead to subjective discomfort, strain on the surgical incision, and myocardial ischemia related to increased myocardial oxygen demand (3).

The most common methods used to rewarm patients after mild intraoperative hypothermia rely on peripheral warming devices, such as forced-air convection, heating blankets, circulating water-warming blankets, and infrared heating lamps. With such methods, the rate of intraoperative surface rewarming is approximately 0.7 °C/hr and depends inversely on body surface area (3). Active rewarming to ward off shivering in this setting is generally felt to be desirable. However, when reversing deeper levels of therapeutic hypothermia in patients with cerebral pathology, there is reasonably good evidence that active rewarming can be dangerous and should be avoided. For example, in a primate model of middle cerebral infarction treated with moderate hypothermia, active rewarming with heating blankets consistently resulted in hypotension, rebound brain edema, ICP elevation, and death (4).

Passive rewarming refers to the practice of allowing body temperature to normalize without the application of a heating device. In our experience, the application of uncontrolled passive rewarming in human stroke patients—analogous to simply turning off the cooling device and allowing body temperature to normalize on its own—can also result in severe cerebral side effects, mainly rebound brain swelling and ICP overshooting (Fig. 2). When a human body is cooled down to 32°C, it will rewarm passively within less than 24 hr after active cooling is interrupted, and, in some cases, this process can take as little as 6–8 hr.

An alternative to uncontrolled passive rewarming is controlled passive rewarming. This technique involves a gradual "tapering off" of active cooling. The cooling device remains active, but the target body temperature is gradually increased in small increments, resulting in a slow increase in body temperature (Fig. 1). Although controlling this process may be safer than uncontrolled passive rewarming, the optimal rewarming period and the rate of reversal still remain uncertain. Among the small numbers of clinical studies available, the rewarming schedule has varied between 4 hr and 5 days.

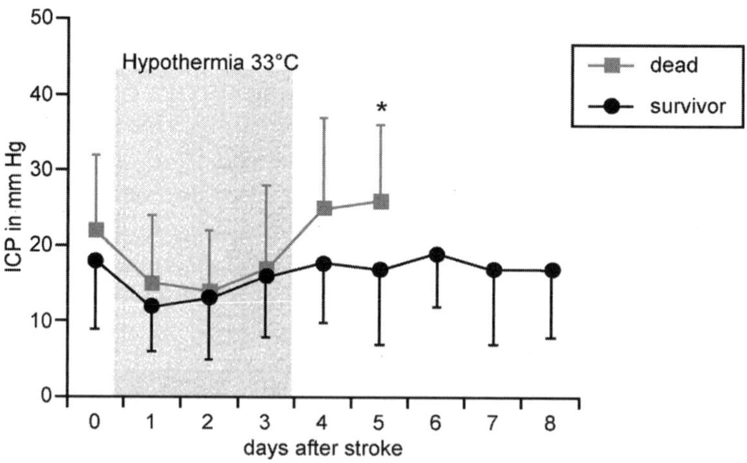

Figure 2 Time course of daily maximum ICP values in patients with MCA infarction treated with hypothermia who survived and those who subsequently died. $*P < 0.05$. ICP values were significantly higher among nonsurvivors during and after the rewarming period. (From Ref. 3.)

The stepwise rewarming rates commonly used vary between 0.1°C/hr and 0.5°C/hr.

A final approach is controlled rewarming, but at a very slow rate such as 0.05–0.1°C/hr. Several devices now offer this level of control and may well prove to be the safest and easiest approach.

Cerebral Side Effects

Rewarming after mild to moderate hypothermia (32–34°C) presents a challenge to clinicians caring for patients treated with therapeutic hypothermia in the ICU setting. Rebound increases of ICP and hyperthermic overshoot are the major concerns.

Rebound Edema and ICP Elevation

Human Studies

In a series of pioneering studies conducted in the 1960s, Bloch (5) was the first to document elevations in ICP during rewarming after moderate hypothermia in humans. In these experiments, 71 episodes of prolonged cooling (30–198 hr at 29–33°C) were induced in 25 conscious, unanesthesized patients who were treated with radiation therapy under hypothermic conditions following decompressive craniotomy. Rewarming was controlled with intermittent cooling in 10 instances, passive cooling in 50, and active (using electric heating blankets) cooling in 11 cases. In the majority of cases (90%), rewarming was associated with a reduction in level of consciousness (lethargy or stupor), which was most severe and prolonged in those who were maintained at hypothermia for longer periods, or who underwent active rewarming. Lumbar cerebrospinal fluid (CSF) pressure was examined during and after cooling in 30 cases and was increased during rewarming in half; these ICP elevations coincided with changes in level of consciousness (Fig. 3).

Although rapid deterioration during rewarming had been described previously, these observations were the first to directly implicate rebound brain edema during rewarming

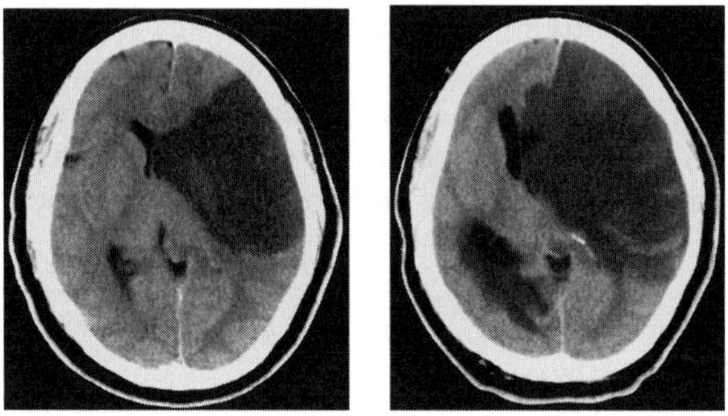

Figure 3 Rebound edema and infarct extension in a 55-year-old man with left middle cerebral infarction treated with hypothermia (33°C for 24 hr). Left panel: computed tomography (CT) obtained 55 hr after stroke onset and 4 hr prior to cooling, at the time of deterioration to stupor. Right panel: CT obtained 95 hr after the onset of cooling, demonstrating postrewarming rebound cerebral edema with extension of infarction involving the left anterior cerebral artery and posterior MCA territories, profound midline shift, and trapping of the contralateral ventricle with transependymal edema. The condition subsequently progressed to brain death. (Courtesy of Dr. Stephan A. Mayer.)

after hypothermia. Earlier studies had simply identified the rewarming phase as a period of high risk. In 1958, Lazorthes and Campan reported the use of hypothermia in 47 comatose patients with severe traumatic brain injury (TBI), and they found that 10 deteriorated abruptly and died immediately after rewarming (6). In 1960, Walsh (7) reported a similar experience, stating that "...even after prolonged hypothermia, the patient's condition may again deteriorate when the temperature is allowed to rise."

More recent studies have shown that during the cooling period, the effect of hypothermic treatment on elevated ICP is beneficial. Intracranial pressure control with hypothermia has been well described in trauma and middle cerebral artery (MCA) infarction patients (see Chapters 13 and 14) (8–11). However, these studies have also confirmed that rewarming can lead to a secondary increase in ICP, which requires additional therapy. In some cases, ICP levels higher than the initial values have been observed (8,11,12). In the first study on the use of hypothermia in patients with malignant MCA infarction reported by Schwab et al. (8), 5 of 11 patients who died had uncontrollable intracranial hypertension during rewarming (45%). Moreover, mean ICP values overall were significantly greater (25 vs. 18 mm Hg) and cerebral perfusion pressure (CPP) values were less (56 vs. 78 mm Hg) in those who died than in those who survived. A follow-up multicenter study of 50 patients with large hemispheric stroke revealed that of the 19 patients who died, 15 (79%) died during or immediately after rewarming, and all were related to brain edema and herniation (12). Importantly, a shorter period of rewarming (<16 hr) was associated with higher posttreatment ICP levels. Thus it seems possible to avoid ICP overshooting by performing rewarming in a slow and controlled fashion.

Steiner et al. (13) studied 13 patients during controlled rewarming. This was achieved by predefining the speed of temperature rise in steps of 0.1–0.2°C every 2–4 hr. This range was chosen because of the limits of the technical equipment at that time. To slow passive rewarming, the cooling blanket was intermittently switched off and on, just before a patient had reached the aimed target temperature. Compared with 10 patients in whom rewarming took place passively in an uncontrolled fashion, controlled rewarming led to a significant prolongation of rewarming. The mean duration of controlled rewarming was 59 hr (26–88 hr) compared to 24 hr or less in patients in whom rewarming was administered passively. Controlled rewarming led to a significant decrease of fluctuations of ICP and CPP. Nonetheless, two patients died of ICP overshooting and the number of infectious complications was high: 12 of 13 patients developed pneumonia, 3 developed sepsis syndrome, and 1 developed pancreatitis; all except one of these complications were reversible. The number of patients was too small to draw any conclusion on mortality rate or neurological outcome. However, it was sufficient to show that controlled rewarming may be used to decrease the problem of ICP overshooting during rewarming.

Today, controlled rewarming is much easier to perform with intravascular or surface cooling systems that employ temperature feedback systems. These systems automatically adjust the cooling temperature of the device to maintain a predetermined core temperature of the patient (see Chapter 10). The main concern regarding ICP increases during rewarming is to maintain a sufficient CPP. The importance of maintaining CPP levels of at least 60–70 mm Hg to prevent secondary increases in ICP (plateau waves) in neurocritical care patients is widely accepted. There is good evidence to suggest that this should apply both during and after the application of therapeutic hypothermia. In an experimental study in cats, Aoki et al. (14) demonstrated that CPP levels of <60 mm Hg during rewarming caused relative ischemia. Moreover, it is known from studies of deep hypothermic circulatory arrest that metabolic needs may outstrip oxygen delivery at various temperatures during rewarming (15). These lines of evidence suggest that CPP insufficiency might be one of the crucial factors for neurological deterioration during the rewarming period.

Abnormal cerebral autoregulation might enhance the susceptibility of the brain to ischemic injury related to decreases in CPP during rewarming. Metz et al. (16) found no correlation between changes in CBF and cerebral metabolic rate of oxygen ($CMRO_2$) in trauma patients treated with hypothermia (33°C), suggesting an uncoupling of CBF and metabolism. By contrast, the presence of intact pressure autoregulation may place patients with low CPP and marginal perfusion at risk for compensatory vasodilation, which can lead to increases in cerebral blood volume and ICP (the vasodilatory cascade model). Despite some conflicting evidence, cerebral autoregulation during hypothermia and rewarming has been found to be preserved in most studies of animals and humans (17,18) (see Chapter 5).

The fact that ICP increases after therapeutic hypothermia suggests that hypothermia only temporarily delays the deleterious effects of brain swelling after stroke or trauma. In a large study of TBI patients, Clifton et al. (9) found no benefit on outcome when cooling was initiated within 6 hr of injury.

Several factors have been identified to explain the negative results of this study (see Chapter 13 for further discussion). One of the more intriguing aspects of these is the observation that mean CPP was mildly, but significantly, less in hypothermic patients on the day of rewarming than in the normothermic ones.

Not all studies have found a relationship between rewarming and cerebral complications after hypothermia. Diephuis et al. (19) examined the effect of rewarming on cerebral blood flow (CBF) in cardiopulmonary bypass surgery. No difference was seen between slow and rapid rewarming regarding CBF levels. This may reflect the fact that rebound cerebral edema or ischemia may be more likely to occur in brain-injured patients than in those with normal brain physiology.

Animal Studies

Animal research aiming to evaluate the influence of hypothermia and rewarming on CBF was first undertaken by Michenfelder and Theye (20) and Steen et al. (21). In their seminal 1968 study, Michenfelder and Theye found that 48 hr of moderate hypothermia (29°C) was consistently lethal in primates subjected to MCA infarction due to massive cerebral edema and other systemic complications, which occurred within 3 hr of the initiation of active rewarming (20). The animals developed uncontrolled pressor-resistant hypotension and, at necropsy, had hemorrhagic pulmonary edema, a syndrome suggestive of SIRS and adult respiratory distress syndrome.

In later studies, Steen et al. (4,21) similarly described cardiovascular collapse and severe tissue hypoxia with acidosis coincident with active rewarming with heat lamps and heating blankets over 2–3 hr in primates and cats subjected to 24 hr of moderate (29°C) hypothermia. Hemodynamic measurements demonstrated a marked increase in systemic vascular resistance during cooling, which failed to normalize during rewarming; this was associated with inadequate and inhomogeneous perfusion of both brain and skeletal muscles. The investigators further noted that CBF did not rise as extensively as the cerebral metabolic rate for oxygen during rewarming, with consequent depletion of brain energy stores [adenosine triphosphate (ATP)]. Similar findings indicating that active rewarming from moderate hypothermia can lead to hypotension, rebound brain edema, and death have been reported in dogs (22) and rats (23). It was on the basis of these observations that Steen et al. (4) first proposed the concept of passive controlled rewarming as a means to reduce the deleterious effects of hypothermia and rewarming.

Temperature Regulation After Rewarming

After peripheral rewarming of hypothermic patients, both a hyperthermic overshoot and a temperature afterdrop may develop. Hayward et al. studied cardiovascular physiological changes in humans subjected to cold-water immersion, followed by one of three methods of rewarming (external bath rewarming, warm air inhalation, and passive rewarming). External rewarming resulted in the most rapid rate of temperature increase, as well as a postrewarming temperature afterdrop of 0.5–0.7 °C, which was associated with moderate decreases in blood pressure and peripheral vascular resistance (24). In a follow-up study (25), they found that inhibition of shivering with meperidine both prolonged the duration of rewarming and increased the degree of postrewarming afterdrop (1.1 °C vs. 0.4 °C). This observation indicates that shivering-related heat production both potentiates rewarming and attenuates the core temperature afterdrop that occurs after active rewarming. Patients rendered hypothermic intraoperatively, even to a mild degree, appear to be at increased risk for postrewarming temperature afterdrops. This has been attributed to thermoregulatory vasoconstriction, which limits the ability of surface techniques such as forced-air warming to effectively transfer heat between body compartments (3).

In other scenarios, temperature overshoot may occur after rewarming. Krieger et al. (26) reported the occurrence of fever after controlled rewarming in 3 of 10 patients cooled to 33 °C for ischemic stroke. They concluded that this was most likely due to the underlying disease or an underlying febrile response to infection, rather than a side effect of hypothermia or the rewarming process per se. Postrewarming hyperthermia can also occur after a period of afterdrop hypothermia. Baker et al. (27) compared postoperative body temperature in patients undergoing craniotomy who were treated with normothermic and hypothermic management and found that the hypothermic patents had significantly lower temperatures upon arrival at the ICU (35.8°C vs. 37.1°C), yet had slightly higher temperatures 10–12 hr thereafter. When hypothermia is induced clinically, close monitoring and control of body temperature are just as important after rewarming as they are during the cooling period.

Extracerebral Side Effects of Rewarming

Infection Risk

Because systemic hypothermia and rewarming affect the entire body, extracerebral as well as cerebral side effects can occur. Pneumonia is probably the most common and important extracerebral side effect of therapeutic hypothermia (see Chapter 6). In a meta-analysis of hypothermia treatment for TBI, cooling was associated with a 95% increase in the odds ratio for pulmonary infection (28). Several authors have suggested that rewarming is an even bigger risk factor for developing pneumonia than cooling per se. Schwab et al. (8) reported pneumonia in 10 of 25 stroke patients undergoing hypothermia, and most of them (60%) developed pneumonia during rewarming. Similar data were published by Metz et al. (11), who found pneumonic lung infiltration in 50% of hypothermic TBI patients, with most cases (80%) diagnosed during rewarming. It is unclear, however, whether more gradual controlled rewarming can reduce the frequency of pneumonia. Even very slow controlled rewarming is associated with frequent pulmonary infection, perhaps because slow rewarming prolongs the total duration of hypothermia (13).

A general concern in the critical care unit is the development of bloodstream infections. Hypothermic patients are not only vulnerable to focal infections such as pneumonia, but also to bacteremia and sepsis syndrome. In 25 stroke patients undergoing hypothermia, for example, sepsis developed in seven (8).

Cardiopulmonary Effects

Nonuniform cooling or rewarming may also cause regional heterogeneity of conduction, action potential duration, and refractory periods of the heart. This favors unidirectional conduction block and reentrant dysrhythmias (29,30). Although serious cardiac rhythm disturbances such as atrial and ventricular fibrillations occur most frequently when patients are cooled to levels below 30 °C, there is some evidence that these complications can also occur during rewarming (29). This again underlines the potential importance of controlled rewarming. Hypothermia and rewarming can cause an elevation of catecholamine serum levels. This may potentially cause cardiac arrhythmia, hypertension, and myocardial ischemia (30). Responsiveness to catecholamines during hypothermia and rewarming may be reduced (3), which may in turn aggravate hypotension related to peripheral vasodilatation during rewarming, as described in humans (24) and dogs (21).

In the pioneering studies of Bloch on astrocytoma patients, florid pulmonary edema was described during rewarming from mild hypothermia in a small number of cases (5). This effect was attributed to a central mechanism and may reflect vasodilation and changes in vascular permeability of the pulmonary microcirculation.

Hematologic Effects

Hypothermia-induced coagulation disorders include reversible platelet sequestration and dysfunction, enhanced fibrinolytic activity, and slowing of enzymatic activity required for clotting (31). Little data exist on how coagulation is affected by rewarming after hypothermia. In neonatal cold injury, rewarming deaths have been attributed to hyperaggregation of platelets and resultant massive thrombosis (19). In hypothermic stroke (8,12) and TBI (16) patients, decreased platelet counts developed during hypothermia, and this suppression was sustained during and after rewarming.

Basal Metabolism and Electrolyte Balance

Metabolic needs during rewarming may outstrip oxygen delivery at various temperatures (15). This might be due to a systemic hypermetabolic response, as has been described after hypothermic cardiopulmonary bypass surgery (32). In this study, the authors found that basal metabolic rate peaked during maximum spontaneous rewarming after anesthesia. Similarly, Rodriguez et al. (33) demonstrated that postoperative oxygen consumption increases during rewarming, and they related this finding to shivering. Finally, mild hypothermia shifts potassium intracellularly and predisposes the patient to hypokalemia, as well as hypocalcemia, hypomagnesemia, and hypophosphatemia. During rewarming, rebound increases of these electrolytes may occur, particularly if they are replaced excessively during the cooling period (34).

FUTURE DIRECTIONS

Based on promising results in animal models of stroke and TBI (Chapter 4) and the positive findings of induced hypothermia in human clinical trials after cardiac arrest (Chapter 15), the clinical application of hypothermia in the emergency department and ICU is likely to become increasingly common. Although the feasibility of systemic cooling has been demonstrated, one major problem remaining relates to our ability to control complications related to this procedure. Considerable evidence suggests that rewarming represents the critical period of risk for brain-injured patients treated with hypothermia. Our lack of understanding of how rewarming leads to cerebral and extracerebral complications, and how these complications can be controlled, is a major issue that continues to hamper our ability to induce hypothermia as safely as possible.

More randomized clinical studies are needed to evaluate the physiological effects of hypothermia and rewarming. The optimal method and time frame for hypothermic treatment and the rewarming period have not yet been determined. Based on our current understanding from animal and clinical studies, hypothermia should start as soon as possible after the onset of injury. However, the optimal length and depth of hypothermic treatment and the following rewarming period remain unclear. In rats, prolonged hypothermia after transient focal ischemia has a greater benefit on outcome than brief hypothermia (35). The critical question that remains is whether these benefits outweigh the risk of complications that might result from a longer period of cooling.

A large body of evidence indicates that only controlled rewarming should be applied to patients treated with mild to moderate hypothermia, at rates in the range from 0.1°C/hr to 0.2°C/hr (13). Rapid passive rewarming appears to harm the patient and probably worsens neurological outcome. Active rewarming from moderate hypothermia with external heating has been associated with disastrous outcomes in animals (4,20,21) and humans (5), and should be avoided at nearly all costs in brain-injured patients who are treated with hypothermia. Patients with normal brain physiology who are recovering from anesthesia-related hypothermia remain the primary exception to this rule.

The appearance and severity of side effects related to hypothermia and rewarming need to be better elucidated. It is not fully understood whether side effects during the rewarming process are related to increasing body temperature, or if they constitute a delayed effect of hypothermic treatment. Careful physiological studies should help to shed light on this important area of therapeutic hypothermia.

REFERENCES

1. Harris OA, Colford JM, Good MC, Matz PG. The role of hypothermia in the management of severe brain injury. A meta-analysis. Arch Neurol 2002; 59:1077–1083.
2. Fay T. Early experiences with local and generalized refrigeration of the human brain. J Neurosurg 1959; 16:239–260.
3. Schubert A. Side effects of mild hypothermia. J Neurosurg Anesthesiol 1995; 7:139–147.

4. Steen PA, Soule EH, Michenfelder JD. Detrimental effect of prolonged hypothermia in cats and monkeys with and without regional cerebral ischemia. Stroke 1979; 10:522–529.

5. Bloch M. Cerebral side effects of rewarming following prolonged hypothermia: significance for the management of severe cranio-cerebral injury and acute pyrexia. Brain 1967; 90:769–784.

6. Lazorthes G, Campan L. Hypothermia in the treatment of craniocerebral traumatism. J Neurosurg 1958; 15:162–168.

7. Walsh LS. In: Cooper KE, Ross DN, eds. Hypothermia in Surgical Practice. London: Cassell, 1960:76.

8. Schwab S, Schwarz S, Spranger M, Keller E, Bertram M, Hacke W. Moderate hypothermia in the treatment of patients with severe middle cerebral artery infarction. Stroke 1998; 29:2461–2466.

9. Clifton GL, Miller ER, Choi SC, Levin HS, McCauley S, Smith KR, Muizelaar JP, Wagner FC, Marion DW, Luerssen TG, Chestnut RM, Schwartz M. Lack of effect of induction of hypothermia after acute brain injury. N Engl J Med 2001; 344:556–563.

10. Marion DW, Penrod LE, Kelsey SFK, Obrist WD, Kochanek PM, Palmer AM, Wisniewski SR, DeKosy ST. Treatment of traumatic brain injury with moderate hypothermia. N Engl J Med 1997; 336:540–546.

11. Metz C, Holzschuh M, Bein T, Woertgen C, Frey A, Frey I, Taeger K, Brawanski A. Moderate hypothermia in patients with severe head injury: cerebral and extracerebral effects. J Neurosurg 1996; 85:533–541.

12. Schwab S, Georgiadis D, Berrouschot J, Schellinger PD, Graffagnino C, Mayer SA. Feasibility and safety of moderate hypothermia after massive hemispheric infarction. Stroke 2001; 32:2033–2035.

13. Steiner T, Friede T, Aschoff A, Schellinger P, Schwab S, Hacke W. Effect and feasibility of controlled rewarming after moderate hypothermia in stroke patients with malignant infarctions of the middle cerebral artery. Stroke 2001; 32:2833–2835.

14. Aoki A, Mori K, Maeda M. Adequate cerebral perfusion pres-

sure during rewarming to prevent ischemic deterioration after therapeutic hypothermia. Neurol Res 2002; 24:271–278.

15. Ausman JI, McCormick PW, Stewart M, Lewis G, Dujovny M, Balakreshnan G, Malik GM, Ghaly RF. Cerebral oxygen metabolism during hypothermic circulatory arrest in humans. J Neurosurg 1993; 79:810–815.
16. Metz C, Holzschuh M, Bein T, Woertgen C, Frey A, Frey I, Taeger K, Brawanski A. Moderate hypothermia in patients with severe head injury: cerebral and extracerebral effects. J Neurosurg 1996; 85:533–541.
17. Verhaegen MJ, Todd MM, Hindman BJ, Warner DS. Cerebral autoregulation during moderate hypothermia in rats. Stroke 1993; 24:407–414.
18. Georgiadis D, Schwarz S, Evans DH, Schwab S, Baumgartner RW. Cerebral autoregulation under moderate hypothermia in patients with acute stroke. Stroke 2002; 33:3026–3032.
19. Diephuis JC, Balt J, Van Dijk D, Moons KGM, Knape JTA. Effect of rewarming speed during hypothermic cardiopulmonary bypass on cerebral pressure–flow relation. Acta Anaesthesiol Scand 2002; 46:283–288.
20. Michenfelder JD, Theye RA. Hypothermia: effects of anesthesia and hypothermia on canine brain and whole-body metabolism. Anesthesiology 1968; 30:1107–1112.
21. Steen PA, Milde JH, Michenfelder JD. The detrimental effects of prolonged hypothermia and rewarming in the dog. Anesthesiology 1980; 52:224–230.
22. Blair E, Montgomery AV, Swan H. Post-hypothermia circulatory failure: I. Physiologic observations on the circulation. Circulation 1956; 13:909–915.
23. Popovic V. Lethargic hypothermia in hibernators and nonhibernators. Ann NY Acad Sci 1959; 80:320–331.
24. Hayward JS, Eckerson JD, Kemma D. Thermal and cardiovascular changes during three methods of resuscitation from mild hypothermia. Resuscitation 1984; 11:21–23.
25. Giesbrecht GG, Goheen MS, Johnston CE, Kenny GP, Bristow GK, Hayward JS. Inhibition of shivering increases core

temperature afterdrop and attenuates rewarming in hypothermic humans. J Appl Physiol 1997; 83:1630–1634.

26. Krieger DW, De Georgia MA, Abou-Chebl A, Andrefsky JC, Sila CA, Katzan IL, Mayberg MR, Furlan AJ. Cooling for acute ischemic brain damage (Cool Aid). An open pilot study of induced hypothermia in acute ischemic stroke. Stroke 2001; 32:1847–1854.
27. Baker KZ, Young WL, Stone JG, Kader A, Baker CJ, Solomon RA. Deliberate mild intraoperative hypothermia for craniotomy. Anesthesiology 1994; 81:361–367.
28. Gadkary CS, Alderson P, Signorini DF. Therapeutic hypothermia for head injury (Cochrane Review). In: The Cochrane Library. Issue 4. Oxford: Update Software, 2002.
29. Cohen IJ. Room-temperature ADP-induced first stage hyperaggregation of human platelets: the cause of rewarming deaths by thrombocytopenia in neonatal cold injury. Pediatr Hematol Oncol 1991; 8:61–67.
30. MacKenzie MA, Aengevaeren WR, Hermus AR, Van Der Werf T, Pieters GF, Smals AG, Kloppenborg PW. Electrocardiographic changes during steady mild hypothermia and normothermia in patients with poikilothermia. Clin Sci 1992; 82:39–45.
31. Rohrer MJ, Natale AM. Effect of hypothermia on the coagulation cascade. Crit Care Med 1992; 20:1402–1405.
32. Chiara O, Giomarelli PP, Biagioli B, Rosi R, Gattinoni L. Hypermetabolic response after hypothermic cardiopulmonary bypass. Crit Care Med 1987; 15:995–1000.
33. Rodriguez J, Weissman C, Damask MC. Physiological requirements during rewarming; suppression of the shivering response. Crit Care Med 1983; 11:490–497.
34. Polderman KH, Peerdeman SM, Girbes ARJ. Hypophosphatemia and hypomagnesemia induced by cooling in patients with severe head injury. J Neurosurg 2001; 94:853–858.
35. Aronowski J, Strong R, Grotta JC. Reperfusion injury: demonstration of brain damage produced by reperfusion after transient focal ischemia in rats. J Cereb Blood Flow Metab 1997; 17:1048–1056.

8

Defeating Thermoregulatory Defenses Against Hypothermia

DANIEL I. SESSLER

Outcomes Research™ Institute
and Department of Anesthesiology
and Perioperative Medicine,
University of Louisville,
Louisville, Kentucky, U.S.A.

BACKGROUND

As detailed in Chapter 4, there is overwhelming animal evidence that mild hypothermia provides marked protection against hypoxia and ischemia in numerous tissues (1–4). Available human data are encouraging and suggest that mild hypothermia will prove protective in at least some conditions (5,6). However, the extent to which hypothermia becomes a valued therapeutic option will depend on the clinician's ability to rapidly and safely reduce core body temperature.

Various factors complicate induction of hypothermia. First is choosing a suitable thermal manipulation device, recognizing that the most effective ones (7) are generally more invasive and, therefore, more prone to complications than surface methods (8). The second is preventing or moderating the physiological consequences of hypothermia per se, including reduced resistance to infection (9) and coagulopathy (10). Issues related to complications of hypothermia and rewarming are explored in Chapters 6 and 7, respectively.

The third aspect of inducing therapeutic hypothermia, and perhaps the most challenging, is defeating thermoregulatory defenses that normally maintain core temperature. The reason that defeating thermoregulatory defenses is so important is that these responses are both highly effective in resisting any attempt to cool and potentially harmful in some patients. The reason that they are difficult to defeat is that core temperature is a fundamental parameter in mammals and is maintained by numerous independent and redundant systems. This chapter will thus focus on the efficacy and consequences of defense activation, along with methods to defeat or moderate thermoregulatory defenses.

REVIEW

Thermoregulatory Defenses

Thermoregulatory control is among the phylogenetically oldest physiological functions and is well developed in all mammals. Core temperature is also remarkably well maintained by behavioral responses in reptiles and fish (11). Induction of therapeutic hypothermia is thus complicated both by the efficacy of thermoregulatory defenses and because activation of these defenses may, per se, be harmful in some patients. In this section, I will review both issues.

Efficacy of Defenses

Behavior

Normally, the most important thermoregulatory defense against hypothermia is behavioral compensation, which includes seeking shelter and warmth. Without behavioral defenses, the range of environments in which humans could live would be considerably restricted. Behavioral thermoregulation is mediated by thermal discomfort. That is, conscious recognition that a given environment is too warm or too cold is followed by volitional actions to moderate the environment. Behavioral thermoregulation can thus be defeated by drugs that restrict people's ability to sense or response to their thermal environment. Accidental hypothermia, for example, is often associated with alcohol intoxication (12). However, even substantial doses of alcohol only slightly impair autonomic thermoregulation (13), whereas intoxication markedly reduces the efficacy of behavioral responses. Thus inadequate behavioral defenses are primarily responsible for the hypothermia that so often accompanies intoxication.

The efficacy of behavioral thermoregulatory defenses can be nearly completely defeated simply by preventing patients from modifying their thermal environments. An example of this would be restricting patients to a hospital bed and insisting on the use of cooling devices. Such maneuvers, though, will not prevent thermal discomfort, which can be intense. (Postoperative patients often remember hypothermia as being more uncomfortable than surgical pain.) Discomfort may even lead patients to withdraw authorization for hypothermic treatment (14).

Vasoconstriction

The primary autonomic defenses against cold are arteriovenous shunt vasoconstriction and shivering. The threshold (triggering core temperature) for vasoconstriction is 1°C greater than for shivering. Vasoconstriction is the first autonomic defense against hypothermia and is typically activated numerous times each day as people move to slightly cooler environments. Unlike the other two major autonomic thermoregulatory defenses, sweating and shivering, vasoconstriction does not cost the body in terms of fluid or energy. The normal threshold for vasoconstriction is $\approx 36.5°C$ (15).

Thermoregulatory vasoconstriction occurs in arteriovenous shunts, which are 100-μm diameter vessels located primarily in the fingers and toes. Thermoregulatory vasomotion alters fingertip flow roughly 10-fold (Fig. 1). The gold standard

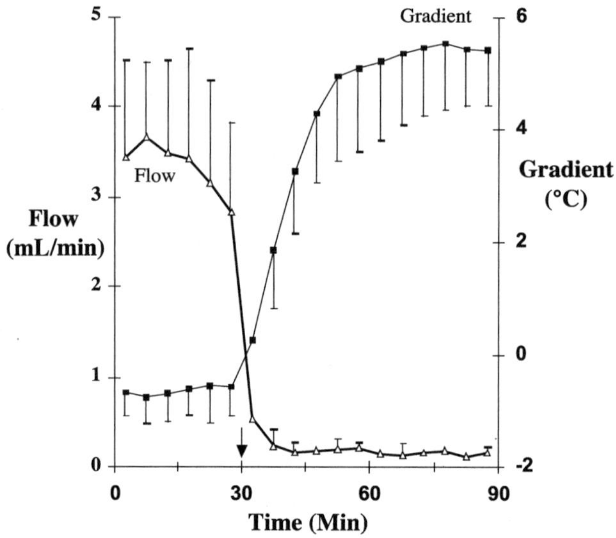

Figure 1 Changes in fingertip blood flow and skin-surface temperature gradients (forearm minus fingertip temperature) before and after thermoregulatory vasoconstriction was triggered at 30 elapsed min by infusion of cold saline (arrow). Fingertip blood flow decreased ≈10-fold within a few minutes and continued to decrease for an additional 5–10 min. Skin-temperature gradients also increased to ≥0°C (a value that defines vasoconstriction) within a few minutes. Results are presented as means ± S.D.s. (From Ref. 18.)

for quantifying flow is volume plethysmography (16). This method does not require sophisticated equipment, but is relatively tricky to perform. Fortunately, flow can be accurately estimated by simply subtracting fingertip skin temperature from forearm temperature (17). Values exceeding 0°C indicate vasoconstriction.

Despite the limited distribution of arteriovenous shunts, shunt vasomotion has substantial thermoregulatory effects. As one might expect, thermoregulatory vasoconstriction reduces cutaneous heat loss. Although there is a major regional decrease in the distal extremities, these areas constitute a relatively small fraction of the body surface area. Nonetheless, heat loss does decrease throughout the extremities—including the proximal segments—because the entire limb cools when shunt flow is obliterated. In contrast, heat loss from the trunk decreases only slightly (Fig. 2). The overall reduction in heat loss that results from thermoregulatory vasoconstriction is ≈25% (18), which is similar to that provided by a single layer of most any insulator (19). Whereas reducing heat loss by one-fourth is not trivial, it may be less important than the other effect of vasoconstriction: altering flow and distribution of heat within the body.

Unlike core temperature, which is maintained within a few tenths of a degree Celsius (15), peripheral tissue temperature is allowed to fluctuate by many degrees Celsius. The

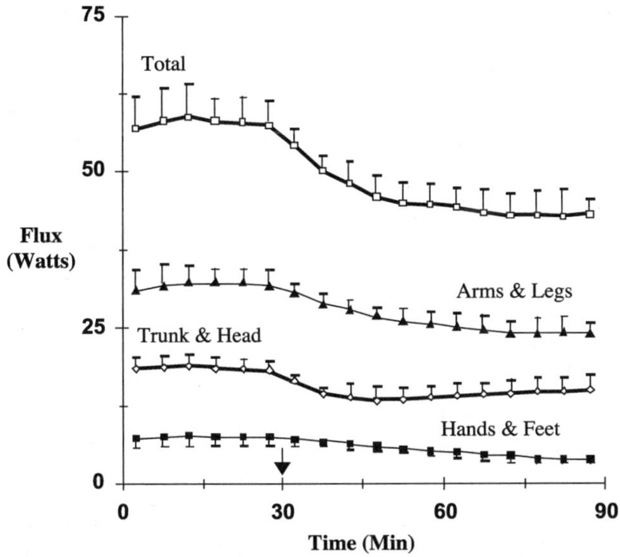

Figure 2 Cutaneous heat flux (heat loss) from the head and trunk (head, back, chest, and abdomen), legs and arms (upper arm, lower arm, thigh, and calf), and hands and feet. Total heat flux and flux from the arms and legs decreased ≈25% after vasoconstriction was triggered by infusion of cold fluid at 30 elapsed min (arrow). Heat loss from the trunk and head decreased only 17%. In contrast, loss from the hands and feet decreased ≈50%. Heat losses indicated in the lower three curves (Arms & Legs, Trunk & Head, and Hands & Feet) comprise the Total loss indicated at the top of the Figure. Results are presented as means ± S.D.s. (From Ref. 18.)

amount of variation depends on ambient temperature, conduction–convection of heat within the body, and the efficacy of thermoregulatory vasoconstriction. But in practice, the core-to-peripheral tissue-temperature gradient ranges from $-4°C$ to $+4°C$ in fairly extreme environments such as during active surface warming or cooling (20). The peripheral thermal compartment thus serves to buffer the core. There is considerable teleological value in this arrangement because during transitions from a warm to cool environment, or the reverse, peripheral tissues can dissipate or absorb heat—often for many hours—before activating the more costly responses such as sweating or shivering. The peripheral thermal compartment is about half the body mass (about 35 kg in a typical adult) (21). Since the specific heat of humans is roughly 0.83 kcal kg^{-1} $°C^{-1}$(22), each degree centigrade change in the peripheral compartment temperature dissipates or absorbs 29 kcal. What this means is that the body heat content can, at least transiently, vary by more than 200 kcal without altering core temperature.

Shivering

Shivering, in contrast to vasoconstriction, is a "last-resort" response that is activated only when behavioral responses and vasoconstriction fail to maintain an adequate core temperature. The normal threshold for shivering is $\approx 35.5°C$ (15). Nonshivering thermogenesis in brown adipose tissue augments metabolic rate only slightly (23,24), if at all (25), in adult humans. Shivering can transiently increase metabolic rate four- or five-fold (26). However, sustained shivering roughly doubles metabolic rate (27), and even that intensity can only be maintained for a limited time. Shivering usually starts in the pectoralis muscles, but most shivering thermogenesis occurs in the extremities where the largest muscles are located. The muscular activity of shivering does not perform any work, so all expended energy is converted into heat. The process is thus thermodynamically efficient. However, the ability of shivering thermogenesis to protect core temperature is limited by two factors. The first is that active muscle must be supplied with oxygen and metabolic substrates, both of which are conveyed by blood. This need for blood flow in distal muscles counteracts the efforts of vasoconstriction to constrain metabolic heat to the core thermal compartment and thus establish a large core-to-peripheral tissue-temperature gradient. The second limitation of shivering is that most heat is generated peripherally—and thus easily dissipated to the environment. The physiology and pharmacology of shivering has been reviewed recently (28).

Consequences of Defense Activation

A major purpose of thermoregulatory vasoconstriction is to isolate core tissues from the environment and thus restrict peripheral-to-core heat transfer. Normally, this is beneficial because it limits dissipation of metabolic heat, which is largely generated in the core, to peripheral tissues and from there to the environment. In the context of active warming or cooling, though, thermoregulatory vasoconstriction slows transfer of heat from the skin surface to the core by trapping heat in peripheral tissues (Fig. 3) (29).

The clinical importance of vasoconstriction insulating the core and restricting heat transfer to the core thermal compartment depends largely on where heat transfer occurs. Its importance can be substantial, though, when heat exchange is attempted through the skin surface. Under the best of circumstances (i.e., perfect intercompartmental flow of heat), peripheral tissues must be heated or cooled at least as much as the core. But in the presence of effective vasoconstriction, peripheral tissues must be heated or cooled far more than core tissues (29). A further complication is that cutaneous cooling activates the thermoregulatory system, thus aggravating vasoconstriction. Intravascular heat exchangers, in contrast, remove or transfer heat directly with the core thermal compartment. They thus may not only transfer more heat than available surface systems, but also exchange heat directly with the core—therefore bypassing the need to first modulate peripheral tissue temperature.

An obvious consequence of shivering is increased metabolic rate. This increase, which is analogous to exercise, pro-

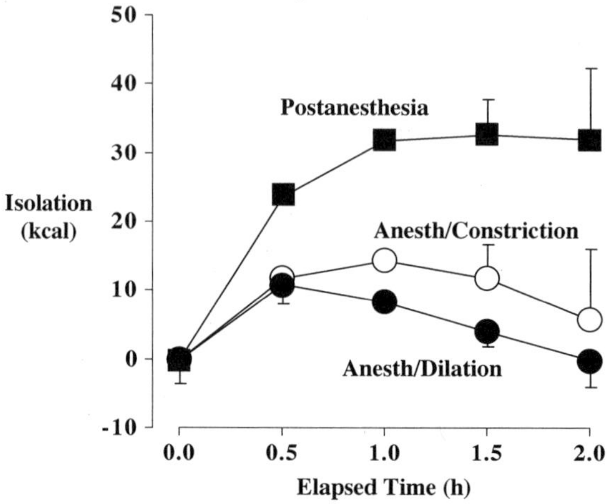

Figure 3 This figure illustrates the amount of heat that is trapped in peripheral tissues of volunteers who were actively warmed with forced air at 43°C (started at elapsed time zero). When the volunteers were unanesthetized ("Postanesthesia"), more than 30 kcal was trapped in peripheral tissues, meaning that core temperature was a full degree Celsius cooler than would have been expected based on systemic heat balance. In contrast, little heat was trapped peripherally during anesthesia, and the constraint was transient. Interestingly, it made little difference whether arteriovenous shunts were constricted ("Anesth/Constriction") or dilated ("Anesth/Dilation") during anesthesia, presumably because general anesthetics dilate arterioles and other vessels. Although constraint of applied heat is illustrated here, a similar delay in peripheral-to-core heat transfer would be observed with active surface cooling. Results are presented as means ± S.D.s. (From Ref. 29.)

vokes a substantial adrenergic response. For example, a reduction in core temperature of only 0.7°C increases norepinephrine concentration by 400% and oxygen consumption by 30%. When core temperature decreases 1.3°C, norepinephrine concentration increases 700% and oxygen consumption doubles. As might be expected, shivering is associated with peripheral vasoconstriction and hypertension—although heart rate remains unchanged, as do plasma epinephrine and cortisol concentrations (30).

It is difficult to provoke shivering in vasodilated patients because the vasoconstriction threshold usually exceeds the shivering threshold by a full degree centigrade (15). By contrast, it is easy to induce vasoconstriction without shivering, either by maintaining core temperature between the two thresholds or by blocking shivering with muscle relaxants. In fact, much of the hemodynamic response associated with shivering actually results from thermoregulatory vasoconstriction. Thermoregulatory vasoconstriction, for example, increases mean arterial pressure 14 $\pm$ 5 (S.D.) mm Hg even without shivering (Fig. 4) (31). Consistent with this theory, morbid postoperative myocardial events caused by hypothermia are not associated with shivering and appear, instead, to result from the adrenergic and hemodynamic responses to vasoconstriction (32). It thus seems likely that vasoconstriction, which is the primary defense against hypothermia in humans, is also the proximal cause for most of the hypertensive and hormonal response to hypothermia.

Induction of Thermoregulatory Tolerance

Nonpharmacological Treatments

An alternative to pharmacological treatment of shivering is surface warming. For example, Sweney et al. (33) recently reported that focal hand warming suppresses shivering in mildly hypothermic volunteers. The same group also reported that shivering can be suppressed by warming of the lower face combined with inhalation of heated and humidified air (34). Others have also reported that facial warming reduces shivering (35), as does radiant heating of the face and upper chest (36–38). However, the face and arms are only a small portion of the total skin surface. As might thus be expected, isolated hand or face warming only trivially reduces the shivering threshold (Fig. 5) (39). The difficulty with these observations is that treatments reducing the shivering threshold only a couple tenths of a degree centigrade (40) may be effective in volunteers or postoperative patients (41,42), but completely inadequate for the induction of therapeutic hypothermia.

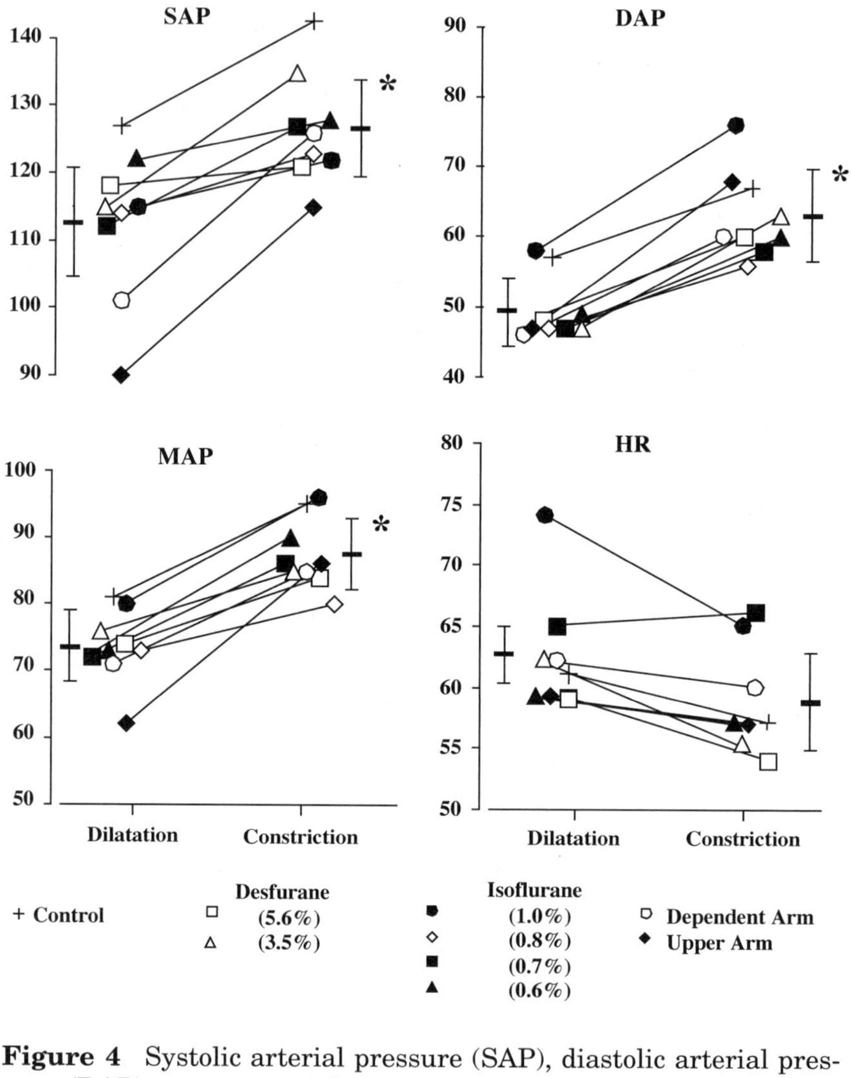

Figure 4 Systolic arterial pressure (SAP), diastolic arterial pressure (DAP), mean arterial pressure (MAP), and heart rate (HR) before and after vasoconstriction. Each symbol represents one group of study subjects without anesthesia or with various concentrations of isoflurane or desflurane. Data are represented as means of the individual studies, with the average and standard deviations for the entire study population also shown. Asterisks (*) identify statistically significant differences from vasodilatation ($P < 0.001$). (From Ref. 31.)

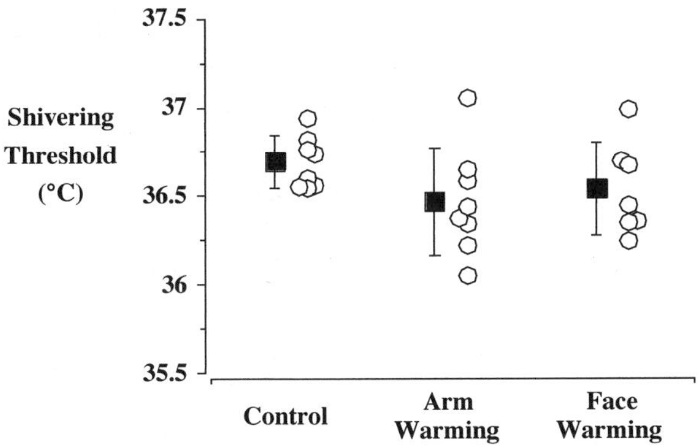

Figure 5 Individual values (○) for the shivering thresholds without warming, with arm and hand warming, and with facial and airway warming. Means (■) ± S.D.s for each day are also indicated. The thresholds did not differ significantly on the 3 treatment days. The shivering threshold was higher in this study than it usually is because skin temperature was controlled to 31°C, which is about 3°C less than normal. (From Ref. 39.)

Skin temperature contributes about 20% to autonomic control of shivering, with the remainder being derived from core temperature (43). Nonetheless, the 20% contribution of skin temperature to thermoregulatory control suggests that autonomic responses to direct core cooling (as with intervascular heat exchangers) can be moderated by simultaneous cutaneous warming. For example, a 4°C increase in mean skin temperature compensates for 1°C of core hypothermia (43). The difficulty, of course, is that warming systems that can maintain high skin temperatures eventually transfer considerable heat to the core. Nonetheless, this strategy has been used with considerable success in clinical trials, although simultaneous pharmacological intervention was required.

Fever is a special type of *regulated* hyperthermia that synchronously increases all thermoregulatory response thresholds. Fever thus represents an increase in the body's temperature set point. Fever is common among patients with neurological injury and is associated with worsened outcome from stroke (44), although fever probably improves infectious outcomes (45). Fever is unusual among medical syndromes in that it is better understood on a molecular than a clinical level. Little is known about appropriate management of fever because human research has been confounded by the sporadic onset, variable magnitude, and unpredictable duration of fever. Consequently, optimal treatment strategies for fever have yet to be established.

The first- and second-line treatments for fever are amelioration of the underlying cause and administration of antipyretic medications. The first treatment strategy often fails because the etiology of fever remains unknown; alternatively, the source may be known but unresponsive. The second strategy also often fails or is only partially effective, perhaps because some fever is mediated by mechanisms that bypass conventional antipyretics (46). The third-line treatment, active cooling, is especially likely to be used in these patients.

Although active cooling of febrile patients makes intuitive sense, it is often either ineffective or counterproductive. This is principally because the febrile target set by the hypothalamus is in terms of mean body temperature, not core temperature. Weighted mean body temperature (for thermoregulatory purposes) is a linear combination of core and skin temperatures, with the skin contributing ≈20% (43). Decreasing skin temperature 4°C will thus increase the target core temperature ≈1°C. In intact patients, thermoregulatory defense is more powerful than most types of surface cooling. The result is that active cooling fails to reduce core temperature (Fig. 6), but does make patients highly uncomfortable, increases plasma catecholamine concentrations, augments metabolic rate, and provokes hypertension (47).

The situation is very different, though, in patients with impaired thermoregulatory control—whether from disease or pharmacological intervention. [Even moderate strokes usually do not impair much thermoregulatory control (14).] In patients with restricted thermoregulatory defenses, surface cooling is an effective treatment for fever (48,49).

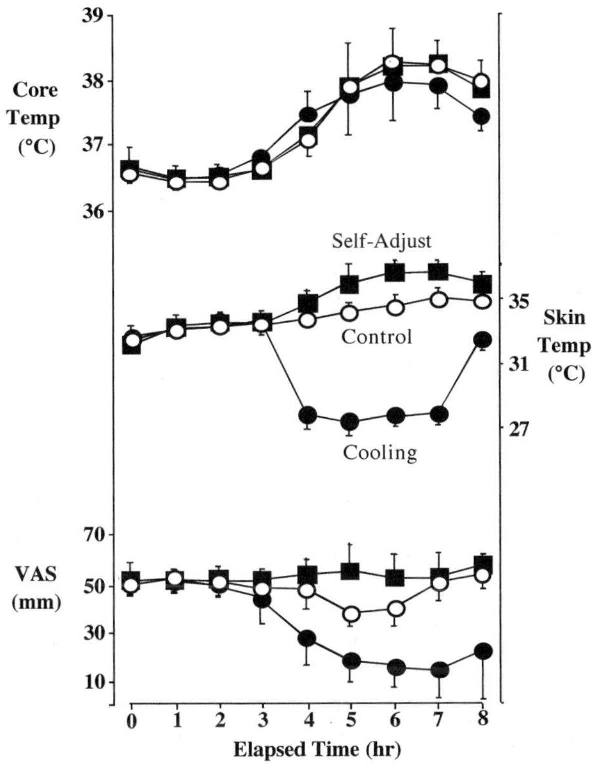

Figure 6 Change in core and skin temperature and thermal comfort after fever was induced by administration of interleukin-2, starting at elapsed time zero. The designated thermal management started after 3 elapsed hr and continued for 5 hr. This consisted of no treatment (control), self-adjustment per the subjects' comfort (self-adjust), and forced-air cooling (cooling). Thermal comfort is reported as millimeters on a visual analog scale (VAS), with 0 mm indicating the worst imaginable cold, 50 mm identifying thermoneutrality, and 100 mm being the worst imaginable heat. Active cooling made the subjects feel miserably cold, but did not reduce core temperature. Data are presented as means ± S.D.s. (From Ref. 47.)

Pharmacological Treatments

Anesthetics and Muscle Relaxants

The most powerful known inhibitors of thermoregulation are general anesthetics. These drugs have been used for decades to facilitate induction of hypothermia for cardiac surgery and, more recently, to facilitate induction of hypothermia during neurosurgery. In sufficient doses, especially when combined with neuromuscular blockers, anesthetics can essentially obliterate defenses against hypothermia. It is thus relatively easy to cool patients during surgery. In fact, the typical clinical problem in surgical patients is maintaining normothermia in a relatively cool operating room environment. The effects of anesthetics on thermoregulation and perioperative heat balance have been reviewed recently (50).

Volatile anesthetics, such as desflurane and sevoflurane, have relatively little effect on sweating: even full anesthetic doses increase the sweating threshold only about 0.5°C. In contrast, anesthetic gases markedly reduce the vasoconstriction and shivering thresholds. Interestingly, the threshold for each major cold defense is reduced synchronously, as if they are similarly controlled. This turns out to be a general feature of drug-induced thermoregulatory inhibition observed with nearly all agents. The volatile anesthetics reduce the vasoconstriction and shivering thresholds nonlinearly, with higher concentrations producing proportionately greater effect (51). In contrast, intravenous anesthetics (52), opioids (53), and sedatives (54) linearly impair thermoregulatory control. The effects of various drugs are illustrated in Fig. 7.

Neuraxial anesthetics, such as spinal or epidural anesthesia, also impair central thermoregulatory control (55). Why peripherally administered local anesthetics alter central control remains unclear. The pattern of inhibition is similar to that observed during general anesthesia, but the magnitude is much smaller, with neuraxial anesthesia typically reducing the vasoconstriction and shivering thresholds only ≈0.6°C (55). Per se, this small reduction is unlikely to facilitate induction of therapeutic hypothermia by much. However, a consequence of regional anesthesia is that it obliterates ther-

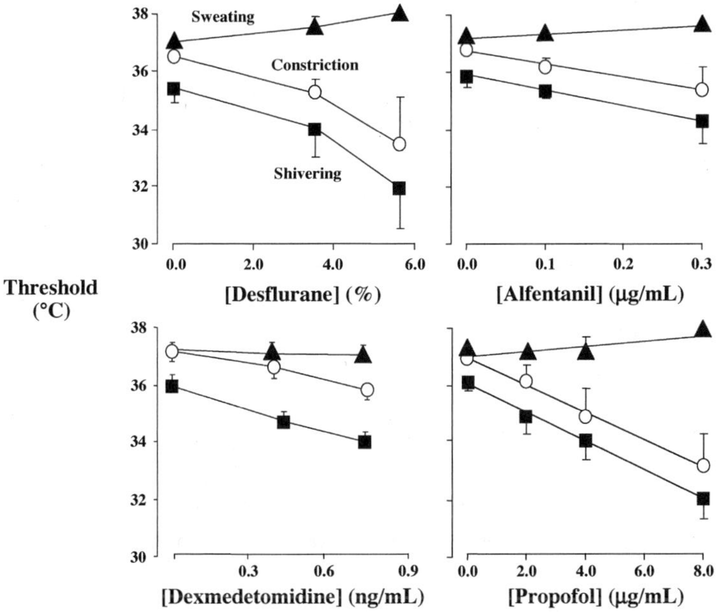

Figure 7 Concentration-dependent thermoregulatory inhibition by desflurane and isoflurane (halogenated volatile anesthetics), propofol (an intravenous anesthetic), and alfentanil (a μ-agonist opioid). General anesthetics are the most powerful known inhibitors of thermoregulatory control. The horizontal axis, in each case, spans a clinically relevant concentration range. The sweating (triangles), vasoconstriction (circles), and shivering (squares) thresholds are expressed in terms of core temperature at a designated mean skin temperature of 34 °C. Anesthesia linearly, but slightly, increases the sweating threshold. In contrast, anesthesia produces substantial and comparable linear or nonlinear decreases in the vasoconstriction and shivering thresholds. Typical anesthetic concentrations thus increase the interthreshold range (difference between the sweating and vasoconstriction thresholds) approximately 20-fold from its normal value near 0.2 °C. Patients do not activate autonomic thermoregulatory defenses unless body temperature exceeds the interthreshold range; surgical patients are thus poikilothermic over a 3–5 °C range of core temperatures. Isoflurane, 1%, and desflurane, 6%, have comparable anesthetic potency. Error bars smaller than the data markers have been deleted. (From Ref. 50.)

mal sensation from the blocked area (56). Regional anesthesia thus presumably blocks the cutaneous contribution to control of vasoconstriction and shivering that normally accompanies cutaneous cooling. Consequently, regional anesthesia has been used to block cutaneous thermal sensation in thermoregulatory studies of core-temperature response thresholds (57). However, given the risks and difficulty of implementing neuraxial anesthesia, this technique is unlikely to prove a clinically useful adjunct for induction of therapeutic hypothermia.

Neuromuscular blockers such as pancuronium are not anesthetics (58) and are not believed to have any effect on central control of thermoregulatory responses. However, they obviously cause paralysis and thus prevent shivering. It is equally obvious though that muscle relaxants can only be given in the context of general anesthesia or substantial sedation and that paralyzed patients require mechanical ventilation. It also remains unclear whether paralysis at the neuromuscular junction prevents the increase in cerebral metabolic rate of glucose and oxygen consumption that typically occurs with shivering. Muscle relaxants are a suitable treatment for shivering only in the context of an intensive care unit and should usually be restricted to patients in whom there are other indications for intubation and mechanical ventilation.

A special type of muscle relaxant is dantrolene, which has been recognized as a specific treatment for malignant hyperthermia crises since 1975 (59). Dantrolene, however, is increasingly being used for emergency treatment of life-threatening hyperthermia that is unresponsive to conventional treatments. For example, the drug has been used with some success for acute treatment of life-threatening hyperthermia resulting from neuroleptic malignant syndrome (60,61) and hyperthermia associated with overdoses of various drugs. It has also been used for treatment of various other types of hyperthermia (62,63).

Anecdotal observations of dantrolene's efficacy for fever suggest that the drug might induce a measure of thermoregulatory tolerance. However, conventional doses of the drug have no effect on the sweating or vasoconstriction thresholds and decrease the shivering threshold only $\approx 0.4°C$. What dantrolene does do, though, is reduce the gain of shivering by 40% (Fig. 8) (64). Reduced gain will moderate shivering-induced thermogenesis, but dantrolene will be considerably less effective than a conventional muscle relaxant, which obliterates shivering, and dantrolene is considerably more expensive. It thus seems unlikely that dantrolene will prove to be a clinically useful adjunct to induction of therapeutic hypothermia.

Sedatives

Muscarinic antagonists such as atropine, which are often given in conjunction with anesthesia or sedatives to reduce salivary secretions, are slightly sedating. Atropine premedication increases the incidence of postoperative shivering (65), as does glycopyrrolate (66). Anticholinergic toxicity can also be associated with severe or even lethal hyperthermia, a condition

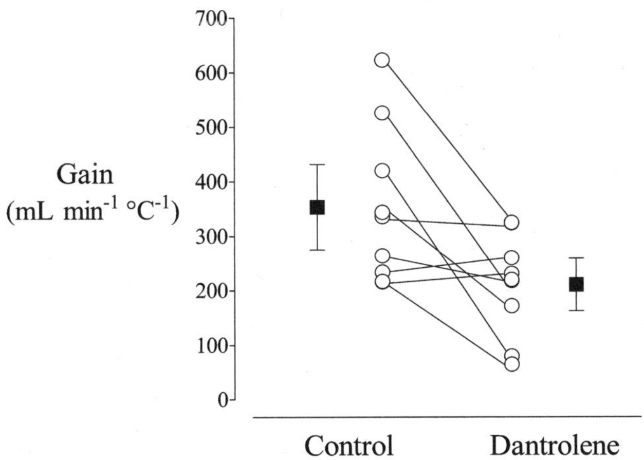

Figure 8 The gain of shivering during dantrolene ($\approx$2.5 mg/kg) administration. The open circles show the gain for each volunteer on the Control and Dantrolene days; the filled squares are the group means ($\pm$S.D.s). Gain was reduced 40% on the Dantrolene day: 211 $\pm$ 93 vs. 353 $\pm$ 144 mL min^{-1} °C^{-1}. While this reduction is highly statistically significant and clinically important, it is important to recognize that a conventional neuromuscular blocker would obliterate shivering. Dantrolene is thus a relatively expensive and risky treatment for shivering. (From Ref. 64.)

known as the "central cholinergic syndrome" (67). In contrast, physostigmine induces cold defenses at neutral temperatures and provokes hyperthermia (68). Furthermore, postanesthetic shivering is prevented by application of central cholinergic agonists in mice (69). Consistent with these observations, physostigmine is an effective treatment for shivering in humans (70).

As might thus be expected, atropine administration increases the thresholds for sweating, vasoconstriction, and shivering (71). Furthermore, these threshold increases are synchronous; that is, each is equally elevated. Atropine thus increases the "set point," rather than decreasing the precision of thermoregulatory control. This thermoregulatory pattern shares some characteristics with fever, but differs distinctly from other anesthetics and opioids, which reduce the precision of thermoregulatory control. Anticholinergic medications should thus be avoided in patients selected for therapeutic hypothermia.

Midazolam is a sedative and amnestic medication that is frequently given to perioperative and critical-care patients. It slightly decreases the sweating, vasoconstriction, and shivering thresholds. However, it reduces the sweating threshold less than the cold responses and therefore does not simply reduce the set point. Since the vasoconstriction and shivering thresholds are only reduced $\approx 0.6°C$ at a substantial plasma concentration of 0.3 μg/mL (72), it is unsurprising that midazolam produces only small amounts of hypothermia in perioperative patients (73). Midazolam will thus only slightly facilitate induction of hypothermia.

Dozens of drugs have been evaluated as potential treatments for postoperative shivering (28,74), including meperidine (75), clonidine (76), nefopam (77), doxapram (78–80), ketanserin (76), physostigmine (70), and tramadol (81). Aside from muscle relaxants, effective drugs presumably stop shivering by reducing the shivering threshold to below the actual core temperature. Fortunately, shivering postoperative patients are often only a few tenths of a degree Celsius below the shivering threshold; this makes postoperative shivering relatively easy to treat. Consequently, drugs that are quite effective for treating postoperative shivering may only slightly reduce the shivering threshold. For example, clonidine (a central alpha-2 receptor agonist) is considered among the most effective treatments for perioperative shivering. However, even substantial doses only slightly increase the threshold for sweating (82) and only slightly reduce the vasoconstriction and shivering thresholds (40). The related drug, dexmedetomidine, produces somewhat more thermoregulatory inhibition (54); however, the amount of inhibition would be insufficient to markedly facilitate induction of therapeutic hypothermia as a single agent. Tramadol (which primarily inhibits norepinephrine neuronal reuptake), similarly, only slightly reduces the vasoconstriction and shivering thresholds (83).

Nefopam is a benzoxazocine compound that is structurally related to orphenadrine and diphenhydramine (84). It is a centrally acting analgesic (84,85) with both supraspinal (86,87) and spinal sites of action (88,89). Nefopam is neither an opiate nor a nonsteroidal noninflammatory drug (90). Nefopam does not induce respiratory depression, even in postoperative patients (91). Nefopam differs from other tested drugs in reducing the shivering threshold without altering the vasoconstriction or sweating thresholds. Thus aside from muscle relaxants, it is the only drug that inhibits shivering without apparently otherwise impairing thermoregulation (92). The reduction was only about 1°C at a plasma concentration of 55 ng/mL, but is nonetheless encouraging because this is a relatively small concentration of the drug and the drug appears to have few side effects. Unfortunately, nefopam is available in some European countries, but is not approved by the Food and Drug Administration in the United States.

Opioids

Mu-receptor opioid agonists inhibit thermoregulation with an inhibition pattern similar to that produced by intravenous anesthetics: little effect on sweating combined with a linear and synchronous reduction in the vasoconstriction and shivering thresholds. However, the treatment-effect size is relatively small. For example, even 300 ng/mL of alfentanil—which is a large concentration—reduces the shivering threshold only to 34.3°C (53). Other mu-receptor agonists have yet to be tested in humans, but presumably cause similar relative amounts of inhibition. These drugs may thus facilitate induction of hypothermia, but are insufficiently powerful by themselves in patients who are expected to breathe spontaneously.

Meperidine is among the most effective treatments for postoperative shivering (74,93,94) and shivering associated with fever (95) and is far more effective than equianalgesic doses of other opioids (75). Meperidine differs from other opioids and, in fact, all other drugs so far tested in reducing the shivering threshold twice as much as the vasoconstriction threshold (Fig. 9) (96). In contrast, the gain of shivering re-

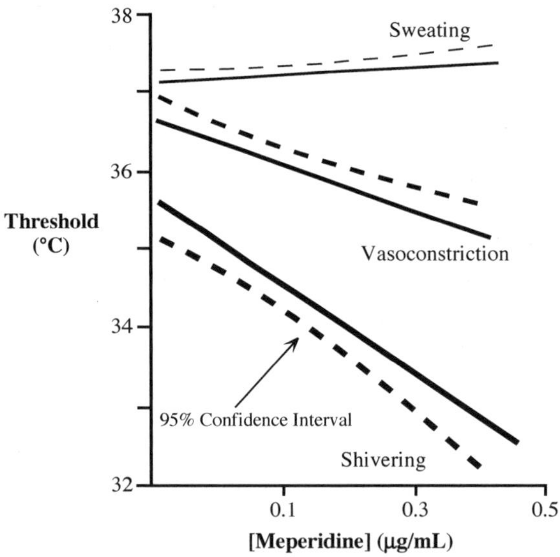

Figure 9 The sweating threshold increased as a function of unbound plasma meperidine concentration: Sweating = 0.5 [Meperidine (°C μg^{-1} mL)] + 37.1, r^2 = 0.10. In contrast, meperidine produced a linear decrease in the core temperature triggering vasoconstriction: Vasoconstriction = −3.0 [Meperidine (°C μg^{-1} mL)] + 36.6, r^2 = 0.54. Meperidine decreased the shivering threshold nearly twice as much as the vasoconstriction threshold: Shivering = −5.6 [Meperidine (°C μg^{-1} mL)] + 35.6, r^2 = 0.62. Dashed lines indicate 95% confidence intervals. (From Ref. 96.)

mains unchanged by meperidine (97). The extent to which shivering inhibition exceeds inhibition of vasoconstriction is considered the drug's "special antishivering property."

Meperidine differs from most drugs in having numerous pharmacological actions. Presumably, one or more account for its remarkable antishivering efficacy. The special antishivering action of meperidine might, in part, be mediated by its agonist activity at kappa-receptors. Kappa activity constitutes about 10% of meperidine's total opioid action (98). A clinically important contribution of kappa-receptors is supported by the observation that meperidine reduces the intensity of cold-induced shivering even in the presence of moderate doses of naloxone that presumably block mu-receptors while having little effect on the relatively resistant kappa-receptors (99). Kappa agonists have also been shown to produce hypothermia and inhibit cold defenses under a variety of circumstances (100). Furthermore, kappa agonist nalbuphine reportedly treats postoperative shivering as effectively as meperidine (94). Nonetheless, nalbuphine turns out to be a relatively poor inhibitor of shivering and does not disproportionately reduce the shivering threshold (71).

Other aspects of meperidine's pharmacology might also be responsible for the drug's special antishivering action. Unlike other opioids, meperidine produces generalized electroencephalographic activation, apparently via inhibition of central cholinergic receptors (101). Monoamine oxidase inhibitors combined with meperidine, but not other opioids, produce a potentially lethal hyperthermia syndrome (102). Gamma-amino butyric acid (GABA)-mimetic drugs reduce the antinociceptive effect of meperidine, but enhance the potency of fentanyl (103). Finally, meperidine has local anesthetic properties not shared by other opioids (104).

One of the most important nonopioid actions of meperidine is the drug's central anticholinergic activity (101); but as noted above, anticholinergic medications increase the vasoconstriction and shivering thresholds rather than reduce them. Another potential explanation for meperidine's special antishivering activity is a recently described activation of alpha-2b adrenoreceptors (105). This is important because, as noted above, alpha-2 receptor agonists such as clonidine (40) and dexmedetomidine (54) synchronously reduce the vasoconstriction and shivering thresholds. As might be expected, alpha-2 agonists are thus effective treatments for postoperative shivering (106). Meperidine's special antishivering action may be similarly mediated. Alternatively, it may result from a yet-to-be determined aspect of meperidine pharmacology—or from a combination of factors.

A limitation of meperidine is that the drug is, in part, metabolized to normeperidine. Normeperidine is neurotoxic and can cause seizures. It is thus prudent to restrict high-dose meperidine administration to a relatively short period such as 24 hr or less—especially in patients at risk for seizures.

Drug Combinations

Even meperidine, the single best antishivering medication, does not completely prevent shivering during induction of therapeutic hypothermia. However, a combination of meperidine and another drug may sufficiently reduce the shivering threshold without provoking excessive side effects. One such combination is meperidine with dexmedetomidine. Meperidine alone (at a plasma concentration of 0.3 μg/mL) reduces the shivering threshold 1.1°C. Dexmedetomidine (at a plasma concentration of 0.3 ng/mL) reduces the shivering threshold 0.7°C. The combination decreases the shivering threshold by 1.9°C, which indicates that the interaction between the two drugs is additive (Fig. 10) (107). These data thus indicate that combining meperidine and dexmedetomidine produces exactly the expected reduction in the shivering threshold. Combinations such as this one may prove clinically valuable because the major toxicities of the two drugs (respiratory depression and hypotension) are unlikely to be additive. In other words, adding dexmedetomidine to meperidine increases thermoregulatory inhibition without increasing the incidence and severity of drug-related side effects by much.

The only known combination of drugs that synergistically impairs shivering is that of meperidine and buspirone (a serotonin-1A partial agonist). Meperidine (at a plasma concentration of 0.6 μg/mL) reduces the shivering threshold by 2.3°C.

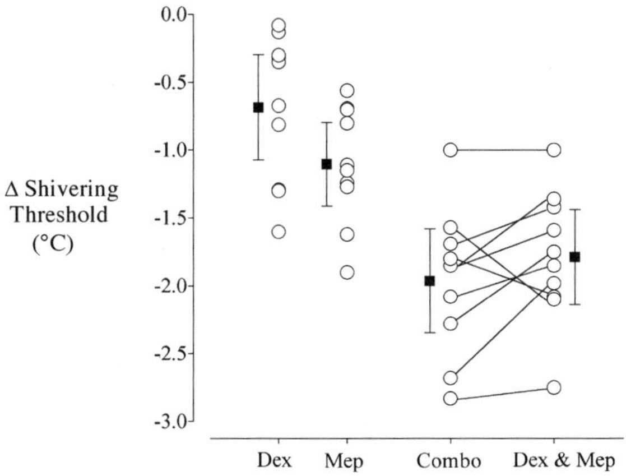

Figure 10 Reductions in the shivering threshold (compared with the Control day) for the dexmedetomidine (Dex), meperidine (Mep), and combination of the two drugs (Combo) days. The plasma concentrations of meperidine (0.3 mg/mL) and dexmedetomidine (0.3 ng/mL) were identical on each treatment day; the volunteers were thus given a full dose of each drug on the combination day. Also shown is the expected reduction for the combination of dexmedetomidine and meperidine assuming an additive effect, calculated as the sum of the individual effects of dexmedetomidine and meperidine (Dex & Mep). Results are shown as means ± S.D.s. Factorial analysis did not show any significant interaction between the two drugs on the shivering threshold. (From Ref. 107.)

Buspirone (60 mg orally) reduces the shivering threshold by 0.7°C. However, when a half dose of each drug is combined, the shivering threshold is reduced 2.3°C, which is significantly more than the expected 1.5°C decrease (Fig. 11) (108). A limitation of buspirone is that the drug is only available orally and requires about 1 hr after ingestion to reach peak plasma concentrations. The combination of buspirone and meperidine has nonetheless proven clinically useful and was the antishivering regimen used in a large multicentral study of therapeutic hypothermia for treatment of acute myocardial infarction. Short of general anesthesia, this combination is the best treatment for shivering currently available.

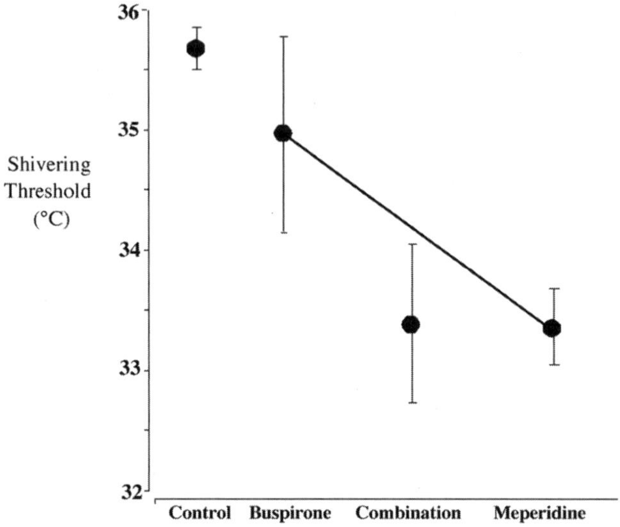

Figure 11 The shivering threshold without drugs ("Control"), with 60 mg of buspirone ("Buspirone"), with meperidine at a target plasma concentration of 0.8 μg/mL ("Meperidine"), and the combination of 30 mg buspirone and meperidine at a target plasma concentration of 0.4 μg/mL ("Combination"). Data are shown as means ± S.D.s. The shivering threshold with a combination of low-dose meperidine and low-dose buspirone was similar to that with a full dose of meperidine. Furthermore, the combination threshold was significantly less than expected from the regression between the thresholds observed with the high doses of each drug alone (i.e., if the effects of each drug were additive) ($P = 0.006$). This Figure thus indicates that the combination synergistically reduces the shivering threshold. (From Ref. 108.)

FUTURE DIRECTIONS

Existing devices, especially intravascular heat exchangers, rapidly extract heat from patients. However, even a small amount of hypothermia triggers vasoconstriction and shivering. These effective thermoregulatory defenses reduce the rate at which hypothermia can be induced and they can be detrimental.

The only existing drugs or drug combinations that induce nearly full thermoregulatory tolerance are general anesthetics. Anesthetics are required for operations and certainly facilitate induction of therapeutic hypothermia during neurosurgery. However, surgery is not usually required in the largest populations likely to benefit from hypothermia: acute myocardial infarction, postcardiac arrest, stroke, and brain-injured patients. Adaptation of therapeutic hypothermia will thus require development of techniques that reduce core temperature without requiring critical care. Some progress has been made toward this goal in recent years. For example, shivering can be prevented to core temperatures as low as 33°C by the combination of meperidine and buspirone. However, adequate plasma concentrations are associated with moderate sedation and at least some respiratory depression. Furthermore, buspirone is an oral drug (and therefore has a slow onset of action) and meperidine should not be given for prolonged periods to avoid accumulation of its toxic metabolite normeperidine.

We have yet to develop or identify drugs or drug combinations that defeat thermoregulatory defenses against hypothermia without causing excessive sedation, respiratory depression, or other serious toxicity. Pharmacological induction of thermoregulatory tolerance thus remains an elusive goal. Much work remains to be done.

REFERENCES

1. Sakai F, Amaha K. The effects of hypothermia on a cloned human brain glutamate transporter (hGLT-1) expressed in Chinese hamster ovary cells: -[3H]L-glutamate uptake study. Anesth Analg 1999; 89:1546–1550.

2. Schwartz LM, Verbinski SG, Vander Heide RS, Reimer KA. Epicardial temperature is a major predictor of myocardial infarct size in dogs. J Mol Cell Cardiol 1997; 29:1577–1583.

3. Churn SB, Taft WC, Billingsley MS, Blair RE, DeLorenzo RJ. Temperature modulation of ischemic neuronal death and

inhibition of calcium/calmodulin-dependent protein kinase II in gerbils. Stroke 1990; 21:1715–1721.

4. Busto R, Dietrich WD, Globus MY-T, Valdés I, Scheinberg P, Ginsberg MD. Small differences in intraischemic brain temperature critically determine the extent of ischemic neuronal injury. J Cereb Blood Flow Metab 1987; 7:729–738.

5. Bernard SA, Gray TW, Buist MD, Jones BM, Silvester W, Gutteridge G, Smith K. Treatment of comatose survivors of out-of-hospital cardiac arrest with induced hypothermia. N Engl J Med 2002; 346:557–563.

6. Hypothermia after Cardiac Arrest Study Group. Mild therapeutic hypothermia to improve the neurologic outcome after cardiac arrest. N Engl J Med 2002; 346:549–556.

7. Doufas AG, Akça O, Barry A, Petrusca DA, Suleman MI, Morioka N, Guarnaschelli JJ, Sessler DI. Initial experience with a novel heat-exchanging catheter in neurosurgical patients. Anesth Analg 2002; 95:1752–1756.

8. Kurz A, Sessler DI, Birnbauer F, Illievich U, Spiss C. Thermoregulatory vasoconstriction impairs active core cooling. Anesthesiology 1995; 82:870–876.

9. Kurz A, Sessler DI, Lenhardt RA and Study of Wound Infections and Temperature Group. Perioperative normothermia to reduce the incidence of surgical-wound infection and shorten hospitalization. N Engl J Med 1996; 334:1209–1215.

10. Schmied H, Kurz A, Sessler DI, Kozek S, Reiter A. Mild intraoperative hypothermia increases blood loss and allogeneic transfusion requirements during total hip arthroplasty. Lancet 1996; 347:289–292.

11. Crawshaw LI, Wollmuth LP, O'Connor CS, Rausch RN, Simpson L. Body temperature regulation in vertebrates: Comparative aspects and neuronal elements. In: Schönbaum E, Lomax P, eds. Thermoregulation: Physiology and Biochemistry. New York: Pergamon Press, 1990:209–220.

12. Steele M, Nelson MJ, Sessler DI, Fraker L, Bunney B, Watson WA, Robinson WA. Forced-air speeds rewarming in victims of accidental hypothermia. Ann Emerg Med 1996; 27:479–484.

13. Johnston CE, Bristow GK, Elias DA, Giesbrecht GG. Alcohol

lowers the vasoconstriction threshold in humans without affecting core cooling rate during mild cold exposure. Eur J Appl Physiol Occup Physiol 1996; 74:293–295.

14. Zweifler RM, Sessler DI, Zivin JA. Thermoregulatory vasoconstriction and shivering impede therapeutic hypothermia in acute ischemic stroke victims. J Stroke Cerebrovasc Dis 1997; 6:100–104.
15. Lopez M, Sessler DI, Walter K, Emerick T, Ozaki M. Rate and gender dependence of the sweating, vasoconstriction, and shivering thresholds in humans. Anesthesiology 1994; 80:780–788.
16. Burch GE, Cohn AE, Neumann C. A study by quantitative methods of the spontaneous variations in volume of the finger tip, toe tip, and postero-superior portion of the pinna of resting normal white adults. Am J Physiol 1942; 136:433–447.
17. Rubinstein EH, Sessler DI. Skin-surface temperature gradients correlate with fingertip blood flow in humans. Anesthesiology 1990; 73:541–545.
18. Sessler DI, Moayeri A, Støen R, Glosten B, Hynson J, McGuire J. Thermoregulatory vasoconstriction decreases cutaneous heat loss. Anesthesiology 1990; 73:656–660.
19. Sessler DI, McGuire J, Sessler AM. Perioperative thermal insulation. Anesthesiology 1991; 74:875–879.
20. Matsukawa T, Sessler DI, Sessler AM, Schroeder M, Ozaki M, Kurz A, Cheng C. Heat flow and distribution during induction of general anesthesia. Anesthesiology 1995; 82:662–673.
21. Kurz A, Sessler DI, Christensen R, Dechert M. Heat balance and distribution during the core-temperature plateau in anesthetized humans. Anesthesiology 1995; 83:491–499.
22. Burton AC. Human calorimetry: The average temperature of the tissues of the body. J Nutr 1935; 9:261–280.
23. Jessen K. An assessment of human regulatory nonshivering thermogenesis. Acta Anaesthesiol Scand 1980; 24:138–143.
24. Jessen K, Rabøl A, Winkler K. Total body and splanchnic thermogenesis in curarized man during a short exposure to cold. Acta Anaesthesiol Scand 1980; 24:339–344.
25. Hynson JM, Sessler DI, Moayeri A, McGuire J. Absence of

nonshivering thermogenesis in anesthetized humans. Anesthesiology 1993; 79:695–703.

26. Just B, Delva E, Camus Y, Lienhart A. Oxygen uptake during recovery following naloxone. Anesthesiology 1992; 76:60–64.
27. Horvath SM, Spurr GB, Hutt BK, Hamilton LH. Metabolic cost of shivering. J Appl Physiol 1956; 8:595–602.
28. De Witte J, Sessler DI. Perioperative shivering: Physiology and pharmacology. Anesthesiology 2002; 96:467–484.
29. Plattner O, Ikeda T, Sessler DI, Christensen R, Turakhia M. Postanesthetic vasoconstriction slows postanesthetic peripheral-to-core transfer of cutaneous heat, thereby isolating the core thermal compartment. Anesth Analg 1997; 85:899–906.
30. Frank SM, Higgins MS, Fleisher LA, Sitzmann JV, Raff H, Breslow MJ. Adrenergic, respiratory, and cardiovascular effects of core cooling in humans. Am J Physiol 1997; 272:R557–R562.
31. Greif R, Laciny S, Rajek A, Doufas AG, Sessler DI. Blood pressure response to thermoregulatory vasoconstriction during isoflurane and desflurane anesthesia. Acta Anaesthesiol Scand, 2003; 47:847–853.
32. Frank SM, Fleisher LA, Breslow MJ, Higgins MS, Olson KF, Kelly S, Beattie C. Perioperative maintenance of normothermia reduces the incidence of morbid cardiac events: A randomized clinical trial. JAMA 1997; 277:1127–1134.
33. Sweney MT, Sigg DC, Tahvildari S, Iaizzo PA. Shiver suppression using focal hand warming in unanesthetized normal subjects. Anesthesiology 2001; 95:1089–1095.
34. Iaizzo PA, Jeon YM, Sigg DC. Facial warming increases the threshold for shivering. J Neurosurg Anesthesiol 1999; 11: 231–239.
35. Mekjavic IB, Eiken O. Inhibition of shivering in man by thermal stimulation of the facial area. Acta Physiol Scand 1985; 125:633–637.
36. Murphy MT, Lipton JM, Loughran P, Giesecke AH Jr. Postanesthetic shivering in primates: Inhibition by peripheral heating and by taurine. Anesthesiology 1985; 63:161–165.

37. Sharkey A, Lipton JM, Murphy MT, Giesecke AH. Inhibition of postanesthetic shivering with radiant heat. Anesthesiology 1987; 66:249–252.

38. Sharkey A, Gulden RH, Lipton JM, Giesecke AH. Effect of radiant heat on the metabolic cost of postoperative shivering. Br J Anaesth 1993; 70:449–450.

39. Doufas AG, Wadhwa A, Lin C-M, Shah YM, Hanni K, Sessler DI. Neither arm nor face warming reduces the shivering threshold in unanesthetized humans. Stroke 2003; 34:1736–1740.

40. Delaunay L, Bonnet F, Liu N, Beydon L, Catoire P, Sessler DI. Clonidine comparably decreases the thermoregulatory thresholds for vasoconstriction and shivering in humans. Anesthesiology 1993; 79:470–474.

41. Delaunay L, Bonnet F, Duvaldestin P. Clonidine decreases postoperative oxygen consumption in patients recovering from general anaesthesia. Br J Anaesth 1991; 67:397–401.

42. Horn E-P, Sessler DI, Standl T, Schroeder F, Bartz H-J, Beyer J-C, Schulte am Esch J. Non-thermoregulatory shivering in patients recovering from isoflurane or desflurane anesthesia. Anesthesiology 1998; 89:878–886.

43. Cheng C, Matsukawa T, Sessler DI, Kurz A, Merrifield B, Lin H, Olofsson P. Increasing mean skin temperature linearly reduces the core-temperature thresholds for vasoconstriction and shivering in humans. Anesthesiology 1995; 82:1160–1168.

44. Ginsberg MD, Busto R. Combating hyperthermia in acute stroke: A significant clinical concern. Stroke 1998; 29:529–534.

45. Kluger MJ. Is fever beneficial? Yale J Biol Med 1986; 59:89–95.

46. Davatelis G, Wolpe SD, Sherry B, Dayer JM, Chicheportiche R, Cerami A. Macrophage inflammatory protein-1: A prostaglandin-independent endogenous pyrogen. Science 1989; 243:1066–1068.

47. Lenhardt R, Negishi C, Sessler DI, Vuong K, Bastanmehr H, Kim J-S, Bjorksten AR. The effects of physical treatment on induced fever in humans. Am J Med 1999; 106:550–555.

48. Poblete B, Romand J-A, Pichard C, König P, Suter PM. Metabolic effects of i.v. propacetamol, metamizol or external

cooling in critically ill febrile sedated patients. Br J Anaesth 1997; 78:123–127.

49. Manthous CA, Hall JB, Olson D, Singh M, Chatila W, Pohlman A, Kushner R, Schmidt GA, Wood LD. Effect of cooling on oxygen consumption in febrile critically ill patients. Am J Respir Crit Care Med 1995; 151:10–14.

50. Sessler DI. Perioperative hypothermia. N Engl J Med 1997; 336:1730–1737.

51. Annadata RS, Sessler DI, Tayefeh F, Kurz A, Dechert M. Desflurane slightly increases the sweating threshold, but produces marked, non-linear decreases in the vasoconstriction and shivering thresholds. Anesthesiology 1995; 83:1205–1211.

52. Matsukawa T, Kurz A, Sessler DI, Bjorksten AR, Merrifield B, Cheng C. Propofol linearly reduces the vasoconstriction and shivering thresholds. Anesthesiology 1995; 82:1169–1180.

53. Kurz A, Go JC, Sessler DI, Kaer K, Larson M, Bjorksten AR. Alfentanil slightly increases the sweating threshold and markedly reduces the vasoconstriction and shivering thresholds. Anesthesiology 1995; 83:293–299.

54. Talke P, Tayefeh F, Sessler DI, Jeffrey R, Noursalehi M, Richardson C. Dexmedetomidine does not alter the sweating threshold, but comparably and linearly reduces the vasoconstriction and shivering thresholds. Anesthesiology 1997; 87:835–841.

55. Ozaki M, Kurz A, Sessler DI, Lenhardt R, Schroeder M, Moayeri A, Noyes KM, Rotheneder E. Thermoregulatory thresholds during spinal and epidural anesthesia. Anesthesiology 1994; 81:282–288.

56. Rajek A, Greif R, Sessler DI. Effects of epidural anesthesia on thermal sensation. Reg Anesth Pain Med 2001; 26:527–531.

57. Leslie K, Sessler DI, Bjorksten A, Ozaki M, Matsukawa T, Schroeder M, Lin S. Propofol causes a dose-dependent decrease in the thermoregulatory threshold for vasoconstriction, but has little effect on sweating. Anesthesiology 1994; 81:353–360.

58. Fahey MR, Sessler DI, Cannon JE, Brady K, Støen R, Miller RD. Atracurium, vecuronium, and pancuronium do not alter

the minimum alveolar concentration of halothane in humans. Anesthesiology 1989; 71:53–56.

59. Harrison G. Control of the malignant hyperpyrexic syndrome in MHS swine by dantrolene sodium. Br J Anaesth 1975; 47:62–65.

60. Goulon M, de Rohan-Chabot P, Elkharrat D, Gajdos P, Bismuth C, Conso F. Beneficial effects of dantrolene in the treatment of neuroleptic malignant syndrome: A report of two cases. Neurology 1983; 33:516–518.

61. Granato JE, Stern BJ, Ringel A, Karim AH, Krumholz A, Coyle J, Adler S. Neuroleptic malignant syndrome: Successful treatment with dantrolene and bromocriptine. Ann Neurol 1983; 14:89–90.

62. Guze BH, Baxter LR Jr. Current concepts. Neuroleptic malignant syndrome. N Engl J Med 1985; 313:163–166.

63. Tanii H, Taniguchi N, Niigawa H, Hosono T, Ikura Y, Sakamoto S, Kudo T, Nishimura T, Takeda M. Development of an animal model for neuroleptic malignant syndrome: Heat-exposed rabbits with haloperidol and atropine administration exhibit increased muscle activity, hyperthermia, and high serum creatine phosphokinase level. Brain Res 1996; 743:263–270.

64. Lin CM, Neeru S, Doufas AG, Liem E, Muneer Shah Y, Wadhwa A, Lenhardt R, Bjorksten A, Taguchi A, Kabon B, Sessler DI, Kurz A. Dantrolene reduces the threshold and gain for shivering. Anesth Analg 2004; 98:1318–1324.

65. Lyons B, Taylor A, Power C, Casey W. Postanaesthetic shivering in children. Anaesthesia 1996; 51:442–445.

66. Baxendale BR, Mahajan RP, Crossley AWA. Anticholinergic premedication influences the incidence of postoperative shivering. Br J Anaesth 1994; 72:291–294.

67. Gordon CJ. Thermoregulation in laboratory mammals and humans exposed to anticholinesterase agents. Neurotoxicol Teratol 1994; 16:427–453.

68. Johnson KG. Thermoregulatory changes induced by cholinomimetic substances introduced into the cerebral ventricles of sheep. Br J Pharmacol 1975; 53:489–497.

69. Nikki P. Influence of some cholinomimetic and cholinolytic drugs on halothane shivering in mice. Ann Med Exp Biol Fenn 1968; 46:521–530.
70. Horn E-P, Standl T, Sessler DI, von Knobelsdorff G, Büchs C, Schulte am Esch J. Physostigmine prevents postanesthetic shivering as does meperidine or clonidine. Anesthesiology 1998; 88:108–113.
71. Greif R, Laciny S, Rajek AM, Larson MD, Bjorksten AR, Doufas AG, Bakhshandeh M, Mokhtarani M, Sessler DI. Neither nalbuphine nor atropine posses special antishivering activity. Anesth Analg 2001; 93:620–627.
72. Kurz A, Sessler DI, Annadata R, Dechert M, Christensen R. Midazolam minimally impairs thermoregulatory control. Anesth Analg 1995; 81:393–398.
73. Matsukawa T, Hanagata K, Ozaki M, Iwashita H, Koshimizu M, Kumazawa T. I.M. midazolam as premedication produces a concentration dependent decrease in core temperature in male volunteers. Br J Anaesth 1997; 78:396–399.
74. Kranke P, Eberhart LH, Roewer N, Tramer MR. Pharmacological treatment of postoperative shivering: A quantitative systematic review of randomized controlled trials. Anesth Analg 2002; 94:453–460.
75. Alfonsi P, Sessler DI, Du Manoir B, Levron J-C, Le Moing J-P, Chauvin M. The effects of meperidine and sufentanil on the shivering threshold in postoperative patients. Anesthesiology 1998; 89:43–48.
76. Joris J, Banache M, Bonnet F, Sessler DI, Lamy M. Clonidine and ketanserin both are effective treatments for postanesthetic shivering. Anesthesiology 1993; 79:532–539.
77. Piper SN, Suttner SW, Schmidt CC, Maleck WH, Kumle B, Boldt J. Nefopam and clonidine in the prevention of postanaesthetic shivering. Anaesthesia 1999; 54:695–699.
78. Singh P, Dimitriou V, Mahajan RP, Crossley AW. Double-blind comparison between doxapram and pethidine in the treatment of postanaesthetic shivering. Br J Anaesth 1993; 71:685–688.

79. Gautier H. Doxapram and shivering. Anaesthesia 1991; 46:1092–1093.

80. Sarma V, Fry EN. Doxapram after general anaesthesia. Its role in stopping shivering during recovery. Anaesthesia 1991; 46:460–461.

81. De Witte J, Deloof T, De Veylder J, Housmans PR. Tramadol in the treatment of postanesthetic shivering. Acta Anaesthesiol Scand 1997; 41:506–510.

82. Delaunay L, Herail T, Sessler DI, Lienhart A, Bonnet F. Clonidine increases the sweating threshold, but does not reduce the gain of sweating. Anesth Analg 1996; 83:844–848.

83. De Witte JL, Kim J-S, Sessler DI, Bastanmehr H, Björksten AR. Tramadol reduces the sweating, vasoconstriction, and shivering thresholds. Anesth Analg 1998; 87:173–179.

84. Heel RC, Brogden RN, Pakes GE, Speight TM, Avery GS. Nefopam: A review of its pharmacological properties and therapeutic efficacy. Drugs 1980; 19:249–267.

85. Guirimand F, Dupont X, Bouhassira D, Brasseur L, Chauvin M. Nefopam strongly depresses the nociceptive flexion (R(III)) reflex in humans. Pain 1999; 80:399–404.

86. Ohkubo Y, Nomura K, Yamaguchi I. Involvement of dopamine in the mechanism of action of FR64822, a novel non-opioid antinociceptive compound. Eur J Pharmacol 1991; 204:121–125.

87. Fuller RW, Snoddy HD. Evaluation of nefopam as a monoamine uptake inhibitor in vivo in mice. Neuropharmacology 1993; 32:995–999.

88. Buritova J, Besson JM. Effects of nefopam on the spinal nociceptive processes: A c-Fos protein study in the rat. Eur J Pharmacol 2002; 441:67–74.

89. Gray AM, Nevinson MJ, Sewell RD. The involvement of opioidergic and noradrenergic mechanisms in nefopam antinociception. Eur J Pharmacol 1999; 365:149–157.

90. Dordoni PL, Della Ventura M, Stefanelli A, Iannace E, Paparella P, Rocca B, Accorra F. Effect of ketorolac, ketoprofen and nefopam on platelet function. Anaesthesia 1994; 49:1046–1049.

91. Bhatt AM, Pleuvry BJ, Maddison SE. Respiratory and metabolic effects of oral nefopam in human volunteers. Br J Clin Pharmacol 1981; 11:209–211.

92. Alfonsi P, Adam F, Passard A, Guignard B, Sessler DI, Chauvin M. Nefopam, a non-sedative benzoxazocine analgesic, selectively reduces the shivering threshold. Anesthesiology, 2004; 100:37–43.

93. Tsai Y-C, Chu K-S. A comparison of tramadol, amitriptyline, and meperidine for postepidural anesthetic shivering in Parturients. Anesth Analg 2001; 93:1288–1292.

94. Wang JJ, Ho ST, Lee SC, Liu YC. A comparison among nalbuphine, meperidine, and placebo for treating postanesthetic shivering. Anesth Analg 1999; 88:686–689.

95. Burks L, Aisner J, Fortner CL, Wiernik PH. Meperidine for the treatment of shaking chills and fever. Arch Intern Med 1980; 140:483–484.

96. Kurz A, Ikeda T, Sessler DI, Larson M, Bjorksten AR, Dechert M, Christensen R. Meperidine decreases the shivering threshold twice as much as the vasoconstriction threshold. Anesthesiology 1997; 86:1046–1054.

97. Ikeda T, Sessler DI, Tayefeh F, Negishi C, Turakhia M, Marder D, Bjorksten AR, Larson MD. Meperidine and alfentanil do not reduce the gain or maximum intensity of shivering. Anesthesiology 1998; 88:858–865.

98. Magnan J, Paterson SJ, Tavani A, Kosterlitz HW. The binding spectrum of narcotic analgesic drugs with different agonist and antagonist properties. Naunyn-Schmiedeberg's Arch Pharmacol 1982; 319:197–205.

99. Kurz M, Belani K, Sessler DI, Kurz A, Larson M, Blanchard D, Schroeder M. Naloxone, meperidine, and shivering. Anesthesiology 1993; 79:1193–1201.

100. Adler MW, Bradley E, Martinez R, Geller EB. Production of hypothermia in the guinea pig by a kappa-agonist opioid alone and in combination with chlorpromazine. Pharmacol Biochem Behav 1991; 40:129–132.

101. Votava Z, Elliott HW. The effect of morphine, meperidine, and methadone on the cholinergic EEG and behavioral activation

in rabbits. In: Sabelli HC, ed. Chemical Modulation of Brain Function. New York: Raven Press, 1973:123–135.

102. Mackenzie JE, Frank LW. Influence of pretreatment with a monoamine oxidase inhibitor (phenelzine) on the effects of buprenorphine and pethidine in the conscious rabbit. Br J Anaesth 1988; 60:216–221.

103. Wynn RL, Bergman SA, Rudo FG, Leventer M. GABA mimetics diminish antinociception of meperidine under conditions which enhance other opioid μ-agonists. Arch Int Pharmacodyn 1990; 304:136–146.

104. Wagner LE Jr, Eaton M, Sabnis SS, Gingrich KJ. Meperidine and lidocaine block of recombinant voltage-dependent Na^+ channels: Evidence that meperidine is a local anesthetic. Anesthesiology 1999; 91:1481–1490.

105. Takada K, Clark DJ, Davies MF, Tonner PH, Krause TK, Bertaccini E, Maze M. Meperidine exerts agonist activity at the alpha(2B)-adrenoceptor subtype. Anesthesiology 2002; 96:1420–1426.

106. Horn E-P, Werner C, Sessler DI, Steinfath M, Schulte am Esch J. Late intraoperative administration of clonidine prevents postanesthetic shivering after total intravenous or volatile anesthesia. Anesth Analg 1997; 84:613–617.

107. Doufas AG, Lin CM, Suleman MI, Liem EB, Lenhardt R, Morioka N, Akça O, Shah YM, Bjorksten AR, Sessler DI. Dexmedetomidine and meperidine additively reduce the shivering threshold in humans. Stroke 2003; 34:1218–1223.

108. Mokhtarani M, Mahgob AN, Morioka N, Doufas AG, Sessler DI. Buspirone and meperidine synergistically reduce the shivering threshold. Anesth Analg 2001; 93:1233–1239.

9

Thermodynamics and Heat Transfer

THOMAS L. MERRILL
Biomedical Engineering Department,
Wyeth Research, Princeton,
New Jersey, U.S.A.

BACKGROUND

Thermodynamics and heat transfer provide the language and the concepts to understand the fundamental nature of temperature and how it can be controlled (1–5). For scientists and engineers, these concepts are necessary tools to analyze and develop therapeutic temperature modulation technologies. Examples of temperature control are ubiquitous, from the ice cream freezers in your grocery store to the comfortable passenger cabins inside jet airliners.

Stripped to its core, thermodynamics studies energy from four perspectives: generation, storage, transfer, and dissipation. More specifically, the first law of thermodynamics, a natural law, provides the starting point for all thermal problems. From a first law perspective, the problem of jet airliner cabin temperature control is no different than patient temperature control.

Thermodynamics, however, inherently deals with equilibrium states—states without temperature gradients. For example, although the first law can tell you the rate or the amount of heat transfer needed to maintain comfortable living conditions in a building, it is silent on what insulation should be selected.

The science of heat transfer provides an essential missing link—linking the rate of heat transfer to temperature gradients and material properties. For example, consider the heating load for a home. Two important temperatures are needed: the desired indoor temperature and the range of outdoor temperatures. Taking these temperatures and the building design and materials into consideration, heat transfer concepts enable us to calculate the expected heat losses and the resultant internal heat generation needed for adequate temperature control. These loss calculations are based on four different modes of heat transfer: conduction, convection, radiation, and advection. Figure 1 illustrates these different modes

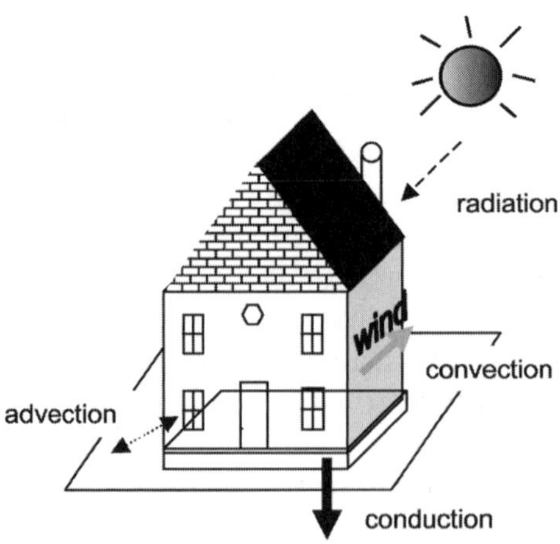

Figure 1 The various heat transfer processes to consider when calculating the heating load for a building.

of heat transfer: radiation from the sun, convection from blowing winds, conduction from the soil in contact with the foundation, and, finally, advection of energy through leaks or open windows. For each mode, laws based on empirical evidence, such Fourier's law of conduction, are used to estimate the heat loss associated with a particular type of heat transfer.

The goal of this chapter is to provide a primer for these two interesting thermal science fields. First, this work will present an overview of classical thermodynamics, followed by a more in-depth review of heat transfer, particularly focusing on how it applies to therapeutic temperature control. Using familiar examples and the human body, this work will emphasize two

Table 1 Nomenclature

Symbol	Name
A	Area
β	Volumetric thermal expansion coefficient
c	Specific heat
E	Total energy
g	Acceleration of gravity
H	Enthalpy
h	Specific enthalpy or heat transfer coefficient
k	Thermal conductivity
l or L	Length scale
m	Mass
P	Pressure or perimeter
Q	Amount of heat transfer
$\dot{Q}$	Rate of heat transfer
Q''	Rate of heat flux
Q'''	Rate of volumetric heat generation
r	Radius
R	Thermal resistance
ρ	Mass density
σ	Stefan–Boltzmann constant
T	Temperature
U	Internal energy
V	Volume or velocity
W	Work
Z	Elevation
∞	Ambient or free stream

core themes: first, the identification of various heat transfer modes, and, second, the design process for temperature control devices. Thermal sciences are complex, so although this chapter will not explore interesting advanced topics or subtleties of each field, it will provide insights into how thermal science can be used to optimize patient temperature control techniques and technologies. To help keep track of the nomenclature used in this chapter, please refer to Table 1.

REVIEW

An Overview of Thermodynamics

The fundamental question thermodynamics helps us answer is: What amount of heat transfer is needed to meet patient hypothermia cooling goals? The core theme of this entire chapter is the conservation of energy, also called the first law of thermodynamics. Before examining the first law, however, an understanding of some basic thermodynamic concepts is needed. This discussion will begin with basic thermodynamic properties and the concept of system boundaries. Then this work will take a close look at the first law of thermodynamics in terms of fundamental equations, new properties, and example applications.

Basic Concepts and Definitions

Classical thermodynamics focuses on macroscopical characteristics. It is interested in the bulk or averaged effects from molecular behavior. These effects are directly quantifiable through measurements of thermodynamic properties such as pressure, temperature, and density. Pressure represents the aggregate effect of the time-averaged momentum exchange of molecules hitting the walls of a container. Temperature represents the aggregate effect of molecular thermal energy or molecular motion. Density is the amount of mass inside a volume with dimensions far greater than molecular length scales. All together, these directly measurable properties, along with other properties that are not measurable, form the thermodynamic coordinates used to distinguish one system state from another. Table 2 shows typical units for these properties.

In addition to thermodynamic properties, to begin a thermal analysis, we also need to distinguish between the entity of interest (such as a turbine, a compressor, or a human body) and its surroundings. We do this by creating an imaginary boundary or artificial envelope. For an entity that does not have mass flowing into or out of it, this envelope is called a system boundary, and this configuration is considered a closed system. For open systems, mass does flow across these imaginary boundaries, and we call these boundaries control surfaces, creating a control volume. Figure 2a and b shows these boundaries for closed and open systems, respectively. For the closed system, imagine a freight elevator, where gas is confined inside an insulated chamber and piston assembly. For the open system, imagine a steam turbine, like those used in power generation plants, where steam continually flows into and out of the control volume. Either system, open or closed, can be used for thermal analysis of the human body.

Connecting these two core concepts, boundaries and properties, is the idea of equilibrium. When we say that a system is in equilibrium, we make two assumptions: (a) the properties of a system apply uniformly throughout the system, and (b) there is no tendency for these properties to change with time. This is an underlying assumption to most classical thermodynamic analyses. As we will see, however, although the first assump-

Table 2 Thermodynamic Properties and Energy Terms

Property	Nominal units	Other units or conversions
Temperature	K	= 5/9°R = 5/9(°F + 459.67) = °C + 273.15
Pressure	mm Hg	= 1.36 cm H_2O = 0.0193 psi
Density	g/cm^3	= 62.43 lb/ft^3
Energy or work	cal	= 4.1868 J = 0.00397 BTU
Power or rate of work or energy transfer	cal/sec	= 4.184 W = 14.285 BTU/hr

tion of uniformity always holds, the second assumption of time dependence is sometimes relaxed.

The First Law of Thermodynamics for a Closed System

With some initial properties and the idea of imaginary boundaries established, the first law of thermodynamics not only gives the word *energy* meaning, but it is also a formal statement that energy is conserved. Mathematically, the first law for a closed system going from state 1 to state 2 is expressed as:

$$Q_{1-2} - W_{1-2} = E_2 - E_1 \tag{1}$$

In words, Eq. 1 says that the total system energy change from state 1 to state 2 ($E_2 - E_1$) depends on two terms: Q, which is the net heat transfer across the system boundary, and W, which is the work that is either done on the system or by the system. The first law is analogous to a company's financial balance sheet. Like the first law, this balance sheet shows the company's performance by quantifying and summing the financial transactions that interact with the company.

Let us look at each of the three terms in the first law more closely. Energy, like money, has many forms. The term E in Eq. 1 represents the total energy of the system: potential energy, kinetic energy, and internal energy. Whereas potential energy and kinetic energy are related to some reference frame, internal energy, usually shown with the variable U, is based on bulk or average molecular behavior, making it a property of the system just like pressure or temperature. The first law does not tell us absolute values for internal energy—only the change in internal energy. The net heat transfer term Q represents the net energy transferred as a result of temperature differences. Without a temperature difference, there is no net heat transfer. In terms of a sign convention, heat transfer into the system is positive and heat transfer from the system is negative. Furthermore, there is an important distinction to make. A system does not contain heat; it contains internal energy. "The First Law of Thermodynamics for an Open System" will probe energy or heat transfer in much greater detail. In its simplest form, the term *work* presents a force located at the boundary of system acting through some displacement. Like heat transfer, work is another way by which energy crosses boundaries. An easy example is a moving piston, but it can also involve magnetic or electrical work. To understand the first law better, let us look at an example.

Example 1 A freight elevator used to move a truck (refer to Fig. 2a).

- System initial conditions (state 1)
  - Pressure: 105 kPa
  - Volume: 160 m^3
- System final conditions (state 2)
  - Pressure: 105 kPa
  - Volume: 630 m^3
- Process: Heat is added to an insulated gas-filled chamber moving a frictionless piston slowly to a higher position. The amount of heat added is 200 MJ.
- Using the first law of thermodynamics (Eq. 1), find the work done and the change in total energy.

The work done by the system (a positive work term) is calculated by the integral of the pressure volume product from state 1 to state 2. The first law is then used to calculate the change in total system energy:

$$W_{1-2} = P(V_2 - V_1) = 105\ \text{kPa}(630\ \text{m}^3 - 160\ \text{m}^3)$$

$$= 49.4\ \text{MJ}$$

$$\Delta E = Q_{1-2} - W_{1-2} = 200\ \text{MJ} - 49.4\ \text{MJ} = 150.6\ \text{MJ}$$

The increase in the total system energy reflects the rise in elevation of the truck and the increase in temperature of the gas that pushes the piston.

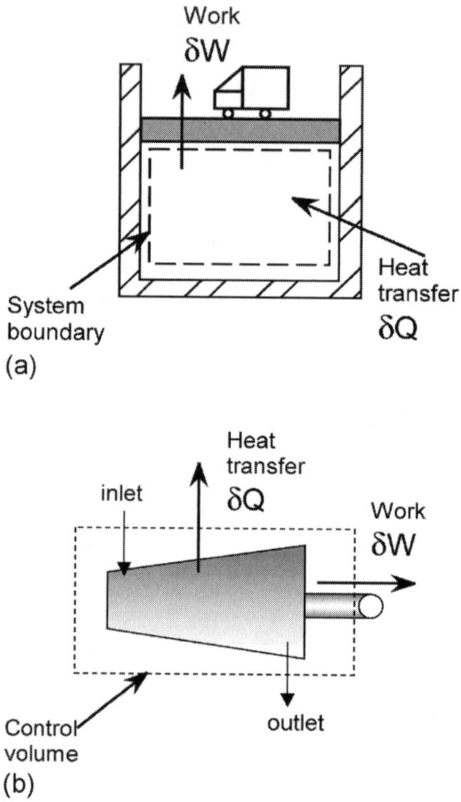

Figure 2 (a) An example of a closed system where mass does not cross the system boundary. (b) An example of an open system where mass does cross the control surfaces. The control surfaces form a control volume. In this case, the control volume surrounds a steam turbine.

For therapeutic temperature control, we can also assume that the human body is a closed system. For this case, the first law can be rewritten to include the internal heat generation term resulting from metabolic reactions inside the body:

$$Q_{1-2} + Q_{\mathrm{g}} - W_{1-2} = E_2 - E_1 \tag{2}$$

where Q_{g} is the internal heat generation term from metabolic activity. When a system has a steady rate of energy transfer, it is convenient to express the first law in rate format, where the rates of energy change, generation, and transfer are related:

$$\dot{Q} + \dot{Q}_{\mathrm{g}} - \dot{W} = \dot{E} \tag{3}$$

The next example shows how Eq. 3 can be used.

Example 2 Rate of temperature rise in a person who lacks heat exchange with the environment.

Assume that the resting metabolic rate is 72 kcal/hr for a 70-kg person. If no work is performed, determine how quickly the body temperature will rise if there is no heat exchange with the environment. Assume that the average specific heat of the human body is 0.83 kcal/kg/°C:

$$\dot{E} = \dot{Q}_{\mathrm{g}}$$

$$mc\frac{\mathrm{d}T}{\mathrm{d}t} = \dot{Q}_{\mathrm{g}}$$

$$\frac{\mathrm{d}T}{\mathrm{d}t} = \frac{\dot{Q}_{\mathrm{g}}}{mc} = \frac{72\ \mathrm{kcal/hr}}{70\ \mathrm{kg} \times 0.83\ \mathrm{kcal/kg/^{\circ}C}} = 1.24\frac{^{\circ}\mathrm{C}}{\mathrm{hr}}$$

$$= 2.23\frac{^{\circ}\mathrm{F}}{\mathrm{hr}}$$

Based on these first law calculations with no heat transfer and no work taking place, the human body temperature will rise relatively rapidly, over 2°F each hour.

Another important thermodynamic property was introduced in this example—c, the specific heat or heat capacity. It quantifies the energy required to raise 1 kg of tissue by 1°C without phase change. Values for water and air are 1.0 and

0.24 kcal/kg/°C, respectively. The specific heat is defined by the following equation:

$$c \equiv \frac{1}{m}\frac{\delta Q}{\delta T}, \tag{4}$$

The specific heat is linked to another key thermodynamic property—enthalpy. Enthalpy is a especially useful property, with first law applications with open systems discussed in "The First Law of Thermodynamics for an Open System." Enthalpy arises in thermodynamics out of the need to simplify: it is a simple grouping of other variables. It is defined this way:

$$H \equiv U - PV, \tag{5}$$

with units of energy. For liquids, we can write the following differential form:

$$\mathrm{d}H = \mathrm{d}U = mc\mathrm{d}T \tag{6}$$

where both enthalpy and internal energy are related to the differential temperature $\mathrm{d}T$.

The First Law of Thermodynamics for an Open System

Looking at Fig. 2b, an open system, we see that energy can cross the control surface in three forms: work, heat transfer, and bulk motion of matter with its own energy, also called advection. The first law for this type of problem is typically written as:

$$\begin{aligned} &\dot{Q}_{\mathrm{cv}} + \sum \dot{m}_i\left(h_i + \frac{V_i^2}{2} + gZ_i\right) + \dot{Q}_{\mathrm{g}} - \dot{W}_{\mathrm{cv}} \\ &\quad = \dot{E}_{\mathrm{cv}} + \sum \dot{m}_{\mathrm{e}}\left(h_{\mathrm{e}} + \frac{V_{\mathrm{e}}^2}{2} + gZ_{\mathrm{e}}\right), \end{aligned} \tag{7}$$

where h is the specific enthalpy or enthalpy per unit mass (H/mass), V is the velocity, g is the acceleration of gravity, and Z is the elevation. The subscripts "i" and "e" represent inlet and exit, respectively. The other terms with the control volume subscript "cv" are consistent with those found in Eq. 3. The summation sign says multiple inlets and outlets may be present on the control volume. In words, Eq. 7 says a lot. It says that the net heat transfer into the control volume, together with the incoming flow of energy, the internal energy generation, and the work done on or by the control volume, matches the change in internal energy and the exiting flow energy from the control volume. Here is an example of how Eq. 7 may be used.

Example 3 Rate of cooling with chilled saline infusion.

A patient is suffering from an ischemic stroke. To cool the patient quickly, a physician suggests infusing saline at 5°C at a rate 500 mL/hr. How quickly will the patient cool if we make the following assumptions?

- The rate of heat transfer loss is increased slightly to 20% above the resting metabolic rate, 86 kcal/hr. There is no work being performed.
- The average rate of energy generation inside the body is maintained at 72 kcal/hr with antishivering drugs.
- The patient weights 70 kg and, for simplicity, we assume that the patient is able to excrete water at the same rate as cold saline infusion.

With these assumptions, Eq. 7 is simplified in the following fashion:

$$\dot{Q}_{\mathrm{cv}} + \dot{Q}_{\mathrm{g}} + \dot{m}_{\mathrm{infusion}}(h_{\mathrm{in}} - h_{\mathrm{out}})_{\mathrm{cv}} = m_{\mathrm{body}}c\frac{\mathrm{d}T}{\mathrm{d}t}$$

$$\frac{\dot{Q}_{\mathrm{cv}} + \dot{Q}_{\mathrm{g}} + \dot{m}_{\mathrm{infusion}}(h_{\mathrm{in}} - h_{\mathrm{out}})_{\mathrm{cv}}}{m_{\mathrm{body}}c} = \frac{\mathrm{d}T}{\mathrm{d}t},$$

and (now with direct substitution)

$$\frac{-86\ \text{kcal/hr} + 72\ \text{kcal/hr} + 0.5\ \text{kg/hr} * (5\ \text{kcal/kg} - 37\ \text{kcal/kg})}{70\ \text{kg} \times 0.83\ \text{kcal/kg/}^\circ\text{C}}$$

$$= \frac{dT}{dt}$$

$$\frac{dT}{dt} = -0.52^\circ\text{C/hr}.$$

These calculations show that cold infusion does not lead to rapid body cooling. Even if the infusion rate could be safely doubled to 1000 mL/hr, the rate of temperature decrease in this example would only change to −0.76°C/hr. Current endovascular cooling devices have a much higher cooling capacity, as much as −5.0°C/hr to −6.0°C/hr (1,2). From a different perspective, note that if the rate of cooling was defined, Eq. 7 could also be used to determine the required amount of net heat transfer.

A Summary of Thermodynamics

Using the basic concepts of equilibrium, control volumes, and the first law of thermodynamics, we can calculate important patient temperature control parameters. Once a system like the human body is identified, properties such as pressure and temperature define the state of the system. This state is nothing more than a thermodynamic coordinate from which other states may move to or from. Not only does the first law quantify energy change, it also provides a tool to determine the energy that crosses boundaries: through work, through heat transfer, and through the bulk motion of matter, which we call advection.

Nevertheless, thermodynamics leaves many practical temperature control questions unanswered. For example, using Eq. 7, we can determine the rate of cooling necessary to achieve a desired rate of patient body temperature cooling. Yet, thermodynamics does not tell you how to achieve that level of cooling. To get that answer, you must go into a new area—an area that thermodynamics does not explore—where temperature gradients or nonequilibrium conditions exist and where temperature can be a function of space and time.

Heat Transfer

Combining what we know about physiology and thermodynamics, we can define two important patient temperature control factors:

1. The preferred level of hypothermia (or the patient target temperature)
2. The heat transfer rate required to achieve a preferred cooling rate (or, in other words, the rate at which the target temperature is achieved).

What remains unknown is the most effective approach to bringing about those conditions in patients. Heat transfer, together with our understanding of thermoregulation, helps us create that approach. For example, medical device companies, using heat transfer concepts, have developed two categories of patient temperature control devices: internal devices and external devices. In both cases, the development of the technology required, first, the identification of the heat transfer mode(s) and, second, the ability to identify and reduce the rate-limiting heat transfer resistance.

To begin this section, each of the three modes of heat transfer—conduction, convection, and radiation—will be presented. Cooling through phase change or evaporation will also be briefly discussed. With these concepts in place, this work will present the concept of multimode heat transfer and the steps used to design effective heat exchange devices, such as cooling blankets and endovascular cooling catheters.

Conduction

Conduction heat transfer is a molecular or atomic event. Consider your car window defrosting. As the temperature rises inside your car, the inside glass surface temperature also rises. Energy is then transferred by way of conduction from the warmer inside surface to the cooler outside surface, raising its temperature above the water melting point. If you could look at this glass at the microscopical level, you would make two interesting observations: (a) the activity level of the molecules, measured as temperature, is not uniform throughout the glass; and (b) the more energetic molecules are able to transfer their energy to less energetic molecules, without a change in the average position of those molecules. In other words, heat conduction involves the diffusion of molecular energy through matter without bulk molecular motion.

The ability of different materials to conduct heat varies widely. A good example of that phenomenon is the feeling you have when you pick up two objects both at room temperature, but one is made of pine and the other is made of carbon steel. Right away, the steel object feels much cooler. It is not. The reason why it feels colder is because it can transfer heat, away from your hand, by conduction much faster. To explain and quantify this difference, a thermophysical property called thermal conductivity was created. A particular law used to relate this property to temperature gradients and to the rate of heat transfer was also created. The law is Fourier's law of conduction:

$$\dot{Q}''_{\text{conduction}} = k\frac{T_1 - T_2}{l}, \tag{8}$$

where $Q''_{\text{conduction}}$ is the heat flux or heat transfer per unit area [W/m^2], k is the thermal conductivity [W/m/°C], l is the thickness of the material [m], and $T_1 - T_2$ is the temperature difference from one point to another on or in the material of interest. Figure 3 describes one-dimensional conduction in the x-direction inside a homogeneous solid material.

Table 3 shows typical thermal conductivities of various materials at 37°C. The difference in thermal conductivities from vapor to solid is largely due to the differences in molecular distances: as spacing increases, the ability to diffuse thermal energy through conduction decreases.

Coupled with the first law of thermodynamics, often Fourier's law is used to determine the temperature distribution inside a material or collection of materials. For example, a rather complicated-looking partial differential equation, known

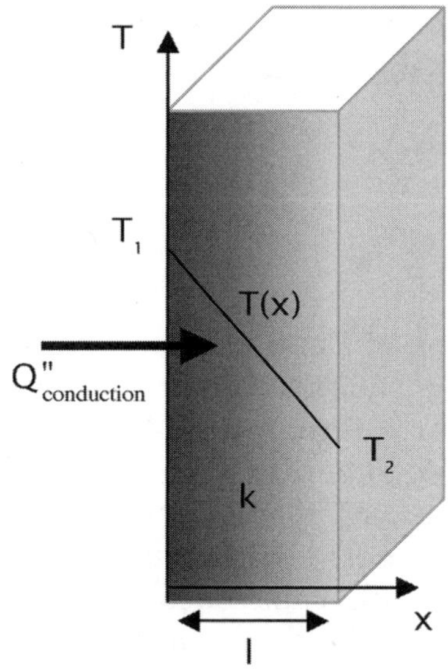

Figure 3 Heat transfer by conduction inside a homogenous solid.

Table 3 Thermal Conductivities for Various Materials at 37°C

Material	Thermal conductivity [W/m/K]
Air	0.026
Wood pine	0.11
Fat	0.20
Teflon	0.36
Blood	0.55
Skin and brain tissue	0.62
Water	0.63
Carbon steel	63.3

Source: Refs. 5 and 6.

as the heat diffusion equation or heat equation, can be used to determine this internal temperature distribution:

$$\frac{\partial}{\partial x}\left(k\frac{\partial T}{\partial x}\right)+\frac{\partial}{\partial y}\left(k\frac{\partial T}{\partial y}\right)+\frac{\partial}{\partial z}\left(k\frac{\partial T}{\partial z}\right)+Q'''_{\text{gen}}=\rho c\frac{\partial T}{\partial t}. \tag{9}$$

This equation is a differential version of Eq. 3. The first three terms on the left-hand side describe the net conductive heat transfer in three directions. The fourth term on the left-hand side is the amount of internal heat generation in terms of energy per unit volume. Finally, the last term on the right-hand side is the change of internal energy within a system. When there is interest in localized hypothermia, such as inside a specific region of the brain, equations like this, modified to account for blood perfusion through tissue, allow us to calculate discrete tissue temperatures (2–4).

Convection

Although conduction does not address heat transfer with bulk motion of matter, convection does. Bulk motion is the movement of matter over large distances relative to molecular dimensions; it is motion at the macroscopical level where you can easily visualize or feel that movement. How that bulk motion arises distinguishes the type of convection. If the bulk motion arises from density gradients that arise from temperature gradients, with buoyancy forces causing flows, the heat transfer process is called free or natural convection heat transfer. This is the mode of heat transfer from a patient lying in still cool air. If the bulk motion arises from an external source, a pump or a fan, the heat transfer process is called forced convection heat transfer. This is the mode of heat transfer from a patient lying near a circulation fan or ventilation duct. If the bulk motion arises from liquid droplet to vapor phase, this is called evaporative heat transfer. This is the mode of heat transfer that occurs when there is sweat on a person's skin. All of these types of convective heat transfer may occur simultaneously.

Figure 4a and b shows the typical velocity and temperature profiles near an external solid flat surface that is hotter than an adjacent fluid. The subscript ∞ indicates the undisturbed fluid property, where the fluid properties and flow conditions are not affected by the solid surface. The distance measured from the solid surface to this undisturbed region is called the boundary layer. As you can see at the solid–fluid interface, the velocity goes to zero; this is called the no-slip boundary condition. A good example of this boundary layer is the fine dust that accumulates on a spinning fan blade. The velocity at the blade–air interface is not great enough to create the drag forces necessary to remove dust particles from the spinning fan blade. This boundary condition says something special about convective heat transfer. Convective heat transfer has two parts; it is a superpositioning of two phenomena. The first part is conductive heat transfer with no bulk motion near the solid interface—purely diffusion of molecular energy. The second part is advection of fluid particles from regions of similar internal energies to regions of dissimilar internal energies. If the fluid flow is sufficiently unstable, which is particularly likely with higher flow rates, we say that the flow is turbulent. In this case, the advection component of convective heat transfer becomes more vigorous with the advent of swirling spinning fluid motions, also called turbulent mixing eddies.

Because convection involves the flow of matter or fluid mechanics, this mode of heat transfer is inherently more complex than conduction. There is a wide range of flow conditions and there are numerous parameters that can affect these flow conditions. As a result, many analysis techniques for convection are empirical. These empirical works are based on another particular law or rate equation, called Newton's law of cooling:

$$Q''_{\text{convection}} = h(T_{\text{s}} - T_{\infty}), \tag{10}$$

where $Q''_{\text{convection}}$ is the convective heat flux [W/m^2], h is the convection heat transfer coefficient [W/m^2/°C] (not to be confused with the enthalpy term used in the "The First Law of Thermodynamics for an Open System"), T_{s} is the surface

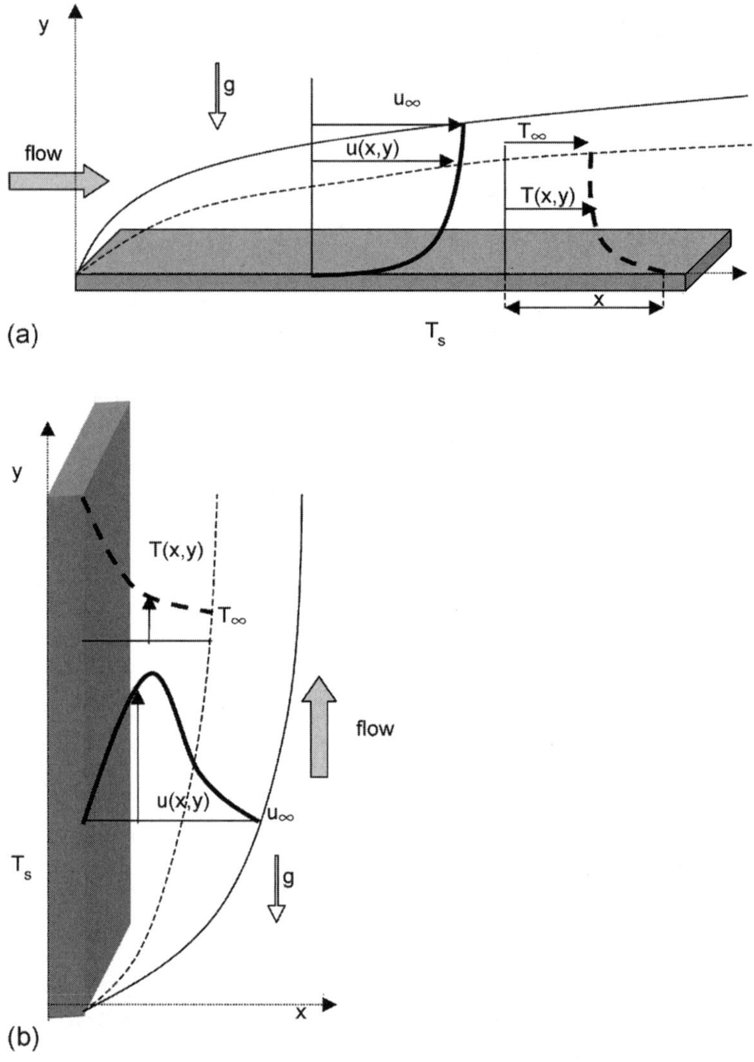

Figure 4 (a) An example of forced convection velocity and (b) temperature profiles that result as fluid is pumped across a flat plate.

temperature, and T_∞ is the bulk fluid temperature. With the effective heat exchange surface area at T_s, Eq. 9 is used to calculate the rate of heat transfer (W) due to convection: $\dot{Q} = Q'' \times \text{Area}$.

When we know fluid and surface temperatures, determining convective heat fluxes is reduced to finding the correct heat transfer coefficient h for Eq. 10. To simplify the experimental analysis of h, special property groupings have been created to reduce the number of independent properties. They are called nondimensional numbers because, when grouped together, they are dimensionless. Here are some of the key nondimensional numbers used for convective heat transfer analysis:

$$Nu = \frac{hL}{k} \text{ (the Nusselt number)}$$

$$Re = \frac{\rho VL}{\mu} \text{ (the Reynolds number)}$$

$$Pr = \frac{c\mu}{k} \text{ (the Prandtl number)}$$

$$Gr = \frac{g\beta(T_s - T_\infty)}{\nu^2} \text{ (the Grashof number).}$$

Each of these of numbers has an interesting physical interpretation. The Nusselt number Nu represents a dimensionless or a normalized temperature gradient in the fluid adjacent to a solid surface. The Reynolds number Re represents the ratio of inertial to viscous forces. This number is used to determine whether or not the flow conditions are turbulent, laminar, or somewhere in between. The Prandtl number Pr represents the ratio of momentum transport to thermal energy transport. Finally, the Grashof number Gr represents the ratio of buoyancy forces to viscous forces. Properties used in these numbers are shown in Table 1 and values for different fluids can be found in Ref. 3.

Equation 11 is an example of a convective heat transfer correlation determined empirically for free convection from the upper surface of a heated horizontal flat plate:

$$Nu_L = 0.54(Gr_L \times Pr)^{1/4}, \tag{11}$$

where L is defined by surface area divided by the perimeter of the flat plate A_s/P. To accurately use correlations like this, the key is to evaluate the necessary properties at the correct conditions while at the same time being aware of the expected accuracy levels.

Table 4 shows typical heat transfer coefficients for three different types of convective heat transfer. They represent expected heat transfer coefficients that may occur near a human body in water and air. The large difference in heat transfer coefficient values between air and water results from the significantly higher water property values for thermal conductivity and specific heat. Table 4 also shows that free convection and forced convection have similar magnitudes at an air speed of 1 mile/hr or 0.45 m/sec. Below this value, free convection dominates the convective heat transfer process and, above this value, forced convection dominates. Furthermore, evaporation may easily dominate either free or forced convection because of one simple fact: the heat vaporization of water (h_{fg}) is quite large at about 2400 J/g.

Table 4 Typical Convective Heat Transfer Coefficients in Water and Air

Experimental conditions	Heat transfer coefficient h [W/m²/K]	Reference
Free convection		(3) (p. 498, Eq. 9.31)
Water (21°C)	675	
Air (21°C)	4.5	
Forced convection[a]		
0.45 m/sec or 1 m/hr		
Water (21°C)	1500 or ($3000v^{0.8}$)	(3) (p. 369, Eq. 7.55b)
Air (21°C)	4.0 or ($7.0v^{0.6}$)	
Evaporative heat transfer[b]	$11.3v^{0.25}$	(5) (p. 116, Table 5.11)

[a] v equals the velocity of flow [m/sec].
[b] Units for evaporative heat transfer coefficient [W/m²/mm Hg], where the evaporative heat transfer = $h \times \text{Area}(P_s - P_\infty)$, where P_s and P_∞ equal the water partial pressure at the surface and the ambient conditions.

Radiation

Before presenting the rate equation for radiation, there are several interesting radiation fundamentals worth noting. Although convection and conduction require matter between two bodies with dissimilar temperatures to transfer heat, radiation does not. Consider the sun's energy transfer through 93 million miles of empty space. Radiation, unlike the other modes of heat transfer, originates at a subatomic event, resulting from energy transitions of electrons inside molecules. Unlike the other modes of heat transfer, radiative heat transfer is proportional to the absolute temperature raised to the fourth power. All materials whose temperatures exceed 0 K or absolute zero emit thermal radiation. So the challenge with radiation calculations is to develop an approach to calculate the net heat exchange from one body to another. In addition to temperature differences, several other factors influence the amount net radiative heat transfer: amount of surface area, type of material surfaces, orientation of surfaces, and, finally, the medium that separates the two surfaces. Fortunately, analysis of radiation heat exchange with the human body usually does not require this level of complexity.

Similar to previous modes of heat transfer, radiation has a particular law or rate equation—the Stephan–Boltzmann equation:

$$Q''_{\text{radiation}} = \sigma T^4, \tag{12}$$

where $Q''_{\text{radiation}}$ represents the radiated heat flux [W/m^2] from a black body at an absolute temperature T [K]. The symbol σ is the Stefan–Boltzmann constant, 5.67×10^{-8} [W/m^2/K^4]. A black body is a concept, an idealization; it represents a body that absorbs all incident radiation, reflecting no radiation. This is a reasonable assumption to make when analyzing human body heat transfer between surroundings. The surface property, emissivity, provides an indication of how accurate that assumption is, and its range is from 0 to 1.0. A black body has an emissivity of 1.0 and most room-temperature or nonmetallic materials have similar values. The emissivity for human skin (of any visible coloration) is around 0.99 (4). The net heat exchange between a body and its environment can be written as:

$$\dot{Q} = \sigma A_{\text{body}}(T^4_{\text{body}} - T^4_{\text{surroundings}}), \tag{13}$$

where the temperatures, again, are absolute and A_{body} is the area of the body where radiation occurs, typically around 1.8 m^2 (5). To make Eq. 13 consistent with the previous heat transfer rate equations (Eqs. 8 and 10), we can also write this equation as:

$$\dot{Q} = h_{\text{rad}} A_{\text{body}}(T_{\text{body}} - T_{\text{surroundings}}), \tag{14}$$

where h_{rad} incorporates σ and a numeric value that arises from the factorial expansion of $(T^4_{\text{body}} - T^4_{\text{surroundings}})$. This is a reasonable approach because the factor that is combined inside h_{rad} is a function of temperatures that are based on the absolute temperature scale and they typically do not change significantly. Cooney (5) shows that a typical value for h_{rad} is about 8.1 $W/m^2/K$.

Taking a step back, all of the rate equations used to compute heat transfer to or from the human body have been presented (Eqs. 8, 10, and 14). Patient temperature control strategies, however, are more complex and they must consider multimode heat transfer.

Multimode Heat Transfer and Heat Exchanger Design

Where does this entire thermal science discussion lead us? The answer is simple: hardware. That hardware is called a heat exchanger—a device that can be used to carefully and precisely control the amount of thermal energy leaving or entering a system, in this case the human body. In Chapter 10, both surface and endovascular heat exchangers will be presented. Let us first outline how these heat exchangers may be developed.

To get started, many initial design specifications are needed. Some of these include body target temperature, rate of body cooling, minimum body fluid temperature, blood-side pressure drop, and material biocompatibility. These criteria are based on our understanding of thermodynamics, hypothermia, and physiology. They tell us what we need to achieve—not how to achieve it.

Following this groundwork, the heat exchanger designer would envision where the heat exchanger would be used and what it might look like. Identifying the heat transfer modes is next. Using initial design specifications and sizing the device to meet practical implementation constraints, heat transfer resistances can be determined. Heat transfer resistance is analogous to electrical resistance. Each mode of heat transfer can be expressed as a separate resistor limiting the flow of heat transfer from one temperature to another temperature. Figure 5 shows a simple electrical circuit with heat transfer analogous pairs in parenthesis. Here are the thermal resistances for conduction, convection, and radiation heat transfer in cylindrical coordinates (6):

$$R_{\mathrm{cond}} = \frac{\ln \frac{r_\mathrm{o}}{r_\mathrm{i}}}{2\pi k l},$$

$$R_{\mathrm{conv_o}} = \frac{l}{h_\mathrm{o} 2\pi r_\mathrm{o} l},$$

$$R_{\mathrm{rad_o}} = \frac{l}{h_\mathrm{r} 2\pi r_\mathrm{o} l},$$

where the subscripts "o" and "i" represent the outside and inside of the cylinder. These resistances are particularly rele-

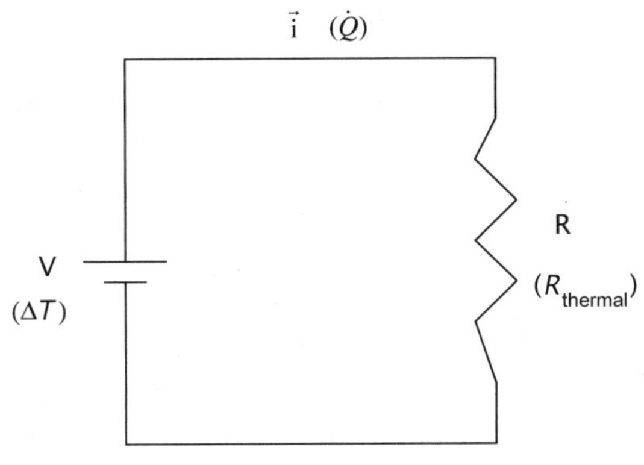

Figure 5 The analogy between electricity and heat transfer.

vant for endovascular cooling devices that are generally cylindrical. Similar to electrical resistors, these thermal resistances can be shown to act in series or in parallel. For example, the combined effects of radiation heat loss and evaporative heat loss from a patient can be illustrated as two thermal resistances in parallel.

Using the idea of thermal resistance, an estimate of the expected overall heat transfer rate can be determined with the following equation:

$$\dot{Q} = \frac{\Delta T}{\sum R_{\text{thermal}}} \quad (15)$$

where ΔT is the overall temperature difference between the coolant and the body. The denominator is the sum of all thermal resistances either in series or in parallel.

Consider a specific device. Suppose we wanted to build an endovascular device and we had established the design specifications that were mentioned above, namely the cooling rate and the allowable blood-side pressure drop (Fig. 6). The basic design has a coolant that is circulated through a flexible insertable catheter. Heat is first transferred from the warm blood to the cool catheter outer wall by convection. Next, heat travels by way of conduction across the catheter wall that separates the blood from the coolant, typically a thin biocompatible polymer. Finally, the heat finishes its journey by traveling from the inner wall of the flexible catheter to the circulating coolant by way of convection. The coolant is then pumped externally through a cooling console and resupplied to the catheter at the specified coolant inlet temperature.

Prior to animal testing of this device, careful bench testing would most likely reveal a rate-limiting or dominant heat transfer resistance. Suppose the initial bench tests showed the following thermal resistance breakdown for the flow of heat from the patient to the coolant inside the endovascular device: conduction through the catheter wall 12%, coolant-side convection 18%, and blood-side convection 70%. The key conclusion would be to focus the heat transfer enhancement or efforts to reduce the resistance on blood-side convection—the domi-

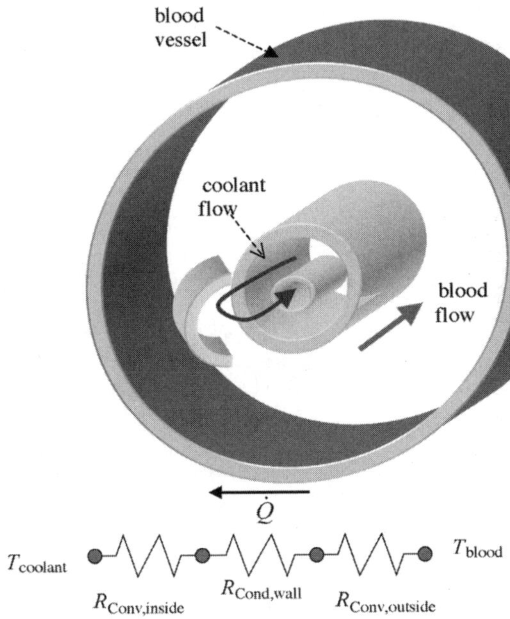

Figure 6 A simple endovascular catheter and its heat transfer circuit.

nant or rate-limiting heat transfer resistance. Figure 7 illustrates how the heat transfer rate would change if either the coolant-side or the blood-side resistance were altered. For example, if the initial prototype testing showed that the cooling capacity fell below the design specifications by 20%, the most effective way to achieve that cooling capacity would be to decrease the blood-side resistance by 30%. No amount of coolant-side resistance reduction would allow you to meet your design specifications.

To reduce this dominant resistance, you would need to carefully choose an enhancement method that would achieve your desired heat transfer resistance reductions without adversely impacting other aspects of the prototype performance, namely, the blood-side pressure drop and the ability to easily insert the catheter. For example, Innercool Therapies Incorporated, makers of an endovascular device discussed in Chap-

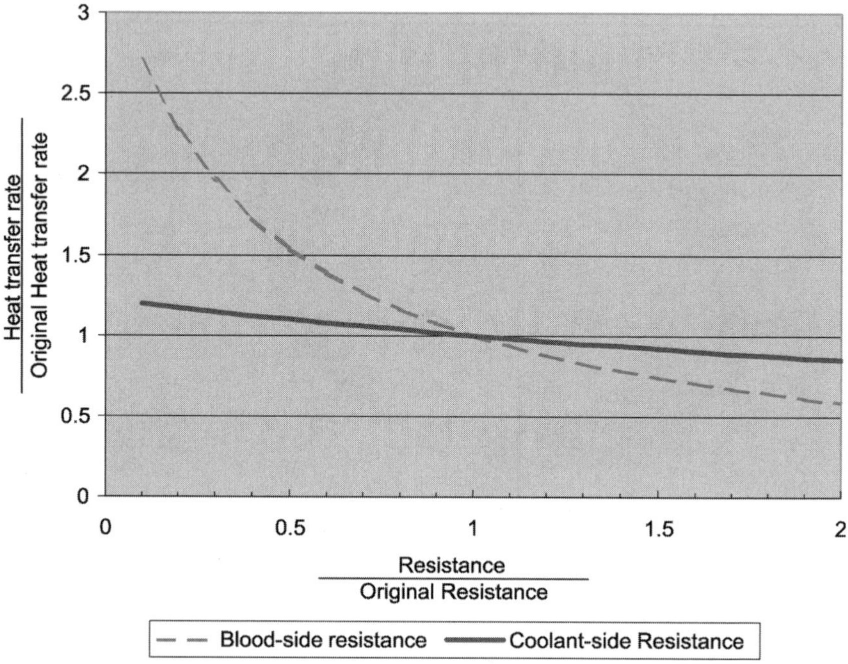

Figure 7 The effect of changing coolant-side and blood-side resistances, individually.

ter 10, have creatively chosen an enhanced blood-side surface. This surface not only increases the surface area for heat transfer, but it also generates turbulence near the device, increasing the convective heat transfer coefficient significantly. From the definition of the convective heat transfer resistance, these combined effects significantly reduce the blood-side resistance. For an in-depth review of heat transfer enhancement concepts and how they work, refer to Webb (7).

A Summary of Heat Transfer

Therapeutic temperature control begins with an understanding of hypothermia physiology and thermodynamics. Heat transfer brings closure, providing the tools to physically design and implement a temperature control solution, with real materials, flows, and temperatures.

We began by discussing the three different heat transfer modes. Whereas conduction and convection require matter to transfer heat from a system, radiation does not. Whereas conduction and convection originate on a molecular or atomic level, radiation originates on a subatomic level, resulting from electron energy transitions. Each of the modes was reduced to a rate equation that related temperature and material properties to rates of heat transfer. This work also showed the enormous amount of energy used to vaporize water during the evaporation process.

To show heat transfer at work, multimode heat transfer and heat exchanger design were explored. A simple endovascular heat exchanger was used to develop the concept of thermal resistances. Using this example, this work showed how target cooling rates may be reached after the rate-limiting or dominant resistance is identified and carefully reduced.

FUTURE DIRECTIONS

Chapter 10 will discuss devices currently available for therapeutic temperature modulation. These devices are based on the thermal science tools discussed in this chapter; future devices will be as well. In many ways, we are just at a starting point in our development of therapeutic temperature modulation technologies.

Fortunately, the field of thermal sciences is vast and constantly changing. Thermal technology applications are everywhere, including systems to cool more and more powerful laptop computers, systems to carefully maintain frozen cells for drug discovery, and systems to power satellites to explore distant parts of our solar system. To reach solutions to these technology challenges and others, emerging ideas such as microchannel heat exchangers, miniature heat pipes, or even nanoscale heat transfer may be used.

In the future, concepts such as these will play a role in therapeutic temperature modulation. Future heat exchange devices will be smaller, less intrusive, and with higher heat transfer capacities. Not only will there be improved heat exchange rates, but there will also be improved temperature-sensing and control systems. In the end, the refinement of our current technology will broaden the field of therapeutic hypothermia applications, beyond global or whole-body cooling and toward more localized or organ-specific cooling.

REFERENCES

1. Innercool Therapies Incorporated. http://www.innercool.com/technology/index.htm. Accessed August 19, 2003.
2. Doufas AG, Akça O, Barry A, Petrusca DA, Suleman MI, Morioka N, Guarnaschelli JJ, Sessler DI. Initial experience with a novel heat-exchanging catheter in neurosurgical patients. Anesth Analg 2002; 95:1752–1756.
3. Incorpera FP, DeWitt DP. Fundamentals of Heat and Mass Transfer. 4th ed. New York: John Wiley and Sons, 1996:827–849.
4. Yang W. Biothermal Fluid Sciences. New York: Hemisphere Publishing Corp., 1989:388–389.
5. Cooney DO. Biomedical Engineering Principles: An Introduction to Fluid, Heat, and Mass Transport Processes. New York: Marcel Dekker, Inc., 1976:105–106.
6. Incorpera FP, DeWitt DP. Fundamentals of Heat and Mass Transfer. 4th ed. New York: John Wiley and Sons, 1996:90–93.
7. Webb RL. Principles of Enhanced Heat Transfer. New York: John Wiley and Sons, 1994.

10

Methods to Induce Hypothermia

MICHAEL DE GEORGIA

Neurological Intensive Care Unit,
Cleveland Clinic Foundation,
Cleveland, Ohio, U.S.A.

ANUPA DEOGAONKAR

Cleveland Clinic Foundation,
Cleveland, Ohio, U.S.A.

THOMAS L. MERRILL

Biomedical Engineering Department,
Wyeth Research, Princeton,
New Jersey, U.S.A.

BACKGROUND

Induced hypothermia is one of the most widely accepted ways available to protect tissue against ischemia. The term "hypothermia" was first coined in 1941 (1) and was first used to treat brain injury in 1943 (2). Hypothermia during experimental circulatory arrest was first reported in 1950 (3) and first applied, with surface cooling, during cardiac surgery in 1953 (4). In 1957, Rosamoff showed a reduction in brain infarct size in animals immersed in ice water (5). Endovascular ("central") cooling was first described in the early 1950s by Delorme of Edinburgh (6) and Boerema of Holland (7). By the late 1960s, deep hypothermia (less than 20°C) using cardiac bypass machines was widely applied during surgery for complex intracranial aneurysms (8,9).

The last two decades have seen renewed interest in induced hypothermia and with it the development of more sophisticated cooling methods for achieving hypothermia. The following is a review of the most common methods used to attain systemic hypothermia; methods for localized brain cooling are reviewed in Chapter 11.

REVIEW

Normal Thermoregulation

An understanding of how the body normally maintains a constant temperature is necessary before considering methods to reduce temperature. Despite changes in environmental temperature, humans maintain a constant body temperature of approximately 37°C. This extraordinary temperature stability requires the integration of temperature sensing, central processing, and efferent responses to precisely balance heat loss and heat production.

Both cold and warm receptors are widely distributed on the skin, particularly on the anterior chest and face. Cold receptors are the free nerve endings of myelinated A-delta fibers (the same endings responsible for "fast pain"), whereas warm receptors are the nerve endings of unmyelinated C fibers (the same endings responsible for "slow pain"). Central processing occurs in the hypothalamus. When the hypothalamus senses cold below a certain threshold (the setpoint), a strong sympathetic nervous system response occurs, causing vasoconstriction of skin vessels to conserve heat and increased muscle tension and shivering to produce heat. Warmth above the setpoint temperature produces sweating and peripheral vasodilatation to promote heat loss. Induced hypothermia requires heat loss to exceed heat production. For a more complete review of temperature regulation, see Chapter 1.

Thermodynamic and Heat Transfer Principles

The science of thermodynamics and heat transfer help us quantify two important questions regarding therapeutic hypothermia. First, what amount of cooling is necessary to bring about a specific level of hypothermia? Cooling can be quantified both in terms of the amount of heat transferred, or *cooling capacity*, and the rate of heat transfer, which is measured in watts. Second, what is the most effective way to bring about that cooling? This question involves specific aspects of heat transfer such as heat exchanger design. Heat can be transferred in three basic ways: radiation, conduction, and convection.

Radiation originates as a subatomic event, resulting from energy transitions of electrons inside molecules. All materials emit thermal radiation. The degree of radiation depends on the temperature difference between the material and its surrounding, the type of material and its surface area, the orientation of the surfaces, and the medium that separates the two surfaces. This is the mode of heat transfer that occurs between a hot fireplace and the surrounding room.

Conduction is heat transfer by diffusion of molecular energy, from more energetic higher temperature regions to less energetic lower temperature regions. However, conduction occurs without a change in the average position of the molecules (i.e., without bulk motion of molecules). Heat transfer by conduction depends on the temperature difference between the two surfaces multiplied by the intrinsic thermal conductivity of the material divided by the thickness of the material. This is the mode of heat transfer that occurs when you place your hand against a cool or warm object.

Convection is heat transfer based on the bulk motion of molecules. There are two kinds of convection. *Free* or *natural convection* occurs when bulk motion results from buoyancy forces. These buoyancy forces arise from density gradients that are driven by temperature gradients. This is the mode of heat transfer occurring when a patient is lying in still cool air. *Forced convection* occurs when bulk motion results from air being moved by a pump or a fan (such as with forced-air cooling blankets).

Evaporation occurs when the bulk motion of heat transfer involves liquids becoming gases, such as with sweating. This highly effective method of surface cooling is the principal method by which humans dissipate excess heat. For a more complete review of thermodynamic and heat transfer principles, please see Chapter 9.

Methods Used to Induce Hypothermia

Surface Cooling

Surface cooling is the simplest and most intuitive approach to inducing hypothermia. Ninety percent of all heat loss occurs through the skin (10). Transfer is directly proportional to the skin surface area, which averages around 1.8 m^2, and the difference between skin temperature and that of an adjacent surface (in the case of conduction) or ambient air (in the case of radiation).

In the setting of anesthesia (perioperative setting), alpha-mediated vasoconstriction is attenuated and redistribution of heat from the core to the periphery occurs. During the first hour of surface cooling, this redistribution is the main determinant of core temperature. Subsequently, rapid reduction in core temperature occurs as more heat is lost and less is produced. Without anesthesia, peripheral vasoconstriction causes a plateau in the core temperature by constraining metabolic heat to the core thermal compartment and shivering is triggered, generating heat. At this point, it becomes difficult to achieve core temperatures below 34°C without general anesthesia and neuromuscular blocking agents.

Ice Packs and Alcohol Rubs

Immersion in ice water is the oldest method of surface cooling. Usually, a plastic sheet is placed under the patient and crushed ice is poured over the patient. The toes and fingers are normally held out of the bath to prevent frostbite (Fig. 1). This is an efficient way to transfer heat for several reasons. First, there is direct contact between the coolant and the skin; there are no thermal barriers. Second, immersion affects most of the

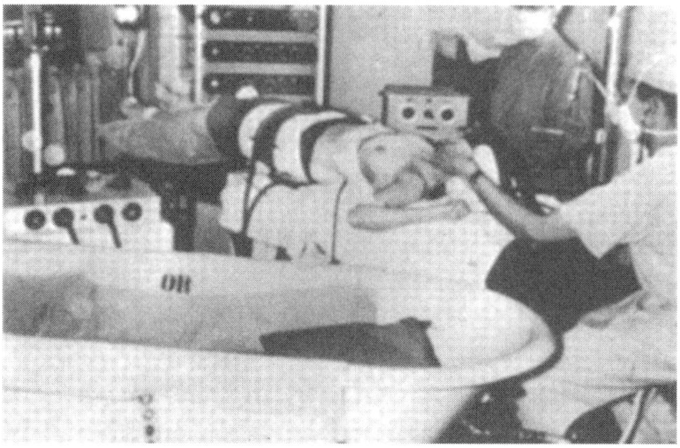

Figure 1 Induction of hypothermia through immersion in ice-water bath.

available skin surface area. Third, latent heat in the form of the heat of fusion is absorbed as the ice melts. Although less efficient than complete immersion in water, rubbing the patient with alcohol and applying ice packs also reduces temperature and is easier to perform. Ice packs can be placed over the whole body or placed strategically over the groin, neck, and axillae. Covering the whole body with ice packs and inducing evaporative cooling, in addition to conductive cooling, have been shown to produce higher cooling rates than strategically placing ice packs over the neck, groin, and axillae (11).

Water-Circulating Cooling Blankets

Liquid-circulating cooling blankets address the ease of application difficulty discussed in the previous section. All liquid-circulating cooling blankets are composed of a reservoir filled with water or alcohol, a cooler/heater (with most capable of temperatures between 4° and 42°C), a circulating pump to circulate the fluid through the blanket, and a microprocessor board to control temperature. The rate of heat transfer for these blankets is determined by five factors: (1) the temperature difference between the two surfaces, (2) the thermal conductivity of the materials separating the skin and the coolant, (3) the thickness of these materials, (4) the skin surface area over which the blanket is applied, and (5) the convective heat transfer coefficient found inside the liquid blanket. This coefficient depends on the coolant flow rate and flow patterns inside the blanket. An additional factor that applies for all surface-cooling techniques is insulation by peripheral tissues, which changes as a function of thermoregulatory vascular tone.

Although, typically, cooling blankets have been positioned beneath patients, for several reasons it may be more efficient to place the blanket on top of them. The back is a relatively small fraction of the total body surface area, and the dependent capillaries may be compressed by the patient's own weight, restricting cutaneous blood flow and slowing the process of cooling even further. Sandwiching the patient between two blankets or wraparound types of blankets may be best.

There are a number of commercially available liquid-circulating cooling blankets on the market. The following is a brief review of the more common ones; it is not meant to be a complete list.

The CSZ Blanketrol® II (Cincinnati Sub-zero, Cincinnati, OH) (Fig. 2) pumps ice-cold water from the unit at a flow rate of 32 gal/hr (2 L/min) to either a single-use vinyl blanket (Maxi-Therm® or Maxi-Therm Lite®) or reusable urethane blanket (PlastiPad®). Both blankets have random flow patterns that are claimed to evenly distribute the temperature and thus enhance the efficiency of heat transfer. The Blanketrol II has a feedback mechanism that, when combined with a patient temperature monitor, can be programmed to achieve a specific patient temperature. This system also has an automatic shut-down feature when the temperature increases more than 1°C from the setpoint (to avoid skin burns).

The Medi-Therm III®, MTA 6900 (Gaymar Industries, Orchard Park, NY) (Fig. 3) is a similar liquid circulating cooling system. Like the Blanketrol II, water is cooled and pumped from the unit into either a single-use, lightweight, polymer blanket (DHP600, 700, 800) or a durable reusable blanket (HP7010, 7020). The Medi-Therm III can be used with Rapr·Round® Hyper/Hypothermia Blankets that completely encircle the patient's legs and torso to maximize the surface area covered. The flow rate of the Medi-Therm III is 16 gal/hr (1 L/min). It does not have a feedback mechanism and cannot be programmed to achieve a desired body temperature.

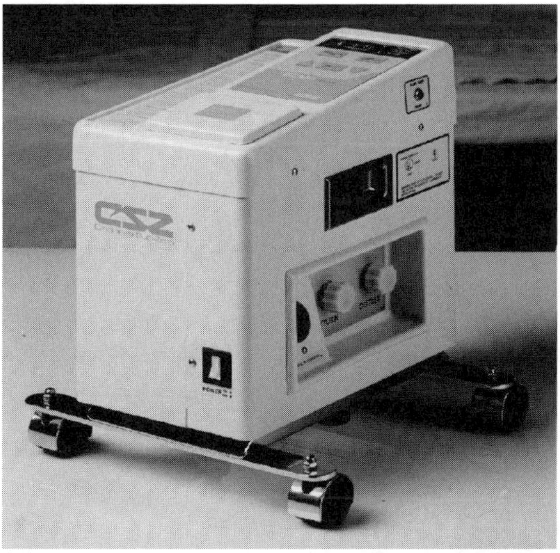

(a)

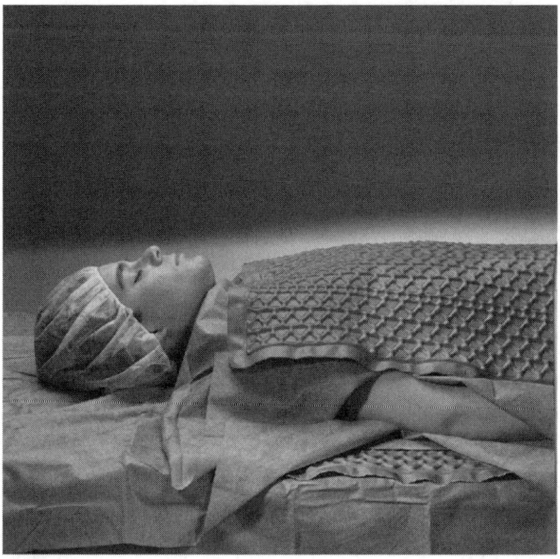

(b)

Figure 2 (a) CSZ Blanketrol II (Cincinnati Sub-zero). (b) Maxi-Therm blanket (Cincinnati Sub-zero).

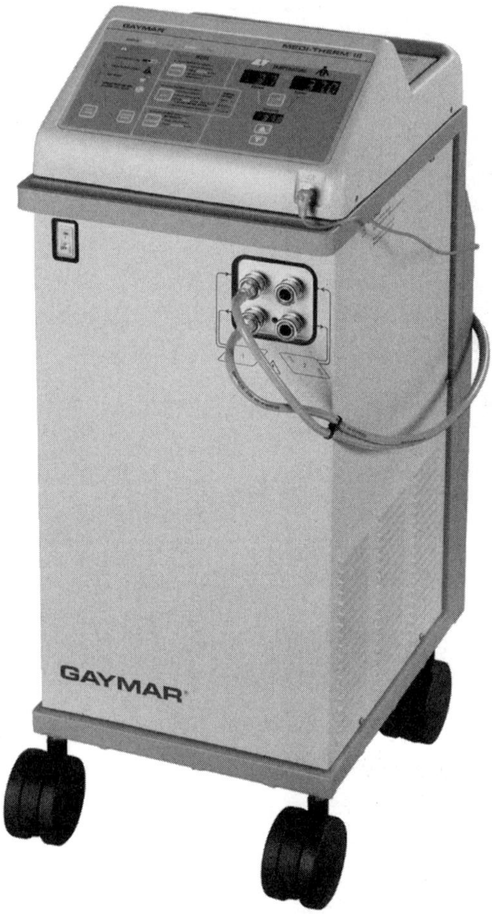

(a)

Figure 3 (a) Medi-Therm III, MTA 6900 (Gaymar Industries). (b) DHP600/800 blanket (Gaymar Industries).

The Arctic Sun Temperature Management System® (Medivance, Louisville, CO) (Fig. 4) is unique in that the blanket (Energy Transfer Pad™) has an adhesive biodegradable hydrogel on the inner surface facing the patient's skin. This gel has a relatively high thermal conductivity, significantly reducing the large contact resistance that normally exists between the cold blanket surface and the skin. The blanket is flexible, adheres tightly to the skin, and is worn on the anterior

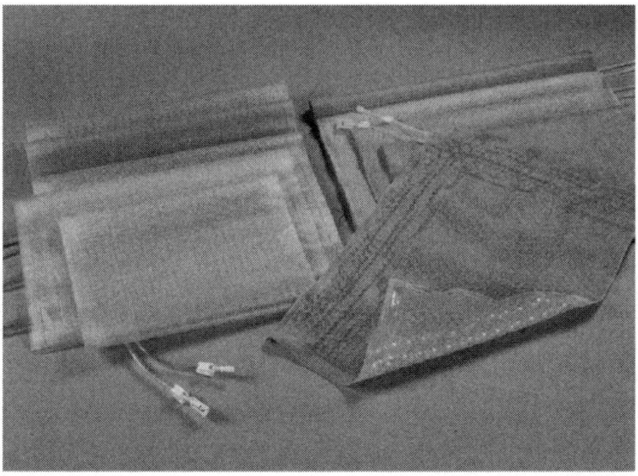

(b)

Figure 3 Continued.

chest, back, and on both thighs. The outer surface has a layer of insulation that prevents heat loss of the pad to the environment. The Arctic Sun system is also unique in that it circulates water under "negative pressure," that is the pump "pulls" cold water into the blanket rather than "pushes" it in. One theoretical advantage of this approach is that the blanket does not become distended or expanded by the pressure of the circulating water that may maximize flow rates, which are listed as ranging from 8 to 80 gal/hr (0.5 to 5 L/min). Circulating the water under negative pressure also achieves inherent sealing at the edges of the blanket, and in case of accidental puncture, air enters the blanket instead of water leaking out. The control module has a temperature feedback system that monitors and automatically adjusts the temperature of circulating water.

Finally, the ALLON 2001 (M.T.R.E. Advanced Technologies, Or-Akiva Industrial Park, Israel) (Fig. 5) supplies water that circulates at the rate of 16 to 19 gal/hr (1 to 1.2 L/min) into a garmentlike disposable ThermoWrap™ worn by the patient. The ThermoWrap is made of polypropylene nonwoven fabric with an inner layer of polyethylene film used as water barrier; it covers between 45% and 70% of body surface area. The unit has a temperature feedback system to allow a consistent level of body temperature.

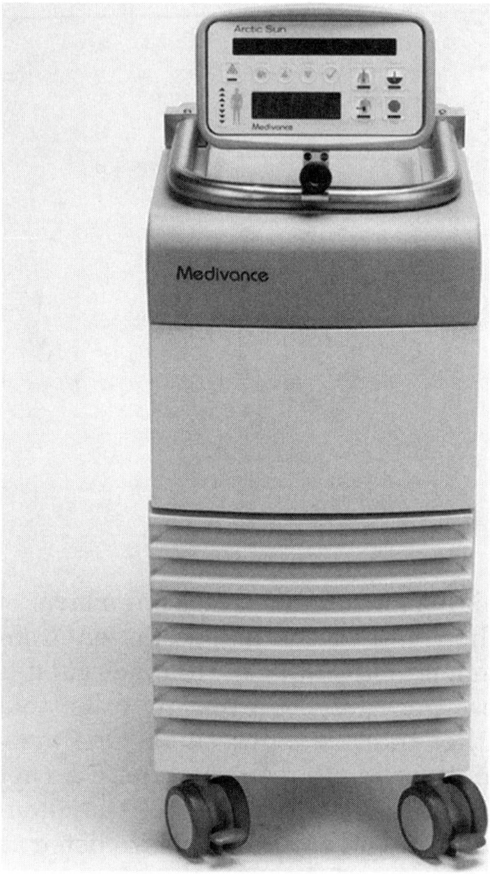

(a)

Figure 4 (a) Arctic Sun Temperature Management System (Medivance). (b) Arctic Sun Energy Transfer Pads, front (Medivance). (c) Arctic Sun Energy Transfer Pads, back (Medivance).

Forced-Air Cooling

This method of surface cooling uses convective heat transfer to lower patient temperature. Forced-air cooling systems consist of an electrically powered blower unit in different sizes and configurations.

Air has a very low thermal conductivity (water's thermal conductivity is 24 times that of air), making it a good thermal insulator. Also the specific heat of air, the ability of air to store

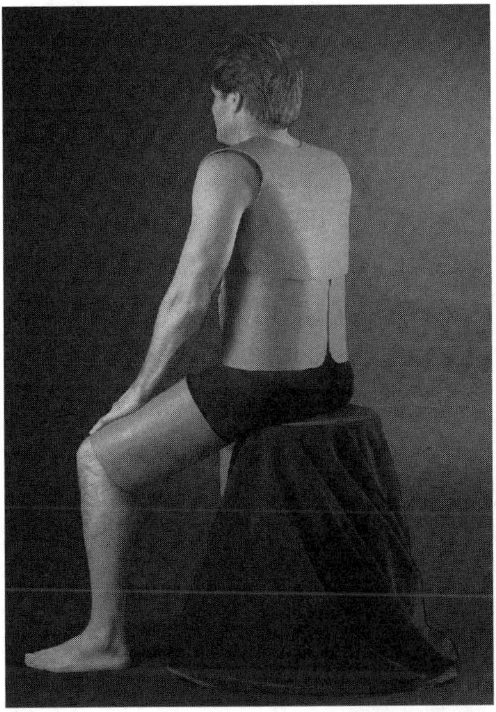

(b)

Figure 4 Continued.

heat, is very low, only one-fourth that of water; therefore, heat transfer per unit area is relatively low with forced air. Although the Bair Hugger Polar Air Cooling System (Arizant, Eden Prairie, MN) is no longer produced, many are still in use and have been used in several surface-cooling studies. Currently, there are no forced-air cooling systems on the market.

The Bair Hugger Polar Air system consisted of a disposable blanket made of paper with parallel hollow tubes that had rounded upper surfaces and flattened lower surfaces. The geometric design allowed it to self-erect when inflated. The blanket was positioned above the patient and directed cold air ($\approx 10°C$) onto the patient through small holes in the undersurface. Air pressure from the exit ports raised the blanket slightly above the patient so that none of the tubes was in direct

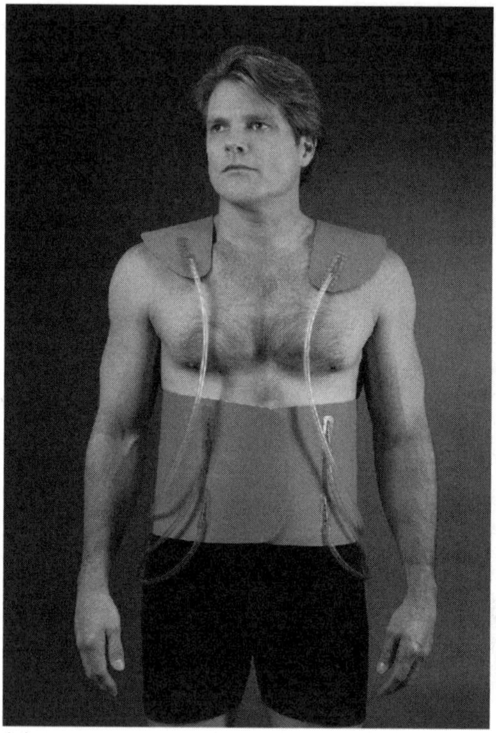

(c)

Figure 4 Continued.

contact with the skin surface. This gap between the patient and blanket facilitated circulation of cold air.

Most forced-air blanket systems currently in production (Bear Hugger system, Arizant; Warm Touch system, Mallinckrodt, St. Louis, MO; and others) focus on patient warming and do not have cooled air settings. Although all of these systems can be set to deliver ambient unwarmed air, even if ambient temperature is as low as 20°C (such as in an operating room), forced-air convection provides only slight cooling compared to simply exposing the patient to room air.

Advantages and Disadvantages of Surface Cooling

Surface cooling is simple. To achieve mild hypothermia (34–36°C) often requires only ice water, ice packs, or a cooling blanket. Kammersgaard and coworkers found forced-air cooling

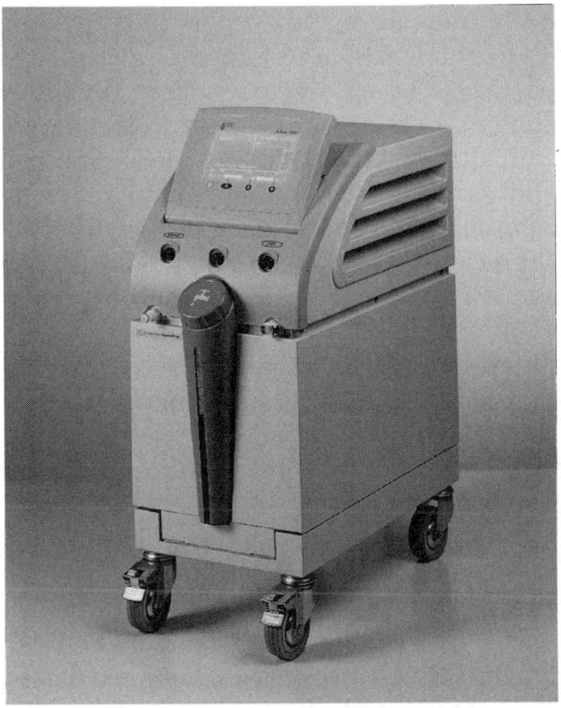

(a)

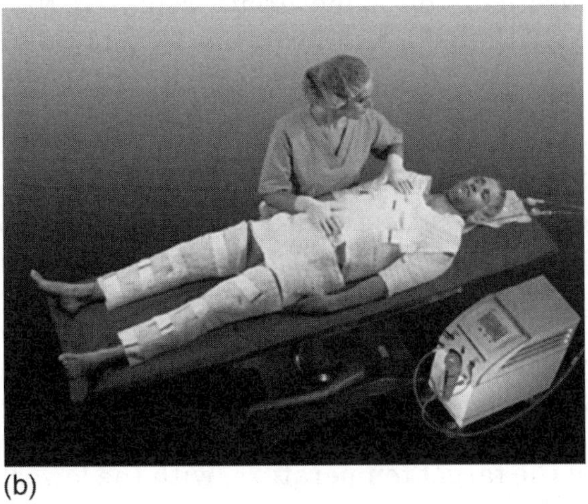

(b)

Figure 5 (a) ALLON 2001 (M.T.R.E. Advanced Technologies). (b) ThermoWrap™ (M.T.R.E. Advanced Technologies).

could be relatively easily done to achieve mild hypothermia (35.5°C) in patients with ischemic stroke, as long as shivering was adequately suppressed (12). Mayer and coworkers similarly found that surface cooling was easy to implement in the neurological intensive care unit, although the forced-air cooling method was not significantly better than acetaminophen in reducing temperature in febrile patients (13). To achieve deeper levels of moderate hypothermia quickly (below 34°C), deep sedation and neuromuscular blockade are often required, a major disadvantage that limits its use and increases the risk of complications.

Even with these methods to minimize reflexive vasoconstriction and shivering, the rate of cooling with surface cooling is relatively slow, with the possible exception of complete ice-water immersion. In one study of normal volunteers under general anesthesia, immersion in ice water decreased the core temperature by 9.7 ± 4.4°C/hr compared with a decrease of 1.7 ± 0.5°C/hr with forced-air cooling and 1.6 ± 1.1°C/hr with liquid-circulating cooling (14). The slow rate of induction with cooling blankets was also demonstrated in a study by Schwab and coworkers, in which 3.5 to 6.2 hr were required to achieve a core temperature of 33°C with forced-air cooling blankets (15). In a follow-up study using a combination of forced-air cooling and evaporative convection, the same group reported that cooling took between 3.5 and 11 hr (mean 6.5 hr) (16). The main reason for the slowness of cooling (and the requirement of anesthesia and neuromuscular blockade) is the intense shivering and generation of heat that occurs when skin temperature receptors are stimulated.

In the Cooling for Acute Ischemia Brain Damage (COOL AID) I study, we achieved a target temperature of 32°C at a mean of 3.6 hr using the combination of immersion (alcohol/ice packs initially) and liquid-circulating cooling blankets (Aqua K-Thermia, American Medical Systems, Belleville, OH) applied both underneath and on top of the patient. This was very labor-intensive, however, and most of our patients (90%) experienced overshoot of the target temperature, with the lowest being 28°C (17) (Fig. 6). This overshoot can be minimized by using a system with a closed-loop, feedback-control feature. The slow rate of surface cooling seems to be particularly relevant in obese patients. Obesity decreases the ratio of

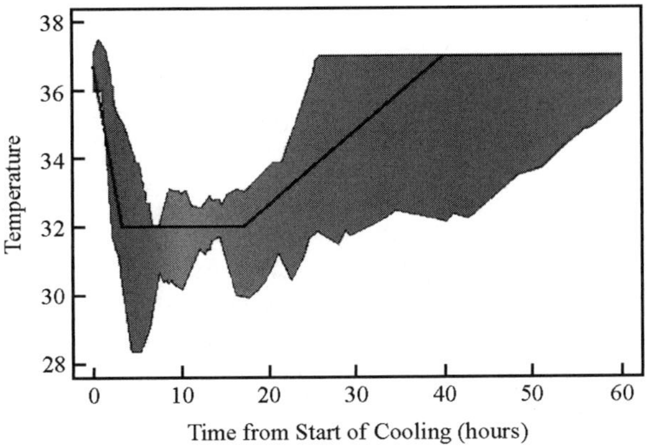

Figure 6 Temperature curve using surface cooling from COOL AID I. (From Ref. 17.)

surface area to mass and increases the size of the peripheral compartment. From a control dynamics perspective, there is simply more thermal inertia with obese patients. Hindmann and coworkers, in a multicenter pilot clinical trial of intraoperative hypothermia during cerebral aneurysm surgery, found that 12% of subjects could not reach a core temperature below 34.5°C mainly because of obesity (18). These patients have a reduced ability to dissipate internal energy because of the low thermal conductivity of their layers of fat.

Finally, thermal injury can occur when there is direct contact between the cooling blanket and skin (conductive methods of cooling). The combination of cold temperature and direct pressure can result in thermal skin injury, especially among the elderly whose thin skin is more susceptible to pressure necrosis and cold burns. Examples of reversible thermal skin injury resulting from excessive dermal vascoconstriction have also been described in patients cooled with Medivance Arctic Sun Cooling System who were treated with multiple vasopressors for vasodilatory shock (Dr. S. Mayer, personal communication). For conventional water-circulating cooling blankets, a sheet is often placed between the body and blankets (e.g., vinyl blankets) to minimize the risk of skin injury, at the price of interfering with heat transfer and limiting the effectiveness of cooling.

Endovascular Cooling

Hypothermia by endovascular cooling results from direct cooling of the blood. This is a potentially more powerful approach, by directly cooling the core and circumventing skin cold receptors, which play a large role in triggering reflexive vasoconstriction and shivering. Although extracorporeal cooling methods (such as cardiopulmonary bypass and extracorporeal membrane oxygenation) can be considered forms of direct blood cooling, we will focus mainly on infusion of ice-cold fluids and countercurrent exchange catheters that can be inserted into a vein or artery. Much like surface cooling, endovascular cooling must also be combined with methods to reduce shivering, such as the administration of buspirone, a 5-HT1a partial agonist, and meperidine (Chapter 8, Defeating Thermoregulatory Defenses Against Hypothermia) (19).

Cooled Intravenous Fluids

Administration of ice-cold intravenous fluids has been shown to be an effective way of reducing core temperature. After central venous infusion of 40 mL/kg of cold normal saline (20°C) over 30 min, Rajek and coworkers found that the core temperature decreased by 1.4 ± 0.2°C. When the temperature of the fluid was ice-cold (4°C), the core temperature decreased almost twice as fast, 2.5 ± 0.4°C (20). In a recent study on patients with out-of-hospital cardiac arrest, Bernard and coworkers infused 30 mL/kg of ice-cold (4°C) lactated Ringer's solution (in addition to applying ice packs to the skin surface). The authors reported a decrease in median core temperature from 35.5° to 33.8°C (21). Baumgardner and coworkers infused 5 mL/kg of ice-cold (1–6°C) 5% albumin very rapidly ($>$100 mL/min) to avoid heat gains in standard IV tubing (22). Whereas this approach can be effective, it is limited by the large volumes of fluid that must be given to substantially reduce core temperature.

Endovascular Countercurrent Heat Exchangers

Recently, internal heat-exchange catheters have been developed to induce therapeutic hypothermia. Several systems have European Union (CE) approval, along with United States

Food and Drug Administration (FDA) approval. The heat-exchange catheter precisely controls the amount of thermal energy entering or leaving a patient. The basic principle is that instead of removing blood and circulating it through a heat exchanger (as in cardiopulmonary bypass or extracorporeal membrane oxygenation), the heat exchanger can be inserted into the body as a catheter and blood can circulate round it. The catheter is cooled by a circulating coolant (usually water) and is inserted into a large central vein. These catheters are considered countercurrent heat exchangers because the coolant circulates in the opposite direction of the blood flow as the blood passes over the catheter surface. Compared to a parallel flow configuration where both the blood and the coolant flow in the same direction, this countercurrent orientation maintains a higher average temperature difference, resulting in higher cooling capacities.

There are several steps in the endovascular cooling process. First, heat is transferred from the warm blood to the outer wall of the cool catheter by convection. Next, heat travels by conduction across the catheter wall (typically a thin biocompatible polymer) that separates the blood from the coolant. The heat then travels from the inner wall of the catheter to the circulating coolant, again, by convection. The coolant is then pumped externally through a cooling console and resupplied to the catheter at the specified coolant inlet temperature.

Designing an endovascular catheter involves many careful design choices. Ultimately, the goal for each design is to meet the cooling requirements based on our understanding of hypothermia while minimizing the physiological side effects. For example, increasing the radius of a cooling catheter may facilitate heat transfer in two ways, first, by increasing the heat exchanger surface area and, second, by increasing the blood velocity going past the cooling catheter, assuming the blood flow rate remains constant. Too large a radius, however, and the assumption that the blood flow rate remains constant loses validity. In this case the form drag, resulting from pressure forces, and the friction drag, because of shear stresses, of the catheter impedes blood flow, reducing the cooling capacity of the catheter. As a result, existing cooling catheters carefully select heat exchange surfaces that are designed for optimal heat transfer performance without negative impacts on hemodynamics. The following is a review of the heat exchange catheters that are currently available or are under development.

The Reprieve™ Endovascular Temperature Therapy System (Radiant Medical, Redwood City, CA) (Fig. 7) uses several creative design ideas. It consists of a triple-lobed,

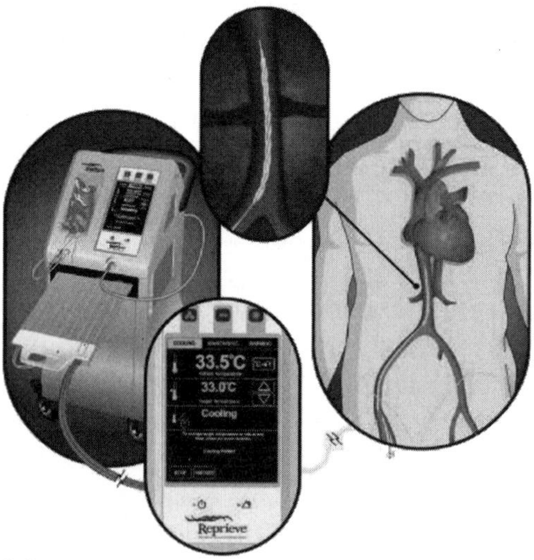

(a)

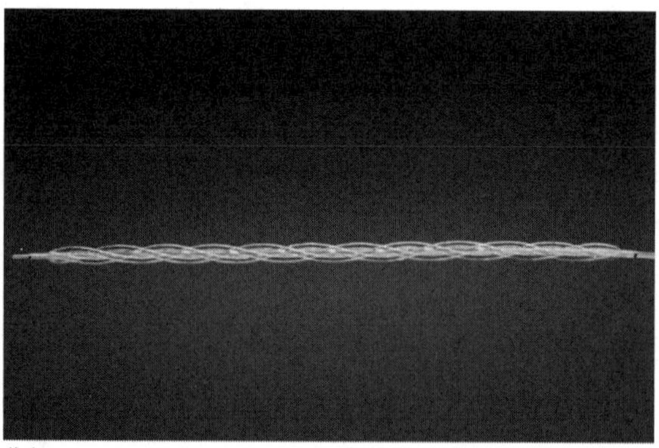

(b)

Figure 7 (a) Reprieve™ Endovascular Temperature Therapy System (Radiant Medical). (b) Reprieve catheter (Radiant Medical).

helically wound, balloon catheter that is placed in the inferior vena cava via the femoral vein and a microprocessor-driven controller that cools or warms normal saline. During insertion, the balloon is unexpanded, keeping the insertion size to a minimum. The catheter with the unexpanded balloon has a 9.2 F diameter and is inserted through a 10 F femoral introducer sheath until the distal tip of the catheter is positioned at the level of the diaphragm. To begin the cooling process, coolant flow is started, expanding the balloon. The device surface area dramatically increases (by 400%), sharply reducing the convective thermal resistances on both the coolant and the blood pathways. The helical nature of the balloon geometry also helps create local mixing of the passing blood near the cold catheter balloon surface. To ensure the maximum possible temperature difference between coolant and blood, carefully selected coolant pathways are used. The catheter is connected via insulated lines to a peripheral cassette consisting of a pump that circulates the saline and a thin-walled heat-exchange bag that lies on a thermal transfer plate. This cools or warms the saline circulating through the cassette and catheter. The catheter is heparin coated to prevent thrombus formation.

The Cool Line™ system (Alsius, Irving, CA) (Fig. 8) consists of a catheter with two MicroTherm™ balloons and a microprocessor-driven controller (Cool Gard system). This functions similarly to the Reprieve catheter in that the balloons are perfused with cold sterile normal saline via a closed-loop tubing system. The Cool Line Catheter is designed to be inserted into the superior vena cava just like a standard central venous catheter and can function as a standard triple-lumen central venous catheter. The Cool Line Catheter may be most useful for maintaining normothermia in the ICU setting. The Icy™ system (Alsius) is a similar catheter, but instead of two MicroTherm balloons there are three for added surface area. The Icy catheter is designed to be inserted in the inferior vena cava via the femoral vein. The catheter size has an 8.5 F diameter, a single infusion lumen and one additional lumen.

The Celsius Control™ System (Innercool, San Diego, CA) (Fig. 9) is different from the previous two balloon designs. It consists of a thin, flexible metallic catheter that is also placed in the inferior vena cava via the femoral vein. The tip of the

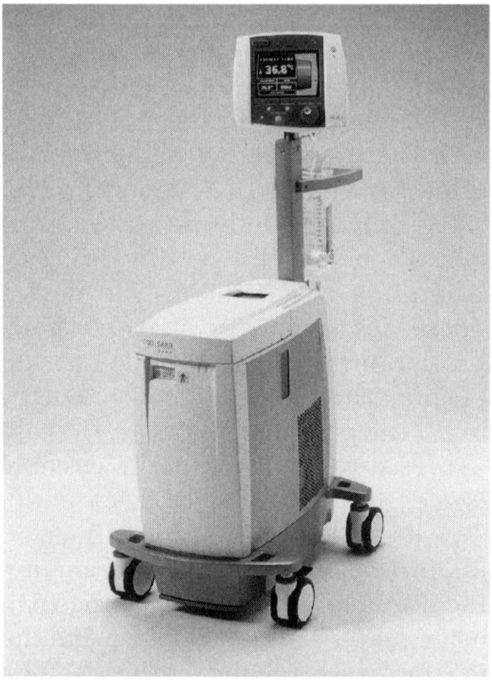

(a)

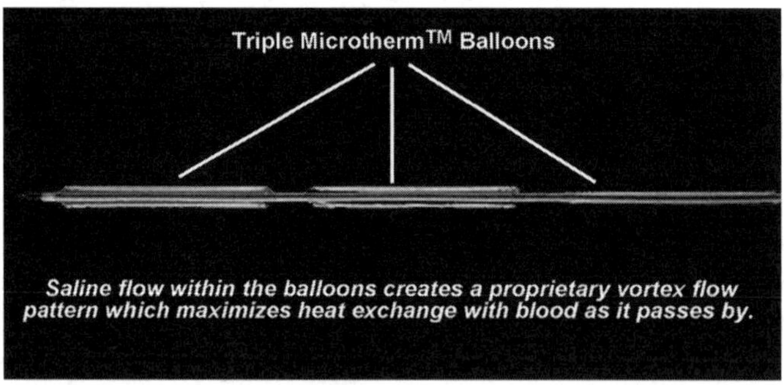

(b)

Figure 8 (a) Icy system (Alsius). (b) Icy catheter (Alsius).

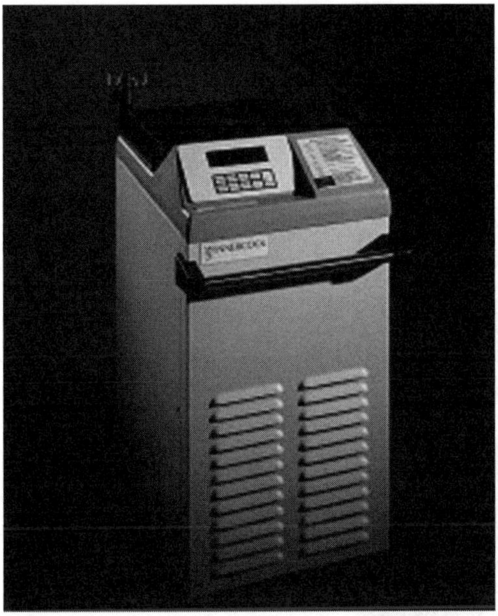

(a)

Figure 9 (a) Celsius Control System (Innercool). (b) Celsius catheter (Innercool).

catheter incorporates a flexible, alloy-based temperature control element (TCE) that can be cooled or warmed with saline solution circulated from the controller. The advantage of this approach is that metal is highly conductive (most metals have thermal conductivities that are two orders of magnitude greater than most plastics). In addition, unlike the other devices, the Celsius system uses an enhanced heat exchanger surface area, also called an articulated surface area, that not only increases the surface area, but also promotes blood mixing.

Advantages and Disadvantages of Endovascular Cooling

The main advantage of endovascular cooling is the rapid rate of induction that is possible and the precision of temperature control it allows. Early animal studies by Dae and coworkers in large pigs using the Reprieve device showed that core temperature can be quickly reduced and precisely maintained with endovascular cooling (23). Inderbitzen and co-

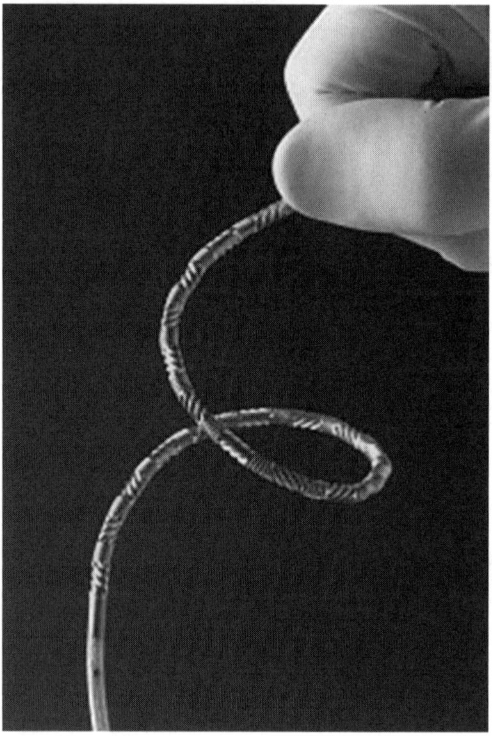

(b)

Figure 9 Continued.

workers, using the Celsius Control System to induce hypothermia in large pigs, found that cooling from 36.2° to 32.0°C was rapid and uniform (mean 7.3 ± 0.7°C/hr), with animals reaching the target temperature within 60 min (24). Clinical studies have confirmed this precision of temperature control. The Reprieve system was demonstrated to effectively cool patients undergoing neurosurgical procedures; cooling was linear and occurred at a rate of 3.9 ± 1.6°C/hr. Once the target temperature was reached, it was maintained within a few tenths of a degree. Rewarming was similarly linear and precise, increasing at 2.0 ± 0.5 °C/hr (25). Our group, also using the Reprieve device, found that a target temperature of 33°C could be achieved quickly (mean of 77 ± 44 min) and safely in patients with ischemic stroke in the COOL AID II study (Fig. 10). Unlike our

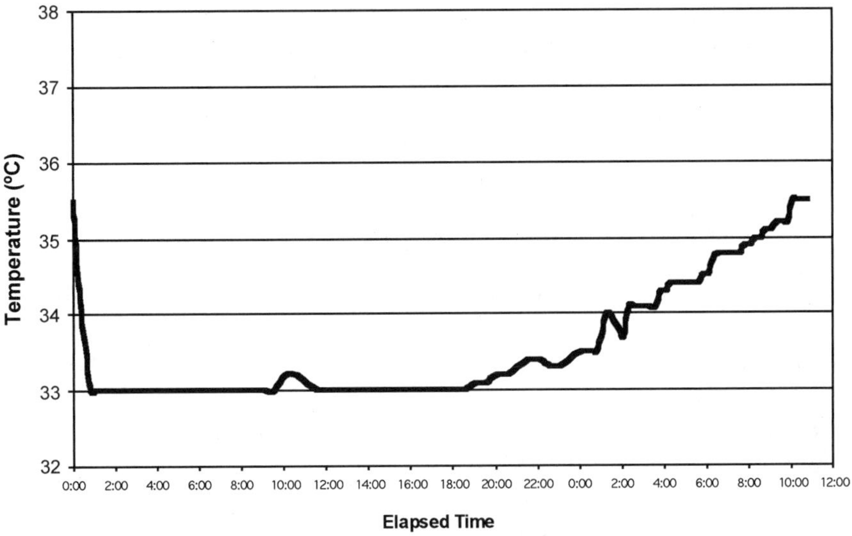

Figure 10 Temperature curve using endovascular cooling from COOL AID II. (From Ref. 26.)

previous surface-cooling experience, we had no overshoot with endovascular cooling (26).

Dixon and coworkers, in a feasibility and safety study of the Reprieve system for endovascular cooling during primary percutaneous coronary intervention for acute myocardial infarction, showed similar results (COOL MI study) (27). It is possible with endovascular cooling to cool patients to 32–33°C without deep sedation or neuromuscular blockade, which is a critical advantage for those with neurological disease who require close clinical monitoring. In the COOL AID and COOL MI studies, shivering was suppressed by using the combination of oral buspirone, intravenous meperidine, and an air convection heating blanket to warm the skin. In both studies, all patients tolerated hypothermia well and there were no major adverse events. (See Chapter 8 for details of defeating thermoregulatory defenses against induction of hypothermia.)

An additional advantage of endovascular cooling is that little staff effort is required once the catheter is inserted.

Schmutzhard and coworkers used the Cool Line system in a pilot study of 51 patients in the intensive care unit to maintain normothermia (36.5°C). They found that the COOL Line system was easy to insert and incorporate into the usual ICU routine (28). Subsequently, Georgiadis and coworkers cooled six patients with severe ischemic stroke to 33°C using the Icy system and similarly found this approach less cumbersome than surface cooling (29).

The main disadvantage is the invasiveness of the procedure. Although central venous access is a common procedure in the intensive care unit, it still requires training and caution. In a pilot study using the Celsius Control System to control fever in subarachnoid hemorrhage patients, two of nine patients developed deep vein thromboses distal to the catheter system, which required treatment with inferior vena cava filters (30). In contrast, no serious adverse events have been observed with the Reprieve system.

Other Cooling Methods

Peritoneal and Gastric Cooling

Peritoneal cooling and gastric cooling are sometimes combined with surface cooling. In peritoneal cooling, up to 2 L of iced Ringer's lactate solution is instilled into the peritoneal cavity with a catheter through a small incision below the umbilicus. The fluid is usually left to dwell for 5 min and then drained by gravity. Continuous peritoneal lavage at the rate of 250 mL/min has also been reported but is less commonly used (31,32). Peritoneal lavage has been extensively used to warm the patients with accidental hypothermia but few studies have examined induced hypothermia. The obvious invasiveness makes this approach less attractive than other methods.

Gastric lavage has been used effectively in the past for treatment of heat stroke. Approximately 500 mL of sterile cold water is instilled through a double lumen oral or nasogastric tube into the stomach and aspirated after 5 min. Iced saline may be used in place of water. Central cooling rates were reported to be 5–6 times faster when this method is used as adjunctive cooling technique, but side effects include abdominal cramping and diarrhea (14).

Extracorporeal Cooling

Extracorporeal cooling, literally cooling outside the body, is used to attain deep hypothermia (≤26°C) for patients undergoing high-risk aneurysm repair procedures in combination with cardiopulmonary bypass and temporary circulatory arrest. By providing profound hypothermia and a bloodless operative field, this approach became widely used for complicated aneurysm surgery in the 1960s (33,34), fell out of favor in the 1970s as complications were reported, and was revitalized in the late 1980s as advances in neuroanesthesia and perioperative monitoring made it safer (35).

Cardiopulmonary bypass begins with femoral venous and arterial cannulation. The venous catheter is advanced to the level of the right atrium while the arterial catheter is advanced to the aorta. Blood is then withdrawn from the venous catheter (usually at a rate of 40 mL/kg per minute), cooled in a countercurrent heat exchanger, oxygenated, and returned to the arterial catheter, thereby bypassing the heart and lungs. With this technique, even profound hypothermia (core temperatures of less than 20°C) can be achieved. The heart can be stopped temporarily with potassium chloride, allowing for mobilization, ligation, and clipping of the aneurysm (usually 15–20 min). Rewarming is done slowly, and between 23° to 28°C spontaneous cardiac activity occurs. Patients are usually taken off bypass when adequate cardiac function has returned and the core temperature is ≥36°C.

Extracorporeal membrane oxygenation (ECMO) is an alternative to the conventional cardiopulmonary bypass technique. It requires only femoral venous and arterial cannulation, rather than intrathoracic cannulation, which makes it suitable for use in the ICU.

FUTURE DIRECTIONS

There is considerable animal and clinical support for the protective effects of hypothermia in the setting of reduced blood flow and ischemia. Surface cooling, the oldest and simplest approach, can be used to achieve hypothermia and most studies in the literature have used surface cooling. With the exception of ice-water immersion, surface cooling often requires several hours to reach 32° to 33°C. Nevertheless, it is relatively straightforward and widely available in most hospitals.

Endovascular cooling is an exciting newer approach that has several potential advantages over surface cooling, especially if core temperatures as low as 32–33°C are desired. For example, target temperature can be achieved more quickly than with surface cooling and temperature can be more precisely controlled. It is invasive, however, and thus requires special training.

Future devices will continue to move in the direction of increased cooling capacity with reduced physiological impact. Building on emerging technologies that arise within the thermal sciences, such as microchannel heat transfer, future devices used to induce hypothermia will enable physicians to turn their attention to more selective and localized cooling within the body. These devices may enable rapid temperature control at specific sites within the body, eliminating the inherent complications associated with systemic hypothermia.

REFERENCES

1. Tablott JH. N Engl J Med 1941; 224:30.
2. Fay T. Observations on generalised refrigeration in cases of severe cerebral trauma. Assoc Res Nerv Ment Dis Proc 1943; 24:6.
3. Bigelow WG, Lindsay WK, Greenwood WF. Hypothermia its possible role in cardiac surgery. Ann Surg 1950; 132.
4. Lewis FJ, Tauffic M. Closure of atrial septal defect with the aid of hypothermia. Surgery 1953; 33:52–59.
5. Rosamoff HL. Hypothermia and cerebral vascular lesions II. Experimental middle cerebral artery interruption followed by induction of hypothermia. Arch Neurol Psychiatry 1957; 78: 454–464.
6. Delorme EJ. Experimental cooling of the blood-stream. Lancet 1952; 2:914–915.
7. Boerema IA, Germs R, Blickman JR. Artificial stenosis of the aorta. Arch Chir Neerl 1951; 3:123–127.

8. Adams J, Wylie EJ. Value of hypothermia and arterial occlusion in the treatment of intracranial aneurysms. Surg Gynecol Obstet 1959; 108:631–663.

9. Connolly JE, Boyd RJ, Calvin JW. The protective effect of hypothermia in cerebral ischemia experimental and clinical application by selective brain cooling in the human. Surgery 1962; 51:15–23.

10. Sessler DI. Perioperative thermoregulation and heat balance. Ann N Y Acad Sci 1997; 813:757–777.

11. Kielblock AJ, Van Rensburg JP, Franz RM. Body cooling as a method for reducing hyperthermia. An evaluation of techniques. S Afr Med J 1986; 69:378–380.

12. Kammersgaard LP, Rasmussen BH, Jorgensen HS, Reith J, Weber U, Olsen TS. Feasibility and safety of inducing modest hypothermia in awake patients with acute stroke through surface cooling: a case–control study: the Copenhagen Stroke Study. Stroke 2000; 31:2251–2256.

13. Mayer S, Commichau C, Scarmeas N, Presciutti M, Bates J, Copeland D. Clinical trial of an air-circulating cooling blanket for fever control in critically ill neurologic patients [comment]. Neurology 2001; 56:292–298.

14. Plattner O, Kurz A, Sessler DI, Ikeda T, Christensen R, Marder D, Clough D. Efficacy of intraoperative cooling methods. Anesthesiology 1997; 87:1089–1095.

15. Schwab S, Schwarz S, Aschoff A, Keller E, Hacke W. Moderate hypothermia and brain temperature in patients with severe middle cerebral artery infarction. Acta Neurochir Suppl 1998; 71:131–134.

16. Schwab S, Georgiadis D, Berrouschot J, Schellinger PD, Graffagnino C, Mayer SA. Feasibility and safety of moderate hypothermia after massive hemispheric infarction [comment]. Stroke 2001; 32:2033–2035.

17. Krieger DW, De Georgia MA, Abou-Chebl A, Andrefsky JC, Sila CA, Katzen IL, Mayberg MR, Furlan AJ. Cooling for Acute Ischemic Brain Damage (COOL AID): an open pilot study of induced hypothermia for acute ischemic stroke. Stroke 2001; 9:28–33.

18. Hindman BJ, Todd MM, Gelb AW, Loftus CM, Craen RA,

Schubert A, Mahla ME, Torner JC. Mild hypothermia as a protective therapy during intracranial aneurysm surgery: a randomized prospective pilot trial. Neurosurgery 1999; 44:23–32. Discussion 32–33.

19. Mokhtarani M, Mahgoub AN, Morioka N, Doufas AG, Dae M, Shaughnessy TE, Bjorksten AR, Sessler DI. Buspirone and meperidine synergistically reduce the shivering threshold. Anesth Analg 2001; 93:1233–1239.

20. Rajek A, Greif R, Sessler DI, Baumgardner J, Laciny S, Bastanmehr H. Core cooling by central venous infusion of ice-cold (4 degrees C and 20 degrees C) fluid: isolation of core and peripheral thermal compartments. Anesthesiology 2000; 93:629–637.

21. Bernard S, Buist M, Monteiro O, Smith K. Induced hypothermia using large volume, ice-cold intravenous fluid in comatose survivors of out-of hospital cardiac arrest: A preliminary report. Resuscitation 2003; 56:9–10.

22. Baumgardner JE, Baranov D, Smith DS, Zager EL. The effectiveness of rapidly infused intravenous fluids for inducing moderate hypothermia in neurosurgical patients. Anesth Analg 1999; 89:163–169.

23. Dae MW, Gao DW, Sessler DI, Chair K, Stillson CA. Effect of endovascular cooling on myocardial temperature, infarct size, and cardiac output in human-sized pigs. Am J Physiol Heart Circ Physiol 2002; 282:H1584–H1591.

24. Inderbitzen B, Yon S, Lasheras J, Dobak J, Perl J, Steinberg GK. Safety and performance of a novel intravascular catheter for induction and reversal of hypothermia in a porcine model. Neurosurgery 2002; 50:364–370.

25. Doufas AG, Akca O, Barry A, Petrusca DA, Sulemann M, Morioka N, Guaraschelli JJ, Sessler DI. Initial experience with a novel heat-exchanging catheter in neurosurgical patients. Anesth Analg 2002; 95:1752–1756.

26. De Georgia MA, Abou-Chebl A, Krieger DW, Andrefsky JC, Sila CC, Furlan AJ. Endovascular cooling for acute ischemic stroke. Stroke 2002; 33:410A.

27. Dixon SR, Whitbourn RJ, Dae MW, Grube E, Sherman W,

Schaer GL, Jenkins S, Baim DS, Gibbons RJ, Kuntz RE, Popma JJ, Nguyen TT, O'Neil WW. Induction of mild systemic hypothermia with endovascular cooling during primary percutaneous coronary intervention for acute myocardial infarction. J Am Coll Cardiol 2002; 40:1928–1934.

28. Schmutzhard E, Engelhardt K, Beer R, Broessner G, Pflauser B, Spiss H, Unterberger I, Kampfl A. Safety and efficacy of a novel intravascular cooling device to control body temperature in neurologic intensive care patients: a prospective pilot study. Crit Care Med 2002; 30:2481–2488.

29. Georgiadis D, Schwartz S, Kollmar R, Scwab S. Endovascular cooling for moderate hypothermia in patients with acute stroke. Stroke 2001; 32:2550–2553.

30. Badjatia N, O'Donnell J, Baker JR, Huamg DY, Ayata C, Greer DM, McDonald CT, Carter BS, Ogilvy CS. Achieving normothermia in febrile subarachnoid hemorrhage patients: feasibility of a novel intravascular cooling catheter [abstr]. Crit Care Med 2003; 30(suppl):A5.

31. Sterz F, Zeiner A, Kurkciyan I, Janata K, Mullner M, Domanovits H, Safar P. Mild resuscitative hypothermia and outcome after cardiopulmonary resuscitation. J Neurosurg Anesthesiol 1996; 8:88–89.

32. Xiao F, Safar P, Alexander HL. Peritoneal cooling for mild cerebral hypothermia after cardiac arrest in dogs. Resuscitation 1995; 30:51–59.

33. Patterson RH, Ray B. Profound hypothermia for intracranial surgery: laboratory and clinical experience with extracorporeal circulation by peripheral cannulation. Ann Surg 1963; 156: 377–39.

34. Michenfelder JD, Kirklin JW, Uihlein A. Clinical experience with a closed-chest technique of profound hypothermia and total circulatory arrest in neurosurgery. Ann Surg 1964; 159: 125–130.

35. Spetzler RF, Hadley MN, Rigamonti D. Aneurysms of the basilar artery treated with circulatory arrest, hypothermia and barbiturate cerebral protection. J Neuorosurg 1988; 68: 868–879.

11

Direct Brain Cooling

BRIDGET A. HARRIS
Western General Hospital,
University of Edinburgh,
Edinburgh, Scotland

PETER J.D. ANDREWS
Anaesthetics, Pain Medicine, and Intensive Care,
Western General Hospital,
Edinburgh, Scotland

INTRODUCTION

Two general approaches to direct brain cooling predominate. The first approach is to reduce brain temperature independently from body temperature (*isolated brain cooling*). To maintain trunk normothermia with isolated brain cooling, active body warming may be necessary to prevent cool venous blood from the brain from lowering core temperature (cool head/warm body methods). A related term, "selective brain cooling," is defined as *natural* cooling of parts of the brain or the whole brain below aortic (arterial blood) temperature (1,2). The second approach is to cool the head and allow secondary cooling of the body to occur (*brain-directed systemic cooling*). Sometimes, body warming is used with head cooling to prevent trunk temperature from becoming as low as brain temperature, thus making the cooling relatively brain-selective (cool body/cooler head methods).

Direct Brain Cooling Methods

Different methods for direct brain cooling are shown in Table 1. A distinction has been made between invasive and noninvasive methods, in part because invasive methods require more skill to perform and may be riskier, and are therefore less likely to be suitable for out-of-hospital use. Restriction to hospital use is important because the speed of initiation of cooling after brain insult presumably influences outcome (3).

Brain and Core Body Temperature

At the risk of stating the obvious, it is brain temperature rather than core body temperature that is important in cerebral protection from injury. Busto et al. (4,5), for example, demonstrated this in rats when they studied the effect of isolated brain cooling during and after an ischemic injury. With rectal

Table 1 Methods for Direct Brain Cooling

Noninvasive methods
Heat loss from the upper airways
Nasal gas flow (convection)
Nasal fluid lavage (conduction)
Heat loss through the skull
Fanning, cooling hoods (convection)
Ice packs, cooling caps, and helmets (conduction)
Invasive methods (all conduction)
Anterograde cerebral perfusion
Intracarotid flush
Open irrigation of the brain surface
Semiclosed and closed irrigation of the brain surface and ventricles
Contact cooling of specific areas of the brain

temperature held constant at 37°C, they found that hypothermic brain temperatures significantly reduced infarct volume. Despite this, most of the studies of cooling in humans after brain injury have used systemic hypothermia rather than direct brain cooling. The reasons are not altogether clear, but probably include the practical problems of attaining and maintaining brain temperature below trunk temperature and concern over increased temperature gradients. As a consequence, very little is known about the effects of direct brain cooling after brain injury in humans compared to systemic hypothermia. But because a cool brain is the therapeutic goal, there is logic in targeting cooling of the brain.

There is evidence that the difference between brain and core body temperatures varies between individuals after brain injury. Human studies have found differences ranging from −0.3°C to 2.1°C between frontal lobe and rectal temperatures (6) and from −0.7°C to 2.3°C between ventricular and pulmonary artery temperatures (7). Therefore, to know whether cooling is affecting brain temperature, it follows that measurement of brain temperature after injury is important, particularly when direct brain cooling methods are employed (8).

REVIEW

Human brain cooling mechanisms and the nature of brain temperature elevations that commonly occur after injury are briefly reviewed to facilitate understanding of the overall advantages and disadvantages of direct brain cooling. Different methods of direct brain cooling are then described in detail and their cooling effectiveness and particular advantages and disadvantages are discussed.

Brain Cooling Mechanisms in Humans

The human brain is believed to have three cooling mechanisms: cooling of venous blood by the skin, which in turn cools the arterial blood supply to the brain; heat loss through the skull; and heat loss from the upper airways (which is abolished by endotracheal intubation) (9,10). The last two can produce natural selective brain cooling. Even if arterial blood temperature remains the major determinant of brain temperature, the other mechanisms are potentially clinically important because factors that enhance or inhibit them will have an effect on brain temperature.

Zenker and Kubik (11) have explained how it is anatomically possible for heat loss from the skull and upper airways to cause brain cooling in humans. Evaporation of sweat from the scalp and face and of secretions from the nose cools blood in the diploic and emissary veins. This blood is transferred via the dural venous sinuses to the dura mater. The dura mater may transmit the cooling to the cerebrospinal fluid, which in turn influences parenchymal temperature by direct contact and via arteries within the subarachnoid space, on the pial surface, and in the brain parenchyma. Some authors believe that the cavernous sinus, which is cooled by veins from the face and by heat loss from the upper airways, is involved in brain cooling by countercurrent heat exchange with the internal carotid, which changes direction in the sinus thus augmenting the surface available for heat exchange (12–16). du Boulay et al. (15) have speculated that the proximity of the carotid artery to the trachea, larynx, and pharynx is also a factor, and that "vertebral artery blood to the brainstem might . . . be cooled by proximity to the vertebral venous plexus conducting cooled blood from around the pharynx (15)." Brain cooling by heat loss through the skull and the upper airways appear to be anatomically complementary because, between them, the brain is nearly completely encircled with cool venous blood and cool air (10) (Fig. 1).

Human Evidence For Brain Cooling By Heat Loss Through the Skull

Cabanac and Brinnel (13) have demonstrated that blood in the mainly valveless emissary veins flows from the skin to the brain in moderately hyperthermic humans, delivering blood cooled by evaporation from the sweating face and scalp. In normothermia, the flow was either undetectable or reversed (i.e., from brain to scalp) and much slower. Caputa et al. (17) and Hirashita et al. (18) have shown similar flow patterns in the angularis oculi and ophthalmic veins.

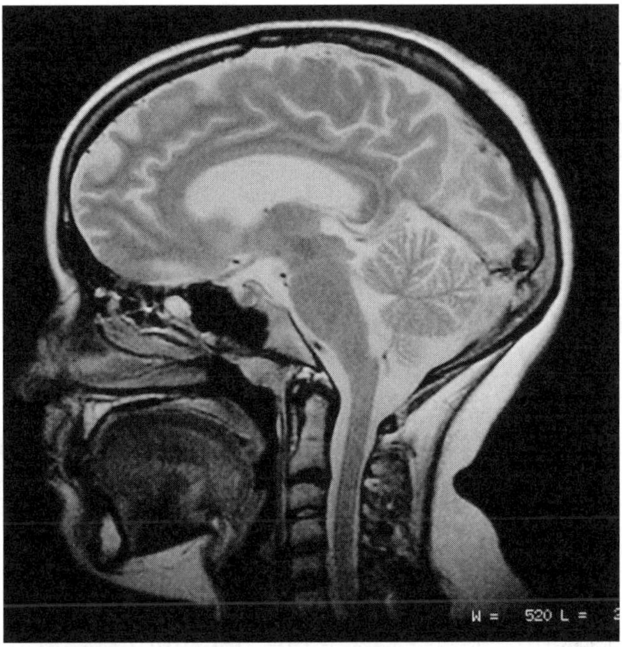

Figure 1 The anatomy that makes heat loss through the skull possible. The dural venous sinuses surround the brain under the skull from the front round to, and into, the back of the brain. Under the base of the brain are the anatomical structures for cooling via the upper airways, i.e., the nose, paranasal sinuses, and cavernous sinus. The vertebral venous plexus surrounds the brainstem.

Human Evidence For Brain Cooling By Heat Loss From the Upper Airways

Mariak et al. (19) demonstrated that selective brain cooling (i.e., natural cooling of the brain, or parts of it) by heat loss from the upper airways can occur in humans. They measured intracranial temperature on the midline between the cribriform plate and the frontal lobes in four conscious, intubated patients with esophageal temperatures ranging from 36.9 °C to 37.5 °C. When airflow through the upper respiratory tract was reinstated by extubation, brain temperature above the cribriform plate fell by between 0.4°C and 0.9°C, and in three patients intracranial temperature decreased to less than esophageal temperature. Once their temperatures had stabilized, the patients were asked to breathe deeply for 3 min, in through their noses and out through their mouths. This caused an additional 0.2–0.3°C reduction in temperature above the cribriform plate.

Advantages and Disadvantages of Direct Brain Cooling

The general advantages and disadvantages of direct brain cooling are discussed here. The advantages and disadvantages of each individual method are discussed later.

Neuroprotection

Direct Brain Cooling vs. Normothermia

Direct brain cooling confers ischemic neuroprotection in animals. Compared to normothermia, direct brain cooling methods with maintenance of normothermic rectal temperature (cool head/warm body) have been shown to convey neuroprotection in rats, rabbits, cats, and dogs (4,20–25), and in cats with no body warming (cool body/cooler head) (26).

However, we have found only two published studies containing data on direct brain cooling methods in humans. Battin et al. (27) used a cool body/cooler head approach in infants with hypoxic–ischemic injury. They were treated with circulating-water cooling caps to produce four different levels of systemic hypothermia ranging from 36°C to 34.5°C (n = 6 or 7 per group). Although the primary aim was to assess safety, the authors concluded that infants with moderate to severe encephalopathy who were cooled had a tendency toward better outcome at 18 months. These investigators are currently conducting a multicenter trial powered to assess long-term functional outcome (28).

Hachimi-Idrissi et al. (29) studied patients after cardiac arrest due to asystole or pulseless electrical activity, who remained unconscious after restoration of spontaneous circulation. Sixteen patients were randomized to head cooling with a noncirculating cooling cap for 4 hr or until their bladder temperature reached 34°C, whichever occurred sooner. One patient did not achieve a bladder temperature of 34°C within 4 hr. Fourteen patients were randomized to normothermia; they were passively rewarmed if hypothermic, whereas temperatures exceeding 38°C were treated with acetaminophen.

This study has methodological problems that make interpretation of the results difficult. At the start of the study, the median tympanic temperature in the hypothermic group was 35.8°C (range 33.7–38.2°C), and it took a median of 180 min (range 70–240) to reach a bladder temperature of 34°C (the baseline bladder temperature was not reported). Therefore the time that patients was hypothermic and the time they spent at target temperature varied. The median tympanic temperature in the normothermic group at the start of the study was 35.5°C (range 33.6–37.5°C), but neither tympanic nor bladder temperature at the end of the study was reported in this group. Therefore it is not known if the normothermic group was in fact normothermic by the end of 4 hr, or how successful the investigators were in maintaining normothermia in this group. The primary purpose of this study was to test the feasibility and speed of cooling of the cap, not patient outcome. Three of 16 patients (18%) in the hypothermic group survived, compared to one of the 14 patients (7%) in the normothermic group. The authors attributed the high overall mortality rate to the poor prognosis associated with cardiac arrest.

Direct Brain Cooling vs. Systemic Cooling

Three animal studies have compared direct brain cooling to systemic hypothermia (8,30–32), but only two of these evaluated histological neuronal damage (30,31).

Minamisawa et al. (30) assessed histopathological brain damage following forebrain ischemia in rats. They compared rats maintained at systemic temperatures of 37°C and 38°C (n = 10 per group) with rats allowed to become systemically hypothermic to 33°C and 35°C (n = 10 per group) *before* ischemia (protective cooling), as well as with rats whose brain temperatures were allowed to drop to 32°C (n = 8) as a *result* of ischemia (preservative cooling), but with body temperature maintained at 37°C (i.e., cool head/warm body). Neuroprotection was afforded by both these cooling methods but the quantitative data shows that the damage reduction to neurons in the hippocampus CA1 sector with isolated brain cooling was more similar to that provided by systemic hypothermia at 35°C than at 33°C. However, it is not possible to deduce from this that systemic cooling produced better neuroprotection than isolated brain cooling because systemic cooling was induced prior to the insult and isolated brain cooling was induced during the insult. The apparently reduced protection afforded by isolated brain cooling, even with lower brain temperatures of 32°C, could therefore reflect the difference between protective and preservative cooling.

Park et al. (31) compared the effects of normothermia, systemic hypothermia, and isolated brain cooling on infarction volume and edema in rats ($n = 6$ per group) after permanent left middle cerebral artery occlusion. Occlusion of the middle cerebral artery reduced cerebral blood flow (CBF) (laser–Doppler flowmetry) to about 40% of baseline in the ischemic area in all three groups. Cooling was started 15 min after occlusion to reduce brain temperature to 32°C. How cooling was achieved is not specified. The rats having isolated brain cooling had their rectal temperatures maintained between 36.6°C and 37.0°C (cool head/warm body).

In comparison with normothermic controls, infarction volume was reduced by 49% with systemic hypothermia and by 27% with isolated head cooling. The volume of brain edema was reduced by 24% with systemic hypothermia and by only 8% with isolated brain cooling. During rewarming, the reductions in CBF were maintained in the normothermic and systemic hypothermia groups, whereas in the brain-selective cooling group, CBF increased to about 70% of baseline. All these results were statistically significant ($P < 0.05$). The authors concluded that "mild systemic hypothermia has much stronger protective effects against focal cerebral infarction and edema than selective brain cooling. The lack of protective effects of selective brain cooling may be caused by postcooling cerebral hyperemia in the ischemic area" (31). It is conceivable that the hyperemia was due to an influx of warm blood from the body during rewarming.

The effect of cerebral hyperemia on brain temperature was evaluated in two isolated brain cooling experiments using cooling caps and body warming to achieve brain hypothermia with normothermic rectal temperatures (cool brain/warm body). During resuscitation of piglets after cardiac arrest, Gelman et al. (32) found a temporary increase in brain temperatures early in reperfusion in the isolated brain cooling group ($n = 7$), which did not occur in the normothermia group ($n = 7$). Interestingly, this increase was greater in the deep structures than in superficial brain tissue. They attributed this to an increase in CBF causing "a net influx of heat from warm arterial blood to brain." Laptook et al. (8) compared isolated brain cooling with systemic hypothermia in piglets ($n = 8$) using a crossover design and found that both methods decreased CBF to a similar degree. When hypoxia was superimposed on cooling, CBF increased equally in both groups but brain temperatures increased only in the isolated brain cooling group. Again, this was presumably because there was an influx of blood from the warm body. Gelman et al. (32) suggest that the effect of the influx of warmed blood to the brain may be even greater in larger mammals.

In summary, it appears that although direct brain cooling using cool head/warm body techniques does convey neuroprotection after brain injury, it may not provide neuroprotection equivalent to that provided by systemic hypothermia. This may be due in part to the "rebound" increases in brain temperature that can occur as warm blood from the body flows into the brain with rewarming when cool brain/warm body techniques are used.

Cerebral Blood Flow, Oxygen Consumption, and Metabolism with Direct Brain Cooling

As with neuroprotection, relatively few experimental studies have examined the effect of direct brain cooling on CBF. The results are not entirely consistent, but this is also true of studies of CBF in systemic hypothermia (21). Compared to normothermia, six studies of direct brain cooling showed a reduction in CBF (8,23,24,33–35), two showed an increase (36,37), and one showed no change (32). These studies used cool head/warm body methods, with the exception of Miyake et al. (36) and Schwartz et al. (34) who used cool body/cooler head. Five of the studies were in brain-injured animals: hypoxic injury (8) and ischemic injury due to cardiac arrest (32,36), bilateral carotid artery ligation (33), and transient middle cerebral artery occlusion (24). It has been suggested that the inconsistency in results may be due to differences in cerebrovascular responses to cooling between species or age groups (35,37), or to the cooling methods used (i.e., whether the brain is cooled from the inside out or the outside in) (35). The presence or absence of brain injury, as well as the type of injury, might also account for some of the inconsistency of these results. Although currently available data does not support this.

Mustafa and Thulesius (38) found that in vitro cooling induces vasodilation in isolated rabbit carotid artery preparations, that the degree of dilation is inversely proportional to temperature, and that the vasoconstrictive effect of norepinephrine and potassium chloride is reduced with cooling. They suggested that in vivo carotid cooling might therefore increase CBF. However, this theory was not confirmed by the three studies that used carotid cooling and measured CBF (34–36), only one of which showed an increase (36).

Three animal studies measured cerebral oxygen consumption and all found reductions with isolated brain cooling (8,32,35). Others have shown that cerebral energy metabolite depletion and lactate accumulation with ischemia are not different with direct brain cooling compared to normothermia (4,25). Ibayashi et al. (33) reported similar results except that cerebral adenosine triphosphate was significantly higher with brain cooling than with normothermia.

Hachimi-Idrissi (29) reported that in humans, after reaching a bladder temperature of 34°C with head cooling, "the mixed venous oxygen content was significantly higher, whereas arterial lactate concentration and the oxygen extraction ratio were significantly lower" in hypothermic ($n = 16$) cardiac arrest patients compared to normothermic patients (n = 14). Lactate was also reduced in the hypothermic group compared to baseline. However, as explained earlier, the time spent at target temperatures varied between and within groups in this study.

Reduction of the Complications of Systemic Hypothermia

The reason most commonly given for using direct head cooling is that it may have fewer side effects than systemic hypothermia (8,39–41). The side effects of systemic hypothermia at temperatures of 33°C to 35°C may include cardiac arrhythmias, pulmonary edema, rebound increases in ICP with rewarming, higher temperatures post hypothermia, coagulation abnormalities, metabolic effects, and immune suppression (see Chapter 6) (42).

The reporting and definition of complications in clinical trials of systemic hypothermia is variable, which makes assessing their impact difficult. Nevertheless, systematic reviews of trials of systemic hypothermia after brain injury have shown that the odds ratios for prothrombin time (but not partial thromboplastin time) (43), cardiac arrhythmias (43), and pneumonia (43,44) are increased with hypothermia.

Ishikawa et al. (45) retrospectively assessed characteristics of infection and leukocyte count in brain-injured patients treated with mild systemic hypothermia (n = 41), compared to controls treated with barbiturates (n = 25) and no barbiturates (n = 25). They found that the incidence of bacteraemia was greater in patients treated with hypothermia compared to controls, that pneumonia, although not more common, was more severe, and that total leukocyte count was considerably lower over the first 2 weeks after hypothermia.

Coagulation Abnormalities

It is unclear whether coagulation abnormalities are reduced with direct brain cooling. Thoresen et al. (41) used a cooling cap combined with body warming to maintain the rectal temperatures of piglets (n = 9) at 33–34°C with deep-brain temperatures around 5°C lower. They found no clotting problems or gross hemorrhages as a result of temperature-probe insertion with "moderate to severe hypothermia of the brain surface." The time over which cooling was maintained was 6 hr at most, and the piglets were systemically hypothermic, although their brain temperatures were lower than their rectal temperatures.

Hachimi-Idrissi et al. (29) found no change in clotting times or platelet counts in humans (n = 16) cooled with a cooling cap to a bladder temperature of 34°C for up to 4 hr after cardiac arrest (29). The cooling time was short and variable, the patients were systemically hypothermic, and their intracerebral temperatures were not measured. However, if the head is cool and the body warm, blood will be cooled and warmed as it circulates and this may affect clotting. Rats exposed to repeated cold stress (fluctuations in air temperature) over several days can develop thrombocytopenia and reduced platelet aggregation (46).

In humans, cooling the forearm from which blood samples were taken for clotting studies resulted in a decrease in clotting time as temperature was reduced from 37°C to 22°C. By 22°C, clotting time was three times longer than at 37°C (47). This suggests that it may not be safe to assume that coagulation abnormalities will be avoided with direct brain cooling. Thus, available evidence suggests that hypothermic coagulopathy depends largely on *local* temperature.

Cardiovascular Effects

Polderman et al. (48) have proposed that cardiac arrhythmias result from loss of electrolytes with hypothermia-induced polyuria; it seems possible that if the head alone is cooled, this problem might be reduced. No hazardous cardiovascular effects were reported in infants treated with cooling caps in comparison with those given surface cooling of the trunk (49) (n = 9) and with normothermia (27,50) (n = 40), provided overcooling and overly rapid rewarming were avoided. However, the direct brain cooling in these infants was not isolated to the head and the infants' rectal temperatures were hypothermic (range approximately 33–34.5°C) (27,49). The response of older people, especially with preexisting cardiac problems, is likely to be different from infants.

Gelman et al. (32) found that isolated brain cooling in piglets after cardiac arrest ($n = 14$) caused "a reduction in intestinal blood flow during reperfusion which persisted even after return to normal brain temperature, as well as a reduction in myocardial blood flow during CPR" as compared to piglets kept normothermic. While mesenteric blood flow reduction has been shown with systemic hypothermia alone in newborn piglets (51), it is a surprising finding with isolated brain cooling. Gelman et al. (32) suggest that "Decreases in brain temperature may alter the release of vasoactive substances by the brain, resulting in redistribution of cardiac output and reduction in splanchnic blood flow." However, Iwata et al. (52) found no ischemic or other abnormalities in the visceral organs of uninjured piglets after direct brain cooling with either cool head/warm body ($n = 3$) or cool body/cooler head ($n = 3$) method. They did not measure intestinal blood flow.

Immune Function

Hypothermic immune suppression may not be ameliorated with isolated brain cooling, because the brain itself controls many immune functions (53,54). Infections such as pneumonia and bacteremia may thus remain serious risks even with isolated brain cooling.

Fever, in response to infection, may have a protective effect and has been shown to correlate with survival from infection (55). Fever is thought to be a protective evolutionary mechanism for enhancing host defenses against infection via a number of mechanisms, including potentiation of immunological responses, activation of T-lymphocytes, stimulation of interferon production, and hypoferraemia (which has a bacteriostatic effect) (55). As far as we are aware, there is no evidence to show that cool head/warm body methods of direct brain cooling result in an improved immunological response to infection compared to systemic hypothermia and no data is available on its impact on brain-mediated immunosuppression.

In summary, there is currently little evidence one way or the other that direct head cooling can ameliorate complications associated with systemic hypothermia.

Reduction of Cooling "Stress" and of Sedation Requirements

We are unaware of any studies examining the effect of direct brain cooling on cooling "stress" and sedation requirements. However, forcing the body to temperatures below its thermoregulatory setpoint is stressful. In piglets subjected to a hypoxic insult under anesthesia (n = 36) and treated with systemic hypothermia (35°C) for 24 hr without sedation or treatment for shivering (n = 18), there was no neuroprotective effect or reduction in posthypoxic seizures compared to normothermic unsedated piglets (n = 18) (56).

The hypothermic piglets showed signs of stress manifested by cortisol levels three times that of the normothermic piglets. Furthermore, the reduction in heart rate that usually accompanies hypothermia did not occur. The authors speculated that "the stress of shivering and feeling cold interfered with the previously shown neuroprotective effect of hypothermia (56)." Cold stress can also induce vasospasm of diseased coronary arteries (57) and myocardial ischemia, probably because of increased noradrenaline release, peripheral vasoconstriction, and increased oxygen consumption due to shivering (58). Shivering can be attenuated with drugs (59) and cutaneous warming (60,61) (see Chapter 8), but other responses to cold stress may not be easily reduced, although they can vary depending on the method of cooling (62).

A stress response to cold may occur even if brain temperature alone is reduced below the setpoint, because cooling of the preoptic area of the hypothalamus is sufficient to cause heat production and retention responses (63,64). Therefore, measures to inhibit thermoregulatory responses to cooling may still be necessary with isolated brain cooling. The extent to which cool brain/warm body cooling can minimize the stress response probably depends on the balance between central and peripheral thermoreceptor inputs into the hypothalamus.

According to Bligh, it is likely "the regulated variable may be some weighted mean body temperature rather than deep body temperature... in some circumstances at least, the input from thermosensors elsewhere in the body are more influential than hypothalamic thermosensors in the control of the thermo-correction effectors, and the stabilization of a body temperature (63)." What happens with direct brain cooling requires investigation.

Intracerebral Temperature Gradients With Direct Brain Cooling

Some direct brain cooling methods have been shown to increase intracerebral temperature gradients compared to normothermia and systemic hypothermia.

Laptook et al. (8) compared systemic hypothermia in piglets with isolated brain cooling using conductive cooling caps and core trunk normothermia. They found that systemic hypothermia did not change brain temperature gradients compared to baseline, but isolated brain cooling resulted in greatly increased gradients between the dura and 2 cm into the brain (mean 7.5°C) (Fig. 2) (65).

Gelman et al. (32) also showed an increased temperature gradient (mean 2.3°C) between the caudate nucleus and superficial parietal cortex in piglets ($n = 14$) with cooling caps and core trunk normothermia ($n = 7$), compared to <0.5°C in normothermic controls ($n = 7$). Caudate nucleus temperature was reduced to about 31°C. A similar study in piglets ($n = 5$) comparing isolated head cooling with systemic hypothermia showed that the average temperature difference across the entire brain was 3.2°C with head cooling compared to 0.5°C with systemic hypothermia (66).

Isolated brain cooling in dogs ($n = 16$) using a convective cooling helmet, with normothermic trunk temperature maintained with cardiopulmonary bypass, produced a mean temperature difference of 1.9°C between probes placed 1 and 2 cm below the dura after 2.5 hr of cooling, compared to a mean 0.1°C difference at normothermic baseline (67).

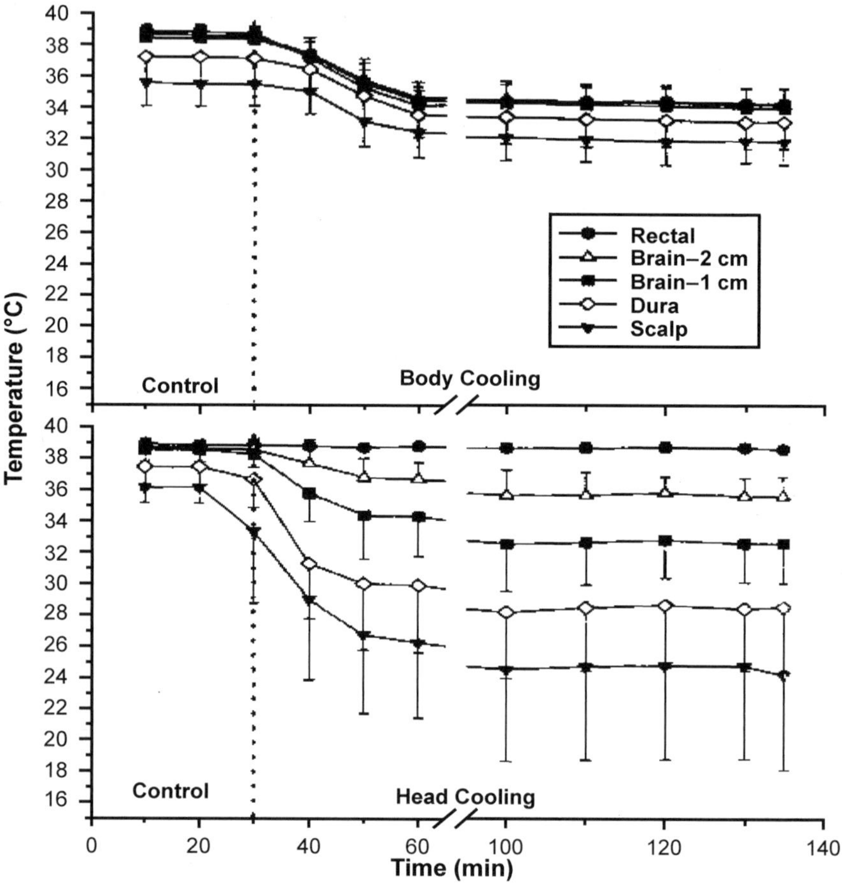

Figure 2 Temperature of the brain, scalp, and rectum before, during, and after whole-body cooling (top panel) or isolated brain cooling with a cooling cap (bottom panel). Temperature was monitored from five sites in each piglet ($n = 9$). Temperatures before and after the break in the time axis represent values during the first 30 min of cooling and during the final 30 min of cooling. (From Ref. 65.)

Ibayashi et al. (33) achieved isolated brain cooling in rats using a metal plate on the scalp cooled by a water-circulating system with core trunk normothermia. Brain temperature was measured every millimeter from 2 mm below the dura to 9 mm below. When temperature at 2 mm was reduced to 33°C ($n = 3$) and 30°C ($n = 3$), temperatures at 9 mm were warmer by 2.5°C and 4°C, respectively (although still below normal). By contrast, this gradient was 0.2°C in controls maintained at normothermia (n = 3).

Although they cool more quickly, anterograde cerebral perfusion methods also produce increased intracerebral temperature gradients. With bilateral carotid perfusion, areas of the brain supplied by the vertebral arteries are slower to cool and do not cool as much as the areas supplied by the carotids. White et al. (68) found in dogs (n = 20) that the frontal lobes were approximately 5°C cooler than the brainstem (duration of cooling not reported). Similarly, Kuhnen et al. (1) found in pigs (n = 8) that the frontal lobes and striatum were cooled the most and the cerebellum the least after 40 min of cooling.

With unilateral carotid perfusion, the side of the brain at which cooling is directed cools more quickly than the contralateral side, causing a gradient between the hemispheres. Mori et al. (69) cooled pigs (n = 6) through the right carotid to a right frontal lobe temperature of about 30°C. After 30 min, the left frontal lobe was still 2.5°C warmer than the right. Schwartz et al. (34) also cooled through the right carotid (n = 12) and after 3 hr had a right to left gradient of only 0.8°C in baboons cooled to <19°C, and 1.2°C in those cooled to <25°C. However, they occluded the external branches of the carotid whereas Mori et al. (69) did not.

Cooling by ventricular perfusion (70) and by carotid flush (71) have also been shown to cause intracerebral temperature gradients of several degrees.

Consequences of Intracerebral Temperature Gradients

It is unclear whether the increased temperature gradients within the brain caused by these methods of direct brain cooling are damaging. Logic suggests that there might be a number of untoward effects. However, cooling the superficial brain to lower temperatures may afford better protection to the more metabolically active and potentially more vulnerable cortex. In the context of neonatal hypoxic–ischemic injury, Laptook and Corbett (65) conclude that it remains to be determined "whether the more homogenous cooling of the brain with whole body cooling is advantageous over the greater cooling of the superficial brain relative to the deep brain with a head cooling approach."

Gelman et al. (32) and Almond et al. (72) have speculated that temperature gradients in the brain might potentially be harmful because of imbalances between flow and metabolism. However, when Gelman et al. compared normothermia with isolated head cooling (cool head/warm body) in piglets, they found that "... the ratio of cerebral blood flow to metabolism was not different between groups at any time point," despite the increase in temperature gradients with cooling. In classic experiments performed by Almond et al., the extent of systemic temperature gradients was found to correlate with brain damage. In dogs ($n = 13$) cooled with cardiopulmonary bypass to an esophageal temperature of 10°C, those with a 4–6°C temperature gradient between the femoral artery and the right atrium had minimal pathological brain damage, with gradients of 13–15°C had moderate damage, and animals with a gradient of ≥20°C died when bypass was terminated and had severe brain damage. However, brain temperature was measured at but a single place is this study, making it impossible to determine the effects of temperature gradients within the brain.

Neuroprotection and Intracerebral Temperature Gradients

Two animal studies using direct brain cooling assessed intracerebral temperature gradients and neuroprotection. Horn et al. (26) compared normothermia with a cool body/cooler head method, using circulating coolant in a head container and no body warming (rectal temperatures dropped to nearly 30°C) in cats ($n = 5$) after cardiac arrest. The maximum thalamic–cerebral cortex temperature gradient was about 7°C. The cooled group had significantly less neuronal damage in two of three assessed brain regions compared to normothermic controls. Natale and D'Alecy (25) used nasal lavage to cool dogs' brains ($n = 21$), maintaining body temperature at normothermia, before and during cardiac arrest. The cooling produced hippocampal–cerebral cortex temperature gradients of 1.5–1.8°C compared to 0.6–1°C in normothermic controls.

Cooled dogs survived to 24 hr and had less neurological deficit than controls, which all had died by 24 hr.

Huh et al. (22) compared two cool body/cooler head regimes (35°C/27°C and 35°C/32°C) with normothermia in rats after temporary middle cerebral artery occlusion. Liquid nitrogen was fanned over the head to achieve the desired temporal muscle temperature and rectal temperature was maintained with a warming blanket. Although intracerebral temperature gradients were not measured, based on Ibayashi et al.'s (33) results, they were likely larger in the 35°C/27°C group. Both cooling regimes provided neuroprotection compared to normothermia, but head cooling to 32°C resulted in greater reductions in cortical and total infarct volumes than cooling to 27°C. The authors suggest this may have been because cooling to 32°C was better tolerated and allowed more rapid recovery from anesthesia, but perhaps smaller intracerebral temperature gradients or a less drastic rewarming effect was also a factor.

In summary, certain methods of direct brain cooling can produce increased intracerebral temperature gradients but there is insufficient evidence to conclude that this is actually damaging and some evidence that neuroprotection still occurs.

Summary: Advantages and Disadvantages of Direct Brain Cooling

There is a particular lack of human evidence on the advantages and disadvantages of direct brain cooling. Although it is commonly believed that isolated brain hypothermia will provide equivalent neuroprotection with fewer complications, there is relatively little evidence to support this assumption.

Methods of Direct Brain Cooling

In this section, we review the effect of the different types of direct brain cooling (Table 1) on brain temperature, along with the advantages and disadvantages of each.

Not all methods of direct brain cooling have been tested in brain-injured subjects or in randomized controlled trials, and much of the work is in animals. Broadly, there are two types of investigation: (1) studies in brain-injured and normal subjects comparing the cooling efficacy of various methods; and (2) studies in brain-injured subjects that, in addition to evaluating cooling efficacy, also evaluate side effects and neuroprotection. With the exception of Battin et al.'s (27) study of direct brain cooling in infants with hypoxic–ischemic injury, none of the methods have been tested in a long-term outcome trial.

In assessing the effectiveness of different methods, we have considered the following points when information is available: type and purpose of study (e.g., controlled trial or uncontrolled experiment/observation), subjects, whether the method has been tried in brain injury, reduction of brain temperature (or trunk temperature if brain temperature was not measured), the speed of cooling, and particular advantages and disadvantages of the methods, such as ease of use and side effects. With the exception of a study by Einer-Jensen and Khorooshi (73), studies on rats have not been included because their small brains are not a good model for the effect of local cooling methods on human brain temperature.

Noninvasive Methods of Direct Brain Cooling

These methods include heat loss from the upper airways and through the skull. Physiological studies of these heat loss mechanisms in normal volunteers using tympanic membrane temperature and auditory-evoked brain stem potentials as indirect measures of brain temperature have been performed (74–76), but these have not been included because they are less relevant to brain injury, and the accuracy of these measurements in reflecting actual changes in brain temperature is debatable.

Heat Loss from the Upper Airways

These studies are classified as follows: those using air or oxygen flow and those using fluid lavage.

Upper airways gas flow: Table 2 shows the results of an animal and two human studies of upper airway oxygen and airflow. The aim of these studies was to assess whether this method can reduce brain temperature; they were not designed to evaluate neuroprotection. Einer-Jensen and Khorooshi's study in rats is included because it was designed to be a model for heat loss from the upper airways in humans (73). Like humans, rats have no carotid rete mirabile, and the oxygen flow rates were proportional to the minute volumes. Brain temperature reduced by flow-dependent amounts up to mean 0.75°C, which may be clinically relevant. Einer-Jensen et al. conducted an additional study in pigs with similar results to their rat study (77), but we have not reported it in detail because pigs have a carotid rete, which can considerably increase brain cooling by heat loss from the upper airways, and are, therefore, not an ideal model for humans. Einer-Jensen's team have also tried nasal oxygen flow in an intubated human and report that brain temperature was reduced (personal communication).

It is surprising, but encouraging, that Mellergård (78) was able to demonstrate even a 0.2°C reduction in brain temperature, because passing the nasal catheter through to the nasopharynx meant that oxygen flow was prevented from contacting the highly vascular nasal cavity, where most of the heat loss in the upper airways occurs as a result of turbulent flow over the turbinates (80). The air only came into contact with mucosa in the nasopharynx.

Our trial investigated replication of normal air intake through the nose in brain-injured, intubated patients, using air at room temperature and humidity with flows equivalent to normal minute volumes (79). We also evaluated safety, and no concerns were identified. However, patients with fractures at sites that could have allowed air to enter the brain were excluded. The flow rates used in this trial did not produce clinically important or statistically significant reductions in brain temperature (mean −0.13°C, SD 0.55°C, 95% CI −0.43–0.17°C).

Heat loss from the upper airways may be impaired by severe brain injury because of increased sympathetic tone, which causes nasal mucosal vasoconstriction and hence re-

Table 2 Animal and Human Studies of Direct Brain Cooling Using Upper Airways Gas Flow

Authors	Type and purpose of study	Subjects	Brain injury	Brain-cooling intervention
Einer-Jensen and Khorooshi, 2000 (73)	Nonrandomized controlled crossover trial of the effect of nasal oxygen flow vs. no flow on brain temperature	11 intubated adult rats	None	250 (normal rat minute vol), 500, 800, and 1000 mL/min oxygen, no added heat or humidity, via bilateral nasal catheters 1.0–1.5 cm into nostrils. 15 min of flow, 15 min without, until all flow rates had been delivered to each rat
Mellergård, 1992 (78)	Observation of the effect of nasopharyngeal oxygen flow on brain temperature	Three intubated adult humans	Trauma or hemorrhage	5–10 L/min of humidified oxygen via foley catheter in one nostril, beyond the posterior choane nasi, with obliquely cut tip in nasopharynx with opening pointing upward and balloon inflated to secure. Cooling applied for ≥2 hr/pt
Andrews and Harris, 2003 (79)	Randomized controlled crossover trial of the effect of nasal airflow vs. no flow on brain temperature	15 intubated adult humans	Trauma or hemorrhage	Air at rates equivalent to normal minute vol at room temperature and humidity via bilateral nasal catheters 1–2 cm into nostrils. 6 hr with airflow, 6 hr without, in random order

N/A = not available.

Brain temperature monitor	Effect of cooling on brain temperature	Core trunk temperature	Speed of cooling
Frontal lobes 5 mm below dura	Flow-dependent reduction from normothermia by a mean of 0.25°C at 250 mL/min to 0.75°C at 1000 mL/min	Placed on a heating pad to maintain rectal temperature. Even so, rectal temperature decreased at higher gas flows but less than brain temperature	Brain temperature started falling almost immediately and continuously dropped during each 15-min cooling period
Lateral ventricle	Max 0.2°C reduction	Slight increase in rectal temperature in two patients	Unclear, but within 2 hr
Frontal lobe or subdural	No significant reduction	No reduction in esophageal temperature	N/A

duced heat loss to inspired air (80,81). Sympathetic tone is greatly increased for some days after brain injury (82); furthermore, all but two patients required noradrenaline infusions. However, Mariak et al. (19) evaluated the effect of extubation on brain temperature in patients who were not severely brain-injured; similarly, the rats were not brain-injured in Einer-Jensen and Khorooshi's study (73).

The higher the flow rate and the lower the temperature and humidity of inspired air, the more heat is transferred from the body. Mariak et al.'s (19) self-ventilating patients were breathing ambient air but when they breathed more intensively this produced a greater decrease in brain temperature than normal breathing. Einer-Jensen and Khorooshi (73) used oxygen with no added heat or humidity in their rat study and showed greater drops in brain temperature with higher flow rates. Therefore, to show clinically relevant heat loss, higher flows of cooler, drier air may be required.

If brain cooling by heat loss from the upper airways and heat loss through the skull via emissary veins are complementary mechanisms (10), then temperature changes because of the former may be detected nearer to the nasopharynx, and changes because of the latter may occur nearer to the skull. There is some support for this theory from Mariak et al. (19) who showed that temperature near to the nasopharynx (between the frontal lobes above the cribriform plate) dropped with extubation, whereas subdural temperature did not. Also, in Einer-Jensen and Khorooshi's study in rats, the brain temperature monitors were 5 mm below the dura (73), which is relatively further into the brain than our human study (79). The position of our brain thermistors in patients may thus have been too far from the nasopharynx to detect changes as a result of nasal airflow. There were, however, temperature changes attributable to heat loss through the skull—although this observation requires substantiation.

Experience with nasal airflow suggests that sedation in humans might not be necessary at flows up to normal minute volume, e.g., in conscious patients with a tracheostomy. With higher, drier, colder flows, though, analgesia and sedation may be required. The sensation is peculiar, rather than painful, but is nonetheless unlikely to be well tolerated. At high flows, attempting to swallow sends air to the tympanic cavity, although in intubated patients the endotracheal tube may prevent complete closure of the mouth on swallowing, thus leaving an alternative escape route for the air. Nevertheless, it is safest to secure the nasal catheters in a manner that allows air to be blown back out of the nostrils if the pressure in the upper airways builds up for any reason.

Bearing in mind that Mariak et al. (19) have shown that human brain temperature drops on extubation, we consider that this is a method of direct brain cooling which, with further development, may have potential to reduce brain temperature in brain-injured humans, although not to cause hypothermia. It has the advantage of being easy and quick to instigate.

Upper airways lavage: The two dog studies shown in Table 3 appear to be the only studies of cooling via the upper airways using fluid lavage. The dog's anatomy is likely to facilitate this method of cooling compared to humans. White et al.'s study (68) combined heat loss from the upper airways with heat loss through the skull; although naso-oral perfusion was used alone for maintenance of cooling. This appears to be the only published study combining both mechanisms.

The dogs in White et al.'s study were not brain-injured; therefore, neuroprotection after injury was not assessed, but all survived the cooling method with no evidence of behavioral change, gross neurological deficit, or damage to eyes or mucous membranes (68). Natale and D'Alecy (25) commented that their control dogs, receiving normothermic nasal lavage, had worse 24-hr survival and neurological deficits than controls who did not receive nasal lavage in a previous study. This may indicate a safety problem with nasal lavage but, as they suggest, it could be because normothermic lavage maintained brain temperature during cardiac arrest more effectively than no lavage, or because it caused transient hyperglycemia compared to cooling lavage.

Both evaporative and convective heat transfer occur in the upper airways (83), and upper airways cooling with liquids will prevent evaporative heat loss. However, water has more heat transfer capacity than air or oxygen, thereby producing far

Table 3 Animal Studies of Direct Brain Cooling Using Upper Airways Lavage

Authors	Type and purpose of study	Subjects	Brain injury	Brain-cooling intervention
White et al., 1983 (68)	Observation of the effect of head immersion in iced water with naso-oral lavage on brain temperature	24 intubated adult dogs	None	Head shaved, placed in container of iced water, head completely submerged. Simultaneous naso-oral perfusion with the same water at 1.5–2.0 L/min. Brain temperature, once cooled, maintained with lavage alone
Natale and D'Alecy, 1989 (25)	Randomized controlled trial of the effect of brain cooling by naso-oral lavage vs. normothermia on cerebral lactate accumulation	Two groups of intubated adult dogs: 11 cases, 10 controls. Within each group were two further groups: (1) Recovery, with survival for 24 hr; (2) Biopsy, for lactate postresuscitation	Cardiac arrest	Nasal lavage with water at 5°C pumped through tubes secured 1.5 cm into nostrils and drained from mouth via funnel. Rectal temperature maintained with warming. Controls: identical but water at approximately 39°C. Lavage begun 10–20 min before arrest and continued for 30 min after

Brain temperature monitor	Effect of cooling on brain temperature	Core trunk temperature	Speed of cooling
Frontal lobe 1–1.5 cm below surface of cortex	Reduced to 14–19°C. Baseline temperature not reported	Normothermic rectal temperature maintained with warming blankets	30°C in 5–12 min, <20°C in 18–40 min
Hippocampus and cerebral cortex	Recovery group: mean hippocampus temperature 32.7–33.5°C (baseline 39.1°C). Mean cortical temperature 34.2–35.3°C (baseline 38.8°C). Biopsy group similar. Controls remained normothermic	Normothermic rectal temperature maintained with heating pad and esophageal heat exchanger	Reduction of approximately 6°C in hippocampus and 4°C in cortex over 40–50 min

greater heat transfer at a given temperature. The practicality of nasal lavage in brain-injured humans is questionable because controlling the outflow would be difficult and fluid could run into the stomach or the lungs if the cuff on the endotracheal tube did not provide an adequate seal. Lavage via catheters passed through the nostrils and out of the mouth is feasible but could cause pressure sores and sinusitis and would be likely to reduce the cooling by preventing good contact with the turbinates and mucous membranes.

Heat Loss Through the Skull

These studies are classified as follows: those using forced convective cooling, i.e., head fanning and cooling hoods, and those using conductive cooling, i.e., ice packs, head containers, and circulating and noncirculating cooling caps.

External forced convective cooling: head fanning and convective cooling helmets: The two studies shown in Table 4 used head fanning and convective cooling helmets, respectively.

Convective cooling by face fanning with ambient air, both with and without evaporative cooling, did not reduce brain temperature in a human subject (84), but it has been suggested that the subject of this report may have had an elevated ICP, which might interfere with the mechanisms for heat loss through the skull (76,85).

On the other hand, a convective cooling helmet worked in dogs, but they had no brain injury, their heads are smaller than humans, and the convective air temperature was considerably lower than ambient air (13°C vs. 22°C) (67). Although cardiopulmonary bypass is not practical after most brain injuries, this study has been included because the head-cooling method could be used on its own or with noninvasive body warming, and has the advantage of being quick and easy to instigate.

External conductive head cooling: ice packs, head containers, and circulating and noncirculating cooling caps: Most of the research on these methods has been in cardiac arrest and infant hypoxic–ischemic encephalopathy

Table 4 Studies in Animals and a Human of Forced Convective Head Cooling

Authors	Type and purpose of study	Subjects	Brain injury	Brain-cooling intervention	Brain temperature monitor	Effect of cooling on brain temperature	Core trunk temperature	Speed of cooling
Wass et al., 1998 (67)	Randomized controlled trial of the effect of a convective cooling helmet on brain temperature during normothermic cardiopulmonary bypass (CPB) with two different anesthetics.	16 intubated dogs: 8 anaesthetized with pentobarbital, 8 with halothane (both groups received the same cooling intervention so the results are not reported separately here)	None	Convective (forced air) cooling helmet, air temperature approximately 13°C, used for 150 min during normothermic CPB	Six sites: bilaterally in parietal epidural space and parenchyma 1 and 2 cm below dura	Max mean drop: epidural 4.5°C, parenchyma 1 cm 3.9°C, 2 cm 2.0°C. Baseline brain temperature 38°C	Baseline 38.0°C maintained with normothermic CPB	Drop of 2°C in epidural temperature and nearly 0.5°C at 2 cm after 10 min. Temperature started to level off at 60 min
Shiraki et al., 1988 (84)	Observation of the effect of face fanning on brain temperature	Conscious, self-ventilating 12-year-old boy	Surgery for a pineal tumor	Face fanning with 25°C (ambient) air, body covered. One convective session and one convective plus evaporative session (body heating with electric blanket to produce facial sweating), each 20 min	Lateral ventricle and 1 cm above ventricle	No convincing effect	Esophageal: essentially unchanged	N/A

N/A = not available.

Table 5 Studies in Adult Animals and Humans of Conductive Head Cooling Using Head Containers, Ice Packs, and Circulating and Non-circulating Cooling Caps

Authors	Type and purpose of study	Subjects	Brain injury	Brain-cooling intervention
Horn et al., 1991 (26)	Pilot, observational study of the effect on brain temperature of a conductive head-cooling container. Part of a larger trial to assess neuronal damage with the head-cooling method vs. normothermia	5 cats with tracheotomy	Cardiovascular suppression with IV pindolol to mimic external cardiac massage	Container of circulating monoethylene–glycol at −25°C, Top made of copper sheet, depressed to contain the head, and coated with heat-conducting gel. Cooling started with CPR and continued for 30 min
Brader et al., 1985 (89)	Trial of the effect of head cooling vs. no head cooling. Randomization not mentioned	12 dogs: 6 controls, 6 cases	Four minutes of cardiac arrest [ventricular fibrillation (VF)], followed by 20 min of CPR	Heads shaved, wetted with saline and packed in ice before cardiac arrest
Leonov et al., 1990 (90)	Pilot study of the effect on brain temperature of head immersion in ice water, mentioned in a report of a larger trial of head cooling and hypothermic CPB in dogs after cardiac arrest	6 large dogs	Cardiac arrest (VF), wait 12.5 min, reversed with defibrillation + CPB	Immersion of head (except snout and pharynx) in an open plastic box filled with ice water for 12.5 min (from start of VF arrest to start of resuscitation).
Tadler et al., 1998 (91)	Randomized controlled trial of the effect on brain	24 adult intubated pigs	Cardiac arrest (VF), wait 8 min, start CPR,	Three plastic bags each with 500 mL ice, applied to sides of head and over

Brain temperature monitor (or proxy)	Effect of cooling on brain temperature	Core trunk temperature	Speed of cooling
Cerebral cortex and thalamus	Thalamus approximately 25°C, cortex approximately 18°C. Baseline approximately 37°C	Baseline rectal temperature approximately 38°C, reduced to nearly 30°C by end of cooling	Over 30 min thalamic temperature dropped approximately 12°C and cortex approximately 19°C
Not measured	N/A	Core temperature (location not stated). Cases: 36.3°C at end CPR, 34.9°C after 1 min of spontaneous circulation. Controls: 36.9°C and 36.5°C, respectively	Not clear because baseline temperature was not reported
Parietal epidural	Parietal epidural reduced from 37.6°C to 35.2°C	Maintained at normothermia for the 12.5 min of VF	Over 12.5 min, mean parietal epidural temperature reduced 2.4°C and hippocampal temperature <1°C
2 cm into parietal cortex	Controls: mean baseline 40.3°C, reduced to 39.7°C. Cases: mean	Esophageal: Controls, little change. Cases: mean baseline	Controls: reduced parietal cortex temperature by 0.6°C over 20 min.

Table 5 Continued

Authors	Type and purpose of study	Subjects	Brain injury	Brain-cooling intervention
	temperature of ice packs applied to the head and neck		continue for 20 min	front of neck at start of CPR
Mellergård, 1992 (78)	Observation of the effect of a gel cooling cap on brain temperature	3 unconscious intubated adults	Trauma or SAH	Hypotherm Gel Kap containing frozen liquid, wrapped around head (no close or direct contact with exposed skin) for approximately 2 hr
Mellergård, 1992 (78)	Observation of the effect of a water-circulating cooling helmet on brain temperature	2 unconscious intubated adults	Trauma or SAH	Water-circulating cooling helmet, water temperature approximately 15°C, for 4–5 hr
Corbett and Laptook, 1998 (92)	Crossover trial of the effect of gel cooling caps on brain temperature. Cap sequence and magnetic resonance spectroscopy measurement sequence alternated between subjects	10 healthy adults	None	Cooling: Two Elasto-gel head caps, inner cap precooled to 4°C and outer to −20°C. Control: Same caps but prewarmed to 34°C (9) or room temperature (1). 50 min with each set of caps
Hachimi-Idrissi et al., 2001 (29)	Randomized controlled trial of the feasibility and cooling speed of an aqueous glycerol cooling helmet	30 unconscious intubated adults: 16 cases, 14 controls	Out-of-hospital cardiac arrest	Cases: Frigicap containing aqueous glycerol at about −4°C, applied over a paper cap and changed every hour to keep temperature

Brain temperature monitor (or proxy)	Effect of cooling on brain temperature	Core trunk temperature	Speed of cooling
	baseline 39.8°C, reduced to 37.7°C	39.8°C, reduced to 38.4°C	Cases: reduced by 2.2°C over 20 min
Lateral ventricle and epidural	Ventricular: "little or no effect." Epidural: maximum drop of 1°C. Baselines not reported	Rectal: little change	Ventricular: N/A. Epidural: immediate and rapid
Lateral ventricle and epidural	Ventricular: Pt 1 0.6°C reduction; Pt 2 slight increase. Epidural: Pt 1 fluctuating by about 0.5°C; Pt 2 unreported. Baselines not reported	Rectal: Pt 1 reduction; Pt 2 not reported	Reduction over approximately 1 hr 40 min of 0.6°C in one patient
Noninvasive proton magnetic resonance spectroscopy of superficial cortex and thalamus	Mean scalp temperature with cooling 15.8°C, without 34.7°C. Mean cortical temperature with cooling 36.8°C, without 37°C. Mean thalamic temperature with cooling 36.6°C, without 36.6°C	Oral and axillary temperatures unchanged by either intervention	Baseline brain temperatures in cooled group not reported but scalp cooled to "lowest value" within 5 min and then rose slowly over 50 min
Tympanic (infrared)	Reduction in tympanic temperature by end of 4-hr study period not reported for either group	Cases: target bladder temperature of 34°C reached by 4 hr in all but one patient. Controls: bladder temperature at end of study period not reported	Median baseline bladder temperature not reported. Median 180 min to bladder temperature 34°C. Median baseline tympanic temperature 35.8°C

Table 5 Continued

Authors	Type and purpose of study	Subjects	Brain injury	Brain-cooling intervention
				low. Cooling started in emergency room and continued until bladder temperature of 34°C reached, or for up to 4 hr. Controls: maintained at normothermia
Callaway et al., 2002 (93)	Randomized controlled trial of the effect of ice packs applied to the head and neck on brain temperature	27 adult humans: 13 controls, 14 cases of which 9 were included (5 did not complete trial)	Out-of-hospital cardiac arrest	Cases: three plastic bags each with 500 mL ice applied to head with one more across neck

patients, in whom direct brain temperature measurement was not recorded. The rationale for cooling in perinatal hypoxic–ischemic encephalopathy is that secondary deterioration may occur some hours after the first insult (27,40).

Studies using modeling to predict brain cooling with ice and cooling caps in adults and infants indicate that cooling would be limited to the superficial regions of the brain if core trunk temperature is normal (86–88). However, these models do not account for natural selective brain cooling mechanisms; indeed it would be difficult to do so because little is known about these mechanisms in humans, particularly after brain injury. More evidence is required before the clinical relevance, or otherwise of these methods can be assessed.

Cooling caps have the advantage of being simple to apply, particularly in the absence of open head wounds or invasive monitoring devices. Noncirculating cooling caps, e.g., containing frozen gel, will thaw and have to be replaced periodically. Circulating cooling caps have the benefit of being maintained

Brain temperature monitor (or proxy)	Effect of cooling on brain temperature	Core trunk temperature	Speed of cooling
			and median 60 min to tympanic temperature 34°C
Cases: nasopharynx. Controls: nasopharynx or tympanic (infrared)	No significant difference between groups	Esophageal: Both groups hypothermic at baseline and no significant change in either group	N/A

at a constant temperature and some allow temperature adjustment. This is potentially important because there is a possibility of tissue freezing and necrosis if scalp temperature is reduced too much. Surprisingly, Gelman et al. (32) found no scalp problems in piglets with a cooling cap at −20°C to −30°C, but Iwata et al. (55) reported pale, blotchy, peeling, blistering scalps in piglets with a cooling cap at 0°C. Some human infants were found to have scalp erythema or edema after cooling caps at 10°C were removed but this resolved quickly (28,50). In human adults, a cooling cap at −4°C applied over a paper cap (and presumably hair) did not cause freezing or necrosis of the scalp (29).

Table 5 includes adult animal and human studies of external conductive head cooling and Table 6 includes infant animal and human studies.

Cooling using head containers worked in dogs (90) and cats (26), and ice packs had some effect in dogs (89) and pigs (91). However, in addition to anatomical and physiological

Table 6 Studies in Infant Animals and Humans of Conductive Head Cooling Using Circulating and Noncirculating Cooling Caps

Authors	Type and purpose of study	Subjects	Brain injury	Brain-cooling intervention
Gelman et al., 1996 (32)	Randomized trial of the effect of head cooling with ethylene glycol cap plus body warming vs. normothermia on brain temperature, regional organ blood flow, cerebral metabolism, and systemic hemodynamics	14 infant tracheotomized piglets: 7 cases, 7 controls	Cardiac arrest (VF) for 6 min, CPR for 6 min, defibrillation, 2 hr reperfusion	Cases: cooling cap filled with 1:1 water and ethylene glycol at −20°C to −30°C. Cooling started during CPR and continued for 45 min of reperfusion, followed by passive rewarming. Controls: normothermia
Laptook et al., 2001 (8)	Randomized crossover trial to compare effect on brain temperature of head cooling with water-circulating cuff vs. systemic hypothermia, with alternating 30-min periods of hypoxia and normoxia	17 tracheotomized miniature piglets with or without hypoxia, plus 8 piglets who had CBF measurement	No hypoxia vs. hypoxia (15 min of 8% oxygen)	Inflatable cuff around top half of head with circulating water at approximately 1°C, rectal temperature maintained with warm water-circulating blanket. Body cooling to 33°C with water-circulating cooling blanket
Thoresen et al., 2001 (41)	Study of the effect of head cooling with water-circulating cooling cap plus body warming on brain temperature	9 intubated newborn piglets	Hypoxic–ischemic insult with FiO_2 4–6% for 45 min	Water-circulating cooling cap at 6°C until rectal temperature 35°C, then adjusted to maintain rectal temperature at 35°C for 20 min with aid of radiant body heating. Group A: four piglets cooled and rewarmed both pre- and postinsult. Group B: 4 piglets cooled and rewarmed only postinsult

Brain temperature monitor (or proxy)	Effect of cooling on brain temperature	Core trunk temperature	Speed of cooling
Parietal cortex and caudate nucleus	Mean parietal cortex 32.8°C and mean caudate 34.9°C after approximately 30 min cooling, 27.8°C and 31.1°C after about 1 hr. Baseline mean 38°C	Rectal temperature maintained at 37.5–38.5°C in cases and controls with radiant heater and heated water blanket	Target brain temperature of 32–33°C achieved in about 30 min
Basal ganglia (1 cm into brain) and cortex (2 cm into brain)	With head cooling: 1 cm brain temperature approximately 32°C, 2 cm 35.5°C. Baseline 38.5°C	Rectal temperature maintained at 38.5°C during head cooling	Head cooling took 70 min to reach steady-state brain temperature, (6.5°C drop at 1 cm and 2.5°C at 2 cm)
Epidural, 0.2 and 1.7 cm laterally into cortex, and 2 cm vertically into gray matter	Lowest median 2 cm brain temperature during cooling: pre-insult, Group A 28.5°C; postinsult, Group A 30.6°C, Group B 29.5°C	Baseline approximately 39°C. Lowest median rectal temperature during cooling: pre-insult, Group A 33.7°C; postinsult, Group A 33.5°C, Group B 33.8°C	About 30 min to achieve target rectal temperature of 35°C, i.e., drop of 4°C

Table 6 Continued

Authors	Type and purpose of study	Subjects	Brain injury	Brain-cooling intervention
Tooley et al., 2002 (94)	Feasibility study of cooling the brain below rectal temperature for 24 hr	8 intubated piglets	Hypoxic–ischemic (45 min of 4–6% oxygen)	Water-circulating cooling cap at 6°C until rectal temperature 35°C, then adjusted to maintain rectal temperature at 34–35°C for 24 hr with aid of radiant body heating.
Iwata et al., 2003 (52)	Investigation of the coolant temperature required to achieve mild brain hypothermia (35°C) and alternatives to invasive brain temperature monitoring	6 tracheotomized newborn piglets	None	Ethylene-glycol-circulating cooling cap set sequentially at 10°C, 0°C, and −10°C
Thoresen and Whitelaw, 2000 (49); Whitelaw and Thoresen, 2001 (95)	Documentation of cardiovascular changes with head cooling using water-circulating cooling cap plus body warming	6 infants, 5 intubated	Hypoxic–ischemic encephalopathy	Water-circulating cooling cap set at 10–15°C to achieve cooling and then adjusted to maintain rectal temperature 34–35°C
Gunn et al., 1998 (50); Battin et al., 2001, 2003 (27,28)	Randomized trial of the practicality and safety of head cooling with increasing levels of systemic hypothermia with dose escalation design	38 infants, some ventilated: 13 uncooled controls, vs. head cooling with minimal (36.5–36.0°C, $n = 6$), mild (35.9–35.5°C, $n = 6$), or moderate (34.5°C, $n = 7$) systemic cooling	Hypoxic–ischemic encephalopathy	Either water-circulating coil around head (secured by bonnet) or commercial water-circulating cooling cap. Water temperature 10°C. Servo-controlled heater used to maintain body temperature at target level. Cooling continued for up to 72 hr

Brain temperature monitor (or proxy)	Effect of cooling on brain temperature	Core trunk temperature	Speed of cooling
Subdural and deep brain (2 cm below surface)	Median subdural temperature about 28°C, 2 cm brain temperature 31.4°C	Rectal temperature maintained at median 35°C	Median time to reach target rectal temperature, 51 min
Superficial brain (depth 0.5 cm) and deep brain (depth 2 cm). Nasopharynx and tympanic membrane	Mean 2 cm brain temperature 34.8°C with cap at 0°C, 35.8°C with cap at 10°C and no body cooling, 35.1°C with cap at 10°C and rectal temperature 1°C below normal. Nasopharynx and tympanic membrane temperatures not reported.	Rectal temperature maintained at 38.5–39°C (n = 3) or 1°C below this (n = 3)	Once cap reached set temperature, brain temperature took 30–75 min to plateau at desired level
None	N/A	Rectal temperature prevented from overshooting desired level with radiant heater. Mean rectal temperature 34.2°C with cooling	30–90 min to cool to target rectal temperature of 34–35°C but baseline not reported
Nasopharynx, in self-ventilating infants only	Mean nasopharyngeal temperature was 34.5°C, 1.2–1.4°C lower than mean rectal temperature in all groups	Target rectal temperatures maintained per protocol	Less than 6 hr

differences, animal brains are smaller than human brains and therefore are probably easier to cool conductively. Corbett and Laptook's trial of gel caps in adult humans, using magnetic resonance spectroscopy to measure temperature, demonstrated relatively superficial cooling only (92). Only Mellergård (78) measured actual brain temperatures in adults with conductive cooling methods. He demonstrated a 0.6°C reduction in ventricular brain temperature in one patient with a water-circulating cooling cap. It is difficult to interpret a single case, but it may be that circulating cooling caps are more effective than noncirculating ones in adult humans. The ease of use and noninvasive nature of circulating cooling caps would be advantageous, if they can be shown to work.

Conductive head cooling with cooling caps appears to be more successful in reducing brain temperature in infants than in adults, although no intracerebral temperature measurements are available in the human infant studies. However, body temperature cannot be maintained at normothermia if adequate temperature reduction is to be achieved in the inner brain, i.e., a cool body/cooler head approach is required.

Although no hazardous cardiovascular events were reported in the trials of cooling caps in infants (27,50,95), inadvertent overcooling or rewarming too quickly can cause hypotension. In clinical practice, to be safe and effective, local head cooling requires careful concomitant control of core body temperature. Thoresen and Whitelaw (49) found in infants that an overhead heater which was servo controlled to abdominal skin temperature was helpful for achieving fine control of core temperature with local cooling (49). With the cool head/warm body approach they used, however, they also encountered hypotension upon rewarming the brain that required treatment with volume and pressors.

Invasive Methods of Direct Brain Cooling

Anterograde Cerebral Perfusion

Anterograde cerebral perfusion techniques were developed in the 1950s and 1960s to achieve profound brain cooling ($\leq$20°C) with only moderate body cooling (around 32°C). The aim was to cool the brain sufficiently to allow either complete circulatory arrest or for partial occlusion of the cerebral circulation for a short time during neurosurgery, while avoiding the life-threatening arrhythmias that could occur with profound systemic hypothermia. Variations of this method have been reported, for example, in dogs (96–98) and monkeys (99) and in some case studies in humans (97,99–101). The most common method seems to have been pumped, unilateral femoral/carotid bypass via a heat exchanger, but unpumped (99), bilateral (99), and proximal/distal carotid bypass (96,100,101) have also been described. Unpumped methods were introduced because of concerns that pumped methods could disrupt cerebral autoregulation (99,102). In humans this method was used for operating on vascular tumors and certain types of aneurysms where more conventional neurosurgery was deemed impossible. Among 10 reported cases in humans, six survived and did well (97,99–101). One death occurred from thrombosis of the internal carotid, which was attributed to using too large a catheter (100).

The purpose of the more recent experimental studies using anterograde cerebral perfusion (Table 7) was to investigate the feasibility of anterograde cerebral perfusion for resuscitation from neurological insults. There appear to be no controlled trials or recent case reports in humans.

The studies in Table 7 show that anterograde cerebral perfusion can produce profound brain cooling with body temperature maintained at mildly hypothermic levels. It therefore should be possible to produce mild cerebral hypothermia with normothermic body temperatures, although this has not been demonstrated.

Anterograde cerebral perfusion will not be suitable for use in all brain injuries simply because it is labor- and skill-intensive, and carries greater risks than noninvasive techniques. Obvious risks include infection, emboli, hemorrhage, vessel damage, vasospasm (104), hemodynamic instability, and overcooling—which can be profound and can happen rapidly (34). Intracerebral temperature gradients occur, as discussed previously, and any abnormalities in the cerebral circulation—for example due to brain injury or vessel dis-

Table 7 Animal Studies of Anterograde Cerebral Perfusion

Authors	Type and purpose of study	Subjects	Brain injury	Brain cooling intervention	Brain temperature monitor	Effect of cooling on brain temperature	Core trunk temperature	Speed of cooling
White et al., 1983 (103)	Observational feasibility study of the cooling method	20 intubated adult dogs	Group 1: 10 dogs with basilar artery ligation. Group 2: 10 dogs with intact cerebral circulation	Bilateral cannulation of proximal and distal carotids, entire blood flow from proximal carotids diverted through water-cooled heat exchanger (no pump) and returned through distal carotids. Heat exchanger reduced flow by 5–10% at baseline and by 45% at end of cooling	Right frontal lobe and brain stem	Group 1 mean brain temperature 13.3°C. Group 2 mean brain temperature 20.0°C. Baseline not reported	Right atrial temperature maintained at >31°C with warming blanket	Mean 17 min to cool to brain temperature of 13.3°C in Group 1 and 20°C in Group 2
Miyake et al., 1984 (36)	Trial of the effect of CPR alone and CPR with carotid cooling	54 intubated adult dogs. Six groups: CPR after 5- or 10-min arrest;	Cardiac arrest (VF), wait either 5 or 10 min, start CPR	Unilateral cannulation of proximal and distal carotid, blood	Neocortex and hippocampus	After 10 min cooling, neocortex temperature was 20.5°C,	No body warming. Rectal temperature reduced to	Baseline not reported, but neocortex temperature was 25°C after

	on cerebral blood flow and brain oxygenation.	CPR with brain cooling for 10 or 30 min after 5-min arrest; CPR with brain cooling for 10 or 30 min after 10-min arrest		pumped from proximal carotid through heat exchanger (10°C) and returned to distal carotid		hippocampus 25°C. After 30 min, neocortex 13.6°C, hippocampus 14.8°C	mean 35.6°C after 10 min cooling and 33.5°C after 30 min	5 min cooling and 13.6°C after 30 min (drop of 11.4°C in 25 min)
Schwartz et al., 1996 (34)	Observational feasibility study of the cooling method	12 intubated baboons, 6 cooled to right cerebral temperature of <19°C for 30 min; 6°C to <25°C for 3 hr	None	Right femoral artery and right common carotid cannulated. Entire blood flow pumped from right femoral artery through cooling water bath and returned to right common carotid with external branches occluded. Pump flow adjusted to keep right carotid pressure equal to systemic blood pressure	Right and left frontal or parietal lobes	At end of cooling: in <19°C group right hemisphere 18.6°C, left 19.4°C. In <25°C group right hemisphere 24.3°C, left 25.5°C	Baseline esophageal temperature 36.4°C, maintained with warming blankets. Esophageal temperature 34.2–34.4°C at end of cooling in both groups	Approximately 9°C drop in brain temperature in 12 min and 15°C in 30 min

Table 7 Continued

Authors	Type and purpose of study	Subjects	Brain injury	Brain cooling intervention	Brain temperature monitor	Effect of cooling on brain temperature	Core trunk temperature	Speed of cooling
Schwartz et al., 1996 (104)	Observational feasibility study of the same cooling method employed by Schwartz et al. (34), but with transfemoral instead of surgical cannulation of carotid artery	4 intubated baboons cooled for 1 hr	None	Cannulation of right femoral artery with introducer sheath with side port, right internal carotid occlusively cannulated under fluoroscopic guidance via the femoral sheath. Blood from femoral artery	Right and left frontal or parietal lobes	After 1 hr mean right hemisphere temperature 23.9°C, mean left 24.6°C	Baseline esophageal temperature 36.7°C, maintained with warming blankets, fell to 33.2°C after 1 hr of cooling	About 9°C drop in brain temperature in 15 min

				pumped via sheath side port through cooling water bath and returned to carotid cannula.				
Mori et al., 2001 (69)	Observational feasibility study of the cooling method	6 intubated pigs cooled for 30 min, target brain temperature 34°C	None	Cannulation of right femoral and carotid arteries, blood pumped 5 mL kg^{-1} min^{-1} from femoral artery through water-cooled heat exchanger at 24°C back to carotid	Right and left frontal lobes	After 30 min cooling right frontal lobe 30.6°C, left 33.1°C	No body warming. Pulmonary artery temperature reduced from mean 37.4°C to 34.6°C after 30 min	Mean 4.3 min to reach target temperature of 34°C in right brain, 16.3°C left brain (drop of 3.2°C)

ease—could make cooling even less uniform. Heparin might be used to prevent thromboembolic complications but could be contraindicated in hemorrhagic brain injuries. Schwartz et al. (34) suggest heparin-coated circuits might be an alternative. White et al. (103) reported bradycardia and hypotension as the brain became colder in dogs, but they used no pump, and significant hemodynamic derangements did not occur in the more recent studies with a pump (34,69,104).

White et al. (103) and Mori et al. (69) did not report mortality. Schwartz et al. (34) had two baboons die. This was attributed to problems with learning the perfusion technique—one had very high pressures and the other was overcooled to 11°C. The surviving baboons were normal on neurological examination. In Schwartz et al.'s second study (104), all four baboons survived without neurological abnormality.

Two studies describe the use of anterograde cerebral perfusion with cardiopulmonary bypass for thoracic aortic surgery (105,106). Use of a dual lumen aortic cannula to achieve cool head/warm body perfusion during cardiopulmonary bypass in pigs has also been reported (107,108). Although these techniques may afford neuroprotection during thoracic and cardiac surgery, the requirement for cardio- pulmonary bypass and the degree of heparinization make them less suitable for use with brain injury.

Ohta et al. (109) tested a technique on dogs (n = 12) for cooling the brain with an infusion of cold Ringer lactate solution delivered through the right vertebral artery. Blood was removed from the left jugular vein and passed through a hemofilter and warming coil to remove the excess fluid and warm the blood again before it was returned to the body. Heparinization was required. During cooling, the left vertebral artery, right jugular vein, and both carotid arteries were temporarily occluded. Frontal lobe brain temperature was reduced to 20°C in a mean of 15.5 min. Rectal temperature was maintained at >32°C with the warming coil in the filter and an electric blanket under the animals. The animals were not brain-injured, no gross neurological or histological evidence of neuronal damage due to the technique itself was evident after 10 weeks.

Kuhnen et al. (1) developed an anterograde cerebral perfusion method in pigs (n = 8) for separately and precisely controlling body and brain temperature in animal experiments. Thalamic brain temperature was controlled at 25°C by connecting the left proximal carotid artery to a heat exchanger and then by Y connector to the two distal carotids. Body temperature (proximal carotid artery) was clamped at 38°C by ligating the distal end of the right jugular vein and connecting the proximal end via a heat exchanger to the right proximal carotid. Heparinization was required.

Other Cerebral Perfusion Techniques

Retrograde (venous) cerebral perfusion is not reviewed here because it is usually only used with cardiopulmonary bypass and profound hypothermic arrest for thoracic aortic surgery and the degree of cerebral protection it affords is controversial (110).

Intracarotid flush: Wolfson and colleagues, in the 1960s and 1970s, conducted a series of studies in animals to develop a technique for direct brain cooling using intracarotid flush (71,111–116). The technique was developed to provide cerebral protection during neurosurgery with circulatory arrest, and there are case reports on five humans undergoing surgery (116,117). A cold solution, usually at 0°C but 2°C, 4°C, and 8°C were also tried (114), was pumped into one common carotid artery for 5 or 6 min at a rate of 10 mL kg^{-1} min^{-1}. Isotonic saline was the solution most commonly used. Blood was also given but resulted in a high mortality rate (113), as was buffered Ringer's solution, which led to longer survival times from ischemic arrest than saline (115). Tham-buffered Ringer's solution at 0°C has been used in humans (116,117). Angiograms with radio-opaque carotid flush showed that the solution perfused the major cerebral arteries and appeared in both external jugular veins (71).

Carotid flush was usually combined with systemic hypothermia at 29–30°C, but in three studies it was used in isolation and these are described in more detail here. Wolfson et al. (71) gave 0°C saline at 10 mL kg^{-1} min^{-1} for 5 min to nine dogs immediately after cardiac arrest (VF), with another 10 mL/kg halfway through the arrest period. The dogs were resuscitated after 20, 30, or 40 min. Brain temperature fell to 20°C and esophageal temperature to 33°C. Body warming was not used. All of the dogs survived without brain damage, but those subjected to 30 and 40 min of circulatory arrest had spinal cord damage.

Bacalzo and Wolfson (114) used carotid flush with ice packs around the head and suggested that this combination might be useful for brain cooling in an emergency such as cardiac arrest. Seven baboons with ice packs around their heads were subjected to 30 min of cardiac arrest (VF) and after 3 min given a right carotid flush with 0°C saline at 10 mL kg^{-1} min^{-1} for 6 min (114). Right brain temperature fell to 16°C and left brain temperature to 21°C (i.e., there was a lateral temperature gradient). Body warming was not used and esophageal temperature fell to 33°C. The baboons survived without detectable gross neurological damage. Although heparin was used, the authors found in other studies that it was not necessary (114). Miyake et al. (118) used a combination of intracarotid dextran, 20% mannitol, methylprednisolone, and heparin in dogs after 5 min of nitrous oxide-induced cardiac arrest. One flush of 30 mL/kg was given at the commencement of resuscitation and a second 15 min later. The temperature of the flush fluid was variously 5°C, 15°C, and 25°C, giving lowest brain temperatures of 22.5°C, 27°C, and 30°C 20 min after the first flush was given (n = 6 or 7 per group). In the absence of body warming, rectal temperature dropped to hypothermic levels in all three groups but not below 33°C. Cerebral oxygen availability and cerebral mitochondrial respiratory activity were improved in the cooled groups compared with the normothermia group.

The volume of fluid delivered with this method is usually large, typically 3.5 L in humans (117), which, in the absence of circulation, ends up in the great veins and heart (71). During circulatory arrest, it is reported that the fluid gradually dissipates out of the vascular system without causing cardiac failure, pulmonary edema, or a massive diuresis (117). Bernard et al. (119) gave ice-cold Ringer's lactate intravenously at 30 mL/kg over 30 min to 22 postcardiac arrest patients without causing pulmonary edema. Nevertheless, problems due to volume overload and hemodilution must be a concern.

Marion et al. (120) report the feasibility of lower volume carotid flush with 0.5–.0 L of Ringer's solution at 4–8°C in humans during resuscitation from cardiac arrest. Carotid puncture was performed, and the fluid was forced in by manual compression of the infusion bag. No outcome data are given and "considerable resistance" from colleagues to the clinical use of this method was reported, which is understandable given the risk of embolism and carotid damage. The attraction of this method lies in the speed of brain cooling which could be afforded in an emergency, although it seems likely that the duration would be short. There is evidence that cooling is of benefit after some types of cardiac arrest in humans (121,122), and if this method was combined with an additional portable method, such as cooling caps or ice packs round the head, the cooling might be prolonged sufficiently to allow time to instigate longer-term solutions. But evidence that the benefits outweigh the risks is needed.

Open irrigation of the brain surface: Cooling by irrigation of the brain surface with normal saline has been successful in cats (24) and humans (123,124), and these authors suggest this method is useful during neurosurgery. Noguchi et al. (24) reduced brain temperature 15 mm into the parenchyma in cats (n = 14) following 1 hr of middle cerebral artery occlusion to about 35°C with saline at 20°C dripped continuously for 4 hr. Iatrou et al. (123) reduced brain temperature 18 mm into the parenchyma in eight patients during craniotomy by a mean of 1.6°C using 1 L of saline at 30°C. In both these studies, body normothermia was maintained with warming.

Semiclosed and closed irrigation of the brain surface and ventricles: Before the advent of antibiotics, Fay (124) used irrigation with cold antiseptics to treat brain infections in humans, apparently with some success. Ommaya and Baldwin (125) report using a combination of subdural and ventricular irrigation and drainage in a woman in status epilepticus, who subsequently died of causes believed to be unrelated to the cooling method. Negrin (126) used a similar method during and after surgery for epilepsy in a boy who survived. White (102) achieved reductions in thalamic temperatures to around 15°C using biventricular irrigation with cold saline at 65 mL/min, with drainage from a cannula in the cisterna magna in 11 normal, anesthetized monkeys. Rectal temperatures reduced only 2–3°C with no body warming. Bradycardia and hypotension occurred with cooling, but the animals survived with no apparent ill effects from the procedure. Costal et al. (70) used various permutations of ventricular perfusion in 20 normal, anesthetized dogs to reduce parenchymal temperature to as low as 12°C with rectal temperature reaching 31°C. Ten deaths occurred because of obstruction in the intracerebral flow of the perfusate or too rapid lowering of brain temperature. Of the survivors, one developed seizures and evidence of meningitis was seen at postmortem in others.

Contact cooling of specific areas of the brain: Ommaya and Baldwin (125) mention methods for selectively cooling parts of the brain rather than the whole brain including circulating cold fluid through open-ended Teflon capsules placed in burr holes, through tubing laid on the brain surface, or by use of sacs filled with gas-cooled liquid directly placed on the brain surface. Fay (124) reports the use of "ice bombs"—cooled metal objects—inserted into the brain after tumor removal to retard regrowth and reduce pain. Similar iterations of these direct brain surface cooling techniques, such as "chiller bolts" and soft flexible "chiller pads" to be left on the brain surface during temporary vessel occlusion during neu-rosurgical procedures, are currently in development (Donald Larnard, Ph.D., personal communication).

FUTURE DIRECTIONS

In two centers, recently, there has been a move to maintain low normothermia (36–37°C) after brain injury (127,128), although the effect of this on outcome has yet to be demonstrated. Tokutomi et al. (129) carried out a retrospective review of 31 patients with traumatic brain injury and Glasgow Coma Scale ≤5 treated with systemic hypothermia of 33°C between 1994 and 1999. Their results suggest that the optimal treatment temperature was 35.0°C to 35.5°C because this can "reduce intracranial hypertension while maintaining sufficient cerebral perfusion pressure without cardiac dysfunction or oxygen debt." Milder cooling may well be the choice for direct brain cooling, because it is not clear that local brain cooling results in fewer complications than systemic hypothermia. Most methods of direct brain cooling have the potential to be used to achieve normothermia or very mild cooling and with some methods it may be necessary to regulate systemic temperature to avoid overshoot or to prevent a febrile response from working against local cooling.

There is a serious dearth of human trials of direct brain cooling methods and no shortage of avenues for research. Noninvasive methods of direct brain cooling are attractive because they carry fewer risks than invasive methods and are relatively quick and easy to instigate; however, there is little evidence to show that they work in brain-injured adult humans. Methods that warrant further investigation include circulating cooling caps and convective cooling hoods. Research is also needed on whether the potential for greater cooling of the vulnerable cortices with external conductive methods outweighs the possible problems of increased intracerebral temperature gradients.

Invasive methods of direct brain cooling carry higher risks of complications, and there are no rigorous human trials evaluating these in brain injury. The more complex and invasive the method, the more skill and attention that are required to deliver it safely. There is a considerable difference between the highly regulated and relatively short application of a method in the operating room or in animal experiments and in the less regulated environment of the intensive care unit. Of the invasive methods reviewed, anterograde cerebral perfusion seems to have the most potential in brain-injured humans. Although cerebral temperatures in animal studies of this technique have been 30°C and lower, and it is debatable whether this amount of cooling is necessary or desirable.

There are two other issues material to direct brain cooling that require further investigation. First, more research on how direct brain cooling affects the normal thermoregulatory physiology of the brain is needed. Second, given the undesirability of placing invasive brain thermistors in humans, further development of noninvasive methods of brain temperature measurement such as magnetic resonance spectroscopy (92,130), multifrequency microwave radiometry (131,132), and zero heat flow (131,133) is needed.

In summary, the benefits of direct brain cooling over systemic cooling remain unclear. Systemic hypothermia has looked promising in animal trials, but with the exception of cardiac arrest (see Chapter 15) improvement in outcome in humans has not been convincingly demonstrated. Direct brain cooling is no different. Methods that work under normal circumstances may not do so with deranged physiology following brain injury. The first step is for investigators to convincingly demonstrate clinically relevant amounts of local brain cooling with a safe regional technique. Randomized controlled outcome trials of direct brain cooling will then be needed in brain-injured humans.

REFERENCES

1. Kuhnen G, Bauer R, Walter B. Controlled brain hypothermia by extracorporeal carotid blood cooling at normothermic trunk temperatures in pigs. J Neurosci Methods 1999; 89:167–174.
2. The Commission for Thermal Physiology of the International Union of Physiological Sciences. Glossary of Terms for Thermal Physiology. 2d ed. Pflügers Arch 1987; 410:567–587.
3. Pulsinelli WA, Jacewicz M, Levy DE, Petito CK, Plum F. Ischemic brain injury and the therapeutic window. Ann N Y Acad Sci 1997; 835:187–193.
4. Busto R, Dietrich WD, Globus MY-T, Valdés I, Scheinberg P, Ginsberg MD. Small differences in intraischemic brain temperature critically determine the extent of ischemic neuronal injury. J Cereb Blood Flow Metab 1987; 7:729–738.
5. Busto R, Dietrich ED, Globus M, Ginsberg MD. The importance of brain temperature in cerebral ischemic injury. Stroke 1989; 20(8):1113–1114.

6. Rumana CS, Gopinath SP, Uzura M, Valadka AB, Robertson CS. Brain temperature exceeds systemic temperature in head-injured patients. Crit Care Med 1998; 28:562–567.
7. Rossi S, Zanier ER, Mauri I, Columbo A, Stocchetti N. Brain temperature, body core temperature, and intracranial pressure in acute cerebral damage. J Neurol Neurosurg Psychiatry 2001; 71:448–454.
8. Laptook AR, Shalak L, Corbett RJ. Differences in brain temperature and cerebral blood flow during selective head versus whole-body cooling. Pediatrics 2001 Nov; 108(5):1103–1110.
9. Cabanac M. Human Selective Brain Cooling. New York: Springer-Verlag, 1995.
10. Harris BA, Andrews PJD. The rationale for human selective brain cooling. In: Vincent J-L, ed. Yearbook of Intensive Care and Emergency Medicine. Berlin: Springer-Verlag, 2002.
11. Zenker W, Kubik S. Brain cooling in humans—anatomical considerations. Anat Embryol (Berl) 1996; 193:1–13.
12. Cabanac M, Caputa M. Natural selective cooling of the human brain: Evidence of its occurrence and magnitude. J Physiol 1979; 286:255–264.
13. Cabanac M, Brinnel H. Blood flow in the emissary veins of the human head during hyperthermia. Eur J Appl Physiol Occup Physiol 1985; 54(2):172–176.
14. du Boulay GH, Lawton M, Wallis A. The story of the internal carotid artery of mammals: from Galen to sudden infant death syndrome. Neuroradiology 1998; 40:697–703.
15. du Boulay G, Lawton M, Wallis A. Selective brain cooling in animals: Internal carotid's significance for sudden infant death syndrome. Ambul Child Health 2000; 6(Suppl 1):36–38.
16. McIntosh DN, Zajonc RB, Vig PS, Emerick SW. Facial movement, breathing, temperature, and affect: implications of the vascular theory of emotional efference. Cogn Emot 1997 Mar; 11(2):171–195.
17. Caputa M, Perrin G, Cabanac M. Ecoulement sanguin réversible dans la veine ophthalmique: mécanisme de refroi-

dissement sélectif du cerveau humain. C R Acad Sci 1978; 287:D1011–D1014.

18. Hirashita M, Shido O, Tanabe M. Blood flow through the ophthalmic veins during exercise in humans. Eur J Appl Physiol 1992; 64:92–97.
19. Mariak Z, White MD, Lewko J, Lyson T, Piekarski P. Direct cooling of the human brain by heat loss from the upper respiratory tract. J Appl Physiol 1999 Nov; 87(5):1609–1613.
20. Kuluz JW, Gregory GA, Yu AC, Chang Y. Selective brain cooling during and after prolonged global ischemia reduces cortical damage in rats. Stroke 1992; 23:1792–1797.
21. Barone FC, Feuerstein GZ, White RF. Brain cooling during transient focal ischemia provides complete neuroprotection. Neurosci Biobehav Rev 1997; 21(1):31–44.
22. Huh PW, Belayev L, Zhao W, Koch S, Busto R, Ginsberg MD. Comparative neuroprotective efficacy of prolonged moderate intraischemic and postischemic hypothermia in focal cerebral ischaemia. J Neurosurg 2000; 92:91–99.
23. Lo EH, Steinberg GK. Effects of hypothermia on evoked potentials, magnetic resonance imaging, and blood flow in focal ischaemia in rabbits. Stroke 1992; 23:889–893.
24. Noguchi Y, Nishio S, Kawauchi M, Asari S, Ohmoto T. A new method of inducing selective brain hypothermia with saline perfusion into the subdural space: effects on transient cerebral ischaemia in cats. Acta Med Okayama 2002; 56(6):279–286.
25. Natale J, D'Alecy L. Protection from cerebral ischemia by brain cooling without reduced lactate accumulation in dogs. Stroke 1989; 20:770–777.
26. Horn M, Schlote W, Henrich HA. Global cerebral ischemia and subsequent selective hypothermia. A neuropathological and morphometrical study on ischemic neuronal damage in cat. Acta Neuropathol 1991; 81:443–449.
27. Battin MR, Dezoete JA, Gunn TR, Gluckman PD, Gunn AJ. Neurodevelopmental outcome of infants treated with head cooling and mild hypothermia after perinatal asphyxia. Pediatrics 2001 Mar; 107(3):480–484.

28. Battin MR, Penrice J, Gunn TR, Gunn AJ. Treatment of term infants with head cooling and mild systemic hypothermia (35.0 °C and 34.5 °C) after perinatal asphyxia. Pediatrics 2003; 111:244–251.

29. Hachimi-Idrissi S, Corne L, Ebinger G, Michotte Y, Huyghens L. Mild hypothermia induced by a helmet device: a clinical feasibility study. Resuscitation 2001; 51:275–281.

30. Minamisawa H, Nordström CH, Smith M-L, Siesjö BK. The influence of mild body and brain hypothermia on ischemic brain damage. J Cereb Blood Flow Metab 1990; 10:365–374.

31. Park CK, Jun SS, Kim MC, Kang JK. Effects of systemic hypothermia and selective brain cooling on ischemic brain damage and swelling. Acta Neurochir Suppl Wien 1998; 71: 225–228.

32. Gelman B, Schleien CL, Lohe A, Kuluz JW. Selective brain cooling in infant piglets after cardiac arrest and resuscitation. Crit Care Med 1996; 24(6):1009–1017.

33. Ibayashi S, Takano K, Ooboshi H, Kitazono T, Sadoshima S, Fujishima M. Effect of selective brain hypothermia on regional cerebral blood flow and tissue metabolism using brain thermo-regulator in spontaneously hypertensive rats. Neurochem Res 2000; 25:369–375.

34. Schwartz AE, Stone JG, Finck AD, Sandhu AA, Mongero LB, Adams DC, Jonassen AE, Young WL, Michler RE. Isolated cerebral hypothermia by single carotid artery perfusion of extracorporeally cooled blood in baboons. Neurosurgery 1996 Sep; 39(3):577–581.

35. Walter B, Bauer R, Kuhnen G, Fritz H, Swiener U. Coupling of cerebral blood flow and oxygen metabolism in infant pigs during selective brain hypothermia. J Cereb Blood Flow Metab 2000; 20:1215–1224.

36. Miyake T, Endo M, Ishii N, Fukuda Y, Kinoshita K, Masuda K. Second report of an experimental study of cerebrocardiopulmonary resuscitation (CCPR) in dogs with reference to a new continuous brain cooling method, using a Resusci Pump TM-1. Resuscitation 1984; 12:9–24.

37. Kuluz JW, Prado R, Chang J, Ginsberg MD, Schleren CL,

Busto R. Selective brain cooling increases cortical cerebral blood flow in rats. Am J Physiol 1993; 265:H824–H827.

38. Mustafa S, Thulesius O. Cooling-induced carotid artery dilatation: An experimental study in isolated vessels. Stroke 2002; 33:256–260.

39. Dietrich WD. The importance of brain temperature in cerebral injury. J Neurotrauma 1992; 9(Suppl 2):S475–S485.

40. Gunn AJ. Cerebral hypothermia for prevention of brain injury following perinatal asphyxia. Curr Opin Pediatr 2000 Apr; 12(2): 111–115 (Review).

41. Thoresen M, Simmonds M, Satas S, Tooley J, Silver IA. Effective selective head cooling during posthypoxic hypothermia in newborn piglets. Pediatr Res 2001; 49:594–599.

42. Schubert AS. Side effects of mild hypothermia. J Neurosurg Anesthesiol 1995; 7:139–147.

43. Harris OA, Colford JM, Good MC, Matz PG. The role of hypothermia in the management of severe brain injury: a meta-analysis. Arch Neurol 2002; 59:1077–1083.

44. Gadkary CS, Alderson P, Signorini DF. Therapeutic hypothermia for head injury (Cochrane Review). The Cochrane Library, Issue 3. Oxford: Update Software, 2002.

45. Ishikawa K, Tanaka H, Shiozaki T, Takaoka M, Ogura H, Kishi M, Shimazu T, Sugimoto H. Characteristics of infection and leukocyte count in severely head-injured patients treated with mild hypothermia. J Trauma 2000; 49:912–922.

46. Hata T, Kawabata A, Itoh E. Platelet hypoaggregability in rats exposed to SART stress (repeated cold stress). Thromb Res 1992; 65(4–5):617–629.

47. Valeri CR, MacGregor H, Cassidy G, Tinney R, Pompei F. Effects of temperature on bleeding time and clotting time in normal male and female volunteers. Crit Care Med 1995 Apr; 23(4):698–704.

48. Polderman KH, Peerdeman SM, Girbes ARJ. Hypophosphatemia and hypomagnesemia induced by cooling in patients with severe head injury. J Neurosurg 2001; 94:697–705.

49. Thoresen M, Whitelaw A. Cardiovascular changes during

mild therapeutic hypothermia and rewarming in infants with hypoxic–ischemic encephalopathy. Pediatrics 2000; 106:92–99.

50. Gunn AJ, Gluckman PD, Gunn TR. Selective head cooling in newborn infants after perinatal asphyxia: A safety study. Pediatrics 1998 Oct; 102(4 Pt 1):885–892.

51. Zayak M, Eyal F. Tolerance of moderate hypothermic therapy: its effect on the neonatal cardiovascular system and particularly pulmonary and intestinal circulation. Arch Pediatr 2002; 9:1104–1106.

52. Iwata O, Iwata S, Tamura M, Nakamura T, Sugiura M, Ogiso Y. Brain temperature in newborn piglets under selective head cooling with minimal systemic hypothermia. Pediatr Int 2003; 45:163–168.

53. Reichlin S. Alternative pathways of neural control of the immune process. In: McCann SM, Lipton JM, Sternberg EM, Chrousos JP, Gold PW, Smith CC, eds. Neuroimmunomodulation: Molecular Aspects, Integrative Systems, and Clinical Advances. Ann N Y Acad Sci 1998; 840:301–306.

54. Reichlin S. Neuroendocrinology of infection and the innate immune system. Recent Prog Horm Res 1999; 54:133–183.

55. Kluger MJ, Kozak W, Mayfield KP. Fever and immunity. In: Ader R, Felten DL, Cohen N, eds. Psychoneuroimmunology. 3rd ed. San Diego: Academic Press, 2001:687–702.

56. Thoresen M, Satas S, Loberg EM, Whitelaw A, Acolet D, Lindgren C, Penrice J, Robertson N, Haug AE, Steen PA. Twenty-four hours of mild hypothermia in unsedated newborn pigs starting after a severe global hypoxic–ischemic insult is not neuroprotective. Pediatr Res 2001; 50:405–411.

57. Mackowiak PA, Plaisance KI. Benefits and risks of antipyretic therapy. Ann N Y Acad Sci 1998; 856:214–223.

58. Wass CT, Lanier WL. Hypothermia-associated protection from ischaemic brain injury: implications for patient management. Int Anesthesiol Clin 1996; 34:95–111.

59. DeWitte J, Sessler DI. Perioperative shivering: Physiology and pharmacology. Anesthesiology 2002; 96:467–484.

60. Iaizzo PA, Jeon YM, Sigg DC. Facial warming increases the

threshold for shivering. J Neurosurg Anesthesiol 1999 Oct; 11(4):231–239.

61. Sweney MT, Sigg DC, Tahvildari S, Iaizzo PA. Shiver suppression using focal hand warming in unanesthetized normal subjects. Anesthesiology 2001 Nov; 95(5):1089–1095.

62. Frank SM, Higgins MS, Fleisher LA, Sitzmann JV, Raff H, Breslow MJ. Adrenergic, respiratory, and cardiovascular effects of core cooling in humans. Am J Physiol 1997; 272:R557–R562.

63. Bligh J. Mammalian homeothermy: An integrative thesis. J Therm Biol 1998; 23(3–4):143–258.

64. Boulant JA. Thermoregulation. In: Mackowiak PA, ed. Fever: Basic mechanisms and Management. 2d ed. Philadelphia: Lippincott-Raven Publishers, 1997:35–58.

65. Laptook AR, Corbett RJT. The effects of temperature on hypoxic–ischemic brain injury. Clin Perinatol 2002; 29:623–649.

66. Gelman B, Schleien CL, Kuluz JW, Pino E, Pinto A. Regional brain temperatures in infant piglets during resuscitation from cardiac arrest: selective brain cooling vs. total body cooling. J Cereb Blood Flow Metab 1997; 17(suppl 1):S45.

67. Wass CT, Waggoner JR III, Cable DG, Schaff HV, Schroeder DR, Lanier WL. Selective convective brain cooling during normothermic cardiopulmonary bypass in dogs. J Thorac Cardiovasc Surg 1998 Jun; 115(6):1350–1357.

68. White RJ, Brown HW, Albin MS, Verdura J. Rapid selective brain-cooling using head immersion and naso-oral perfusion in dogs. Resuscitation 1983; 10:189–191.

69. Mori K, Saito J, Kurata Y, Takeyama Y, Itoh Y, Kaneko M, Asai Y, Renzi FP, Dickson EW. Rapid development of brain hypothermia using femoral-carotid bypass. Acad Emerg Med 2001 Apr; 8(4):303–308.

70. Costal M, Owens G, Woldring S, Butler W, Cody B, Siwirski D. Experimental production of cerebral hypothermia by ventricular perfusion techniques. J Neurosurg 1963; 20:112–117.

71. Wolfson SK, Inouye WY, Kavianian A, Icoz MV, Parkins WM. Preferential cerebral hypothermia for circulatory arrest. Surgery 1965; 57(6):846–855.

72. Almond CH, Jones JC, Snyder HM, Grant SM, Meyer BW. Cooling gradients and brain damage with deep hypothermia. J Thorac Cardiovasc Surg 1964; 48:890–897.

73. Einer-Jensen N, Khorooshi MH. Cooling of the brain through oxygen flushing of the nasal cavities in intubated rats: an alternative model for treatment of brain injury. Exp Brain Res 2000; 130:244–247.

74. Brengelmann GL. Dilemma of body temperature measurement. In: Shiraki K, Yousef MK, eds. Man in Stressful Environments: Thermal and Work Physiology. Springfield, IL: Charles C. Thomas, 1987:75–122.

75. Brinnel H, Cabanac M. Tympanic temperature is a core temperature in humans. J Therm Biol 1989; 14:47–53.

76. Nagasaka T, Brinnel H, Hales JR, Ogawa T. Selective brain cooling in hyperthermia: The mechanisms and medical implications. Med Hypotheses 1998 Mar; 50(3):203–211.

77. Einer-Jensen N, Khorooshi MH, Petersen MB, Svendsen P. Rapid brain cooling in intubated pigs through nasal flushing with oxygen: prevention of brain hyperthermia. Acta Vet Scand 2001; 42(4):459–464.

78. Mellergård P. Changes in human intracerebral temperature in response to different methods of brain cooling. Neurosurgery 1992; 31:671–677.

79. Andrews P, Harris B. A randomised cross-over trial of the effects of airflow through the upper respiratory tract of intubated, brain injured patients on brain temperature and selective brain cooling [online summary], 2003. Available from http://www.show.scot.nhs.uk/cso/Publications/ExecSumms/Jan_March03.htm.

80. Cole P. Upper respiratory airflow. In: Proctor DF, Andersen IB, eds. The Nose: Upper Airway Physiology and the Atmospheric Environment. Oxford: Elsevier Biomedical Press, 1982:163–182.

81. Eccles R. Neurological and pharmacological considerations.

Proctor DF, Andersen IB, eds. The Nose: Upper Airway Physiology and the Atmospheric Environment. Oxford: Elsevier Biomedical Press, 1982:191–214.

82. Naredi S. Cerebral Circulation and the Sympathetic Nervous System in Patients with Traumatic Brain Injury or Subarachnoid Hemorrhage. Goteborg, Sweden: Departments of Anaesthesiology and Intensive Care, Neurosurgery, Clinical Physiology at Goteborg University and the Department of Anaesthesiology and Intensive Care at Umea University, 2000.

83. Houdas Y, Ring E. Human Body Temperature: Its Measurement and Regulation. New York: Plenum Press, 1982:81–103.

84. Shiraki K, Sagawa S, Tajima F, Yokota A, Hashimoto M, Brengelmann GL. Independence of brain and tympanic temperatures in an unanesthetized human. J Appl Physiol 1988; 65:482–486.

85. Cabanac M. Selective brain cooling in humans: "fancy" or fact? FASEB J 1993 Sep; 7(12):1143–1146.

86. vanLeeuwen GMJ, Hand JW, Lagendijk JJW, Azzopardi DV, Edwards AD. Numerical modelling of temperature distributions within the neonatal head. Pediatr Res 2000; 48:351–356.

87. Zhu L, Diao C. Theoretical simulation of temperature distribution in the brain during mild hypothermia treatment for brain injury. Med Biol Eng Comput 2001; 39:681–687.

88. Diao C, Zhu L, Wang H. Cooling and rewarming for brain ischemia or injury: Theoretical analysis. Ann Biomed Eng 2003; 31:353–356.

89. Brader E, Jehle D, Safar P. Protective head cooling during cardiac arrest in dogs. Ann Emerg Med 1985; 14:510.

90. Leonov Y, Sterz F, Safar P, Radovsky A, Oku K, Tisherman S, Stezoski SW. Mild cerebral hypothermia during and after cardiac arrest improves neurologic outcome in dogs. J Cereb Blood Flow Metab 1990; 10:57–70.

91. Tadler S, Callaway C, Menegazzi J. Noninvasive cerebral cooling in a swine model of cardiac arrest. Acad Emerg Med 1998; 5:25–30.

92. Corbett R, Laptook AR. Failure of localised head cooling to reduce the brain temperature in adult humans. NeuroReport 1998; 9:2721–2725.

93. Callaway CW, Tadler SC, Katz LM, Lipinski CL, Brader E. Feasibility of external cranial cooling during out-of-hospital cardiac arrest. Resuscitation 2002 Feb; 52(2):159–165.

94. Tooley J, Satas S, Eagle R, Silver IA, Thoresen M. Significant selective head cooling can be maintained long-term after global hypoxia ischemia in newborn piglets. Pediatrics 2002; 109:643–649.

95. Whitelaw A, Thoresen M. Clinical experience with therapeutic hypothermia in asphyxiated infants. Dev Med Child Neurol Suppl 2001 Mar; 86:30–31.

96. Parkins WM, Jensen JM, Vars HM. Brain cooling in the prevention of brain damage during periods of circulatory occlusion in dogs. Ann Surg 1954; 140(3):284–289.

97. Connolly JE, Boyd RJ, Calvin JW. The protective effect of hypothermia in cerebral ischaemia: experimental and clinical application by selective brain cooling in the human. Surgery 1962; 52(1):15–24.

98. White RJ, Donald DE. Selective hypothermic perfusion and circulatory arrest. Arch Surg 1962; 84:40–48.

99. White RJ, Massopust LA, Wolin LR, Taslitz N, Yashon D. Profound selective cooling and ischaemia of primate brain without pump or oxygenator. Surgery 1969; 66(1):224–232.

100. Kristiansen K, Krog J, Lund I. Experiences with selective cooling of the brain. Acta Chir Scan 1960; 253(suppl):151–161.

101. Kristiansen K. Methods of circulatory arrest. Prog Brain Res 1968; 30:377–382.

102. White RJ. Cerebral hypothermia and circulatory arrest. Mayo Clin Proc 1978; 53:450–458.

103. White RJ, Locke GE, Albin LS. Isolated profound cerebral cooling with a bi-carotid heat exchanger shunt in dogs. Resuscitation 1983; 10:193–195.

104. Schwartz AE, Stone JG, Pile-Spellman J, Finck AD, Sandhu AA, Mongero LB, Michler RE. Selective cerebral hypothermia

by means of transfemoral internal carotid artery catheterisation. Radiology 1996 Nov; 201(2):571–572.

105. Jacobs MJ, deMol BA, Veldman DJ. Aortic arch and proximal supraaortic arterial repair under continuous antegrade cerebral perfusion and moderate hypothermia. Cardiovasc Surg 2001 Aug; 9(4):396–402.

106. Matsuwaka R, Sakakibara T, Hori T, Shinohara N. Initial experience with cool head, warm body perfusion in aortic arch surgery. J Card Surg 1998; 13:463–467.

107. Boston US, Sungurtekin H, McGregor CG, Macoviak JA, Cook DJ. Differential perfusion: A new technique for isolated brain cooling during cardiopulmonary bypass. Ann Thorac Surg May 2000; 69(5):1346–1350.

108. Macoviak JA, Hwang J, Boerjan KL, Deal DD. Comparing dual-stream and standard cardiopulmonary bypass in pigs. Ann Thorac Surg 2002; 73(1):203–208.

109. Ohta T, Kuroiwa T, Sakaguchi I, Sakai N, Moriwaki K, Solomon RA, Hodge CJ, Young W. Selective hypothermic perfusion of canine brain. Neurosurgery 1996; 38(6):1211–1215.

110. Reich DL, Uysal S, Ergin A, Griepp RB. Retrograde cerebral perfusion as a method of neuroprotection during thoracic aortic surgery. Ann Thorac Surg 2001; 72(5):1774–1782. Review.

111. Wolfson SK, Icoz MV, Inouye WY, Parkins WM. Prolonged circulatory arrest with preferential cerebral hypothermia and resuscitation by external cardiac massage. Surg Forum 1964; 15:415–417.

112. Wolfson SK, Icoz MV, Luber S. Preservation of conditioned responses in primates after total circulatory arrest with preferential cerebral hypothermia. Surg Forum 1965; 16:409–411.

113. Icoz MV, Wolfson SK. Tolerance to total ischaemia in dogs after cold blood or cold physiologic saline perfusion of the brain. Surg Forum 1966; 17:403–405.

114. Bacalzo LV, Wolfson SK. Resuscitation after unexpected circulatory arrest: tolerance to cerebral ischaemia provided by cold carotid perfusion. Biom Sci Instrum 1969; 5:75–78.

115. Bacalzo LV, Wolfson SK. Preferential cerebral hypothermia: Tromethamine and Dextran 40 and tolerance to circulatory arrest of 90–120 minutes. Arch Surg 1971; 103:393–397.

116. Wolfson SK, Selker RG. Carotid perfusion hypothermia for brain surgery using cardiac arrest without bypass. J Surg Res 1973; 14:449–458.

117. Selker RG, Wolfson SK, Maroon JC, Steichen FM. Preferential cerebral hypothermia with elective cardiac arrest: resection of "giant" aneurysm. Surg Neurol 1976; 6:173–179.

118. Miyake T, Kinoshita K, Ishii N, Endo M. First report of an experimental study in dogs of cerebrocardiopulmonary resuscitation (CCPR). Resuscitation 1982; 10:105–120.

119. Bernard S, Buist M, Monteiro O, Smith K. Induced hypothermia using large volume, ice-cold intravenous fluid in comatose survivors of out-of-hospital cardiac arrest: a preliminary report. Resuscitation 2003; 56:9–13.

120. Marion DW, Leonov Y, Ginsberg M, Katz LM, Kochanek PM, Lechleuthner A, Nemoto EM, Obrist W, Safar P, Sterz F, Tisherman SA, White RJ, Xiao F, Zar H. Resuscitative hypothermia. Crit Care Med 1996; 24(suppl 2):S81–S89.

121. The Hypothermia After Cardiac Arrest Study Group. Mild therapeutic hypothermia to improve the neurologic outcome after cardiac arrest. N Engl J Med 2002; 346:549–556.

122. Bernard SA, Gray TW, Buist MD, Jones BM, Silvester W, Gutteridge G, Smith K. Treatment of comatose survivors of out-of-hospital cardiac arrest with induced hypothermia. N Engl J Med 2002; 346:557–563.

123. Iatrou CC, Domaingue CM, Thomas RD, Nye DH. The effect of selective brain cooling on intracerebral temperature during craniotomy. Anaesth Intensive Care 2002; 30(2):167–170.

124. Fay T. Early experiences with local and generalized refrigeration of the human brain. J Neurosurg 1959; 16:239–260.

125. Ommaya AK, Baldwin M. Extravascular local cooling of the brain in man. J Neurosurg 1963; 20:8–20.

126. Negrin J. Selective local hypothermia in neurosurgery. N Y State J Med 1961; 61:2951–2954.

127. Knoll T, Wimmer MLJ, Gumpinger F, Haberl RL. The low normothermia concept—maintaining a core body temperature between 36 and 37°C in acute stroke unit patients. J Neurosurg Anesthesiol 2002; 14:304–308.

128. Schmutzhard E, Beer R, Brössner G, Pfausler B. Prophylactic normothermia—A new concept with innovative technology. Int J Intensive Care 2003; 10(1):21–22.

129. Tokutomi T, Morimoto K, Miyagi T, Yamaguchi S, Ishikawa K, Shigemori M. Optimal temperature for the management of severe traumatic brain injury: effect of hypothermia on intracranial pressure, systemic and intracranial hemodynamics, and metabolism. Neurosurgery 2003; 52:102–112.

130. Corbett R, Laptook A, Weatherall P. Noninvasive measurements of human brain temperature using volume-localized proton magnetic resonance spectroscopy. J Cereb Blood Flow Metab 1997; 17:363–369.

131. Togawa T. Body temperature measurement. Clin Phys Physiol Meas 1985; 6:83–108.

132. Maruyma K, Mizushina S, Sugiura T, VanLeeuwen GMJ, Hand JW, Marrocco G, Bardati F, Edwards AD, Azzopardi D, Land D. Feasibility of non-invasive measurement of deep brain temperature in newborn infants by multifrequency microwave radiometry. IEEE Trans Microwave Theor Tech 2000; 48:2141–2147.

133. Lees DE, Kim YD, Macnamara TE. Noninvasive determination of core temperature during anesthesia. South Med J 1980; 73:1322–1324.

12

Prevention and Treatment of Fever in Neurocritical Care

STEPHAN A. MAYER and JAN CLAASSEN

Division of Critical Care Neurology,
Department of Neurology,
Columbia University College of Physicians
and Surgeons, New York, New York, U.S.A.

INTRODUCTION

Body temperature is normally tightly regulated at approximately 37.0°C (98.6°F). The term "fever" is generally used in clinical practice (as well as in this chapter) when body temperature exceeds 38.3°C (101.0°F). Strictly speaking, however, the term "fever" specifically denotes temperature elevation resulting from an increased temperature set point. Set point elevation results from prostaglandin E synthesis in the hypothalamus, which is stimulated by circulating systemic inflammatory (pyrogens) such as tumor necrosis factor or interferon

1β (1). The origin of these mediators is often an infection such as pneumonia, meningitis, or bacteremia, but not always: conditions associated with systemic inflammatory response syndrome (SIRS), drug allergy, deep vein thrombosis, and a variety of other processes can also lead to cytokine elevation and fever (1). Vasoconstriction and shivering are the body's principle means of generating heat when body temperature is lower than the hypothalamic set point.

By contrast, the term "hyperthermia" refers to clinical conditions in which body temperature exceeds the hypothalamic set point (2). This scenario occurs when either an external or an internal source of heat production overwhelms the normal heat-dissipating mechanisms of the body: vasodilation and sweating. The best example of hyperthermia from an external source is heat stroke; prolonged exercise and neuroleptic malignant syndrome are examples of hyperthermia resulting from endogenous heat production. Distinguishing between fever and hyperthermia may have important implications for treatment. Antipyretic nonsteroidal anti-inflammatory agents (NSAIDs) are effective for treating fever, but not hyperthermia. External cooling, by contrast, can result in shivering when used to treat fever, but not hyperthermia. In this chapter, the term "fever" is used generically to denote any type of temperature elevation, even though it remains possible that central fever may involve mechanisms more consistent with hyperthermia in some cases.

Frequency of Fever in the NICU

Fever (≥38.3°C) is frequently encountered in neurological intensive care unit (NICU) patients. It occurs in 25–50% of neurocritically ill patients (3,4), with higher frequencies in more neurosurgically oriented ICUs. Specifically, fever is observed in up to 40% of patients during the first week after ischemic stroke (5), in 33–42% of patients with spontaneous intracerebral hemorrhage (ICH) (3,6), and in 40–70% of patients with severe traumatic brain injury (TBI) (3,7,8) or a subarachnoid aneurysmal hemorrhage (SAH) (3,8,9). Early severe pyrexia (>39.0°C within 12 hr of stroke onset), which is often equated with central fever, occurs in 37% of patients with pontine hemorrhage (10).

Impact of Fever on Outcome

Temperature elevation has consistently been associated with increased neuronal injury in animal models of ischemic stroke (see Chapter 4) (11), and with increased mortality and poor functional outcome in patients with acute brain injuries. In patients with ischemic stroke, mortality is higher and infarct size increases with higher admission body temperatures (12–14); the relative risk for poor functional outcome doubles with each degree Celsius of temperature elevation (12,13). Fever has also been associated with symptomatic vasospasm and poor neurological outcome in SAH patients (9,15,16), with increased mortality and functional disability in patients with ICH (6,10), and with poor outcome after severe TBI (17).

Clinical Epidemiology of Fever in the NICU

Two main categories of fever can be distinguished in the NICU population. About half of cases can be classified as infectious fever, with an identifiable infection diagnosed according to standard criteria (3). Another one-fifth to one-third of cases remains unexplained after an extensive diagnostic workup; many of these patients may be considered to have central fever (3,7,18). In the NICU setting, infectious fevers are most often caused by nosocomial pulmonary infections (Table 1); risk factors include coma, endotracheal intubation, and increased ICU length of stay (1). Depressed level of consciousness may predispose to fever because of impaired thermoregulation related to brain injury, whereas the association with intubation almost certainly reflects the high rate of aspiration and ventilator-associated pneumonia in these patients. Increased ICU length of stay has previously been associated with fever in neurosurgical patients (4); however, it remains unclear whether fever per se is a cause or effect of increased ICU length of stay.

Acute brain injury can also lead to spontaneous temperature elevations in the absence of infection or a systemic inflammatory response—a condition known as central fever. The

Table 1 Site-Specific Incidence Rates for Nosocomial Infections in Neurosurgical ICU Patients

	Incidence per 100 patients	Incidence density per 1000 days (procedure)
Pneumonia	9.0	15.1 (ventilator days)
Urinary tract infection	7.3	8.5 (urinary catheters)
Blood stream infection	1.0	0.9 (central line days)
Meningitis	1.1	NC
Brain abscess/ventriculitis	0.7	NC
Other[a]	1.7	NC
Total	20.7	NC

NC = not calculated.
[a] Most often wound infection, bronchitis, local intravenous cellulitis, and diarrhea.
Source: (Ref. 19.)

diagnosis of central fever has inherent methodological problems and is generally one of exclusion, which partly accounts for the limited amount of data available on this clinical entity. Animal studies suggesting a relationship between intraventricular hemorrhage (IVH) and central fever (20,21) have been corroborated by the observation that external ventricular drain placement (usually for IVH) is a risk factor for unexplained fever in NICU patients (3). The mechanism by which acute brain injury triggers central fever is poorly understood; direct hemotoxic damage to thermoregulatory centers in the preoptic region, interference with tonic inhibitory inputs from the lower midbrain that ordinarily suppress thermogenesis, and stimulation of central prostaglandin production with subsequent elevation of the temperature set point have all been invoked (22). Like infectious fever, unexplained fever in NICU patients is associated with increased ICU length of stay (1). Unexplained and, presumably, central fevers tend to occur earlier than infection-related fevers (23).

Fever Control in the NICU

Increasing awareness of the deleterious effects of fever on neurological outcome in patients with acute brain injury is driving the search for safe and effective measures to suppress fever in this population. For many years, the nearly universal approach to treating fever has been the administration of an antipyretic agent (acetaminophen or other NSAIDs), followed by the application of conventional water-circulating cooling blankets (24). Unfortunately, the effectiveness of these interventions in neurological patients is limited, with success rates in the range of 30–40% (25,26).

This chapter will review both established and newer treatment approaches for fever control in patients with acute brain injury. As clinicians continue to test induced hypothermia as a means of providing neuroprotection in NICU patients, there has also been increasing interest in the concept of induced prophylactic normothermia in patients at risk for temperature-related brain injury. Novel external and endovascular cooling devices that may improve our ability to combat fever in patients at risk for temperature-related brain injury are currently in development. If normothermia can be effectively maintained in these patients, it then remains to be seen if this type of intervention can improve survival or functional outcome.

REVIEW

There are three main strategies for reducing fever in the ICU setting: (1) elimination of fever source, (2) antipyretic therapy, and (3) active body cooling. Infectious fever should initially be treated with an antibiotic agent. Selection of the antibiotic should be guided by identification of the infection-causing pathogen and empiric clinical experience (24). Antibiotic therapy alone is rarely effective for reducing infection-related fever in the first hours to days, however; hence, if fever control is an important goal, antipyretic medication and active cooling are usually required (Table 2). Relatively few randomized controlled trials have been completed to test the feasibility and efficacy of different approaches of fever treatment in neurological patients. One of the obstacles in comparing the efficacy of different approaches for fever control is that the study end

Table 2 Therapeutic Interventions for Fever

Antibiotics
Antipyretic medications (reduce hypothalamic set point)
  Acetaminophen
  Other nonsteroidal anti-inflammatory agents
Cooling interventions (no effect on hypothalamic set point)
  Surface cooling
    Evaporation
      Water sprays
      Sponge baths
    Conduction
      Ice packs
      Immersion
      Water-circulating cooling blankets (i.e., Blanketrol System; Cincinnati Sub-Zero)
      Water-circulating hydrogel-coated pads (i.e., Arctic Sun System; Medivance, Inc.)
    Convection
      Fans
      Air-circulating cooling blankets (i.e., Polar Air; Augustine Medical)
    Radiation
      Skin exposure
  Intravascular catheter cooling (circulates cooled saline via closed loop within catheter)
    Balloon-tipped design (Cool Line; Alsius Corp.)
    Helical design (Set Point System; Radiant Medical, Inc.)
    Metallic heat exchange element (Celsius Control System; Innercool Therapies, Inc.)

points vary widely: these include attaining a desired target temperature or not surpassing a given threshold, the rate of temperature reduction, and the calculation of fever burden over a specific time interval. The results of retrospective studies that defined treatment end points post hoc are, in some cases, particularly difficult to interpret.

Antipyretic Agents

Antipyretic medications lower the hypothalamic set point, which is increased in pyrogen-induced fever (1,27,28). Nonsteroidal anti-inflammatory drugs are the standard first-line drugs for fever in the ICU. Acetaminophen, the most widely used NSAID for fever control, is a strong inhibitor of central nervous system biosynthesis of prostaglandins, with both analgesic and antipyretic properties. Other NSAIDs, such as acetylsalicylic acid and ibuprofen, also lower the hypothalamic set point, but the relative efficacy of different NSAIDs for treating fever in NICU patients is largely unknown. Prior reports indicate that there are only minor differences in efficacy between different NSAIDs for reducing fever (27,29).

NSAID Prophylaxis of Fever After Acute Stroke

Six studies have investigated the antipyretic effects of NSAIDs in the prevention or treatment of fever in patients with acute neurological diseases (Table 3), all of which primarily focused on the feasibility of NSAIDs to maintain lower body temperatures (30–35). None of these studies was designed to demonstrate a benefit on outcome. The best data come from four studies that compared different dosages of prophylactic acetaminophen to placebo to lower body temperature in nonfebrile patients with stroke (30–33). All four of these prospective studies agreed that acetaminophen could be safely administered to patients. However, they also found that the magnitude of the effect of acetaminophen on body temperature was small. In two studies involving a total of 151 ischemic stroke patients conducted by Dippel et al. (31,32), high-dose acetaminophen (1000 mg every 4 hr) lowered body temperature by only 0.3–0.4°C at 24 hr compared to controls. A meta-analysis of these two trials found that this effect on temperature was present at 4 hr, and remained fairly constant over the following 20 hr (Fig. 1) (36). Ibuprofen (2400 mg/day) was also evaluated in the second of these studies, and had no effect. In another trial of 42 ischemic stroke patients, Koennecke and Leistner (30) found that subjects who received 4000 mg of acetaminophen daily were significantly less likely to develop temperature elevations exceeding 37.5°C during the first 5 days (5% vs. 36%). By contrast, Kasner et al. (33) found that 3900 mg of acetaminophen daily had no significant effect on body temperature during the first 24 hr of treatment.

Table 3 Studies of Antipyretic Agents for Fever Prevention and Control in the Neurological ICU

Reference	Patients	n	Study design	Intervention (daily dose)	Primary outcome measure	Results
(30)	INF	42	P/p	Acetaminophen 4 g vs. placebo for 5 days	$T > 37.5°C$ within 5 days of admission	T less often >37.5°C (5% vs. 36%) with treatment
(31)	INF	76	P/p	Acetaminophen 6 g vs. 3 g vs. placebo for 5 days	T at 24 hr after start of diagnosis	Mild (0.4°C) T decrease with high dose vs. placebo
(33)	INF/ICH	39	P/p	Acetaminophen 3.9 g vs. placebo	T during first 24 hr	Trend for T <36.5°C with treatment (14% vs. 5%), otherwise no effect
(35)	SAH/TBI	12	C/r	Diclofenac low-dose infusions (no control group)	T at days 1 and 2	Effective and safe, no control group
(34)	TBI	66	C/r	NSAIDs (no control group)	Mean T before vs. after intervention	NSAIDs lowered T slightly (0.6°C) and caused small drop in CPP
(32)	INF	75	P/p	Acetaminophen 6 g vs. ibuprofen 2.4 g vs. placebo for 5 days	T during first 5 days	No overall effect over 5 days; mild T (0.3°C) reduction at 24 hr with high dose vs. placebo

All medications are given as grams per day.
T = temperature; C = fever control; NA = not available; NSAID = nonsteroidal anti-inflammatory drug; P = fever prophylaxis; p = prospective; r = retrospective; SAH = subarachnoid hemorrhage; TBI = traumatic brain injury; ICH = intracerebral hemorrhage; INF = cerebral infarction.

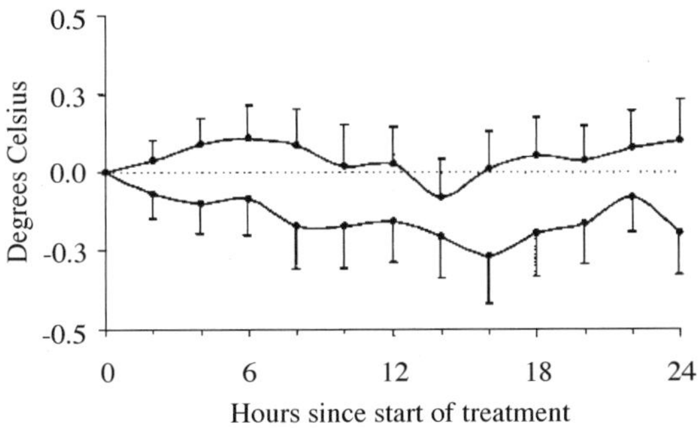

Figure 1 Mean difference between follow-up temperature and temperature at start of treatment at 2-hr time points for ischemic stroke patients receiving placebo (upper line) or acetaminophen (lower line). Vertical lines indicate two SE. (From Ref. 36.)

NSAID Therapy for Fever Reduction

Less evidence is available regarding the effectiveness of NSAIDs for reducing established fever in patients with acute neurological diseases. In a clinical trial that compared acetaminophen alone to acetaminophen plus external air convection cooling in a general NICU population, about one-third of patients remained febrile in both study arms after treatment was initiated (Table 4) (25). Two retrospective studies analyzed the efficacy of NSAIDs on fever in patients with TBI or hemorrhagic stroke (Table 3) (34,35). One of these studies retrospectively identified 63 TBI patients who were treated with NSAIDs, among whom 23 were treated with surface cooling as well (34). Comparing mean body temperature in each patient before and after initiating these interventions, NSAID treatment led to a modest 0.58°C drop in temperature (from 38.7°C to 38.1°C). Importantly, NSAID administration was also associated with a 7-mm Hg drop in cerebral perfusion pressure. The authors admitted that despite attaining statistical significance, the effect of NSAIDs on temperature was clinically negligible in most cases. These findings are difficult to interpret due to the retrospective nature of the study, lack of controls, and possible treatment biases. The other study

Table 4 Surface Cooling for Fever Control in the Neurological ICU

Reference	Patients	n	Study design	Intervention (daily dose)	Primary outcome measure	Results
(25)	NICU	220	P/r	Acetaminophen (3.9 g) alone vs. added Polar Air air-circulating cooling blanket	Within 24 hr: ≤37.2°C success; sustained ≥38.3°C failure	Polar Air had no significant effect
(55)	NICU	21	P/o	Acetaminophen (3.9 g) alone vs. added water sponging or conventional cooling blanket	Time to return to 38°C	Underpowered, no difference found
(54)	MICU	20[a]	R/o	Propacetamol (1 g bolus) vs. metamizol ±0.5 mg bolus) vs. iced water bath	>1°C T reduction within 1 hr	Iced water bath more effective than antipyretics

(26)	MICU	83[b]	R/o	Antipyretics alone vs. added conventional cooling blanket	Rate of T reduction	Cooling blanket no more effective than antipyretics
(56)	NICU	6	P/o	Arctic Sun cooling system	Time to $T \leq 37°C$	Mean time to normothermia 120 min (38.4–37.0°C)
(34)	NICU	26	R/o	NSAID plus conventional cooling blanket	Mean T before vs. after intervention	Small (0.6°C) T reduction after intervention
(53)	NICU	53	P/r	Arctic Sun cooling system vs. conventional cooling blanket	Fever burden over 24 hr	Significant reduction of fever burden with Arctic Sun

T = temperature; P = prospective; R = retrospective; o = observational; r = randomized; NICU = neuro-ICU; MICU = medical ICU.
[a] From a total of 20 patients, only six of these had neurological disease.
[b] From a total of 83 patients, only 16 of these had neurosurgical service.

evaluated the feasibility of treating fever in patients with severe head injury or SAH ($n = 12$) with low-dose diclofenac infusions (36). Although this approach effectively lowered body temperature without major side effects, the efficacy of this approach remains to be shown in a controlled trial.

Clinical Impact

So far, no prospective randomized trial for fever intervention in stroke patients has been powered to evaluate neurological outcome. Functional disability (modified Rankin scale) at discharge (30) or 1 month (31), and neurological status (National Institutes of Health Stroke Scale) at discharge (30,33) did not differ between treatment and placebo groups in the trials comparing prophylactic acetaminophen to placebo in stroke patients. In fact, one study reported slightly worse outcomes in the high-dose acetaminophen group—albeit the difference was nonsignificant; the investigators attributed this to differences in baseline stroke severity (31).

In summary, NSAIDs for fever prophylaxis or reduction in neurocritical care patients can be safely administered, but they are likely to have only a small effect on body temperature. A very large trial would be needed to demonstrate that these relatively modest effects can improve outcome after stroke. A large phase III randomized trial of high-dose acetaminophen in stroke (the PAIS trial) is currently in progress (36). Until these results are available, the routine use of prophylactic NSAIDs to prevent fever in neurocritical care patients remains questionable. However, their use remains a basic standard of care for the reduction of active fever (37–41). Routine NSAID administration may also play a role in the facilitation of therapeutic hypothermia because these agents may minimize elevations of the temperature set point and shivering threshold in response to a pyrogenic stimulus.

Active Cooling

Active cooling reduces body temperature by promoting heat loss without affecting the hypothalamic set point, thus making it an attractive therapeutic approach for treating fever, particularly in the setting of impaired thermoregulation (1). Even though active cooling may be counterproductive in healthy individuals or non-brain-injured ICU patients due to an increase in the metabolic rate and heat-generating defense mechanisms such as shivering (42), it may be beneficial in stroke and brain-injured patients. Active cooling in NICU patients has been tested using external cooling techniques and internal heat exchange catheters inserted into the femoral or subclavian vein.

External Cooling For Fever Control

Techniques

Techniques for external cooling include evaporation, conduction, convection, and radiation (Table 2). The high degree of efficiency of external cooling by evaporation was first demonstrated in an experimental study of exercise-induced hyperpyrexia in normals (43). In addition to vasodilation, sweating-related evaporation is the body's main natural mechanism for heat dissipation when body temperature exceeds the hypothalamic set point (see Chapter 1). Further studies determined that the combination of evaporative and convective cooling with water sprays or sponging and forced airflow was more effective than conduction cooling or either method alone for reducing temperature in patients with hyperthemia induced by exercise or heat exposure (44,45). Water sprays and fans are not feasible for use in ICU environment, however, where electrical equipment predominates and space is usually limited. For this reason, most studies to date that have evaluated external cooling in patients with acute brain injury have relied on conduction cooling with conventional external water-circulating cooling blankets (46–52).

Clinical Studies

Apart from antipyretics, water-circulating cooling blankets are the most commonly prescribed intervention for febrile neurologic patients (26). Efficacy, tolerability, and complication profiles may differ substantially depending on the type of external cooling device used for this indication. Seven studies have investigated the external cooling approach for fever control in neurological patients (25,26,34,53–56), including two prospective randomized controlled trials (Table 4) (25,53). The first of these trials studied the efficacy of an air-circulating convection cooling blanket (Polar Air™; Augustine Medical, Eden Prairie, MN) as first-line therapy for fever in a mixed population of neuro-ICU patients (25). In this study, all patients with fever ≥38.3°C for more than 2 hr received 3.9 g/day acetaminophen, and half were also treated with the air-circulating cooling blanket. The primary study end points were time to treatment success ($T \leq 37.2$°C) or failure ($T \geq 38.3$°C on two consecutive measurements 1 hr apart). External cooling led to a small increase in the proportion of patients with treatment success, and an increase in time to treatment failure, but these differences were not significant (Fig. 2). In

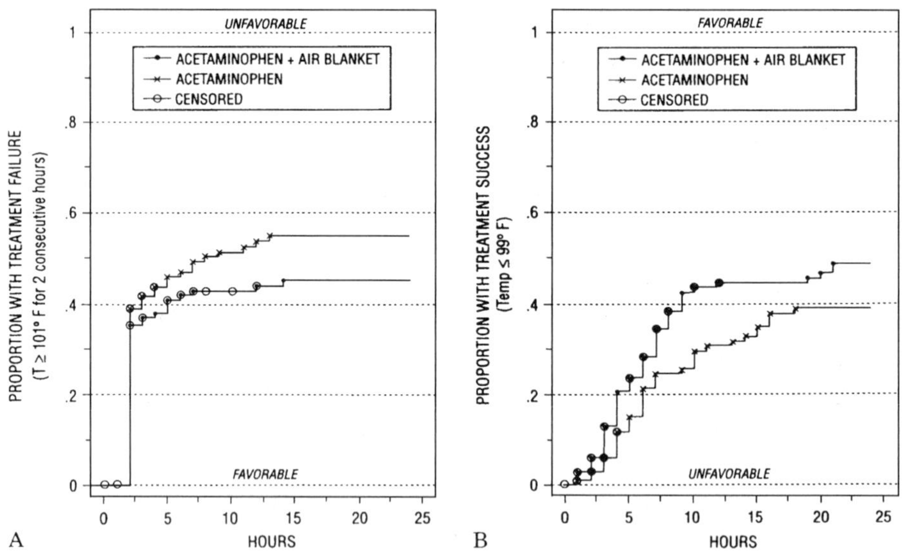

Figure 2 Kaplan–Meier survival curves comparing the proportion of patients with treatment failure (A), defined as $T \geq 38.3$°C for two consecutive hours, or treatment success (B), defined as $T \leq 37.2$°C, in a clinical trial of an air-circulating cooling blanket for new-onset fever in neurocritical care patients. Note that nearly 40% of patients "failed" after the first 2 hr of treatment in both groups. (From Ref. 25.)

fact, the main finding of this study was the inadequacy of either technique: nearly 40% of patients in both groups remained persistently febrile after randomization and "failed" after the first 2 hr of treatment.

The second prospective trial of surface cooling for fever cooling in neurological patients compared the Arctic Sun™ Temperature Management System (Medivance, Inc., Louisville, CO) with a conventional water-circulating cooling blanket (Blanketrol™ Model 420; Cincinnati Sub-Zero Products, Inc., Cincinnati, OH) (53). The Arctic Sun system employs four to five hydrogel-lined water-circulating energy transfer pads applied to the trunk and thighs (see Chapter 10). These patients had persistent fever refractory to acetaminophen (the mean cumulative duration of fever was 24 hr prior to randomization), and the majority were comatose and mechanically ventilated. Compared to patients treated with the Sub-Zero blanket ($n = 24$), Arctic Sun-treated patients ($n = 23$) experienced a 75% reduction in fever burden (median 4.1 vs. 16.1 degree hours, $P = 0.001$) during the 24-hr study period (Fig. 3). Arctic Sun-treated patients also spent less percent time febrile ($T \geq 38.3°C$, 8% vs. 42%, $P < 0.001$) and more percent time normothermic ($T \leq 37.2°C$, 59% vs. 3%, $P < 0.001$), and attained normothermia faster than the Sub-Zero group median (2.4 vs. 8.9 hr, $P = 0.008$). Arctic Sun-treated patients also exhibited a trend toward greater improvement in Glasgow Coma Scale scores during the study period ($P = 0.038$, Generalized Estimating Equation model), although this observation requires confirmation.

Observational studies have also evaluated external cooling in adult ICU patients (Table 4). One small nonrandomized study compared the use of acetaminophen alone with tepid water sponging, or with a water-circulating cooling blanket in 21 febrile neurologic patients, and found no difference between the three treatments. However, this study had important methodological problems and inadequate power to detect differences between the three treatments (55). Another study of 20 febrile patients under sedation, analgesia, and mechanical ventilation found that ice water sponging was superior to NSAIDs (paracetamol and metamazol) in a nonrandomized crossover study (54). This study, however, included only six

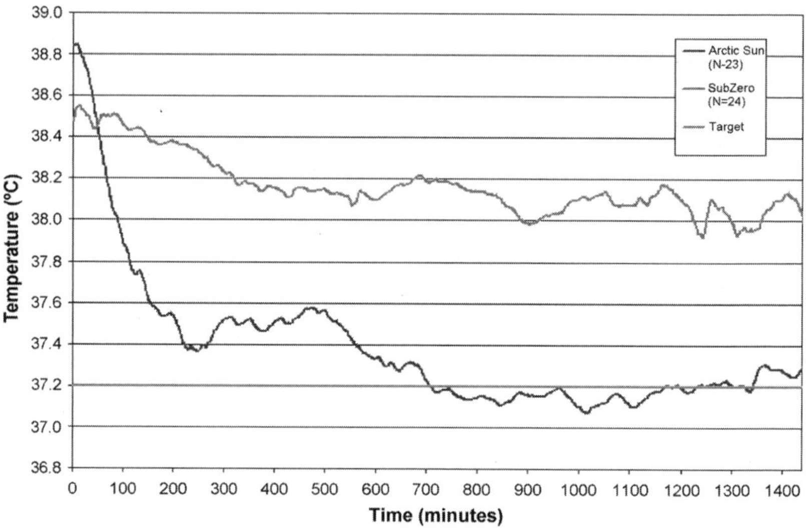

Figure 3 Fifteen-minute moving average of mean core body temperature during the Medivance Arctic Sun vs. Blanketrol Sub-Zero trial. Fever burden (median 4.1°C hr vs. 16.1°C hr; $P = 0.001$) and overall body temperature ($P = 0.008$; GEE repeated-measures analysis) were significantly lower in Arctic Sun-treated patients compared to the Sub-Zero-treated patients. (From Ref. 53.)

patients with an acute neurological problem. A large observational study found no difference in the mean cooling rate in febrile ICU patients treated with or without water-circulating cooling blankets (26). The nonrandomized design of this study, with potential for allocation bias and the lack of a systematic treatment protocol, makes these results difficult to interpret. In a larger multicenter study of 110 patients with TBI and fever (mean temperature, 38.8°C), which found a minimal effect with NSAID therapy (mean temperature reduction, 0.6°C), physical cooling with ice packs, alcohol, and gastric lavage, alone or in combination, added no additional benefit (34). Two small uncontrolled pilot studies of the Arctic Sun system in febrile neurocritical care patients (total $n = 16$) found that temperature normalizes in 2–3 hr and is subsequently "locked in" within a range of ±0.4°C, with faster results if more energy transfer pads are used (56,57).

Shivering with Surface Temperature Control

An important potential limitation of external cooling for the management of fever is reflex shivering and vasoconstriction. Shivering increases body temperature and the basal and cerebral metabolic rate, is uncomfortable, and fights the cooling process, making it less efficient. Because the skin contributes approximately 20% of afferent thermal input into the hypothalamus (58), these side effects may be particularly apparent with external cooling techniques. These problems were illustrated in a study of nine normal volunteers who had fever inducted by interleukin-2 injection. Compared to control patients, forced-air cooling (15°C) resulted in only a trivial degree of temperature reduction (38.1°C vs. 38.4°C) because of shivering, which was associated with significant increases in O_2 consumption, catecholamine levels, and subjective discomfort. This study elegantly illustrates the critical role of adjunctive therapy to blunt the body's thermoregulatory responses to physical cooling.

For reasons that are unclear, shivering appears to be substantially less frequent in NICU patients treated with external cooling for fever. In the previously described cooled air blanket study, shivering occurred in just 7% of patients during the 24-hr trial period and, overall, 12% did not tolerate the treatment, leading to its removal (25). In an uncontrolled pilot study of the Arctic Sun system, shivering occurred in all of six febrile, mechanically ventilated, and sedated patients, and was easily controlled with small doses of meperidine (56). By contrast, shivering occurred in only 39% or Arctic Sun-treated patients in the aforementioned clinical trial (compared to 8% among conventionally treated patients, $P = 0.013$). This lower frequency may reflect the concurrent use of acetaminophen, differences in patient characteristics, or baseline sedative use. Of the nine patients who shivered, it resolved spontaneously or was controlled with skin counterwarming alone in five of nine patients and required pharmacological intervention in four.

Outlook

In summary, there is evidence that external conduction cooling with water-circulating hydrogel-coated pads may offer a highly efficient method for fever treatment in neurocritical care patients. Cooled forced-air and conventional cold water blankets appear to be ineffective. Further research is needed to better understand and improve on adjunctive therapies to facilitate external cooling, and to determine if strict fever control can reduce temperature-related brain injury and improve clinical outcome.

Endovascular Catheter Cooling for Fever Control

Devices

Recently, an alternative to external cooling—intravenous heat exchange catheters—has become available. Currently, there are three main catheter systems being used in animal models and clinical trials: the Set Point™ by Radiant Medical, Inc., the Cool Line™ by Alsius Corp., and the Celsius Control™ by Innercool Therapies, Inc. (Table 1; see also Chapter 10). In all devices, cooled sterile saline flows through the catheter to remove heat from the body without direct contact of saline with blood. Catheters are inserted into the femoral, jugular, or subclavian vein. Saline is cooled and pumped through the catheter by an external heat exchange unit. Heat exchange is facilitated by helical counterflow with Set Point catheter, by two or three small inflatable balloons at the catheter tip of the Cool Line system, and by a combination of counterflow and a variegated metallic heat transfer element at the tip of the Celsius Control catheter.

Theoretically, catheter cooling devices may be more efficient for lowering body temperature than external cooling approaches because they may not be associated with the same degree of shivering and vasoconstriction. Moreover, they may not result in large thermal gradients between the peripheral and core compartments that have been described with overshoot of the target temperature when external cooling is used (59). Animal studies suggest that the risk of local vascular damage from hypothermia with cooling catheters is minimal, and that adverse effects on blood elements and cardiovascular function are limited (60–62). Nevertheless, this therapeutic approach is invasive and may carry a substantial risk for an entry for infection, may be a source of embolism, and may cause mechanical vascular damage.

Clinical Studies

Clinical studies have evaluated the efficacy, safety, and impact on outcome of intravascular cooling. Most were designed to evaluate the efficacy of inducing hypothermia in the ICU or intraoperative setting (63–65). So far, there have been only three studies published on the preliminary experience with cooling catheters in NICU patients (Table 5) (66–68). The first trial focused on the cooling capacity of the Cool Line catheter (target temperature, 36.5°C) in a mixed NICU population (66). This prospective pilot trial found that cooling catheters could effectively control body temperature and were not associated with unexpected complications. The mean fever burden was 4.0°C hr per patient over an average of 152.4 cooling hours, equivalent to 0.6°C hr per patient and day. These results are promising, but are difficult to interpret in the absence of a comparison group in the same ICU setting. The authors anecdotally reported an average fever burden of 4.1°C hr per patient and day in ICH and poor-grade SAH patients prior to the start of the cooling catheter trial. Infectious and non-infectious complications were comparable between patients receiving the Cool Line catheter and historical controls. Interestingly, the cooling catheter was least successful in two obese patients with severe infectious complications.

More recently, a large prospective, randomized, non-blinded trial demonstrated that the same Cool Line catheter was able to reduce the fever burden in a large number of NICU patients (67). This study compared patients who received only the standard of care (defined as a combination of antipyretics and external cooling with water-circulating blankets, ice packs, and gastric lavage) to patients who received the cooling catheter in addition. Eligibility criteria included a body temperature greater than 38°C on two occasions or continuously

Table 5 Intravascular Cooling Catheters for Fever Control in the Neuro-ICU

Reference	Patients	n	Study design	Intervention (daily dose)	Primary outcome	Comment
(66)	NICU	51	P/o	Cool Line catheter (no controls)	Fever burden	Intervention effectively maintained normothermia, no increase in side effects
(67)	NICU	294	P/r	Acetaminophen 4 g, cooling blankets, ice packs and gastric lavage vs. added Alsius Cool Line catheter	Fever burden over 72 hr	Fever burden (>38°C) reduced by 64%, shivering in only 4%
(68)	SAH	9	P/o	Innercool Celsius Control catheter and acetaminophen 4 g (no controls)	Normothermia within 24 hr	Normothermia achieved in 78%; DVT in two patients

P = prospective; o = observational; r = randomized; NICU = neuro-ICU; DVT = deep vein thrombosis; SAH = subarachnoid hemorrhage.

for 4 hr. The primary outcome measure was the fever burden exceeding 38°C for the first 72 hr. Among 296 enrolled patients, fever burden was 7.92°C hr for the first 72 hr with conventional treatment compared to 2.87°C hr in the catheter group (Fig. 4)—a reduction of 64% ($P < 0.001$). Although these results are promising, it is unclear from the data presented whether the device could effectively "lock in" body temperature at 37°C or not. The two groups were matched for baseline characteristics, but the catheter group required significantly less conventional fever interventions such as cooling blankets or antipyretic medications. Again, no increase in complications was reported for the catheter group.

Finally, a small study of nine SAH patients demonstrated the feasibility of using the Innercool Celsius Control catheter to control fever in this population (68). The majority had noninfectious fever (n = 8). Normothermia was attained in seven of nine patients (78%); the two who failed to attain normothermia were not adequately treated for shivering. Faster times to normothermia were attained with a 14-Fr catheter than a 9-Fr catheter. Two occurrences of ipsilateral deep vein thrombosis were detected on lower extremity. These

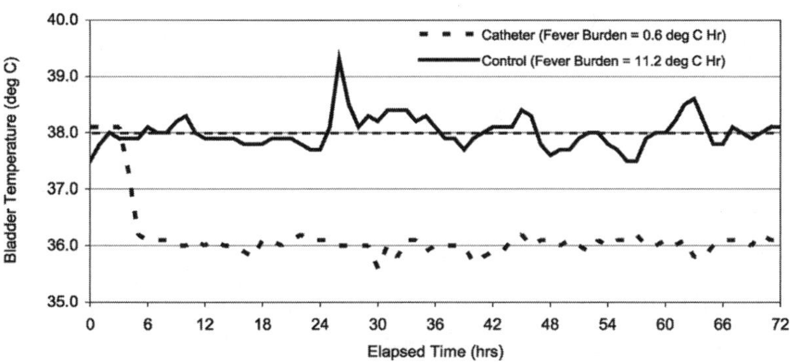

Figure 4 Example of the calculation of fever burden in the Alsius Cool Line trial. Patients in both groups also received standard antipyretic and external cooling blankets. The graph depicts hourly rectal temperature over time. The area under the fever curve that exceeds 38.0°C represents the fever burden. (From Ref. 67.)

were not associated with clinical sequelae, but given the inability to anticoagulate, inferior vena cava filters were placed. No other unanticipated adverse events occurred.

Shivering with Surface Temperature Control

The experience cited above suggests that shivering may be less frequent when fever is controlled with internal cooling, as opposed to external cooling. In the uncontrolled pilot Alsius Cool Line study, mild to moderate shivering occurred in only 1 of 51 patients (2%)—an awake SAH patient—and this was effectively treated with skin-warming blankets (66). In the larger controlled trial of the Alsius device, shivering was noted in only 3.7% (67). For reasons that are unclear, shivering occurred in all nine (100%) of the febrile SAH patients enrolled in the pilot study of the Innercool device (68). Meperidine doses of 573–825 mg/24 hr were required to control shivering among those who were successfully cooled.

Outlook

In summary, catheter-based cooling appears to be a feasible and effective method for attaining fever control in the NICU setting. This technique is still in its infancy. Additional studies are needed to directly compare the efficacy and tolerability of surface and catheter-based systems for fever control, and to determine whether these strategies can improve clinical outcome.

FUTURE DIRECTIONS

Cooling interventions, both for inducing hypothermia as well as for fever control, are promising therapeutic options for patients with acute neurological disease. New technological developments will now enable neurointensivists to precisely control body and brain temperature during the acute phase of illness. A major challenge that remains is optimization of adjunctive pharmacological and nonpharmacological therapies to facilitate these interventions and enhance safety and patient comfort. Whether it is feasible or preferable to "clamp" critically ill neurological patients to normothermia (37°C) or to mild degrees of hypothermia (i.e., –0.5°C, 1.0°C, or 1.5°C) remains an open question. Finally, in addition to stroke and trauma, animal models suggest that other acute neurological disorders such as status epilepticus may also benefit from fever control (69). Well-designed disease-specific outcome studies are warranted to determine the impact on outcome of the different treatment approaches that are available to achieve normothermia.

REFERENCES

1. Holtzclaw BJ. The febrile response in critical care: state of the science. Heart Lung 1992; 21:482–501.
2. Guyton AG. Body temperature, temperature regulation and fever. In: Guyton AG, ed. Textbook of Medical Physiology. 8th ed. Philadelphia: W. B. Saunders, 1991:797–808.
3. Commichau C, Scarmeas N, Mayer SA. Risk factors for fever in the neurological intensive care unit. Neurology 2003; 60:837–841.
4. Kilpatrick MM, Lowry DW, Firlik AD, Yonas H, Marion DW. Hyperthermia in the neurosurgical intensive care unit. Neurosurgery 2000; 47:850–856.
5. Azzimondi G, Bassein L, Nonino F, Fiorani L, Vignatelli L, Re G, D'Alessandro R. Fever in acute stroke worsens prognosis. A prospective study. Stroke 1995; 26:2040–2043.
6. Schwarz S, Hafner K, Aschoff A, Schwab S. Incidence and prognostic significance of fever following intracerebral hemorrhage. Neurology 2000; 54(2):354–361.
7. Circiumaru B, Baldock G, Cohen J. A prospective study of fever in the intensive care unit. Int Care Med 1999; 25:668–673.
8. Albrecht RF II, Wass CT, Lanier WL. Occurrence of potentially detrimental temperature alterations in hospitalized patients at risk for brain injury. Mayo Clin Proc 1998; 73:629–635.
9. Oliveira-Filho J, Ezzeddine MA, Segal AZ, Buonanno FS, Chang Y, Ogilvy CS, Rordorf G, Schwamm LH, Koroshetz WJ, McDonald CT. Fever in subarachnoid hemorrhage: relationship to vasospasm and outcome. Neurology 2001; 56:1299–3304.

10. Wijdicks EF, St Louis E. Clinical profiles predictive of outcome in pontine hemorrhage. Neurology 1997; 49:1342–1346.

11. Ginsberg MD, Busto R. Combating hyperthermia in acute stroke: a significant clinical concern. Stroke 1998; 29:529–534.

12. Castillo J, Martinez F, Leira R, Prieto JM, Lema M, Noya M. Mortality and morbidity of acute cerebral infarction related to temperature and basal analytic parameters. Cerebrovasc Dis 1994; 4:66–71.

13. Reith J, Jorgensen HS, Pedersen PM, Nakayama H, Raaschou HO, Jeppesen LL, Olsen TS. Body temperature in acute stroke: relation to stroke severity, infarct size, mortality, and outcome. Lancet 1996; 347:422–425.

14. Hajat C, Hajat S, Sharma P. Effects of poststroke pyrexia on stroke outcome: a meta-analysis of studies in patients. Stroke 2000; 31:410–441.

15. Mayer SA, Kreiter KT, Huddleston D, Peery S, Fitzsimmons B-F, Yavagal D, Ostapkovich ND, Connolly ES, Kowalski RG. Fever after subarachnoid hemorrhage: predictors and impact on outcome [abstr]. Crit Care Med Suppl 2003; 31:A5.

16. Kreiter KT, Commichau C, Kowalski RG, Ostapkovich N, Huddleston D, Fitzsimmons B-F, Parra A, Connolly ES, Mayer SA. Fever burden and cognitive outcome after subarachnoid hemorrhage [abstr]. Neurology 2003; 60(suppl 1):A230.

17. Tisherman SA, Rodriguez A, Safar P. Therapeutic hypothermia in traumatology. Surg Clin North Am 1999; 79:1269–1289.

18. Georgilis K, Plomaritoglou A, Dafni U, Bassiakos Y, Vemmos K. Aetiology of fever in patients with acute stroke. J Intern Med 1999; 246:203–209.

19. Dettenkofer M, Ebner W, Hans FJ, Forster D, Babikir R, Zentner J, Pelz K, Daschner FD. Nosocomial infections in a neurosurgery intensive care unit. Acta Neurochir 1999; 141:1303–1308.

20. Morimoto A, Murakami N, Nakamori T, Watanabe T. Fever induced in rabbits by intraventricular injection of rabbit and human serum albumin. J Physiol 1987; 390:137–144.

21. Rudy TA, Westergaard JL, Yaksh TL. Hyperthermia produced by simulated intraventricular hemorrhage in the cat. Exp Neurol 1978; 58:296–310.

22. Shibata M. Hyperthermia in brain hemorrhage. Med Hypotheses 1998; 50:185–190.

23. Georgilis K, Plomaritoglou A, Dafni U, Bassiakos Y, Vemmos K. Aetiology of fever in patients with acute stroke. J Inter Med 1999; 246:203–209.

24. Ropper AH, Gress DR, Diringer MN, Green D, Mayer SA, Bleck TP. Fever and infections in the neurological intensive care unit. Neurological and Neurosurgical Intensive Care. 4th ed. Baltimore: Lippincott, Williams and Wilkins, 2003:113–128.

25. Mayer SA, Commichau C, Scarmeas N, Presciutti M, Bates J, Copeland D. Clinical trial of an air-circulating cooling blanket for fever control in critically ill neurologic patients. Neurology 2001; 56:292–298.

26. O'Donnell J, Axelrod P, Fisher C, Lorber B. Use and effectiveness of hypothermia blankets for febrile patients in the intensive care unit. Clin Infect Dis 1997; 24:1208–1213.

27. Ameer B, Greenblatt DJ. Acetaminophen. Ann Intern Med 1977; 87:202–209.

28. Klein NC, Cunha BA. Treatment of fever. Infect Dis Clin North Am 1996; 10:211–216.

29. Done AK. Treatment of fever in 1982: a review. Am J Med 1983; 74:27.

30. Koennecke HC, Leistner S. Prophylactic antipyretic treatment with acetaminophen in acute ischemic stroke: a pilot study. Neurology 2001; 57:2301–2303.

31. Dippel DWJ, van Breda EJ, van Gemert HMA, van der Worp HB, Meijer RJ, Kappelle LJ, Koudstaal PJ. Effect of paracetamol (acetaminophen) on body temperature in acute ischemic stroke: a double-blind, randomized phase II clinical trial. Stroke 2001; 32:1607–1612.

32. Dippel DWJ, van Breda EJ, van Gemert HMA, van der Worp HB, Meijer RJ, Kappelle LJ, Koudstaal PJ; PISA-Investigators. Effect of paracetamol (acetaminophen) and ibuprofen on body temperature in acute ischemic stroke. PISA, a phase II double-blind randomized placebo-controlled trial [abstr]. BMC Cardiovasc Disord 2003; 3:22.

33. Kasner SE, Wein T, Piriyawat P, Villar-Cordova CE, Chalela JA, Kriegar DW, Morgenstern LB, Kimmel SE, Grotta JC. Acetaminophen for altering body temperature in acute stroke: a randomized clinical trial. Stroke 2002; 33:130–135.

34. Stocchetti N, Rossi S, Zanier ER, Colombo A, Beretta L, Citerio G. Pyrexia in head-injured patients admitted to intensive care. Intensive Care Med 2002; 28:1555–1562.

35. Cormio M, Citerio G, Spear S, Fumagalli R, Pesenti A. Control of fever by continuous, low-dose diclofenac sodium infusion in acute cerebral damage patients. Intensive Care Med 2000; 26:552–557.

36. Dippel DWJ, van Breda EJ, van der Worp HB, van Gemert HMA, Kappelle LJ, Algra A, Koudstaal PJ. Timing of the effect of acetaminophen on body temperature in patients with acute ischemic stroke. Neurology 2003; 61:677–679.

37. Adams HP Jr, Brott TG, Crowell RM, Furlan AJ, Gomez CR, Grotta J, Helgason CM, Marler JR, Woolson RF, Zivin JA, et al. Guidelines for the management of patients with acute ischemic stroke. A statement for healthcare professionals from a special writing group of the Stroke Council, American Heart Association. Circulation 1994; 90:1588–1601.

38. Mayberg MR, Batjer HH, Dacey R, Diringer M, Haley EC, Heros RC, Sternau LL, Torner J, Adams HP Jr, Feinberg W, Thies W. Guidelines for the management of aneurysmal subarachnoid hemorrhage. A statement for healthcare professionals from a special writing group of the Stroke Council, American Heart Association. Stroke 1994; 25:2315–2328.

39. Broderick JP, Adams HP Jr, Barsan W, Feinberg W, Feldmann E, Grotta J, Kase C, Krieger D, Mayberg M, Tilley B, Zabramski JM, Zuccarello M. Guidelines for the management of spontaneous intracerebral hemorrhage: a statement for healthcare professionals from a special writing group of the Stroke Council, American Heart Association. Stroke 1999; 30:905–915.

40. Bullock R, Chesnut RM, Clifton G, Ghajar J, Marion DW, Narayan RK, Newell DW, Pitts LH, Rosner MJ, Wilberger JW. Guidelines for the management of severe head injury. Brain Trauma Foundation. Eur J Emerg Med 1996; 3:109–127.

41. O'Grady NP, Barie PS, Bartlett J, Bleck T, Garvey G, Jacobi J,

Linden P, Maki DG, Nam M, Pasculle W, Pasquale MD, Tribett DL, Masur H. Practice parameters for evaluating new fever in critically ill adult patients. Crit Care Med 1998; 26:392–408.

42. Lenhardt R, Negishi C, Sessler DI, Vuong K, Bastanmehr H, Kim JS, Bjorksten AR. The effects of physical treatment on induced fever in humans. Am J Med 1999; 106:550–555.

43. Wyndham CH, Strydom NB, Cooke HM, Maritz JS, Morrison JF, Fleming PW, Ward JS. Methods of cooling subjects with hyperpyrexia. J Appl Physiol 1959; 14:771–776.

44. Weiner JS, Khogali M. A physiological body-cooling unit for treatment of heat stroke. Lancet 1980; 1:507–509.

45. Kielblock AJ, Van Rensburg JP, Franz RM. Body cooling as a method for reducing hyperthermia. An evaluation of techniques. S Afr Med J 1986; 69:378–380.

46. Marion DW, Penrod LE, Kelsey SF, Obrist WD, Kochanek PM, Palmer AM, Wisniewski SR, DeKosky ST. Treatment of traumatic brain injury with moderate hypothermia. N Engl J Med 1997; 336:540–546.

47. Clifton GL, Miller ER, Choi SC, Levin HS, McCauley S, Smith KR Jr, Muizelaar JP, Wagner FC Jr, Marion DW, Luerssen TG, Chesnut RM, Schwartz M. Lack of effect of induction of hypothermia after acute brain injury. N Engl J Med 2001; 344:556–563.

48. Schwab S, Schwarz S, Spranger M, Keller E, Bertram M, Hacke W. Moderate hypothermia in the treatment of patients with severe middle cerebral artery infarction. Stroke 1998; 29:2461–2466.

49. Kammersgaard LP, Rasmussen BH, Jorgensen HS, Reith J, Weber U, Olsen TS. Feasibility and safety of inducing modest hypothermia in awake patients with acute stroke through surface cooling: a case–control study: the Copenhagen Stroke Study. Stroke 2000; 31:2251–2256.

50. Schwab S, Georgiadis D, Berrouschot J, Schellinger PD, Graffagnino C, Mayer SA. Feasibility and safety of moderate hypothermia after massive hemispheric infarction. Stroke 2001; 32:2033–2035.

51. Bernard SA, Gray TW, Buist MD, Jones BM, Silvester W, Gutteridge G, Smith K. Treatment of comatose survivors of out-of-hospital cardiac arrest with induced hypothermia. N Engl J Med 2002; 346:557–563.

52. The Hypothermia after Cardiac Arrest Study Group. Mild therapeutic hypothermia to improve the neurological outcome after cardiac arrest. N Engl J Med 2002; 346:549–556.

53. Mayer SA, Kowalski RG, Presciutti M, Ostapkovich ND, McGann E, Fitzsimmons B-F, Yavagal DY, Du EY, Naidech AM, Janjua N, Claassen J, Kreiter KT, Commichau C, Parra A. Clinical trial of a novel surface cooling system for fever control in neurocritical care patients. Crit Care Med. In press.

54. Poblete B, Romand JA, Pichard C, Konig P, Suter PM. Metabolic effects of i.v. propacetamol, metamizol or external cooling in critically ill febrile sedated patients. Br J Anaesth 1997; 78:123–127.

55. Morgan SP. A comparison of three methods of managing fever in the neurologic patient. J Neurosci Nurs 1990; 22:19–24.

56. Carhuapoma JR, Gupta K, Coplin WM, Muddassir SM, Meratee MM. Treatment of refractory fever in the neurosciences critical care unit with a novel, water-circulating cooling device. J Neurosurg Anesth 2003; 15:313–318.

57. Mayer SA, Kowalski RG, Ostapkovitch N, Fitzsimmons B-F, Yavagal DY. Normalization of body temperature in febrile neuro-ICU patients with the Arctic Sun Temperature Management System [abstr]. Neurology 2002; 58(suppl 3):A93.

58. Lenhardt R, Greif R, Sessler DI, Laciny S, Rajek A, Bastanmehr H. Relative contribution of skin and core temperatures to vasoconstriction and shivering thresholds during isoflurane anesthesia. Anesthesiology 1999; 91:422–429.

59. Krieger DW, De Georgia MA, Abou-Chebl A, Andrefsky JC, Sila CA, Katzan IL, Mayberg MR, Furlan AJ. Cooling for acute ischemic brain damage (cool aid): an open pilot study of induced hypothermia in acute ischemic stroke. Stroke 2001; 32:1847–1854.

60. Inderbitzen B, Yon S, Lasheras J, Dobak J, Perl J, Steinberg GK. Safety and performance of a novel intravascular catheter

for induction and reversal of hypothermia in a porcine model. Neurosurgery 2002; 50:364–370.

61. Dae MW, Gao DW, Ursell PC, Stillson CA, Sessler DI. Safety and efficacy of endovascular cooling and rewarming for induction and reversal of hypothermia in human-sized pigs. Stroke 2003; 34:734–738.

62. Mack WJ, Huang J, Winfree C, Kim G, Oppermann M, Dobak J, Inderbitzen B, Yon S, Popilskis S, Lasheras J, Sciacca RR, Pinsky DJ, Connolly ES Jr. Ultrarapid, convection-enhanced intravascular hypothermia: a feasibility study in nonhuman primate stroke. Stroke 2003; 34:1994–1999.

63. Georgiadis D, Schwarz S, Kollmar R, Schwab S. Endovascular cooling for moderate hypothermia in patients with acute stroke: first results of a novel approach. Stroke 2001; 32:2550–2553.

64. Doufas AG, Akca O, Barry A, Petrusca DA, Suleman MI, Morioka N, Guarnaschelli JJ, Sessler DI. Initial experience with a novel heat-exchanging catheter in neurosurgical patients. Anesth Analg 2002; 95:1752–1756.

65. DeGeorgia M, Abou-Chebl A, Devlin T, Jauss M, Davis S, Krieger D. Endovascular cooling for patients with acute ischemic stroke [abstr]. Neurology 2002; 58(suppl 3):A506.

66. Schmutzhard E, Engelhardt K, Beer R, Brossner G, Pfausler B, Spiss H, Unterberger I, Kampfl A. Safety and efficacy of a novel intravascular cooling device to control body temperature in neurologic intensive care patients: a prospective pilot study. Crit Care Med 2002; 30:2481–2488.

67. Diringer MN. Treatment of fever in the neurologic intensive care unit with a catheter-based heat exchange system. Crit Care Med 2004; 32:559–564.

68. Badjatia N, O'Donnell J, Baker JR, Huang DY, Ayata C, Greer DM, Carter BS, Ogilvy CS, McDonald CT. Achieving normothermia in febrile subarachnoid hemorrhage patients: feasibility and safety of a novel intravascular cooling catheter. Neurocrit Care, 2004; 1:145–156.

69. Lundgren J, Smith ML, Blennow G, Siesjo BK. Hyperthermia aggravates and hypothermia ameliorates epileptic brain damage. Exp Brain Res 1994; 99:43–55.

13

Hypothermia for Traumatic Brain Injury and ICP Control

DONALD W. MARION

The Brain Trauma Foundation,
New York, New York, U.S.A.

BACKGROUND

The use of hypothermia to treat traumatic brain injury was first described more than 60 years ago by Fay (1). In the 1950s, Sedzimir (2) cooled several patients who had severe traumatic brain injury to 27–30°C for 1–5 days and observed "better than expected" outcomes for those patients. These early investigators may have assumed that traumatic brain injury (TBI) was associated with a hypermetabolic state, and that the brain swelling associated with it could be explained by an increase in cerebral blood flow. In uninjured dogs, Rosomoff (3,4) found that both cerebral blood flow and the cerebral metabolic rate for oxygen decreased by 6.7% per 1°C reduction in body temperature between 35°C and 25°C. Stone et al. (5) found that hypothermia to 30°C was associated with a 50% reduction in the cerebral metabolic rate for oxygen and a significantly lower rate of adenosine triphosphate depletion. Lundberg et al. (6) alluded to hypothermia as being as effective as osmotic diuretics for reducing elevated intracranial pressure in his 1959 publication. He also found that hypothermia had a more prolonged effect on ICP reduction than hyperventilation. James et al. (7) studied the effect of hypothermia in 40 patients with severe TBI and reported that cooling led to a reduction of the ICP in half of the patients. The ICP reduction in those patients averaged 51%.

However, none of these investigators conducted clinical trials that prospectively compared hypothermic patients with patients kept normothermic. Consequently, therapeutic hypothermia did not gain wide acceptance. The optimal depth and duration of cooling also was not determined. Surgeons using hypothermia during and after cerebral aneurysm procedures became concerned that this treatment was responsible for an increased incidence of postoperative hemorrhage and other complications, so most neurosurgeons stopped using hypothermia by the mid-1960s.

During the last 20 years, there has been a resurgence of interest in the use of hypothermia to treat TBI, in large part stimulated by preclinical investigations that have clearly established efficacy of the treatment. These studies have described several potential mechanisms through which hypothermia may limit secondary brain injury and have demonstrated how those effects translate into preservation of tissue and improved functional and cognitive outcomes following experimental TBI. Some of the most important preclinical discoveries were that deep hypothermia was not necessary to achieve efficacy and that postinjury treatment could be effective. Clifton et al. (8) performed a series of rodent experiments using standardized cortical contusions and demonstrated that cooling to 32°C for 4 hr, with induction of cooling delayed for 30 min after injury, provided significant tissue preservation when compared with animals kept normothermic. Prior investiga-

Table 1 Effect of Hypothermia on ICP in Clinical TBI Studies

Author (year)	PRCT	No. of patients	Duration of Cooling	Effect on ICP
Shiozaki et al. (1993) (19)	Y	33	48 hr	Decrease
Clifton et al. (1993) (18)	Y	46	48 hr	No Change
Metz et al. (1996) (53)	N	10	25 hr	Decrease
Marion (1997) (20)	Y	82	24 hr	Decrease
Nara et al. (1998) (54)	N	23	?	Decrease
Tateishi et al. (1998) (55)	N	9	1–6 days	Decrease
Clifton et al. (2001) (23)	Y	392	48 hr	Decrease
Takahashi et al. (2000) (56)	N	9[a]	3–21 days	Decrease
Jiang et al. (2000) (21)	Y	87	3–14 days	Decrease
Biswas et al. (2002) (32)	Y	21[a]	48 hr	Decrease
Gal et al. (2002) (57)	Y	30	72 hr	Decrease
Tokutomi et al. (2003) (33)	N	31	48–72 hr	Decrease

PRCT: prospective randomized clinical trial, ICP: intracranial pressure.
[a] Pediatric patients.

tors had established that there was an unacceptable risk of cardiac arrhythmias and coagulopathy associated with body temperatures below 30 °C. Others found that prolonged cooling for several days or more led to a high incidence of pneumonia and other infections.

Most prior studies had focused on the effects of hypothermia during the injury, a paradigm not relevant to treatment of patients with TBI. Subsequent investigations have consistently demonstrated that postinjury treatment with moderate hypothermia results in reduced levels of excitatory amino acids and inflammatory cytokines (9,10), a decrease in the cellular inflammatory response (11), decreased edema (12), tissue preservation (13,14), preservation of energy stores (15), and improved functional outcomes (16). These and other experimental studies of therapeutic moderate hypothermia are described in detail in Chapter 4.

The positive results of numerous experimental studies led to more than 20 clinical trials of this treatment for patients with severe TBI that have been completed during the last 15 years. While the dramatic improvement seen in the preclinical studies has not been observed in some of the clinical trials, there is increasing evidence that therapeutic moderate hypothermia can help reduce elevated ICP and reduce secondary brain injury (Table 1). There is also evidence that only certain subgroups of TBI patients may benefit from this treatment, while others may actually be harmed. This chapter reviews clinical studies of therapeutic moderate hypothermia for severe TBI with an emphasis on prospective studies that compared outcomes between hypothermia and normothermia patients.

REVIEW

Pilot and Feasibility Studies

The first controlled randomized clinical study of the use of therapeutic moderate hypothermia for severe TBI was published in 1993 (17). In this pilot and feasibility study of 40 patients, half were assigned to a group that was cooled to 32 °C as quickly as possible after injury and kept at that temperature for 24 hr. The 20 control patients were maintained at 37–38 °C. Outcomes 3 months after injury compared using the Glasgow Outcome Scale (GOS) and Disability Rating Scale (DRS) scores were similar. This study did find that hypothermia caused a significant reduction of ICP and CBF during the period of cooling, and that it improved cerebral metabolism for at least 5 days after injury.

Later that same year Clifton et al. (18) and Shiozaki et al. (19) also reported clinical trials of the use of hypothermia for TBI patients. In the Clifton study of 46 patients, the 24 patients assigned to the hypothermia group were kept at 32–33 °C for 48 hr rather than 24 hr, and in the Shiozaki study, they were cooled for up to 4 or 5 days. While Clifton attempted to cool the patients as quickly as possible after their injury, Shiozaki assigned 16 patients to be cooled only after they had intracranial hypertension refractory to conventional treatment and compared their outcomes with 17 patients randomized to a normothermic control group. Both studies found a trend toward improved outcomes in the hypothermia groups. All three studies found that therapeutic moderate hypothermia used in this way did not cause cardiac arrythmias or clinically significant coagulopathies, and when its use was limited to 48 hr or less, there was no increase in the incidence of pneumonia or other infectious complications.

Small Efficacy Studies

In 1997, we reported the results of the use of therapeutic moderate hypothermia in a clinical trial of 82 patients with severe TBI (20). Forty patients were cooled to 32 °C within 10 hr of injury and kept at that temperature for 24 hr, followed by controlled passive rewarming at a rate no greater than 1 °C per hour. The 42 control patients were kept at 37–38 °C with active warming. At 3 and 6 months after injury, although not at 12 months, patients in the hypothermia group had significantly better outcomes than did those in the normothermia group. But this effect was only seen in subgroup of patients with an initial GCS of 5–7 and not those with an initial GCS of 3 or 4. Among the patients with scores of 5–7, the adjusted risk ratio for a poor outcome was 0.2 (95% confidence interval: 0.1–0.9). While the mortality rates were similar, the proportion of hypothermia patients who had mild or no disability was significantly greater in the hypothermia group. We again observed a significant decrease in ICP in the hypothermia group, and there were no significant medical complications associated with this treatment.

In a subsequent study, Jiang et al. (21) investigated the use of hypothermia in 87 patients with severe TBI. Forty-three patients were assigned to the hypothermia group and were maintained at 33–35°C for 3–14 days, and their outcomes were compared with 44 patients assigned to the normothermia group. At 1 year after injury, 46% of the hypothermia patients, and only 27% of the normothermia patients, had good outcomes defined as a GOS score of 4 or 5 (independent with no to moderate disability, $P < 0.05$). The hypothermic patients had significantly lower ICPs and a lower frequency of hyperglycemia during their acute care as compared with the normothermia group. However, there was more pneumonia and other infectious complications in the patients who were kept hypothermic more than 3 days.

Large Efficacy Studies

Two large clinical trials of therapeutic moderate hypothermia for TBI were completed in 2001. Clifton et al. (23) reported the results of a multicenter prospective randomized trial that enrolled 392 patients aged 16–65 years. Patients assigned to the hypothermia group were cooled as quickly as possible after injury to 32–33°C for 48 hr, and then slowly rewarmed. The normothermia group was kept at 37–38°C with passive rewarming. Both groups had a similar severity of injury at enrollment, and both received similar medical treatment. At 6 months after injury, 17 patients (4.3%) were not available for follow-up. In the remaining 368 patients, there were no significant differences in functional outcomes between the hypothermia and normothermia groups. Approximately 57% of the patients in both groups were severely disabled, vegetative, or had died, whereas 43% were independent with moderate to no disability. During their acute care, it was observed that the hypothermia patients were significantly less likely to have intracranial hypertension. Among patients 45 years of age and younger, there was a trend toward improved outcomes if the patients had been treated with hypothermia.

Zhi et al. (24) completed a prospective clinical trial of hypothermia in 396 TBI patients. Hypothermia was induced within 24 hr in 198 patients, and they were kept at 32–35 °C for 1–7 days after injury. The control patients were kept at 36.5–37 °C during that time. Patients ranged in age from 15 to 65 years, and the mean age was 43 years. The initial GCS was similar in both groups. All patients had similar initial medical management, and all were cared for at a single trauma center (Tianjin Huanhu Hospital, China). Outcomes for the hypothermia group were significantly better than for the normothermia group: 62% of the hypothermia patients achieved a good outcome (GOS score 4 or 5) compared with 38% of the normothermia patients. The mortality rate for the hypothermia patients was 26%, and for the normothermia patients, it was 36%. Again, a significant decrease in ICP was observed in the hypothermia patients during the time they were cooled.

There are several possible explanations for the conflicting results of the Clifton and Zhi clinical trials. Intercenter differences in the management of patients with severe TBI may have confounded the results in the Clifton trial (26). In this study, there were significant intercenter differences in the incidence of mean arterial blood pressures less than 70 mm Hg ($P < 0.001$), the percentage of patients who were dehydrated ($P < 0.001$), and the frequency of cerebral perfusion pressures (CPPs) less than 50 mm Hg ($P < 0.05$) during the first 5 days after injury in the hypothermia patients. In this and several other studies, CPPs less than 50 mm Hg have been shown to be a powerful independent predictor of poor outcomes. The use of vasopressor agents and morphine also was significantly different between centers in the Clifton study. The Zhi clinical trial was a single center study conducted by a small group of investigators that carefully controlled all of these variables.

Meta-Analyses

In a meta-analysis of eight clinical trials of therapeutic moderate hypothermia for severe TBI published during the 1990s,

Signorini and Alderson (22) concluded that the odds of death or severe disability were significantly lower for patients treated with hypothermia than for those kept normothermic. They found a 61% reduction of death and severe disability in the hypothermia group, with an odds ratio of 0.39 and a 95% confidence interval of 0.02–0.74 ($P = 0.004$).

In July 2002, Harris et al. (25) published a comprehensive review of all clinical studies of the use of therapeutic moderate hypothermia for severe TBI. These investigators carefully searched the six most comprehensive medical literature databases and identified 445 publications. Of those, only seven studies were analyzed because they were the only ones that met predetermined inclusion criteria: a randomized clinical trial comparing the efficacy of hypothermia with normothermia in patients with TBI; all study patients at least 10 years of age; and relative risks (odds ratios, cumulative incidence, or incidence density measures) and 95% confidence intervals, or weighted mean differences and 95% confidence intervals, could be calculated from the data presented in the article. The Zhi study described above was not included in this search because it had not yet been published. In a meta-analysis of the seven studies (excluding the Zhi Study, which had not yet been published), the odds ratios and confidence intervals were calculated for the Glasgow Outcome Score and several medical complications in hypothermia patients vs. normothermia patients. Based on this analysis, they concluded that therapeutic moderate hypothermia did not result in improved outcomes following severe TBI nor was it associated with a significant decrease in ICP. They also found that hypothermia did not cause an increased incidence of pneumonia or cardiac arrhythmias, but that it did cause an increase in the partial thromboplastin time.

However, there are several important features of this study that make its conclusions questionable. The most important is that for the meta-analysis of outcomes, the authors actually only included four studies. One of those studies, the Clifton study (23), contained four times as many patients as the next largest study (20) and twice as many patients as the other three combined. Thus the conclusions of the analysis were heavily weighted toward the outcomes of the Clifton study. In addition, the analysis looked only at crude overall results of each of the seven studies, and this may be misleading. For example, in the Marion et al. (20) study of 82 patients, only those with an initial GCS of 5–7 benefited from hypothermia and not those with an initial GCS of 3 or 4, but Harris et al. looked only at the results in these two groups combined. In the Clifton study of 392 patients, those who were less than 45 years of age were most likely to benefit from hypothermia, and those who were older appeared to have worse outcomes if they were cooled. In a study of 91 patients with severe TBI, Shiozaki et al. (29) found that therapeutic hypothermia was not beneficial for patients who did not have intracranial hypertension. Harris et al. did not evaluate these or other subgroups in their analysis. This issue may be particularly relevant to the effect of hypothermia on ICP. For any meta-analysis to be scientifically valid, the studies included must be similar with regard to characteristics likely to affect the results. In this case, such characteristics would include depth and duration of hypothermia, protocol for induction of hypothermia, and methods used to monitor ICP. Unfortunately, she included studies that were very different in this regard: duration of cooling from 24 hr to 7 or more days, target depth of cooling from 32°C to 35°C, cooling induced as soon as possible after injury vs. induction of cooling only after conventional treatment of intracranial hypertension had failed, and studies that used transducer-tipped white matter ICP monitors combined with studies that used ventriculostomy catheters to measure ICP. To their credit, Harris et al. did include a statistical analysis of the homogeneity of the studies they included in their meta-analysis and found that there was significant heterogeneity among the studies used to determine the effect of hypothermia on ICP ($P < 0.001$). Finally, important clinical trials were not included in her meta-analysis because the published reports of those studies did not include the statistical details she required for inclusion (21). This does not mean that the studies were invalid, and inclusion of those studies may have altered her conclusions. The Zhi study, one of the largest to date and a study that found a significant benefit with therapeutic hypothermia in TBI patients, was not included because it had not yet been published at the time of her analysis (24).

The failure of Harris et al. to find an effect of hypothermia on ICP may also be explained by the relatively long interval during which they evaluated this effect. As previously noted, the reduction in ICP that can occur with cooling after TBI has been observed for nearly 50 years (6), and most modern studies have reported a beneficial effect of hypothermia on ICP (13.1). Once hypothermia is discontinued, however, ICP usually increases and may slightly exceed average levels in normothermic patients. In most of the studies Harris et al. included in their meta-analysis, the effect of hypothermia on ICP was based on data averaged over 5 days or more. For the hypothermia groups, this often included several days of ICP values obtained after the patients had been rewarmed. It is possible that no overall reduction in ICP was observed because 3 days or more of slightly increased ICPs were averaged with 24 or 48 hr when the ICP was significantly reduced.

Confounding Factors

The lack of consistent benefit of hypothermia in TBI trials to date may be explained by confounding variables that also affect functional outcome. Medical complications associated with cooling may be more common than previously recognized (see Chapter 6) and may, in part, also explain the negative results of the Clifton trial because any neuroprotective effect may have been counterbalanced by systemic complications. For example, Polderman et al. (27) observed significant reductions of serum magnesium, phosphate, calcium, and potassium levels during the first 6 hr of cooling in 21 patients who were cooled for 48 hr or more. Ishikawa et al. (28) found that hypothermia caused a higher incidence of bacteremia in patients with severe TBI. Whereas the incidence of pneumonia was not higher in hypothermia patients, it was significantly more severe when it occurred in those patients. Hypothermia was also associated with a lower total leukocyte count during the first 2 weeks after injury.

Age

Age has been suggested as an important variable influencing the effect of hypothermia, with older patients unlikely to benefit or even harmed by the treatment. In the Clifton study, patients over 45 years of age who were assigned to the hypothermia group actually had worse outcomes than patients that age or older who were assigned to the normothermia group (30). Yamamoto et al. (31) examined the influence of age in 35 patients with severe TBI who were cooled to 33–35°C for several days after injury. The mean age for those who achieved a good outcome (mild, moderate, or no disability) was 30.2 years, and for those with a poor outcome (severe disability, vegetative, or dead), it was 45.2 years. All of those older than 50 years had a poor outcome. But Biswas et al. (32) studied the effect of hypothermia in 21 children with severe TBI and found that functional outcomes at 3 and 12 months after injury were similar for hypothermia and normothermia patients. All patients were less than 18 years and the mean age was 5.9–6.5 years. Children assigned to the hypothermia group were cooled to 32–34°C for 48 hr and then rewarmed over 12 hr. Those assigned to the normothermia group were kept at 36.5–37.5°C. In that study, hypothermia was associated with a significant decrease in the severity of intracranial hypertension. Hypothermic patients had ICP values below 20 mm Hg for at least 90% of the duration of their acute care, and hypothermia patients required significantly less treatment for intracranial hypertension during the first 5 days after injury than did the normothermic children.

Depth of Cooling

There are some data to suggest that in the case of TBI, 32–33°C may be too low, and that milder hypothermia (35–36°C) may still provide a benefit while minimizing adverse systemic and cerebral metabolic consequences of the treatment. Tokutomi et al. (33) investigated the physiologic and metabolic consequences of cooling at various temperatures in 31 patients with severe TBI. They found that the ICP decreased significantly from 37°C to 35°C, but that there was no further reduction in

ICP when the brain temperature was reduced below this level. CPP peaked at 35–36°C and decreased when the brain temperature was lower. By contrast, the beneficial effects of hypothermia on cerebral metabolism appear to increase with temperatures below 35°C. Tokutomi et al. found that cerebral oxygen delivery and oxygen consumption progressively decreased when temperatures were reduced below 35°C. Gupta et al. (34) directly measured brain tissue pO_2 in 30 patients with severe TBI cooled to as low as 33°C when clinically indicated. They found that although the brain tissue pO_2 decreased with any degree of cooling, the most significant reduction occurred when the brain temperature was reduced below 35°C.

Extracranial Injury

Hypothermia may have differential effects with regard to cerebral vs. extracranial injury. Gentilello et al. (35) conducted a randomized prospective trial in 57 hypothermic ($T = 34.5$°C), critically injured patients who required pulmonary artery catheterization. Patients were randomly assigned to a group subjected to a rapid rewarming protocol using continuous arteriovenous rewarming or to a standard rewarming group. The mortality rate for the rapid rewarming group was significantly lower: 7% vs. 43% for the standard rewarming group ($P = 0.047$). Of note, however, is that only a small proportion of these patients had a severe TBI, and outcome assessment did not include a GOS or any other determination of functional outcomes.

Spontaneous Hypothermia

It is still not clear if the spontaneous hypothermia that frequently occurs following severe TBI is protective and, if so, whether or how quickly patients who arrive at the trauma center should be rewarmed. Several investigators have examined the effect of admission body temperature on outcomes in patients with severe TBI and found a very strong relationship: the lower the body temperature, the worse the outcome (36,37). In one of these studies, the mortality rate for spontaneously hypothermic patients was 62%, but only 26% if the patient was normothermic (37). However, it is important to recognize that the hypothermic patients in these studies were probably more severely injured. Spontaneous hypothermia is thus very different from induced therapeutic hypothermia. In the Clifton multicenter study, patients in the normothermia group who arrived with a temperature of ≤35°C had a 78% chance of a poor outcome, compared with 52% in subjects who were normothermic on admission ($P < 0.004$) (30). A subanalysis of the Clifton study did find that the speed with which patients were rewarmed appeared to adversely affect outcomes. Those who were rapidly rewarmed had worse outcomes than did those who were allowed to passively rewarm over 12 hr or more. In the Marion study of 82 patients published in 1997, the control group was actively rewarmed if they arrived with body temperatures less than 37°C. This has been used as one possible explanation for the apparent beneficial effect of hypothermia in the Marion study, but not in the later Clifton study in which control patients who arrived hypothermic were passively rewarmed (38). Active cooling of patients with hypothermia on admission may be preferable to passive rewarming: the rate of poor outcomes in this subset was 61% with hypothermia compared with 78% with normothermia, but this difference was nonsignificant.

Fever

It also remains unclear whether fever during the first several days after TBI is detrimental (39). In this regard, it seems possible that the apparent beneficial effects of hypothermia in some of the earlier studies may in fact be due to the prevention of febrile episodes in those patients. Preclinical studies clearly show a detrimental effect of brain temperatures greater than 39°C in ischemic regions of the brain (40). This effect is evident even if fever occurs 24 hr after injury (41). In a meta-analysis of 3790 patients with stroke, Hajat et al. (42) found that there was a highly significant association between fever and morbidity and mortality. Others have found a similar association between fever and poor outcomes in patients with spontaneous intracerebral hemorrhage and subarachnoid hemorrhage (43,44). Moreover, fever is common in the neuro-ICU. We measured rectal temperatures every 4 hr in our neuro-ICU in

428 consecutive patients with stroke, subarachnoid hemorrhage and TBI (45). Febrile episodes occurred in 47% of all patients and 93% of those who were in the ICU for 14 days or more. In addition, studies show that brain temperatures are frequently 1–2°C higher than rectal temperatures following severe TBI (46).

FUTURE DIRECTIONS

Despite the relatively large number of clinical trials already completed, and the rather disappointing results of some of those studies, several questions remain to be answered before we can make any conclusions about the efficacy of therapeutic hypothermia (Table 2). A crucial issue relates to admission body temperature. It seems most likely that spontaneous hypothermia following severe TBI reflects increased severity of brain injury. Patients who arrive at the trauma center with brain temperatures less than 36°C have been shown to have significantly higher levels of glutamate and lactate, well-known mediators of secondary brain injury, compared with those who arrive with normal brain temperatures (36). The observations from the Clifton study certainly do not establish that maintaining hypothermia in those who arrive hypothermic will necessarily improve outcomes. To better address this question, Clifton has organized a new multicenter clinical trial that will focus on patients with severe TBI who arrive at the trauma center hypothermic. Patients will be assigned to a group that is left hypothermic for 48 hr or a group that is slowly rewarmed over 12 hr, and outcomes will be compared 6 months after injury.

Newer methods of cooling need to be applied to TBI hypothermia research. Most of the clinical trials used surface cooling techniques, but with this method of cooling, it takes at least 4–6 hr to reduce the body temperature from 37°C to 32°C. Preclinical studies find that maximum levels of excitatory amino acids, oxygen-free radicals and inflammatory cytokines appear within minutes of the injury. Thus if the mechanism of action of hypothermia is to reduce the levels of

Table 2 Prospective Randomized Clinical Trials of Therapeutic Moderate Hypothermia for Severe TBI

Author (year)	Number of patients	Good outcome (GOS 4 or 5) (%)		Significant differences
		Hypothermia	Normothermia	
Shiozaki et al. (1993) (19)	33	38	6	N
Clifton et al. (1993) (18)	46	52	36	N
Marion et al. (1997) (20)	82	56	33	Y
Jiang et al. (2000) (21)	87	46.5	27	Y
Shiozaki et al. (2001) (29)	91	23	30	N
Clifton et al. (2001) (23)	368	43	43	N
Zhi et al. (2001) (24)	396	62	38	Y

GOS: Glasgow Outcome Scale. Score of 4 or 5 indicates survival with independent lifestyle and moderate to no disability.

these mediators of secondary brain injury, the delay of 4–6 hr before reaching target temperatures may undermine the potential of hypothermia to be effective. Rodent studies have shown that hypothermia is not effective if induced more than 1 hr after a controlled cortical contusion injury (47,48). In the Clifton study, outcomes were not different if target temperature was reached by 6 hr after injury (70% with poor outcomes) compared with those that did not reach target temperature for 11–24 hr after injury (53% with poor outcomes) (38). But even 6 hr may have been too long. Several companies have developed heat exchange indwelling venous catheters that can rapidly reduce body temperature, and future hypothermia trials will likely include their use. This technique of temperature modulation already has been successfully used for fever prevention in the ICU.

Finally, it may be that the optimal treatment for patients with severe TBI will involve a combination of therapies, only one of which is hypothermia. In this regard, we completely agree with Bayir et al. (49) who have concluded that secondary brain injury occurs as a result of multiple mechanisms, and that successful future treatment strategies will have to target several if not all of those mechanisms. Preclinical studies have investigated the combination of hypothermia with 21-aminosteroids (48), FGF-2 (50), cyclosporin A (51), and IL-10 (52). In none of those studies, though, was the combination therapy found to be more efficacious than hypothermia alone.

REFERENCES

1. Fay T. Observations on generalized refrigeration in cases of severe cerebral trauma. Assoc Res Nerv Ment Dis Proc 1943; 24:611–619.
2. Sedzimir CB. Therapeutic hypothermia in cases of head injury. J Neurosurg 1959; 16:407–414.
3. Rosomoff HL, Holaday DA. Cerebral blood flow and cerebral oxygen consumption during hypothermia. Am J Physiol 1954; 179:85–88.

4. Rosomoff HL. Relationship of metabolism to hypothermia. Res Publ Assoc 1966; 41:116–126.

5. Stone HH, Donnelly C, Frobese AS. The effect of lowered body temperature on the cerebral hemodynamics and metabolism of man. Surg Gynecol Obstet 1956; 103:313–322.

6. Lundberg N, Kjallquist A, Bien C. Reduction of increased intracranial pressure by hyperventilation. Acta Psychiatr Scand 1959; 34:4–64.

7. James HE, Langfitt TW, Kumar VS, Ghostine SY. Treatment of intracranial hypertension. Analysis of 105 continuous recordings of intracranial pressure. Acta Neurochir (Wien) 1977; 36:189–200.

8. Clifton GL, Jiang JY, Lyeth BG, Jenkins LW, Hamm RJ, Hayes RL. Marked protection by moderate hypothermia after experimental traumatic brain injury. J Cereb Blood Flow Metab 1991; 11:114–121.

9. Busto R, Globus MYT, Dietrich WD, Martinez E, Valdes I, Ginsberg MD. Effect of mild hypothermia on ischemia-induced release of neurotransmitters and free fatty acids in rat brain. Stroke 1989; 7:904–910.

10. DeKosky ST, Miller PD, Styren S, O'Malley M, Marion DW. Interleukin-1B elevation in CSF following head injury in humans is attenuated by hypothermia. J Neurotrauma 1994; 11:106. Ref Type: Abstract.

11. Chatzipanteli K, Alonso OF, Kraydieh S, Dietrich WD. Importance of posttraumatic hypothermia and hyperthermia on the inflammatory response after fluid percussion brain injury: biochemical and immunocytochemical studies. J Cereb Blood Flow Metab 2000 Mar; 20(3):531–542.

12. Kawai N, Nakamura T, Okauchi M, Nagao S. Effects of hypothermia on intracranial pressure and brain edema formation: studies in a rat acute subdural hematoma model. J Neurotrauma 2000; 17(3):193–202.

13. Busto R, Dietrich WD, Globus MY, Ginsberg MD. Postischemic moderate hypothermia inhibits CA1 hippocampal ischemic neuronal injury. J Cereb Blood Flow Metab 1989; 9(suppl 1):S266.

14. Dietrich WD, Alonso O, Busto R, Globus MYT, Ginsberg MD. Post-traumatic brain hypothermia reduces histopathological damage following concussive brain injury in the rat. Acta Neuropathol 1994; 87:250–258.

15. Kramer RS, Sanders AP, Lesage AM. The effect of profound hypothermia on preservation of cerebral ATP content during circulatory arrest. J Thorac Cardiovasc Surg 1968; 56:699–709.

16. Dixon CE, Markgraf CG, Angileri F, Pike BR, Wolfson B, Newcomb JK, Bismar MM, Blanco AJ, Clifton GL, Hayes RL. Protective effects of moderate hypothermia on behavioral deficits but not necrotic cavitation following cortical impact injury in the rat. J Neurotrauma 1998; 15(2):95–103.

17. Marion DW, Obrist WD, Carlier PM, Penrod LE, Darby JM. The use of moderate therapeutic hypothermia for patients with severe head injuries: a preliminary report. J Neurosurg 1993; 79:354–362.

18. Clifton GL, , Allen S, Barrodale P, Plenger P, Berry J, Koch S, Fletcher J, Hayes RL, Choi SC. A phase II study of moderate hypothermia in severe brain injury. J Neurotrauma 1993; 10:263–271.

19. Shiozaki T, Sugimoto H, Taneda M, Yoshida H, Iwai A, Yoshioka T, Sugimoto T. Effect of mild hypothermia on uncontrollable intracranial hypertension after severe head injury. J Neurosurg 1993; 79:363–368.

20. Marion DW, Penrod LE, Kelsey SF, Obrist WD, Kochanek PM, Palmer AM, Wisniewski SR, Dekoski ST. Treatment of traumatic brain injury with moderate hypothermia. N Engl J Med 1997; 336(8):540–546.

21. Jiang J, Yu M, Zhu C. Effect of long-term mild hypothermia therapy in patients with severe traumatic brain injury: 1-year follow-up review of 87 cases. J Neurosurg 2000; 93(4):546–549.

22. Signorini DF, Alderson P. Therapeutic hypothermia for head injury. Cochrane Database Syst Rev 2000; (2):CD001048.

23. Clifton GL, Miller ER, Choi SC, Levin HS, McCauley S, Smith KR Jr, Muizelaar JP, Wagner FC Jr, Marion DW, Leurssen TG, Chesnut RM, Schwartz M. Lack of effect of induction of

hypothermia after acute brain injury. N Engl J Med 2001; 344(8):556–563.

24. Zhi D, Zhang S, Lin X. Study on the therapeutic mechanism and clinical effect of mild hypothermia in patients with severe head injury. Surg Neurol 2003; 5(59):381–385.
25. Harris OA, Colford JM Jr, Good MC, Matz PG. The role of hypothermia in the management of severe brain injury: a meta-analysis. Arch Neurol 2002; 59(7):1077–1083.
26. Clifton GL, Choi SC, Miller ER, Levin HS, Smith KR Jr, Muizelaar JP, Wagner FC, Marion DW, Luerssen TG. Intercenter variance in clinical trials of head trauma—experience of the National Acute Brain Injury Study: Hypothermia. J Neurosurg 2001; 95(5):751–755.
27. Polderman KH, Peerdeman SM, Girbes AR. Hypophosphatemia and hypomagnesemia induced by cooling in patients with severe head injury. J Neurosurg 2001; 94(5):697–705.
28. Ishikawa K, Tanaka H, Shiozaki T, Takaoka M, Ogura H, Kishi M, Shimazu T, Sugimoto H. Characteristics of infection and leukocyte count in severely head-injured patients treated with mild hypothermia. J Trauma 2000; 49(5):912–922.
29. Shiozaki T, Hayakata T, Taneda M, Nakajima Y, Hashiguchi N, Fujimi S, Nakamer Y, Tameka H, Shimazu T, Sugimoto H. A multicenter prospective randomized controlled trial of the efficacy of mild hypothermia for severely head injured patients with low intracranial pressure. Mild Hypothermia Study Group in Japan. J Neurosurg 2001; 94(1):50–54.
30. Clifton GL, Miller ER, Choi SC, Levin HS, McCauley S, Smith KR Jr, Muizelaar JP, Marion DW, Luerssen TG. Hypothermia on admission in patients with severe brain injury. J Neurotrauma 2002; 19(3):293–301.
31. Yamamoto T, Mori K, Maeda M. Assessment of prognostic factors in severe traumatic brain injury patients treated by mild therapeutic cerebral hypothermia therapy. Neurol Res 2002; 24(8):789–795.
32. Biswas AK, Bruce DA, Sklar FH, Bokovoy JL, Sommerauer JF. Treatment of acute traumatic brain injury in children with moderate hypothermia improves intracranial hypertension. Crit Care Med 2002; 30(12):2742–2751.

33. Tokutomi T, Morimoto K, Miyagi T, Yamaguchi S, Ishikawa K, Shigemori M. Optimal temperature for the management of severe traumatic brain injury: effect of hypothermia on intracranial pressure, systemic and intracranial hemodynamics, and metabolism. Neurosurg 2003; 52(1):102–112.

34. Gupta AK, Al Rawi PG, Hutchinson PJ, Kirkpatrick PJ. Effect of hypothermia on brain tissue oxygenation in patients with severe head injury. Br J Anaesth 2002; 88(2):188–192.

35. Gentilello LM, Jurkovich GJ, Stark MS, Hassantash SA, O'Keefe GE. Is hypothermia in the victim of major trauma protective or harmful? A randomized, prospective study. Ann Surg 1997; 226(4):439–447.

36. Soukup J, Zauner A, Doppenberg EM, Menzel M, Gilman C, Bullock R, Young HF. Relationship between brain temperature, brain chemistry and oxygen delivery after severe human head injury: the effect of mild hypothermia. Neurol Res 2002; 24(2):161–168.

37. Jeremitsky E, Omert L, Dunham CM, Protetch J, Rodriguez A. Harbingers of poor outcome the day after severe brain injury: hypothermia, hypoxia, and hypoperfusion. J Trauma 2003; 54:312–319.

38. Clifton GL, Miller ER, Choi SC, Levin HS, Smith KR, Muizelaar JP, Wagner FC, Marion DW, Luerssen TG, Chesnut RM, Schwartz M. Lack of effect of induction of hypothermia after acute brain injury. N Engl J Med 2001; 344: 556–563.

39. Cairns CJ, Andrews PJ. Management of hyperthermia in traumatic brain injury. Curr Opin Crit Care 2002; 8(2):106–110.

40. Dietrich WD, Alonso O, Halley M, Busto R. Delayed post-traumatic brain hyperthermia worsens outcome after fluid percussion brain injury: a light and electron microscopic study in rats. Neurosurg 1996; 38(3):533–541.

41. Baena RC, Busto R, Dietrich WD, Globus MY, Ginsberg MD. Hyperthermia delayed by 24 hours aggravates neuronal damage in rat hippocampus following global ischemia. Neurol 1997; 48(3):768–773.

42. Hajat C, Hajat S, Sharma P. Effects of poststroke pyrexia on stroke outcome : a meta-analysis of studies in patients. Stroke 2000 Feb; 31(2):410–414.

43. Schwarz S, Hafner K, Aschoff A, Schwab S. Incidence and prognostic significance of fever following intracerebral hemorrhage. Neurology 2000 Jan 25; 54(2):354–361.

44. Oliveira-Filho J, Ezzeddine MA, Segal AZ, Buonanno FS, Chang Y, Ogilvy CS, Rordorf G, Schwamm LH, Koroshetz WJ, McDonald CT. Fever in subarachnoid hemorrhage: relationship to vasospasm and outcome. Neurol 2001; 56(10): 1299–1304.

45. Kilpatrick MM, Lowry DW, Firlik AD, Yonas H, Marion DW. Uncontrolled hyperthermia in the neurosurgical intensive care unit. Neurosurg 2000; 47:850–856.

46. Henker RA, Brown SD, Marion DW. Comparison of brain temperature with bladder and rectal temperatures in adults with severe head injury. Neurosurg 1998; 42(5):1071–1075.

47. Markgraf CG, Clifton GL, Moody MR. Treatment window for hypothermia in brain injury. J Neurosurg 2001; 95(6):979–983.

48. Marion DW, White MJ. Treatment of experimental brain injury with moderate hypothermia and 21-aminosteroids. J Neurotrauma 1996; 13(3):139–147.

49. Bayir H, Clark RS, Kochanek PM. Promising strategies to minimize secondary brain injury after head trauma. Crit Care Med 2003; 31(1):S112–S117.

50. Yan HQ, Yu J, Kline AE, Letart P, Jenkins LW, Marion DW, Dixon CE. Evaluation of combined fibroblast growth factor-2 and moderate hypothermia therapy in traumatically brain injured rats. Brain Res 2000; 887(1):134–143.

51. Li PA, He QP, Siesjo BK. Effects of intracarotid arterial injection of cyclosporin A and spontaneous hypothermia on brain damage incurred after a long period of global ischemia. Brain Res 2001; 890(2):306–313.

52. Kline AE, Bolinger BD, Kochanek PM, Carlos TM, Yan HQ, Jenkins LW, Marion DW, Dixon CE. Acute systemic administration of interleukin-10 suppresses the beneficial effects of moderate hypothermia following traumatic brain injury in rats. Brain Res 2002; 937(1–2):22–31.

53. Metz C, Holzschuh M, Bein T, Woertgen C, Frey A, Frey I, Taeger K, Brawanski A. Moderate hypothermia in patients

with severe head injury: cerebral and extracerebral effects. J Neurosurg 1996; 85:533–541.

54. Nara I, Shiogai T, Hara M, Saito I. Comparative effects of hypothermia, barbiturate, and osmotherapy for cerebral oxygen metabolism, intracranial pressure, and cerebral perfusion pressure in patients with severe head injury. Acta Neurochir Suppl (Wien) 1998; 71:22–26.

55. Tateishi A, Soejima Y, Taira Y, Nakashima K, Fujisawa H, Tsuchida E, Maekawa T, Ito H. Feasibility of the titration method of mild hypothermia in severely head-injured patients with intracranial hypertension. Neurosurg 1998; 42(5):1065–1069.

56. Takahashi I, Kitahara T, Endo M, Ohwada T. Clinical analysis of hypothermia in children with severe head injury. No Shinkei Geka 2000; 28(11):983–989.

57. Gal R, Cundrle I, Zimova I, Smrcka M. Mild hypothermia therapy for patients with severe brain injury. Clin Neurol Neurosurg 2002; 104(4):318–321.

14

Hypothermia for Ischemic Stroke

RAINER KOLLMAR and STEFAN SCHWAB
Department of Neurology,
University of Heidelberg,
Im Neuenheimer Feld,
Heidelberg, Germany

INTRODUCTION

Hypothermia has been found to be neuroprotective in experimental models of acute focal and global cerebral ischemia (1). Even though the neuroprotective mechanisms remain to be fully identified, hypothermia influences a variety of pathophysiological mechanisms during cerebral ischemia (see Chapter 4, "Molecular Mechanisms of Hypothermic Neuroprotection"). The concept of the ischemic core with irreversibly damaged neurons and the surrounding area of hypoperfusion called the "ischemic penumbra" is widely accepted (1–5). Neurons in the penumbra do not perform normally, but remain potentially salvageable if sufficient perfusion is reestablished in time (3,5).

By delaying or preventing the onset of ischemic cell death, the penumbra is the principle site of action through which hypothermia exerts its neuroprotective effects in focal ischemia.

In recent years, it has become apparent that the neuroprotective effects of hypothermia extend far beyond its ability to reduce metabolic demand for oxygen and glucose. Hypothermia also diminishes harmful intracellular proteolytic reactions, disruption of the blood–brain barrier (6), the deleterious inflammatory cascade (7), and the release and production of oxygen free radicals (8). Moreover, the release of excitotoxic neurotransmitters such as glutamate that poison the surrounding neurons is decreased (9). Hypothermia is also capable of reducing delayed or "programmed" cell death by apoptotic mechanisms (10). In contrast, these effects are exacerbated by hyperthermia (1).

One important conclusion that can be drawn from experimental studies of focal ischemia is that hypothermia is more successful when it is started early and maintained relatively long (1,2,10). Consequently, pre- and intraischemic hypothermia leads to better outcomes than postischemic hypothermia (1). Moreover, experimental data show that when initiation of hypothermia is delayed, a longer cooling period results in better neuroprotective effects. For example, in one study, hypothermia initiated after temporary middle cerebral artery occlusion in rats had a protective effect when cooling was sustained for 24 hr, but not for 2 hr (11).

In accordance with experimental data indicating that even small fluctuations in brain temperature can have a powerful effect on the extent of ischemic tissue damage, several clinical studies have emphasized the importance of body temperature on outcome after stroke (12). In 1976, Hintfeldt (13) showed retrospectively in 110 patients that stroke outcome was influenced by body temperature: Patients with a temperature over 37.5°C within the first 24 hr after stroke onset had a worse neurological outcome than normothermic patients. Terent and Anderson (14) found that poor neurological outcome resulted when core temperatures exceeded 38°C, and Castillo et al. (15) retrospectively found a similar correlation in 177 patients. By contrast, the study of Boysen and Christensen could not find a relationship between body temperature within 6 hr of stroke onset and outcome at 3 months (16,17). Azzimondi et al. (18) showed that fever in the first 7 days after stroke was an independent predictor of poor outcome: in 183 patients with acute ischemic or hemorrhagic stroke, fever occurred in 43% during the first week in hospital. Fever was associated with a poor functional outcome, and patients with high fever were more likely to die within the first 10 days of stroke than those with lower temperatures.

Other researchers have similarly shown that lower body temperature is associated with improved outcome after ischemic stroke. Reith et al. (19) demonstrated lower mortality and better outcome in patients with mild hypothermia (<36.5°C) on admission. In this study, 390 patients were classified into three groups according to their admission temperature: hypothermic (<36.5°C), normothermic (>36.5°C to 37.5°C), and hyperthermic (>37.5°C). Using multiple regression analysis, they found body temperature on admission to be highly correlated with clinical outcome and infarct size. In a similar study by Castillo et al. (20), the relative risk for poor outcome was increased by 2.2 for each 1°C increase in body temperature above normal, and an independent relationship between body temperature during the stroke and outcome was still observed after 2 years of follow-up.

The association between body temperature and outcome after cerebral infarction described above was confirmed in a meta-analysis conducted by Hajat et al. (12), who analyzed a total of 3790 patients with stroke reported in nine different studies. A rise in body temperature was highly correlated with stroke mortality and morbidity.

It is not entirely clear how long the time window is for the influence of body temperature on stroke outcome. According to the concept of the ischemic penumbra, it would seem obvious that the initial hours after stroke onset are most important in terms of neuroprotection. This notion was supported by Jorgensen et al. (21), who found a correlation between body temperature and outcome only within the first 12 hr after stroke in 1191 consecutive patients. Similarly, Castillo et al. (22) found a correlation between outcome and body temperature measured within 24 hr of onset, but not when temperature was measured beyond this timepoint.

The association between body temperature and stroke severity described above does not prove that a cause-and-effect relationship exists. However, these studies set the stage and provide a strong rationale for clinical trials designed to determine whether therapeutic hypothermia can improve outcome in patients with acute cerebral infarction. However, before this question can be addressed, important questions remain regarding patient selection, the optimal timing and depth of cooling, and the specifics of protocols designed to minimize hypothermia-related complications. Although early intervention to limit infarct size may be seen as the ultimate goal of therapeutic hypothermia for ischemic stroke, cooling may have beneficial effects even after an infarction is completed. Many of the pathophysiological cascades related to ischemia continue over days (23). Accordingly, delayed hypothermia has been shown to reduce blood–brain barrier disruption and infarct swelling in experimental models of stroke (6). Starting in 1998, most of the initial human pilot and feasibility studies of mild-to-moderate hypothermia for large hemispheric stroke described below were designed with this indication in mind (24). More recent studies have focused on achieving early rapid cooling with the use of newer endovascular and surface cooling devices (see Chapter 10).

REVIEW

Measurement of Brain Temperature: Where and How?

Interest in brain temperature monitoring has increased with recognition of the therapeutic potential of hypothermia as a neuroprotective measure. Busto et al. (25) addressed the importance of precisely measuring brain temperature in experimental cerebral ischemic injury by demonstrating that reductions in ischemic injury depended primarily on intra-ischemic brain temperatures. Although monitoring global brain temperature would be ideal, brain temperature probes can measure only in small areas of the brain. Until now, there is no surrogate for intraparenchymatous temperature monitoring. Several studies that have correlated bladder, rectal, tympanic membrane, esophageal, jugular venous, and pulmonary artery temperature with brain temperature have shown that temperature at these sites does not consistently and reliably reflect brain temperature, which can exceed core temperature by as much as 0.5–2.0°C in certain situations (26–29). In one recent study investigating the effects of hypothermia in patients with severe traumatic brain injury, rectal temperatures were compared to brain temperature assessed with subdural or intraparenchymal monitors. A good correlation between brain and core temperatures was found, but brain temperature consistently exceeded rectal temperature by an average of 0.5 ± 0.3°C (30). Even within the brain, significant temperature gradients have been described. In one study, depending on the depth of insertion, brain temperature was shown to vary of 1.0°C or more (26).

Most studies of brain temperature monitoring to date were performed in neurosurgical patients undergoing craniotomy for head trauma, brain tumor, or large intracerebral hematoma. Studies that have described the relationship between brain and core body temperature in humans with middle cerebral artery (MCA) infarction are described below.

Body-Core Temperature Relationship in Stroke Patients

A study of patients suffering from severe MCA infarction showed a significant gradient between brain temperature and core body temperature. Not only was a disparity between body and brain temperature identified, temperature gradients between infarcted and healthy tissue in the opposite hemisphere were also found in the early phase of ischemia, with temperatures in the infarcted hemisphere exceeding those of the contralateral side by up to 0.8°C (31).

These results confirm the findings of Mellergard and others, who all showed a significant gradient between body-core and brain temperatures in head trauma patients (29,32,33).

The explanation for this may lie in the high metabolic activity of cerebral tissue, which results in considerable production of heat (34–36). Nurse and Corbett (34) postulated an acute phase of locomotor hyperactivity to be the cause of a secondary rise in brain temperature after experimental ischemia in a rat model. Other mechanisms must be sought to explain the finding of initially increased temperatures within the zone of infarction that we found in the first hours after ischemia (31). We have speculated that this finding may be attributable to the release of excitatory neurotransmitters and increased energy (ATP) depletion and lactate accumulation during ischemia (35–38). Another possibility is that in the early stages of infarct formation, a decrease in cerebral blood flow (CBF) may result in a decreased capacity for the blood to carry off heat generated by local cerebral metabolism.

Better characterization of human brain temperature will facilitate the successful implementation of hypothermia as a therapeutic tool in the neurointensive care setting. Invasive brain temperature monitoring is reasonably safe, with a complication rate similar to that of intraparenchymal intracranial pressure monitoring devices (0.5–1.0% risk of bleeding or infection), and is the only practical method currently available to measure brain temperature accurately in humans.

Methods to Control Brain Temperature in Stroke Patients

In animal models, various measures of controlling brain temperature, including fanning, nasopharyngeal cooling, cardiopulmonary bypass, ice water immersion, or simply packing the head in ice have been employed (39–44).To date, several methods—including surface cooling combined with muscle relaxants and anesthesic agents, selective head cooling, internal cooling, endovascular approaches and extracorporal cooling devices—have been used for the induction and maintenance of hypothermia in humans (see Chapter 10). In our initial studies in the mid-1990s, surface cooling with water circulating blankets was initially used to induce mild-to-moderate hypothermia in stroke patients (24). Its effectiveness was limited by a slow cooling rate, limited efficiency in obese patients, and the requirement of muscle relaxants and anesthetic agents (45,46). The combination of hypothermia-related immunosuppression with prolonged immobilization frequently resulted in respiratory infections (45). Even in studies where cooling blankets were combined with alcohol compresses and ice bags to induce and maintain hypothermia (24,45,46), the time to reach the target temperature of 33 °C ranged between 2 and 11 hr. Moreover, hypothermic "overshoot" during cooling occurred frequently, and investigators have described the surface cooling procedure as being highly labor-intensive.

Selective head cooling via a cooling helmet was proved ineffective in adults (43). Internal cooling by intravenous and intraarterial ice-cold saline solutions may be practicable in healthy volunteers (47), and has been shown to be feasible in cardiac arrest patients (48); however, it remains unclear whether critically ill stroke patients can tolerate this method because large volumes are needed.

Recently, the initial results of an endovascular cooling device to cool acute stroke patients were published (49). Moderate hypothermia was induced and maintained in 6 patients with malignant stroke. A circulating temperature-adjusted closed loop system entailing three balloons near the tip of a central line (Figure 1), which dwelled in the inferior vena cava, was able to induce a body temperature of 33 °C within an average of 3 ± 1 hr. Thereafter, hypothermia was easily maintained within a range of 33.4–32.2 °C. Also, passive controlled rewarming was easily accomplished without major temperature overshoots. Apart from the frequently observed side effects of hypothermia such as pulmonary infections and hypotension, singultus was the only device-related complication.

This preliminary experience suggests that the endovascular approach might be superior to external cooling for treating acute stroke, because cooling can be induced more rapidly. The only other method that can attain a comparable speed of cooling—extracorporal heat exchange—was investigated in patients with severe head injury (44). Moderate hypothermia was induced and maintained by a venous extracorporal circulation over a double-lumen cannula in the femoral vein. The goal temperature was reached within 2 ± 1.4 hr. Although the cooling time was fast, this method is extremely elaborate,

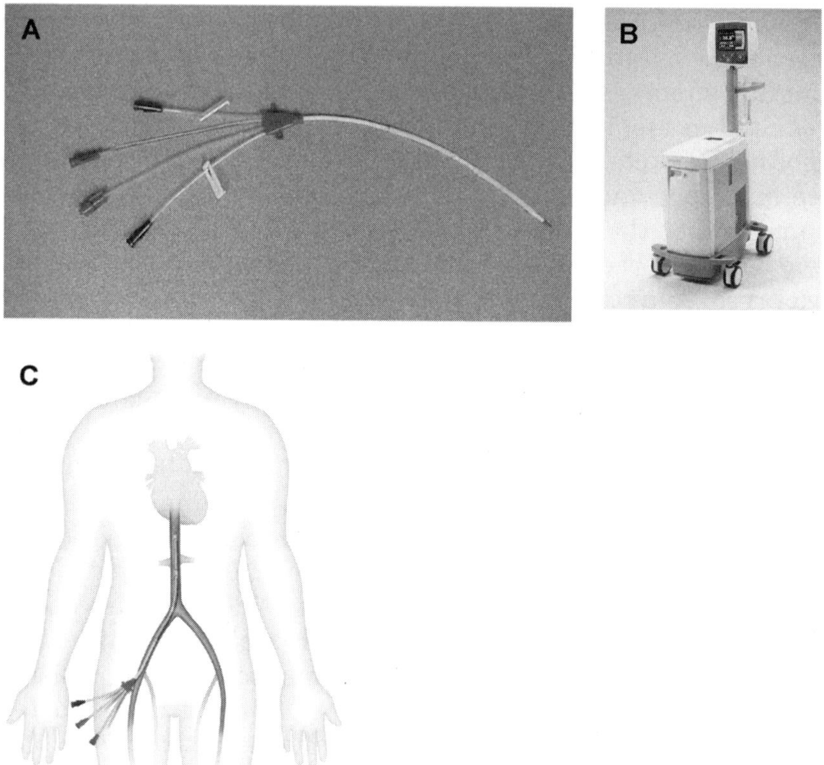

Figure 1 Endovascular cooling technique using the CoolGard System (Alsius Corporation, Irvine, CA), including the endovascular catheter (A), the CoolGard water-cooling control unit (B), and the femoral vein approach (C).

requires special expertise, and poses significant problems regarding its feasibility in the sometimes chaotic setting of the intensive care unit (ICU).

Clinical Experience with Hypothermia in Stroke

Course and Prognosis of Malignant MCA Infarction

The so-called "malignant" MCA stroke presents clinically with hemispheric neurological deficits that include hemiplegia, forced eye and head deviation, and progressive deterioration of consciousness within the first 2 days (51). When this clinical presentation is accompanied by early computer tomography (CT) signs of major infarction during the first 12 hr after stroke and a distal internal carotid artery (ICA) or proximal MCA occlusion is demonstrated, massive hemispheric swelling usually occurs during the next 24–96 hr, which is heralded by unilateral pupillary dilatation. Intracranial pressure (ICP) measurements frequently exceed 30 mm Hg, although intracranial hypertension in this setting often follows clinical deterioration related to transtentorial herniation, and medical therapy to reduce ICP at this point is usually ineffective. The prognosis is poor for malignant MCA territory infarction, with a reported mortality rate as high as 80% (51).

Therapeutic Options for Malignant MCA Infarction

Conventional treatment of raised ICP for malignant MCA infarction consists of artificial ventilation and hyperventilation, osmotherapy, and barbiturate administration. The value and duration of these measures has come into question. Aggressive hyperventilation has been discouraged because the potential decrease in cerebral blood flow resulting from profound hypocarbia ($p\mathrm{CO}_2 < 26$ mm Hg) might exacerbate tissue ischemia (52). Early use of agents such as glycerol or mannitol, at least in theory, may actually hasten tissue shifts and therefore lead to an aggravation of brain edema (53). Barbiturate therapy has not been shown to be of therapeutic benefit in the treatment of postischemic brain edema (54).

More recently, decompressive surgery for control of otherwise intractable elevated ICP has been proposed for a variety of neurological disorders, including head trauma, space-occupying hemispheric infarction, and subdural hematoma. The surgical management of intracranial hypertension is directed at improving cerebral perfusion and preventing ischemic damage and mechanical compression of the brain against various intracranial structures such as the falx, tentorium, or the sphenoid ridge. However, particularly in patients with cerebrovascular accidents, there is still controversy as to when and how to implement this highly invasive procedure (55). Because of the potential adverse effects and general ineffectiveness of conventional medical therapy, and uncertainty regarding the patient selection and timing for neurosurgical intervention, new therapeutic concepts for the treatment of ischemic brain edema are needed. Although hypothermia has been used as a means of providing neuroprotection during surgical procedures and in perioperative management for over 40 years (56), it has only been recently introduced as a primary therapeutic modality in the critical care setting.

Hypothermia for Malignant MCA Infarction

It is known from animal models with global ischemia and traumatic brain injury that moderate hypothermia attenuates ischemic brain damage. Even though hypothermia has potent neuroprotective effects after experimental focal ischemia, there are few clinical studies of hypothermic therapy after MCA infarction in humans.

Because the patient numbers are so small and hypothermia was, in most cases, not compared to a concurrent randomly assigned control group, most studies of hypothermia for MCA infarction can be considered pilot studies for feasibility and safety (Table 1). The earliest modern report was published 1996 and included 4 patients who were cooled within 5 hr after stroke onset for a duration of 3–5 days to 33°C (46). These patients were cooled with cooling blankets and alcohol compresses.

In a study published in 1998, Schwab et al. (45) studied 25 patients with malignant MCA infarction. Hypothermia was induced by cold water applied to the skin, cooling blankets, and cold intravenous fluid infusion within 14 $\pm$ 7 hr after stroke onset and was maintained for 48–72 hr (Figure 2). All patients were sedated, paralyzed, and artificially ventilated during the cooling period. Intracranial pressure (ICP), cerebral perfusion pressure (CPP), and cerebral temperature were monitored, and outcome was assessed at 4 weeks and 3 months using the Scandinavian Stroke Scale and the Barthel index. Mortality in this cohort was 44%, compared to a previously reported rate of 80% among patients treated with barbiturates at the

Table 1 Overview of Studies of Ischemic Stroke and Hypothermia

	Number of patients	Target temperature (°C)	Hours from stroke onset until induction of cooling	Duration of cooling
Severe ischemic stroke				
Naritomi et al. (46)	4	33	<5	3–5 days
Schwab et al. (45)	25	33	14 ± 7	2–3 days
Schwab et al. (60)	50	33	22 ± 9	1–3 days
Georgiadis et al. (49)	6	33	28 ± 17	2–3 days
Georgiadis et al. (50)	19	33	24 (range 18–24)	2–3 days
Moderate ischemic stroke				
Kammersgaard et al. (62)	17	35.5	3 ± 4	6 hrs
Kreiger et al. (63)	6	32 ± 1	6 ± 1	1–4 days

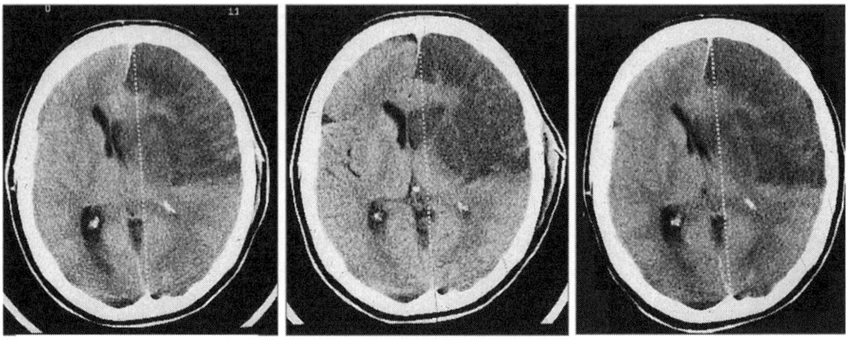

Figure 2 Hypothermia in malignant cerebral infarction, showing three cranial CT scans of a patient with a severe ischemic stroke in the left hemisphere before, during, and after moderate therapeutic hypothermia.

same institution (51). Moreover, hypothermic treatment was able to significantly reduce ICP, which was similar to the results of Shiozaki et al. (57) and Marion et al. (58), who used hypothermia to treat traumatic brain injury. With a minimal effect on mean arterial blood pressure and increased CPP, hypothermic therapy appeared to be beneficial for these patients, as uncontrolled intracranial hypertension is the main cause of death in the first week after stroke. However, rewarming the patients constantly led to a secondary rise of ICP, which required additional ICP therapy with mannitol. In some cases it even exaggerated the initial ICP levels and an association was identified between mortality in this cohort and "rebound" intracranial hypertension during rewarming (Figure 3).

It is known that the rewarming period is a high-risk time for brain injury because metabolic need can outstrip oxygen delivery at various temperatures (see Chapter 7) (59). In our pilot study of 25 patients, 9 of 11 patients who died had untreatable elevated ICP during rewarming. In this study, patients rewarmed passively: the cooling system was simply turned off, with the rewarming process ensuing over 17–24 hr. In a subsequent analysis, Steiner et al. (60) showed a correlation

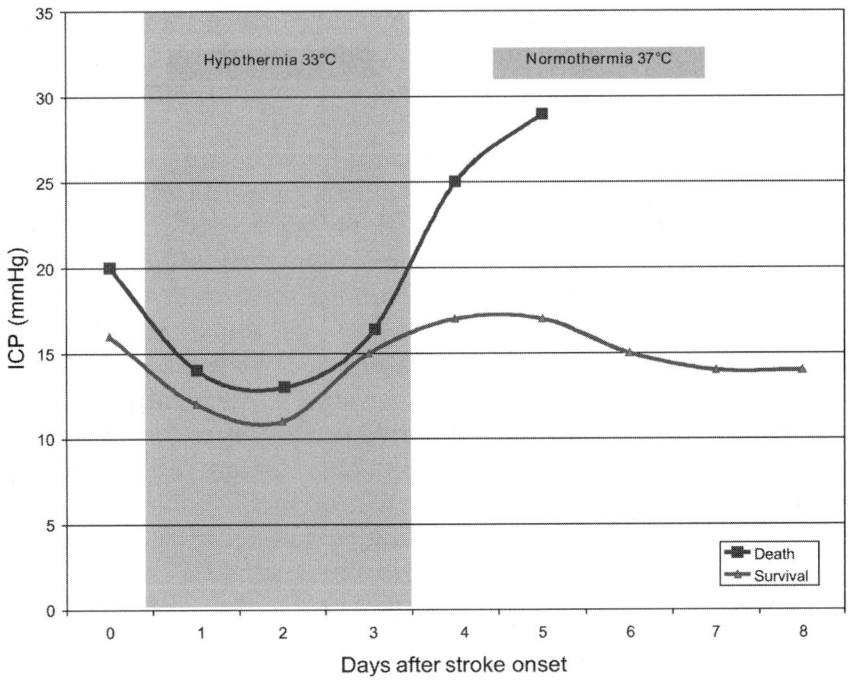

Figure 3 Course of intracranial pressure before, during and after hypothermia in two patients with a severe MCA infarction. One patient had a rebound of ICP during the rewarming period and died on day 5.

between the rewarming rate and the consecutive rise in ICP. They recommend a strategy of controlled passive rewarming for ICP and CPP control after moderate hypothermia.

A more recent study from Georgiadis et al. (49) investigated the method of endovascular cooling (the CoolGard System; Alsius Corporation, Irvine, CA) for inducing and maintaining moderate hypothermia after ischemic stroke. Six patients with malignant MCA infarction were treated by a circulating temperature-adjusted closed loop system entailing three balloons near the tip of a central line, which dwelled in the inferior vena cava. As described in the preceding paragraph, target temperature was reached faster compared to external cooling. Additionally, temperature overshoot and deviations from the target temperatures were minimized. In contrast to former studies, controlled rewarming was performed more easily using the endovascular approach compared to external cooling.

The largest study investigating hypothermia in ischemic stroke was published in 2001 (61). Fifty patients with massive cerebral infarction were included prospectively in this nonrandomized multicenter trial. The average time for induction of hypothermia was 22 ± 9 hr from stroke onset, and cooling was performed using alcohol and ice bags. The duration of the cooling period was 24–72 hr. Afterwards patients were passively rewarmed over a mean duration of 17 hr. Analysis of the data showed that four patients died during hypothermia from severe coagulopathy, cardiac failure, or uncontrollable intracranial hypertension. As discussed later on, 30% of the patients died during or after the rewarming period because of rebound increases in ICP and fatal herniation. Still, ICP was significantly reduced during the cooling period.

These studies show that while hypothermia is feasible in stroke patients, it can be associated with several side effects. These side effects can mostly be handled with meticulous ICU management. The rewarming period itself was identified as the most critical situation in patients with malignant MCA stroke.

Hypothermia for Moderate Cerebral Infarction

Even though hypothermia may be most effective in terms of neuroprotection at early stages of cerebral ischemia, only two studies have investigated its early use (62,63). In the Copenhagen study, 17 patients were cooled with a forced-air cooling blanket (Polar Air, Augustine Medical, Minneapolis, MN) and compared to 56 nonrandomized controls (62). The time from stroke onset was 3 ± 4 hr on the average. Because these patients were awake during the cooling period, intravenous meperidine was used to prevent shivering. In contrast to the other studies, the goal temperature was 35.5°C, which was reached after a mean of 4 hr from the beginning of cooling and maintained for only 6 hr. Because the goal temperature was higher compared to the other studies, infections and other adverse events were not associated with the cooling procedure itself. The outcome of hypothermic patients was not better than that of controls, but the study was not powered to detect an impact on outcome.

The COOL-AID study combined early thrombolysis with moderate hypothermia (63). In the COOL-AID trial, a total of 19 patients were included into the study: 10 were nonrandomized controls and 9 patients were cooled. Hypothermia was performed using water-circulating cooling blankets and alcohol rubs after intubation, paralysis, and opioid infusions. Patients first received intravenous thrombolysis within the 3-hr time window, with hypothermia initiated within 6 hr of stroke onset. The mean duration of hypothermia was 48 ± 20 hr and the target temperature was reached within a mean of 3.5 ± 1.3 hr. As is often the case with external cooling, many patients experienced an overshoot to temperatures below the target of 33°C during the induction phase. Hypothermia seemed to be well tolerated with few complications. Because the absolute patient number in this trail was rather small, no significant benefit in 3-month outcome measured with the modified Rankin Scale was observed.

More recently, these same investigators have reported the preliminary results of the Cool-Aid 2 trial (64), a prospective, randomized pilot-safety study of early hypothermia induced with endovascular cooling (the Set Point System, Radiant Medical, Redwood City, CA). A total of 40 patients with moderate-to-severe stroke were enrolled within 12 hr of onset, with 18 randomized to hypothermia (37°C for 24 hr) and 22 to normothermia. Of the 18 patients assigned to hypothermia, 13 were successfully cooled, with a mean time to reach 33°C of 77 ± 44 min. In the 5 remaining patients, difficulty in reaching or maintaining target temperature resulted from shivering or issues related to catheter placement. Thirty-day clinical outcomes and changes in infarct volumes on MR scans did not differ between the two groups.

Risks of Hypothermia in Stroke Patients

Complications of hypothermia are numerous and can be life-threatening (see Chapter 6). These risks may be particularly considerable in stroke patients, who tend to have more underlying cardiovascular disease than patients with head injury or other conditions. The traditional clinical target for mild-to-moderate hypothermia (33°C) is primarily dictated by cardiac complications that are known to occur at slightly lower temperatures. Below 32°C, prolongation of the P–R interval and QRS complex will occur. It is followed by increased Q–T interval, and finally below 27°C, ventricular ectopy and fibrillation may occur. Besides these cardiac side effects, hematologic perturbations are often seen, primarily thrombocytopenia and clotting disturbances. Abnormalities in clotting mechanisms occur by slowing the enzymatic cascades and by promoting fibrinolysis.

In several animal studies, the most severe side effects of hypothermia were clotting abnormalities and coagulopathy (40,65). In baboons, systemic hypothermia led to platelet dysfunction and increased bleeding times (66). In humans, the enzymatic reactions of the coagulation cascade were shown to be strongly inhibited by hypothermia (67,68). Although a reversible decrease in platelet counts during cooling has been reported in patients treated with hypothermia following head trauma or stroke, severe clotting abnormalities have not been reported so far.

In animals the toxicity from moderate hypothermia increases as the depth and duration of cooling is increased, and virtually every organ system can be affected (69,70). In stroke patients, the most commonly reported serious complication of hypothermia has been pneumonia, with a reported incidence ranging from 10% to 40% (70–72). The risk of developing pneumonia further increases when neurological injury associated with impaired airway reflexes are present at admission to the critical care unit. The extent to which hypothermia further increases the rate of ventilator-associated pneumonia in this high-risk population is unclear. The 40% rate of pneumonia in our multicenter study of hypothermia in stroke patients (61) is comparable to that of Metz and colleagues (73), who observed pneumonia in 50% of their hypothermically treated trauma patients within the first week in the intensive care unit. Finally, pancreatitis with elevated serum amylase and lipase levels has been observed during hypothermic therapy. The cause is poorly understood (74). The condition is rarely symptomatic, and the elevated levels of amylase and lipase are usually completely reversible after rewarming.

Rewarming

Moderate hypothermia has been shown to reduce ICP in patients with malignant MCA infarction during the cooling period itself. However, during the rewarming period, ICP often exceeds baseline levels, with rebound infarct swelling leading to lethal herniation in a large subpopulation of patients (see Chapter 7, "Complications of Rewarming") (45). In the first study from our department, hypothermia was followed by "passive rewarming": the cooling system was turned off, and patients were allowed to rewarm on their own without any cooling or rewarming device over the next 24 hr. A more recent publication from our department showed that in 13 stroke patients the so-called "controlled passive rewarming" at a rate of 0.1–0.2°C over 2–4 hr was safer in terms of ICP and CPP control (60). With the use of endovascular cooling devices, controlled rewarming in this fashion will be relatively easy. Other approaches to rewarming, including adjustment of the rate of rewarming to minimize concurrent changes in ICP and CPP, deserve further study.

Ventilation Strategies During Hypothermia

Mild-to-moderate hypothermia (33°C) usually requires sedation, paralyzing agents, and mechanical ventilation (45). Endotracheal intubation and mechanical ventilation are routinely performed in patients with severe stroke to provide airway protection and as an adjunct for controlling ICP. Additionally, hypothermia usually provokes shivering as a thermoregulatory response, which can be uncomfortable for patients and hinder the cooling process. The use of meperidine (pethidine), paralyzing agents, and other treatments to suppress shivering (see Chapter 8) usually require control of the airway and mechanical ventilation. Alteration of ventilation management during hypothermia influences acid–base status and leads to a different physiological response, which can affect cerebral blood flow (CBF) (75). There are basically two ventilation managements used during hypothermia: "pH-stat" and "alpha-stat" management. During alpha-stat management, the blood gas analysis is performed at a fictional "normal" temperature of 37°C, whereas the blood gas analysis during pH-stat management is corrected for the true lower temperature of the patient. Mechanical ventilation during alpha-stat management aims for an arterial CO_2 tension ($PaCO_2$) of 40 mm Hg when measured at 37°C, whereas pH-stat management aims for a $PaCO_2$ of 40 mm Hg under hypothermic conditions.

As a result of the increased gas solubility during hypothermia, the alpha-stat strategy results in higher pCO_2 levels for any given degree of minute ventilation, and hence relative hyperventilation and a lower CBF than pH-stat management. This relatively diminished CBF during hypothermia with alpha-stat management was found to be beneficial in cardiac surgical patients on cardiopulmonary bypass (76), presumably because the delivery of microemboli was reduced compared to pH-stat management. The optimal ventilation strategy in stroke patients treated with therapeutic hypothermia remains unclear, because most reports have not precisely described their ventilation strategy or analyzed their effects on CBF and outcome.

Experimental studies suggest the possibility that pH-stat management may contribute to the neuroprotective effects of hypothermia for several reasons (77). First, an increase of CBF in marginally perfused penumbral regions might be beneficial. Second, increased CBF might lead to a more homogenous temperature profile (78) throughout the brain, providing better cooling of damaged brain areas. An increase in CBF might also contribute to faster elimination of potentially toxic metabolites such as glutamate and aspartate. On the other hand, it remains unclear whether increased CBF (and cerebral blood volume) with pH-stat management can aggravate intracranial hypertension in patients with malignant cerebral infarction, as is seen in severe head trauma (79).

A single experimental study compares the effects of alpha-stat and pH-stat management after focal cerebral ischemia in rats treated with hypothermia (77). CBF was increased in penumbral regions during pH-stat management and infarct volumes were reduced compared to alpha-stat management (Figures 4 and 5). The major limitations of this study were the short time window from stroke onset to analysis and the lack of an analysis after rewarming, which needs to be addressed in further studies. In conclusion, pH-stat management might be beneficial during hypothermia in stroke, but additional investigations need to be performed to find the optimal ventilation regimen. For a more detailed discussion of the impact of ventilatory and acid–base management on cerebral blood flow and metabolism, please see Chapter 5.

Shivering During Hypothermia in Stroke Patients

Despite the extensive neurological damage that occurs with malignant MCA infarction, thermoregulatory responses to maintain normal body temperature in these patients are generally well maintained (80). Induced hypothermia can lead

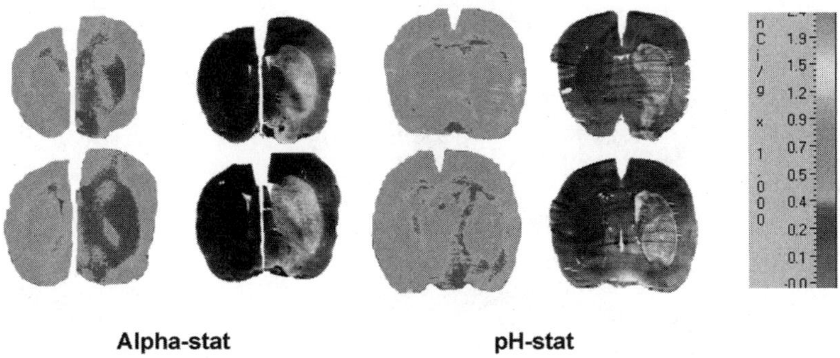

Figure 4 Cerebral blood flow (CBF) during hypothermia and experimental focal cerebral ischemia demonstrating the effect of alpha-stat and pH-stat ventilation. Examples of autoradiographs measured by 4-iodo[M-methyl-14C] antipyrine and silver infarct staining (SIS) are shown. Color variation indicates different regional blood flow as indicated in the scale. In high-contrast silver stains, pale areas indicate infarcted regions. The brain slices under alpha-stat conditions demonstrate lower core CBF levels and larger areas of infarction. (From Ref. 77.)

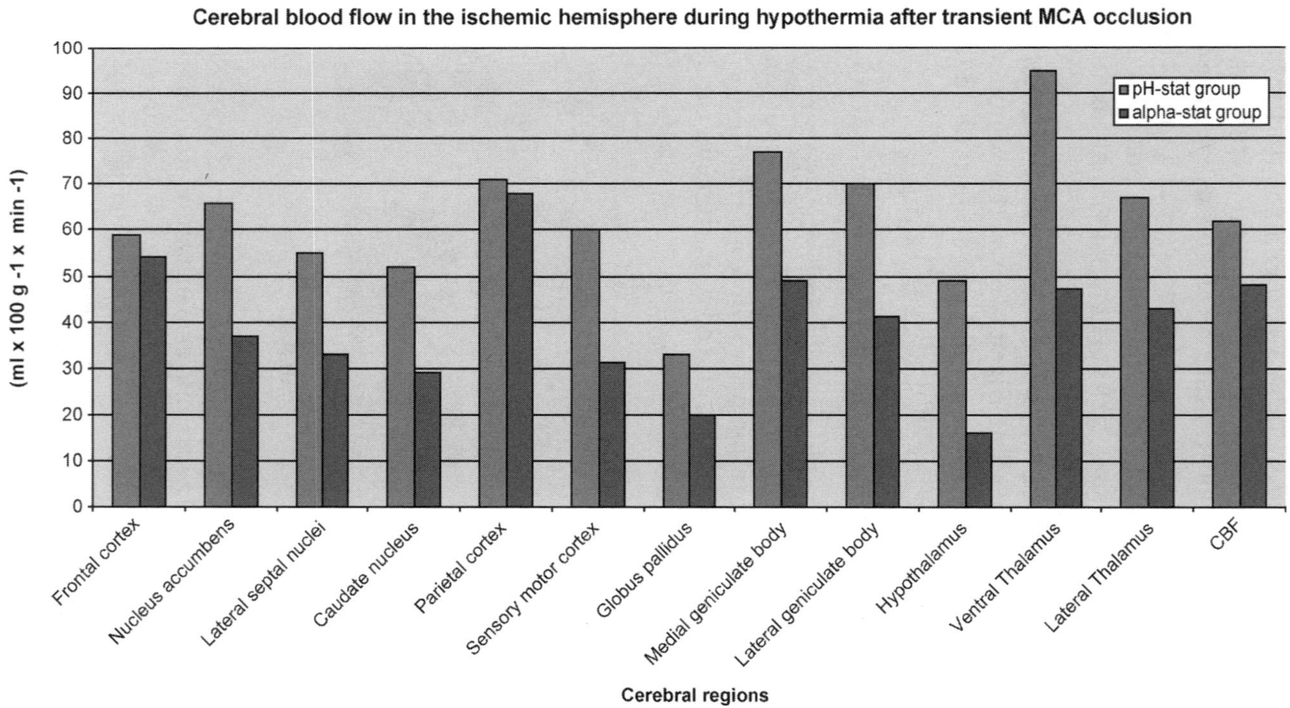

Figure 5 Bar graph comparing cerebral blood flow (CBF) measured by 4-iodo[M-methyl-14C] antipyrine after experimental cerebral ischemia (transient middle cerebral artery occlusion in the rat) during moderate hypothermia at 33°C under two different ventilation strategies. Gray indicates pH-stat, whereas black indicates alpha-stat ventilation.

to thermal discomfort (81), sympathetic nervous system activation, and shivering—all of which may be deleterious in these seriously ill stroke patients. The primary autonomic thermoregulatory defenses against hypothermia are vasoconstriction and shivering. Numerous pharmacologic agents impair these responses, reducing the activation threshold (triggering core temperature) by 2–3 °C; however, most are anesthetics, opioids, or sedative-hypnotic agents that can significantly compromise airway defenses and respiratory drive when given in sufficient doses to suppress shivering (Table 2) (82). More recently, the combination of meperidine and buspirone (a 5-HT_{1C} partial antagonist) (83–85) has been shown to reduce the shivering threshold without producing significant sedative effects. In contrast, focal warming of the face or extremities is ineffective (86).

Although these studies investigated healthy subjects, they imply that at least mild hypothermia may be feasible in stroke patients with smaller infarcts without the requirement of sedation or paralysis and mechanical ventilation. In accordance with this approach, Kammersgaard et al. (61) treated acute stroke victims with mild hypothermia (35.5 °C) by using meperidine to control shivering. The mean dose of meperidine given per patient throughout the 6 hr of hypothermic treatment (core temperature of 35.5 °C) was 241 mg, but was highly variable among patients. Clearly, more work is needed to

Table 2 Overview of Different Pharmacological Antishivering Agents

	Tested in stroke	Dosage
Alfentanil		0.5–3.0 μg/kg/min
Fentanyl	×	0.02–0.07 μg/kg/min
Nalbuphine		0.1–0.2 mg/kg
Meperidine	×	0.25–2.0 mg/kg
Tramadol		0.25–1 mg/kg
Clonidine	×	1–2 μg/kg
Buspirone		30–60 mg q6h
Dexmedetomidine		0.3–0.7 μg/kg/hr

develop optimal strategies for controlling shivering in stroke patients treated with hypothermia.

FUTURE DIRECTIONS

Although hypothermia has been tested as a treatment for acute cerebral ischemia, the results of these studies remain preliminary. Further investigations are required to define the optimal methodology for inducing hypothermia in stroke patients and to evaluate its safety and efficacy. The most pressing issues in terms of methodology relate to patient selection and the timing, depth, and duration of cooling.

Patient Selection

The patients who stand to benefit the most from cooling remain to be identified. Basically, two potential subgroups can be identified from a pathophysiological perspective. The first group of patients treated during the acute period (<6 hr), who have an evolving infarct with a penumbra that might be "rescued" with rapidly administered hypothermic neuroprotection. This approach has yet to be adequately tested and should be the goal of future studies. The second group consists of patients with a large established infarct who are at risk for deterioration because of mass effect and elevated ICP. Most studies of hypothermia for cerebral infarction performed to date have taken this approach, with cooling generally initiated between 12 and 24 hr after onset. Hemicraniectomy may prove to be a better option for "salvaging" these patients, although the combination of hypothermia with hemicraniectomy deserves further attention. Studies are also needed to determine whether hypothermia is useful before, during, or after thrombolysis, because thrombolytic therapy is the only currently established treatment for acute cerebral ischemia. Until now, there is only a single experimental study investigating this combination therapy (87). In particular, experiments are needed to determine whether hypothermia interferes or exaggerates the activity of thrombolytic agents, and to evaluate the effect of cooling on reperfusion injury.

Timing of Cooling

According to the experimental data (see Chapter 4), the benefits of hypothermia for focal ischemia increase the earlier it is applied. Consequently, patients suffering from acute ischemic stroke should be cooled as quickly as possible. This approach requires more efficient cooling techniques than have been widely available up to now. Endovascular heat-exchange catheters (see Chapter 10) offer a promising approach for rapid systemic cooling, but more work in this area is needed (88). This modality may best be supplemented by infusions of cooled intravenous fluids in the ambulance or emergency room, and pharmacological agents such as buspirone or meperidine to prevent shivering. Most of the challenges related to rapid and safe cooling of stroke patients relate to the implementation of new methods for attaining hypothermia.

Depth of Hypothermia

Although mild-to-moderate hypothermia (33°C) has been applied in most studies to date, the issue of the most appropriate target temperature for treating stroke patients remains unresolved. As suggested by the experience of Kammersgaard et al., mild hypothermia may be sufficient for the treatment of mild-to-moderate ischemic strokes, with fewer of side effects than deeper levels of cooling (61). In fact, the same may be the case for patients with larger malignant MCA infarcts. As an example of the type of study that might shed light on this issue, Tokutomi et al. assessed the optimal temperature for the treatment of severe traumatic brain injury (30). Modest hypothermia was capable of reducing ICP significantly, whereas no additional benefit was found at temperatures below 35°C. Moreover, CPP continued to decrease with further temperature reductions below this level. Dose-ranging studies of this type in stroke patients treated with hypothermia are badly needed.

Because fever is a common problem in neurological and neurosurgical intensive care unit patients (84), the feasibility and efficacy of fever control in stroke patients also requires further evaluation (see Chapter 12). This approach was applied in a pilot study by Schmutzhard et al. (88) using an intravascular cooling device with good results. Additional studies of "prophylactic normothermia" in patients with stroke, either alone or following an initial period of more intense cooling, are needed. Ultimately, a temperature control strategy with different target temperatures based on time from onset—an early burst of moderate hypothermia (32°C), followed by 2–3 days of mild hypothermia (35.5°C), and then a fever control approach (37°C)—might be envisioned (Figure 6).

Duration of Cooling

The issue of the optimal duration of cooling is important, because longer cooling periods are associated with a stronger neuroprotective effect in experimental models, but also pose the risk of increased complications. Studies of hypothermia for stroke to date have used cooling periods ranging from 6 hr to 5 days (46,56). Because improved management of complications may allow the cooling period to be safely extended, other critical methodologic questions relate to ventilatory and acid–base management, strategies to minimize infections, and protocols for cardiovascular support and the control of shivering.

Finally, the issue of rewarming must be addressed (see Chapter 7). Hypothermia has been shown to significantly

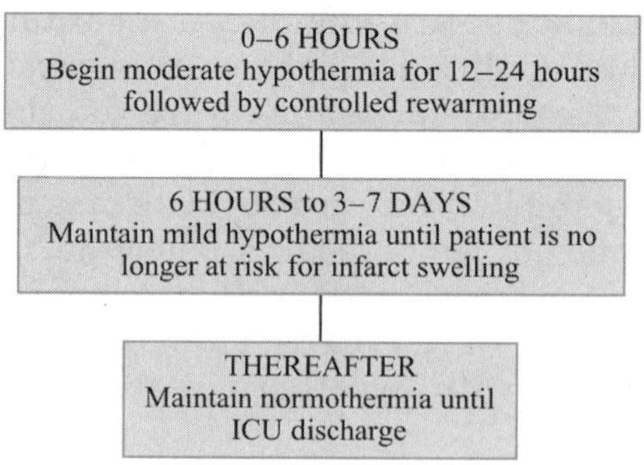

Figure 6 Potential scheme for temperature management for large hemispheric infarction, with varying target temperatures based on time from onset. (Provided courtesy of Dr. Stephan A. Mayer).

decrease ICP levels in patients with mass effect due to malignant cerebral infarction; however, rebound increases in ICP can occur during rewarming and are the main cause of death during this period (45). Potentially, a slower and more controlled increase in brain and body temperature may prevent the rebound of elevated ICP in these critical patients.

Conclusion

In conclusion, there are only two approaches for the treatment of acute cerebral ischemia that have been successfully transferred from the laboratory to the patient: thrombolysis and hypothermia. The recent studies and experiences with hypothermia described in this chapter are just the first steps toward developing an optimal strategy for treating stroke patients. Many questions remain to be solved both clinically and experimentally to ideally use this promising technique in stroke.

REFERENCES

1. Corbett D, Thornhill J. Temperature modulation (hypothermic and hyperthermic conditions) and its influence on histological and behavioral outcomes following cerebral ischemia. Brain Pathol 2000; 10:145–152.
2. Ginsberg MD. Adventures in the pathophysiology of brain ischemia: penumbra, gene expression, neuroprotection: the 2002 Thomas Willis Lecture. Stroke 2003; 34:214–223.
3. Phan TG, Wright PM, Markus R, Howells DW, Davis SM, Donnan GA. Salvaging the ischaemic penumbra: more than just reperfusion? Clin Exp Pharmacol Physiol 2002; 29:1–10.
4. Belayev L, Zhao W, Busto R, Ginsberg MD. Transient middle cerebral artery occlusion by intraluminal suture. I: Three-dimensional autoradiographic image-analysis of local cerebral glucose metabolism-blood flow interrelationships during ischemia and early recirculation. J Cereb Blood Flow Metab 1997; 17:1266–1280.
5. Astrup J, Siesjo BK, Symon L. Thresholds in cerebral ischemia—the ischemic penumbra. Stroke 1981; 12:723–725.

6. Karibe H, Zarow GJ, Graham SH, Weinstein PR. Mild intraischemic hypothermia reduces postischemic hyperperfusion, delayed postischemic hypoperfusion, blood–brain barrier disruption, brain edema, and neuronal damage volume after temporary focal cerebral ischemia in rats. J Cereb Blood Flow Metab 1994; 1:620–627.
7. Wang GJ, Deng HY, Maier CM, Sun GH, Yenari MA. Mild hypothermia reduces ICAM-1 expression, neutrophil infiltration and microglia/monocyte accumulation following experimental stroke. Neuroscience 2002; 114:1081–1090.
8. Maier CM, Sun GH, Cheng D, Yenari MA, Chan PH, Steinberg GK. Effects of mild hypothermia on superoxide anion production, superoxide dismutase expression, and activity following transient focal cerebral ischemia. Neurobiol Dis 2002; 11:28–42.
9. Winfree CJ, Baker CJ, Connolly ES Jr, Fiore AJ, Solomon RA. Mild hypothermia reduces penumbral glutamate levels in the rat permanent focal cerebral ischemia model. Neurosurgery 1996; 38:1216–1222.
10. Maier CM, Ahern K, Cheng ML, Lee JE, Yenari MA, Steinberg GK. Optimal depth and duration of mild hypothermia in a focal model of transient cerebral ischemia: effects on neurologic outcome, infarct size, apoptosis, and inflammation. Stroke 1998; 29:2171–2180.
11. Colbourne F, Corbett D, Zhao Z, Yang J, Buchan AM. Prolonged but delayed postischemic hypothermia: a long-term outcome study in the rat middle cerebral artery occlusion model. J Cereb Blood Flow Metab 2000; 20:1702–1708.
12. Hajat C, Hajat S, Sharma P. Effects of poststroke pyrexia on stroke outcome: a meta-analysis of studies in patients. Stroke 2000; 31:410–414.
13. Hindfelt B. The prognostic significance of subfebrility and fever in ischaemic cerebral infarction. Acta Neurol Scand 1976; 53:72–79.
14. Terent A, Andersson B. Prognosis for patients with cerebrovascular stroke and transient ischaemic attacks. Ups J Med Sci 1981; 86:63–74.
15. Castillo J, Davalos A, Noya M. Progression of ischemic stroke and excitotoxic amino acids. Lancet 1997; 349:79–83.

16. Sharma JC, Ross IN. Antipyretic therapy in acute stroke. Lancet 1998; 352:740–741.

17. MacWalter R, McMahon A, Fraser H, Bruce V, Hendrick S. Does body temperature on admission predict long-term outcome after an acute stroke [abstr]? Cerebrovasc Dis 1998; 8(suppl 4):11.

18. Azzimondi G, Bassein L, Nonino F, Fiorani L, Vignatelli L, Re G, D'Alessandro R. Fever in acute stroke worsens prognosis. Stroke 1995; 26, 2040–2043.

19. Reith J, Jorgensen S, Pedersen PM, Nakayama H, Raaschou HO, Jeppesen LL, Olsen TS. Body temperature in acute stroke: relation to stroke severity, infarct size, mortality, and outcome. Lancet 1996; 347:422–425.

20. Castillo J, Martinez F, Leira R, Prieto JM, Lema M, Noya M. Mortality and morbidity of acute cerebral infarction related to temperature and basal analytic parameters. Cerebrovasc Dis 1994; 4:56–71.

21. Jorgensen HS, Reith J, Pedersen PM, Nakayama H, Olsen TS. Body temperature and outcome in stroke patients [letter]. Lancet 1996; 348:193.

22. Castillo J, Davalos A, Marrugat J, Noya M. Timing for fever-related brain damage in acute ischemic stroke. Stroke 1998; 29:2455–2460.

23. Dirnagl U, Iadecola C, Moskowitz MA. Pathobiology of ischaemic stroke: an integrated view. Trends Neurosci 1999; 22:391–397.

24. Schwab S, Schwarz S, Aschoff A, Keller E, Hacke W. Moderate hypothermia and brain temperature in patients with severe middle cerebral artery infarction. Acta Neurochir Suppl (Wien) 1998; 71:131–134.

25. Busto R, Dietrich D, Globus MYT, Ginsberg MD. The importance of brain temperature in cerebral ischemic injury. Stroke 1989; 20:1113–1114.

26. Stone JG, Goodman RR, Baker KZ, Baker CJ, Solomon RA. Direct intraoperative measurement of human brain temperature. Neurosurgery 1997; 41:20–24.

27. Crowder CM, Tempelhoff R, Therard MA, Cheng MA, Todorov A, Dacey RG. Jugular bulb temperature: comparison with

brain surface and core temperature in neurosurgical patients during mild hypothermia. J Neurosurg 1996; 85:98–103.

28. Henker RA, Brown SD, Marion DW. Comparison of brain temperature with bladder and rectal temperatures in adults with severe head injury. Neurosurgery 1998; 42:1071–1075.

29. Rumana CS, Gopinath SP, Uzura M, Valadka AB, Robertson CS. Brain temperature exceeds systemic temperature in head injured patients. Crit Care Med 1998; 26:562–56710.

30. Tokutomi T, Morimoto K, Miyagi T, Yamaguchi S, Ishikawa K, Shigemori M. Optimal temperature for the management of severe traumatic brain injury: effect of hypothermia on intracranial pressure, systemic and intracranial hemodynamics, and metabolism. Neurosurgery 2003; 52:102–112.

31. Schwab S, Spranger M, Aschoff A, Steiner T, Hacke W. Brain temperature monitoring and modulation in patients with severe MCA infarction. Neurology 1997; 48:762–767.

32. Mellergård P, Nordstroem C-H. Intracerebral temperature in neurosurgical patients. Neurosurgery 1991; 28:709–713.

33. Ko K, Ghajar J, Hariri RJ. A method for monitoring intracranial temperature via tunneled ventricular catheter: technical note. Neurosurgery 1994; 34:927–930.

34. Nurse S, Corbett D. Direct measurement of brain temperature during and after intraischemic hypothermia: correlation with behavioral, physiological, and histological endpoints. J Neurosci 1994; 14:7726–7734.

35. Haraldseth O, Gronas T, Southon T, Thommessen L, Borchgrevink G, Jynge P, Gisvold SE, Unsgard G. The effects of brain temperature on temporary global ischemia in rat brain. A 31 Phosphorous NMR spectroscopy study. Acta Anaesthesiol Scand 1992; 36:393–399.

36. Jiang J, Lyeth B, Clifton G, Jenkins L, Hamm R, Hayes R. Relationship between body and brain temperature in traumatically brain-injured rodents. J Neurosurg 1991; 74:492–496.

37. Sutton LN, Clark BJ, Norwood CR, Woodford EJ, Welsh FA. Global cerebral ischemia in piglets under conditions of mild and deep hypothermia. Stroke 1991; 22:1567–1573.

38. Swain JA, McDonald TJ, Balaban RS, Robbins RC. Metabolism

of the heart and brain during hypothermic cardiopulmonary bypass. Ann Thorac Surg 1991; 51:105–109.

39. Busto R, Globus MY-T, Dietrich WD, Martinez E, Valdes I, Ginsberg MD. Effect of mild hypothermia on ischemia induced release of neurotransmitters and free fatty acids in rat brain. Stroke 1989; 20:904–910.

40. Clifton G, Jiang J, Lyeth B, Jenkins L, Hamm R, Hayes R. Marked protection by moderate hypothermia after experimental traumatic brain injury. J Cereb Blood Flow Metab 1991; 11:114–121.

41. Leonov Y, Sterz F, Safar P, Radovsky A, Oku K, Tisherman S, Stezoski SW. Mild hypothermia during and after cardiac arrest improves neurological outcome in dogs. J Cereb Blood Flow Metab 1990; 10:57–70.

42. Boris-Möller F, Smith ML, Siesjö BK. Effects of hypothermia on ischemic brain damage: a comparison between preischemic and postischemic cooling. Neurosci Res Commun 1989; 5: 87–94.

43. Mellergård P. Changes in human intracerebral temperature in response to different methods of cooling. Neurosurgery 1992; 31:671–677.

44. Piepgras A, Roth H, Schürer L, Tillmans R, Quintel M, Herrmann P, Schmiedek P. Rapid active internal core cooling for induction of moderate hypothermia in head injury by use of an extracorporeal heat exchanger. Neurosurgery 1998; 42:311–317.

45. Schwab S, Schwarz S, Spranger M, Keller E, Bertram M, Hacke W. Moderate hypothermia in the treatment of patients with severe middle cerebral artery infarction. Stroke 1998; 29:2461–2466.

46. Naritomi H, Shimizu T, Oe H. Mild hypothermia therapy in acute embolic stroke: a pilot study. J Stroke Cerebrovasc Dis 1996; 6:193–196.

47. Rajek A, Greif R, Sessler DI, Baumgardner J, Laciny S, Bastanmehr H. Core cooling by central venous infusion of ice-cold (4 degrees C and 20 degrees C) fluid: isolation of core and peripheral thermal compartments. Anesthesiology 2000; 93: 629–637.

48. Bernard SA, Buist MD, Monteiro O, Smith K. Induced hypothermia using large volume, ice-cold intravenous fluid in comatose survivors of out-of-hospital cardiac arrest: a preliminary report. Resuscitation 2003; 56:9–13.

49. Georgiadis D, Schwarz S, Kollmar R, Schwab S. Endovascular cooling for moderate hypothermia in patients with acute stroke: first results of a novel approach. Stroke 2001; 32:2550–2553.

50. Georgiadis D, Schwarz S, Aschoff A, Schwab S. Hemicraniectomy and moderate hypothermia in patients with severe ischemic stroke. Stroke 2002 June; 33(6):1584–1588.

51. Hacke W, Schwab S, Horn M, Spranger M, De Georgia M, von Kummer R. Malignant middle cerebral artery territory infarction: clinical course and prognostic signs. Arch Neurol 1996; 53:309–315.

52. Muizelaar JP, Marmarou A, Ward JD, Kontos HA, Choi SC, Becker DP, Gruemer H, Young HF. Adverse effects of prolonged hyperventilation in patients with severe head injury. A randomized clinical trial. J Neurosurg 1991; 75:731–739.

53. Kaufmann AM, Cardoso ER. Aggravation of vasogenic cerebral edema by multiple-dose mannitol. J Neurosurg 1992; 77: 584–589.

54. Schwab S, Spranger M, Schwarz S, Hacke W. Barbiturate coma in severe hemispheric stroke: useful or obsolete? Neurology 1997; 48:1608–1613.

55. Schwab S, Rieke K, Aschoff A, Albert F, von Kummer R, Hacke W. Hemicraniectomy in space-occupying hemispheric infarction: useful intervention or desperate activism? Cerebrovasc Dis 1996; 6:325–329.

56. Hitchcock CR, Strobel CJA, Haglin JJ, Wilson JA. Use of prolonged moderate hypothermia in postoperative care. Arch Surg 1962; 85:549–556.

57. Shiozaki T, Sugimoto H, Taneda M, Yoshida H, Iwai A, Yoshioka T, Sugimoto T. Effect of mild hypothermia on uncontrollable intracranial hypertension after severe head injury. J Neurosurg 1993; 79:363–368.

58. Marion DW, Penrod LE, Kelsey SF, Obrist WD, Kochanek PM, Palmer AM, Wisniewski SR, DeKosky ST. Treatment of

traumatic brain injury with moderate hypothermia. N Engl J Med 1997; 336:540–546.

59. Ausman JI, McCormick PW, Stewart M, Lewis G, Dujovny M, Balakrishnan G, Malik GM, Ghaly RF. Cerebral oxygen metabolism during hypothermic circulatory arrest in humans. J Neurosurg 1993; 79:810–815.
60. Steiner T, Friede T, Aschoff A, Schellinger PD, Schwab S, Hacke W. Effect and feasibility of controlled rewarming after moderate hypothermia in stroke patients with malignant infarction of the middle cerebral artery. Stroke 2001; 32:2833–2835.
61. Schwab S, Georgiadis D, Berrouschot J, Schellinger PD, Graffagnino C, Mayer SA. Feasibility and safety of moderate hypothermia after massive hemispheric infarction. Stroke 2001; 32:2033–2035.
62. Kammersgaard LP, Rasmussen BH, Jorgensen HS, Reith J, Weber U, Olsen TS. Feasibility and safety of inducing modest hypothermia in awake patients with acute stroke through surface cooling: a case-control study. The Copenhagen Stroke Study. Stroke 2000; 31:2251–2256.
63. Krieger DW, De Georgia MA, Abou-Chebl A, Andrefsky JC, Sila CA, Katzan IL, Mayberg MR, Furlan AJ. Cooling for acute ischemic brain damage (COOL-AID): an open pilot study of induced hypothermia in acute ischemic stroke. Stroke 2001; 32:1847–1854.
64. Krieger DW, De Georgia MA, Devlin T, Jauss M, Rordorf G, Koroshetz WJ, Davis S. Cooling acute ischemic brain damage (COOL AID): a randomized pilot trial of endovascular cooling for patients with acute ischemic stroke [abstr]. Stroke 2001; 34:248.
65. Reed RL, Johnston TD, Hudson JD, Fischer RP. The disparity between hypothermic coagulopathy and clotting studies. J Trauma 1992; 33:, 465–470.
66. Valeri CR, Cassidy G, Khuri S, Feingold H, Rango G, Atschule MD. Hypothermia induced reversible platelet dysfunction. Ann Surg 1987; 205:175–181.
67. Resnick DK, Marion DW, Darby JM. The effect of hypothermia on the incidence of delayed traumatic intracerebral hemorrhage. Neurosurgery 1994; 34:252–256.

68. Rohrer MJ, Natale AM. Effect of hypothermia on the coagulation cascade. Crit Care Med 1992; 20:1402–1405.

69. Steen PA, Soule EH, Michenfelder JD. Detrimental effects of prolonged hypothermia in cats and monkeys with and without regional cerebral ischemia. Stroke 1979; 10:522–529.

70. Michenfelder JD, Milde JH. Failure of prolonged hypocapnia, hypothermia, or hypertension to favorably alter acute stroke in primates. Stroke 1977; 8:87–91.

71. Chevret S, Hemmer M, Carlet J, Langer M. Incidence and risk factors of pneumonia acquired in intensive care units. Results from a multicenter prospective study on 996 patients. Intensive Care Med 1993; 19:256–264.

72. Ruiz-Santana S, Gimenez A, Esteban A. ICU pneumonia: a multi-institutional study. Crit Care Med 1987; 15:930–932.

73. Metz C, Holzschuh M, Bein T, Woertgen C, Frey A, Frey I, Taeger K, Brawanski A. Moderate hypothermia in patients with severe head injury: cerebral and extracerebral effects. J Neurosurg 1996; 85:533–541.

74. Foulis AK. Morphological study of the relation between accidental hypothermia and acute pancreatitis. J Clin Pathol 1982; 35:1244–1248.

75. Frietsch T, Piepgras A, Krafft P, Schwab S, Kuschinsky W, Waschke KF. Acid–base management—is it relevant for the study design of hypothermic neuroprotection? Eur J Anaesthesiol 2002; 19:389–394.

76. Hindman BJ. Choice of alpha-stat or pH-stat management and neurologic outcomes after cardiac surgery: it depends. Anesthesiology 1998; 89:5–7.

77. Kollmar R, Frietsch T, Georgiadis D, Schabitz WR, Waschke KF, Kuschinsky W, Schwab S. Early effects of acid–base management during hypothermia on cerebral infarct volume, edema, and cerebral blood flow in acute focal cerebral ischemia in rats. Anesthesiology 2002; 97:868–874.

78. Kurth CD, O'Rourke MM, O'Hara IB. Comparison of pH-stat and alpha-stat cardiopulmonary bypass on cerebral oxygenation and blood flow in relation to hypothermic circulatory arrest in piglets. Anesthesiology 1998; 89:110–118.

79. Clifton GL, Miller ER, Choi SC, Levin HS, McCauley S, Smith KR Jr, Muizelaar JP, Wagner FC Jr, Marion DW, Luerssen TG, Chesnut RM, Schwartz M. Lack of effect of induction of hypothermia after acute brain injury. N Engl J Med 2001; 344:556–563.

80. Zweifler RM, Sessler DI, Zivin JA. Thermoregulatory vasoconstriction and shivering impede therapeutic hypothermia in acute ischemic stroke victims. J Stroke Cerebrovasc Dis 1997; 6:100–104.

81. Kurz A, Sessler DI, Narzt E, Bekar A, Lenhardt R, Huemer G, Lackner F. Postoperative hemodynamic and thermoregulatory consequences of intraoperative core hypothermia. J Clin Anesth 1995; 7:359–366.

82. Xiong J, Kurz A, Sessler DI, Plattner O, Christensen R, Dechert M, Ikeda T. Isoflurane produces marked and nonlinear decreases in the vasoconstriction and shivering thresholds. Anesthesiology 1996; 85:240–245.

83. Lesch KP, Poten B, Sohnle K, Schulte HM. Pharmacology of the hypothermic response to 5-HT1A receptor activation in humans. Eur J Clin Pharmacol 1990; 39:17–19.

84. Young AH, McShane R, Park SB, Cowen PJ. Buspirone-induced hypothermia in normal male volunteers. Biol Psychiatry 1993; 34:665–666.

85. Mokhtarani M, Mahgoub AN, Morioka N, Doufas AG, Dae M, Shaughnessy TE, Bjorksten AR, Sessler DI. Buspirone and meperidine synergistically reduce the shivering threshold. Anesth Analg 2001; 93:1233–1239.

86. Doufas AG, Wadhwa A, Lin C-M, Shah YM, Hanni K, Sessler DI. Neither arm nor face warming reduces the shivering threshold in unanesthetized humans. Stroke 2003; 34:1736–1740.

87. Meden P, Overgaard K, Pedersen H, Boysen G. Effect of hypothermia and delayed thrombolysis in a rat embolic stroke model. Acta Neurol Scand 1994; 90:91–98.

88. Schmutzhard E, Engelhardt K, Beer R, Brossner G, Pfausler B, Spiss H, Unterberger I, Kampfl A. Safety and efficacy of a novel intravascular cooling device to control body temperature in neurologic intensive care patients: a prospective pilot study. Crit Care Med 2002; 30:2481–2488.

15

Hypothermia for Cardiac Arrest

STEPHEN BERNARD
Intensive Care Unit,
Dandenong Hospital,
Dandenong, Australia

INTRODUCTION

During cardiac arrest, cerebral blood flow ceases and consciousness is lost almost immediately. Permanent neurological injury will begin to occur if spontaneous circulation is not restored within several minutes. When cardiac arrest occurs out of the hospital, resuscitation requires attendance by emergency medical services (EMS) and a "chain-of-survival" for successful return of spontaneous circulation (ROSC) (1). However, even in countries with advanced emergency medical care, EMS takes between 4 and 12 min to respond to patients with suspected cardiac arrest and most patients who are initially resuscitated and transported to hospital suffer significant hypoxic–ischemic neurological injury (2). This neurological injury leads to a high rate of major morbidity and mortality in these patients (3).

Mechanisms of Cellular Injury

The mechanisms by which cardiac arrest and subsequent reperfusion causes neurological injury have been reviewed (4). During cardiac arrest, cerebral blood flow ceases and anaerobic glycolysis predominates, with a marked decrease in the generation of adenosine triphosphate. After several minutes of cerebral ischemia, the supply of adenosine triphosphate is exhausted and cellular metabolism ceases. The failure of the sodium/potassium transmembrane pump leads to persistent depolarization of the cell membrane and the shift of sodium and water leads to neuronal cell swelling. In addition, hydrogen and lactate ions are generated, causing an intracellular metabolic acidosis that is toxic to intracellular enzyme systems.

During reperfusion, intracellular levels of glutamate, an excitatory neurotransmitter released from presynaptic terminals, increases markedly (5). Glutamate activates ion channel complexes including *N*-methyl-D-aspartate receptors and alpha-amino-3-hydroxy-5-methyl-4-isoxazole propionic acid receptors. When activated, these ion channels increase calcium conductance from the extracellular to intracellular fluid, and cells begin to flood with calcium. In addition, multiple biochemical cascades lead to the production of oxygen-free radicals and the activation of proteases, endonucleases, phospholipases, and xanthine oxidase which cause cellular injury. Even if these events are not immediately fatal to the cell, some neurons later undergo programmed cell death (apoptosis).

Even after cardiac resuscitation and restoration of systemic blood pressure, cerebral blood flow may remain abnormally low for some hours (6). After an initial hyperemia resulting from high circulating levels of catecholamines, cerebral blood flow decreases just as the cerebral metabolic rate for oxygen increases. This leads to a prolonged state of relative cerebral ischemia. This abnormal cerebral oxygen balance may be worsened by systemic hypoxemia, hypotension, raised intracranial pressure, and/or seizure activity.

Since a considerable amount of the neurological injury may occur after ROSC, there is the possibility that neurological injury may be decreased by therapies applied immediately following resuscitation.

Neuroprotection for Cardiac Arrest

A number of pharmacological interventions that have shown improved neurological outcome in animal models of global cerebral ischemia have undergone human trials. These include a barbiturate (7), a corticosteroid (8), and the calcium antagonists lidoflazine (9) and nimodipine (10), as well as diazepam (11) and magnesium (11). However, none of these studies found improved neurological or improved overall functional outcome.

In the early 1990s, laboratory studies in animal models provided evidence that induced hypothermia (IH) decreased neurological injury when applied shortly after ROSC (12–15). These studies confirmed that IH improved functional performance and histological appearance compared with animals maintained at normothermia. For example, in a dog model of out-of-hospital cardiac arrest, Stertz et al. (12) induced ventricular fibrillation and maintained "no flow" for 10 min, then provided "low flow" with external cardiac compression for a further 5 min. Following defibrillation and ROSC, the animals were supported for 72 hr when a cerebral performance assessment was made. There were 10 animals maintained at normothermia, 10 underwent mild IH (34°C for 1 hr) commencing after ROSC, and another 10 underwent IH during the "no-flow" period. The outcome of the animals at 72 hr is shown in Table 1. Although it had been known for many years that hypothermia was protective if applied before or during cardiac arrest, these data were the first good evidence that mild IH might be useful in patients when applied after resuscitation from cardiac arrest.

The use of induced hypothermia (IH) is theoretically attractive in the setting of cerebral ischemia since cerebral oxygen demand is decreased by approximately 7% for each 1°C decrease in temperature without a corresponding decrease in cerebral oxygen supply. In addition to improving cerebral oxygen balance, clinical studies in patients with stroke and

Table 1 Outcomes of Mild Hypothermia after Resuscitation from Cardiac Arrest in Dogs

Outcomes	Control	Hypothermia after ROSC	Hypothermia during CPR
Dead			
Comatose	4		
Severe disability	5	5	4
Moderate disability	1	3	2
Normal or mild disability		2	4

ROSC: return of spontaneous circulation. CPR: cardiopulmonary resuscitation.
Source: Ref. 12.

trauma suggest that IH decreases the levels of excitotoxic amino acids in the biochemical cascades involved in the reperfusion injury (5). Whereas IH was used for a wide range of neurological disorders between 1938 and 1959 (16,17), there were few clinical reports of the use of IH for global hypoxic–ischemic brain injury related to cardiac arrest between 1960 and 1997 (18). This was presumably based on fears that hypothermia would be associated with increased complications, such as sepsis and/or cardiac arrhythmias in critically ill adults (18). Nevertheless, preliminary safety and feasibility clinical studies were conducted and the results of these supported the findings of animal models. Subsequently, several prospective, randomized, controlled trials were undertaken in adults with neurological injury following out-of-hospital cardiac arrest.

REVIEW

The first use of IH in adult patients with coma following resuscitation from out-of-hospital cardiac arrest was reported by Bernard et al. (19) in Australia. Hypothermia (33°C) was induced in 22 patients in the Emergency Department using surface cooling with ice packs and maintained for 12 hr in the ICU. In comparison to 22 historical controls, there was a significant increase in the number of patients with good outcome (50% compared with 13%).

This preliminary study also described the hemodynamic and biochemical effects of hypothermia. The IH appeared to be well tolerated, and there was no measurable increase in the rate of complications such as sepsis or cardiac arrhythmias.

Other reports from Europe (20) and Japan (21,22) confirmed that IH (33 °C for 12–72 hr) was feasible and not associated with major complications when used in adults who remained comatose after resuscitation from cardiac arrest.

Three randomized, controlled trials of IH in adults with coma after resuscitation from out-of-hospital cardiac arrest have now been undertaken (23–25), with two of these studies examining the effects of IH on outcome (23,24). Of the two studies examining functional outcome, entry criteria were similar: return of spontaneous circulation (ROSC), patients remaining intubated and ventilated, and persistent coma. The majority of patients in these studies had a minimal Glasgow Coma Scale score of 3, and a small number of patients in the larger European study (n = 10) were actually enrolled after in-hospital arrest. Additional criteria for entry into the European study were witnessed cardiac arrest, a maximal interval of 15 min from onset to first resuscitation attempt, and ROSC within 60 min from collapse. Both studies excluded patients in severe cardiogenic shock.

In an Australian study, Bernard et al. (23) enrolled 77 patients with coma following resuscitation from out-of-hospital ventricular fibrillation. There were 43 patients randomized to IH (33 °C for 12 hr) and 34 patients maintained at normothermia, with no significant differences in the baseline characteristics of the patients at study entry. The primary outcome measure was favorable outcome at hospital discharge (defined as discharge to home or rehabilitation facility). There were 21/43 (49%) in the IH group with good outcome compared with 9/34 (26%) in the control group (relative risk for good outcome: 1.85, 95% confidence interval: 0.97–3.49, $P = 0.046$). Following multivariate analysis for differences at baseline, the odds ratio for good outcome in the hypothermic group improved to 5.25 (95% confidence intervals: 1.47–18.76, $P = 0.011$). In the subgroup of patients with a pulmonary artery catheter derived hemodynamic data, IH was associated with decreased cardiac output and increased systemic vascular resistance. The overall incidence of cardiac arrhythmias, sepsis, lactic acidosis, neutropenia, and thrombocytopenia was similar in both groups. However, this study was relatively small and used an odd–even day randomization.

A larger multicenter clinical trial conducted in Europe of comatose survivors of prehospital cardiac arrest enrolled 273 patients, with 136 patients undergoing IH (33°C for 24 hr) and 137 patients maintained at normothermia (24). The primary outcome measure was a favorable outcome at 6 months, defined as a score of 1 or 2 in a Cerebral Performance Score, which is analogous to survival with independence and no, minimal, or

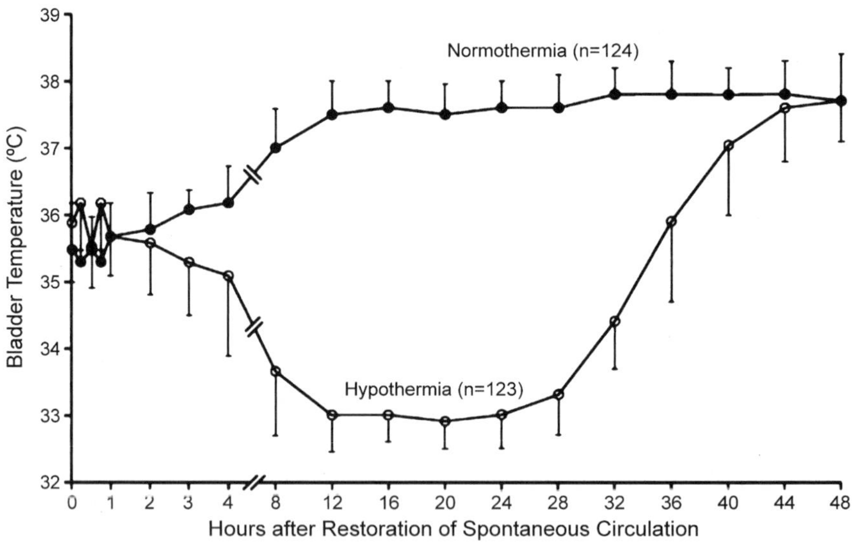

Figure 1 Bladder temperature in the normothermia and hypothermia groups in the HACA trial. The T bars indicate the 75th percentile in the normothermia group and the 25th percentile in the hypothermia group. The target temperature in the hypothermia group was 32–34°C, and the duration of cooling was 24 hr. Only patients with recorded temperatures were included in the analysis. (From Ref. 24.)

moderate disability on the Glasgow Outcome Scale (score of 4 or 5). The hypothermia patients were cooled using cold-air blankets and maintained at 32–34°C for 24 hr. At 6-month follow-up, 55% of the IH patients had a favorable outcome, compared with 39% of normothermic controls (relative risk for good outcome: 1.40, 95% confidence interval: 1.08–1.81). In addition, the mortality rate at 6 months was significantly decreased from 55% to 41% (risk ratio: 0.74, CI: 0.58–0.95). In this study, 6 was the number needed to treat to achieve one good outcome (Fig. 1).

The results of these two randomized, controlled trials appear to provide evidence that IH (33°C) for 12–24 hr is an effective treatment for patients who remain comatose after resuscitation from out-of-hospital cardiac arrest when the initial cardiac rhythm is ventricular fibrillation (26). However, it must be kept in mind that these studies involved a highly selected subgroup of patients, excluding up to 92% of patients screened for eligibility (24) (Fig. 2).

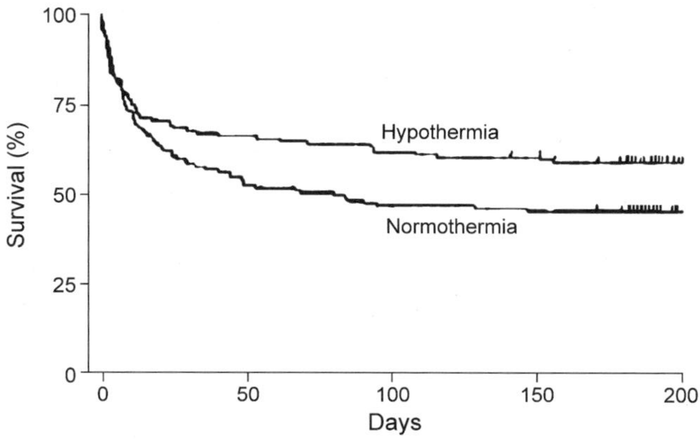

No. at Risk					
Hypothermia	137	92	86	83	11
Normothermia	138	74	66	64	9

Figure 2 Cumulative survival in the normothermia and hypothermia groups in the HACA trial. Censored data are indicated by tick marks. (From Ref. 24.)

Some adverse events occurred more frequently in the hypothermia groups. Although not statistically significant, in the European hypothermia group, there were 22% more complications, including pneumonia, bleeding, and sepsis (24). In the Australian hypothermia group, hypothermia patients experienced more hypoglycemia (23).

In a third prospective, randomized, controlled trial, Hachimi-Idrissi et al. (25) randomized 30 patients with cardiac arrest due to asystole or pulseless electrical activity who remained unconscious after restoration of spontaneous circulation (ROSC) to either hypothermia or normothermia. The primary outcome measure for this study was the efficacy of a cooling helmet device to achieve the core temperature, and the study was not powered to assess an effect on outcome. Therefore this study is discussed further in the following section.

FUTURE DIRECTIONS

Technique of Induction of Hypothermia

There is evidence from animal studies of further improvement in outcome if hypothermia is induced during or immediately after resuscitation (12,14). Therefore, alternative techniques for the rapid induction of hypothermia during or immediately after resuscitation from cardiac arrest will be one important focus of future studies.

Whereas surface cooling with ice packs limited to the head and neck alone appears to be ineffective (27), Hachimi-Idrissi et al. (25) have studied the feasibility and the speed of a cooling helmet device to achieve the target temperature of 34°C in patients who are unconscious after out-of-hospital cardiac arrest. Thirty patients with cardiac arrest due to asystole or pulseless electrical activity (PEA) who remained unconscious after restoration of spontaneous circulation (ROSC) were enrolled in the study. There were 14 randomized to normothermia and 16 to hypothermia. In the latter, a helmet device was used to induce mild hypothermia, and in these patients, the core target temperature of 34°C was achieved after a median time of 180 min after ROSC. The authors concluded that mild hypothermia was able to be easily and inexpensively induced by a helmet device. However, this approach is also relatively slow—probably too slow to be practical. Furthermore, there is no evidence that a cooling helmet specifically cools the brain; instead, it appears to provoke systemic cooling via the scalp.

Most previous studies of the use of IH have used surface cooling with ice packs and/or cold air blankets. Although reasonably feasible and safe (28), this approach has significant limitations for the introduction of IH into routine clinical care. Surface cooling applied to the head, neck, and torso provides for relatively slow core cooling, with a temperature decrease of only 0.3°C per hour in the European study using cold-air cooling (25) and 0.9°C per hour in the Australian study using ice packs (24). In addition, surface cooling with ice packs applied to the torso is inconvenient for medical and nursing staff for the performance of procedures and possibly hazardous for defibrillation. Possible alternatives to surface cooling include the rapid infusion of large volume, ice-cold intravenous fluid, cooling helmets, intravascular cooling devices, and extracorporeal devices.

The effect of large volume, cold fluid intravenous infusion for the induction of moderate hypothermia has been studied in anesthetized volunteers by Rajek et al. (29) who infused 40 mL/kg 0.9% saline solution over 30 min in nine subjects. Using 4°C fluid, the mean decrease in core temperature was 2.5°C (±0.4) which was 0.4°C more than expected if the fluid was distributed evenly.

Although simple, inexpensive, and apparently effective in volunteers, the infusion of a large volume of intravenous fluid into patients who have been resuscitated from cardiac arrest might be expected to result in pulmonary edema. In a study by Bernard et al. (30), 30 mL/kg of ice-cold (4°C) intravenous lactated Ringer's solution was infused at 100 mL/min fluid to induce mild hypothermia in 22 comatose survivors of out-of-hospital cardiac arrest. After initial evaluation in the Emergency Department, a large volume, ice-cold lactated Ringer's solution was infused intravenously over 30 min and vital signs, arterial blood gas, electrolyte, and hematological data were collected immediately before and after the infusion. The infusion significantly decreased core temperature from 35.5°C to 33.9°C and increased mean arterial blood pressure from 90 to 100 mm Hg. There were also improvements in acid–base and renal function. No patient developed pulmonary edema or other adverse effect of the infusion. Currently, a clinical trial of the use of this technique by the EMS in Victoria, Australia, is in progress.

Intravascular cooling devices are now commercially available and preliminary laboratory studies have been conducted which suggest that these are effective for the rapid decrease in core temperature (31). However, the initial and recurrent cost of these devices limits widespread applicability. In addition, personnel with appropriate training are required to be immediately available in the Emergency Room to insert the intravascular catheter. There are similar limitations on the use of extracorporeal techniques for cooling (22,32).

Hypothermia in Patients with Asystole

Previous studies of IH after cardiac arrest have focused on adult patients who present to the EMS with an initial cardiac rhythm of ventricular fibrillation. For patients with an initial cardiac rhythm of asystole or pulseless electrical activity, the role of IH is uncertain. These patients are generally not included in cardiac arrest studies because the outcome is poor. For example, in an Australian study of 778 patients presenting with an initial cardiac rhythm of asystole to an EMS in Victoria, Australia, resuscitation was commenced in 37%; however, there was only one survivor to hospital discharge (33).

Whereas it may be intuitive that some patients with an initial cardiac rhythm of asystole would benefit from IH, it may also be that this treatment only increases the number of patients with severe disability. Further studies are needed.

Hypothermia in Pediatric Patients

Out-of-hospital cardiac arrest in children usually occurs as a result of severe hypoxemia due to asthma, near-drowning, or airway obstruction. When vital signs are absent on arrival of EMS, the survival rate is very low.

One previous observational study of IH in children with neurological injury following near-drowning indicated that this therapy was associated with increased rates of sepsis and adverse outcomes (34). In this study, Bohn et al. (34) used IH in 24 children with anoxic brain injury following near-drowning over a 3-year period. These patients were compared with 16 patients treated over 3 subsequent years with children maintained at normothermia. The authors found that the IH patients had a higher incidence of neutropenia and septicemia, but no improvement in neurological outcome. However, the use of IH in this study was primarily for the control of intracranial hypertension. Whereas the use of early IH for a shorter duration in children with anoxic neurological injury is intuitively attractive, clinical trials with sufficient power to demonstrate improvements in outcome will be difficult to conduct due to the relative rarity of this event in any one city. Therefore, future studies will need to be multicenter to enroll the required numbers of patients.

Hypothermia After Neonatal Birth Asphyxia

Neonates with severe birth asphyxia who are resuscitated from cardiac arrest undergo a similar pathophysiological process of neurological reperfusion injury. Preliminary studies have indicated that the use of mild IH in neonates is feasible (35,36). In a case-control study, Simbruner et al. (37) treated 21 infants suffering neonatal asphyxia with IH. The complications and outcomes were compared with 15 historical controls. Nasopharyngeal temperature in the IH group was maintained at 34–35°C for 72 hr. There were no differences in the rates of complications, and neurological scores at day 5 were significantly improved in the IH group. However, any assessment of efficacy of IH requires long-term follow-up to assess changes in neurological development. Randomized, controlled trials of mild IH in neonates with hypoxic–ischemic encephalopathy are currently underway.

Induced Hypothermia for In-Hospital Cardiac Arrest

Whereas out-of-hospital cardiac arrest is primarily of cardiac origin, most in-hospital cardiac arrests are due to respiratory failure or other noncardiac causes (38). Nevertheless, on the basis of the benefit of IH after out-of-hospital cardiac arrest, it seems intuitive that there would be benefit for the patient who undergoes prolonged resuscitation attempts in the hospital. The only studies of the use of IH after in-hospital cardiac arrest were in the 1950s when Benson et al. (39) reported the use of IH in patients who were resuscitated from in-hospital cardiac arrest using thoracotomy and internal cardiac massage (40). However, this anecdotal use of IH occurred prior to the introduction of external cardiac massage and defibrillation and is therefore of limited relevance to current management.

Neurological Monitoring and the Duration of Induced Hypothermia

Ideally, clinicians managing patients who are at risk of anoxic brain injury after cardiac arrest would have cerebral monitoring to indicate the degree of reperfusion injury and/or cerebral oxygen mismatch. This monitoring would provide information on the required duration of IH and indicate when an increase in cerebral temperature might be appropriate. Currently, there are insufficient data on the optimal duration of hypothermia after resuscitation from cardiac arrest. Neurophysiological monitoring systems which can monitor brain electrical activity, and possibly provide information regarding cerebral metabolic activity and prognosis, are currently in development (Geocadin, MD, personal communication).

REFERENCES

1. Cummins RO, Ornato JP, Thies WH, Pepe PE. Improving survival from sudden cardiac arrest: The "chain of survival" concept. Circulation 1991; 83:1832–1847.
2. Bernard SA. Outcome from prehospital cardiac arrest in Melbourne, Australia. Emerg Med 1998; 10:25–29.
3. Edgren E, Hedstrand U, Kelsey S, Sutton-Tyrrell K, Safar P. Assessment of neurological prognosis of comatose survivors of cardiac arrest. Lancet 1994; 343:1055–1059.

4. Bernard SA. Cerebral resuscitation. In: Cameron P, Jelinek G, Kelly AM, eds. A Textbook of Adult Emergency Medicine. 2nd ed. Churchill Livingstone, 2004.
5. Berger C, Schabitz WR, Georgiadis D, Steiner T, Aschoff A, Schwab S. Effects of hypothermia on excitatory amino acids and metabolism in stroke patients: a microdialysis study. Stroke 2002; 33:519–524.
6. Oku K, Kuboyama K, Safar P, Obrist W, Sterz F, Leonov Y, Tisherman SA. Cerebral and systemic arteriovenous oxygen monitoring after cardiac arrest: inadequate cerebral oxygen delivery. Resuscitation 1994; 27:141–152.
7. The Brain Resuscitation Clinical Trial Study Group. Randomized clinical study of thiopentone loading in comatose survivors of cardiac arrest. N Engl J Med 1986; 314:397–410.
8. The Brain Resuscitation Clinical Trial Study Group. Glucocorticoid treatment does not improve neurologic recovery following cardiac arrest. JAMA 1989; 262:3427–3430.
9. Brain Resuscitation Clinical Trial II Study Group. A randomized clinical study of a calcium-entry blocker (lidoflazine) in the treatment of comatose survivors of cardiac arrest. N Engl J Med 1991; 324:1225–1231.
10. Roine RO, Kaste M, Kinnunen A, Nikki P, Sarna S, Kajaste S. Nimodipine after resuscitation from out-of-hospital ventricular fibrillation. A placebo-controlled, double-blind, randomized trial. JAMA 1990; 264:3171–3177.
11. Longstreth WT Jr, Fahrenbruch CE, Olsufka M, Walsh TR, Copass MK, Cobb LA. Randomized clinical trial of magnesium, diazepam, or both after out-of-hospital cardiac arrest. Neurology 2002; 27:506–514.
12. Stertz F, Safar P, Tisherman SA, Radovsky A, Kuboyama K, Oku K. Mild hypothermic cardiopulmonary resuscitation improves outcome after cardiac arrest in dogs. Crit Care Med 1991; 19:379–389.
13. Weinrauch V, Safar P, Tisherman SA, Kuboyama K, Radovsky A. Cerebral benefit of mild or moderate hypothermia and cardiac risk of deep resuscitative hypothermia after cardiac arrest in dogs. Stroke 1992; 23:1454–1462.

14. Kuboyama K, Safar P, Radovsky A, Tisherman SA, Stezoski SW, Alexander H. Delay in cooling negates the beneficial effect of mild resuscitative cerebral hypothermia after cardiac arrest in dogs: a prospective, randomized study. Crit Care Med 1993; 21:1348–1358.

15. Illievich UM, Zornow MH, Choi KY, Scheller MS, Strnat MA. Effects of hypothermic metabolic suppression on hippocampal glutamate concentrations after transient global cerebral ischemia. Anesth Analg 1994; 78:905–911.

16. Vandam DV, Burnap TK. Hypothermia (Part 1). N Engl J Med 1959; 261:546–553.

17. Vandam DV, Burnap TK. Hypothermia (Part 2). N Engl J Med 1959; 261:595–603.

18. Bernard SA. Induced hypothermia in intensive care medicine: A review. Anaesth Int Care 1996; 24:382–388.

19. Bernard SA, Jones BM, Horne MK. A clinical trial of induced hypothermia in comatose survivors of prehospital cardiac arrest. Ann Emerg Med 1997; 30:146–153.

20. Zeiner A, Holzer M, Stertz F, Behringer W, Schorkhuber W, Mullner M, Frass M, Siostrzonek P, Ratheiser K, Kaff A, Laggner AN. Mild resuscitative hypothermia to improve neurological outcome after cardiac arrest. A clinical feasibility trial. Stroke 2000; 31:86–94.

21. Yanagawa Y, Ishihara S, Norio H, Takino M, Kawakami M, Takasu A, Okamato K, Kaneko N, Terai C, Okada Y. Preliminary clinical outcome study of mild resuscitative hypothermia after out-of-hospital cardiac arrest. Resuscitation 1998; 39:61–66.

22. Nagao K, Hayashi N, Kanmatsuse K, Arima K, Ohtsuki J, Kikushima K, Watanabe I. Cardiopulmonary cerebral resuscitation using emergency cardiopulmonary bypass, coronary reperfusion therapy and mild hypothermia in patients with cardiac arrest outside the hospital. J Am Coll Cardiol 2000; 36:776–783.

23. Bernard SA, Gray TW, Buist MD, Jones BM, Silvester W, Gutteridge G, Smith K. Treatment of comatose survivors of out-of-hospital cardiac arrest with induced hypothermia. N Engl J Med 2002; 346:557–563.

24. The Hypothermia after Cardiac Arrest Study Group. Mild therapeutic hypothermia to improve the neurological outcome after cardiac arrest. N Engl J Med 2002; 346:549–556.

25. Hachimi-Idrissi S, Corne L, Ebinger G, Michotte Y, Huyghens L. Mild hypothermia induced by a helmet device: a clinical feasibility study. Resuscitation 2001; 51:275–281.

26. Smith TL, Bleck TP. Hypothermia and neurologic outcome in patients following cardiac arrest: should we be hot to cool off our patients? Crit Care 2002; 6:377–380.

27. Callaway CW, Tadler SC, Katz LM, Lipinski CL, Brader E. Feasibility of external cranial cooling during out-of-hospital cardiac arrest. Resuscitation 2002; 52:159–165.

28. Felberg RA, Kreiger DW, Chuang R, Persse DE, Burgin WS, Hickenbottom SL, Morgenstern LB, Rosales O, Grotta JC. Hypothermia after cardiac arrest: feasibility and safety of an external cooling protocol. Circulation 2001; 104:1799–1804.

29. Rajek A, Grief R, Sessler DI, Baumgardner J, Laciny S, Bastanmehr H. Core cooling by central venous infusion of ice-cold (4 degrees Celsius or 20 degrees C) fluid: isolation of core and peripheral thermal compartments. Anaesthesiology 2000; 93:629–637.

30. Bernard SA, Buist MD, Monteiro O, Smith K. Induced hypothermia using large volume, ice-cold intravenous fluid in comatose survivors of out-of-hospital cardiac arrest: A preliminary report. Resuscitation 2003; 56:9–13.

31. Dae MW, Gao DW, Ursell PC, Stillson CA, Sessler DI. Safety and efficacy of endovascular cooling and rewarming for induction and reversal of hypothermia in human-sized pigs. Stroke 2003; 34:734–738.

32. Mori K, Saito J, Kurata Y, Takeyama Y, Itoh Y, Kaneko M, Asai Y, Renzi FP, Dickson EW. Rapid development of brain hypothermia using femoral-carotid bypass. Acad Emerg Med 2001; 8:303–308.

33. Meyer A, Bernard SA, Smith KL, McNeil JJ, Cameron PA. Asystolic cardiac arrest in Melbourne, Australia. Emerg Med 2001; 13:186–189.

34. Bohn DJ, Biggar WD, Smith CR, Conn AW, Barker GA.

Influence of hypothermia, barbiturate therapy, and intracranial pressure monitoring on morbidity and mortality after near-drowning. Crit Care Med 1986; 14:529–534.

35. Gunn AJ, Gluckman PD, Gunn TR. Selective head cooling in newborn infants after perinatal asphyxia: a safety study. Paediatrics 1998; 102:885–892.

36. Azzopardi D, Robertson NJ, Cowan FM, Rutherford MA, Rampling M, Edwards AD. Pilot study of treatment with whole body hypothermia for neonatal encephalopathy. Pediatrics 2000; 106:684–694.

37. Simbruner G, Haberi C, Harrison V, Linley L, Willeitner AE. Induced hypothermia in asphyxiated human newborn infants: a retrospective chart analysis of physiological and adverse effects. Int Care Med 1999; 25:1111–1117.

38. Buist MD, Moore GE, Bernard SA, Waxman BP, Anderson JN, Nguyen TV. Effects of a medical emergency team on reduction of incidence of and mortality from unexpected cardiac arrests in hospital: preliminary study. BMJ 2002; 324:1–6.

39. Benson DW, Williams GR, Spencer FC, Yates AJ. The use of hypothermia after cardiac arrest. Anesth Analg 1959; 38:423–428.

40. Williams GR Jr, Spencer FC. Clinical use of hypothermia following cardiac arrest. Ann Surg 1959; 148:462–468.

16

Hypothermia for Acute Myocardial Infarction

SIMON R. DIXON and WILLIAM W. O'NEILL
William Beaumont Hospital,
Royal Oak, Michigan, U.S.A.

INTRODUCTION

Despite advances in reperfusion therapy, acute myocardial infarction remains a major public health problem throughout the world. Following acute coronary artery occlusion, progressive myocardial injury develops in a time-dependent manner that rapidly leads to irreversible cell death (1). Complications such as congestive heart failure, arrhythmia, and death are directly related to the extent of myonecrosis and subsequent pump failure. As left ventricular function is the most important determinant of survival after myocardial infarction, the primary goal of modern therapies is to salvage jeopardized myocardium and limit infarct size (2–7). Recent studies suggest that hypothermia may be cardioprotective during acute myocardial infarction. Although the focus of research on therapeutic hypothermia has been as a neuroprotective strategy, there appears to be an equally sound rationale for using cooling to protect ischemic myocardium. This chapter will review the experimental data that form the scientific basis for applying hypothermia in acute myocardial infarction, as well as recent developments in clinical trials investigating this novel therapy.

REVIEW

Determinants of Myocardial Salvage

Survival of ischemic myocardium is fundamentally dependent on a balance between the blood flow deficit and metabolic demand in the area distal to the coronary occlusion (8) (Table 1). Previous studies have shown that increasing the supply of oxygen and/or substrate to the affected area or decreasing metabolic demand can reduce the size and severity of ischemic injury (9). Since the pathophysiological basis for acute myocardial infarction was established, however, efforts to limit infarct size have predominantly focused on restoring epicardial coronary flow (10). More recently, attention has shifted downstream as the importance of the microcirculation

Table 1 Determinants of Myocardial Salvage in Acute Myocardial Infarction

Determinants of myocardial salvage
Duration of occlusion
Intermittency of occlusion
Maintenance of patency
Myocardial oxygen demand
Extent of collateral circulation

Source: Ref. 8.

and myocardial perfusion has been recognized. Studies performed with intracoronary myocardial contrast echocardiography have demonstrated that up to 30% of patients undergoing primary angioplasty have poor myocardial perfusion or "no-reflow" despite recanalization of the infarct vessel (11–13). Failure to reestablish tissue level perfusion may be due to several different mechanisms, including ischemia-induced microvascular damage, reperfusion injury, and distal embolization from the lesion site (14–20). Regardless of the mechanism, the presence of myocardial "no-reflow" is associated with progressive ventricular dilatation and poor recovery of ventricular function in the infarct zone (21). Thus there is a clear need for new therapeutic strategies to enhance myocyte protection during reperfusion therapy.

Experimental Studies of Hypothermia in Acute Myocardial Infarction

Historical Overview

In the 1950s, hypothermia was considered dangerous when used during evolving myocardial infarction because of a high incidence of ventricular fibrillation in animal models (22–25). However, subsequent investigators found that induction of moderate hypothermia in dogs after coronary occlusion was not associated with an increase in arrhythmia and appeared to be associated with improved hemodynamic recovery after rewarming (26–29). Over the next two decades, hypothermia gained widespread acceptance as a cardioprotective strategy during cardiac surgery; however, there was relatively little research in cooling for acute myocardial infarction. These studies were conducted largely in the prereperfusion era and used moderate, whole-body cooling or hypothermic synchronized retroperfusion in experimental models of coronary occlusion without reperfusion (30–35) (Table 2). Overall, these experiments suggested that moderate hypothermia, induced after coronary occlusion, significantly decreased ischemic injury and was associated with preservation of hemodynamic parameters and left ventricular function during ischemia.

Table 2 Experimental Studies of Moderate Hypothermia in Myocardial Infarction

Author	Model	Target temperature	Technique	Onset of cooling	Duration of cooling	Results
Abendschein et al. (30)	Dog	26°C	Surface	30 min after occlusion	5 or 10 hr	Hypo ↓ 25% ischemic injury at 5 hr
Meerbaum et al. (31)	Dog	20°C[a]	HSRP	30 min after occlusion	3 or 6 hr	↓ Infarct size in HSRP grp (7.5% vs. 47% at 3 hr)
Haendchen et al. (32)	Dog	—	HSRP	30 min after occlusion	2.5 hr	↓ Infarct size in HSRP grp (12% vs. 4.2%). Better EF during occlusion
Voorhees et al. (33)	Dog	26°C	Surface	30 min after occlusion	5 hr	↓ Necrosis with hypothermia
Bergmann et al. (34)	Dog	27°C	Surface	30 min after occlusion	2 hr	Preserved hemodynamic parameters during ischemia in hypothermia grp
Wakida et al. (35)	Dog	15°C[a]	HSRP	30 min after occlusion	3 hr	↓ Infarct size in HSRP grp (6.2% vs. 24.1% at 3.5 hr)

HSRP = Hypothermic synchronized retroperfusion; EF = ejection fraction.
[a] Temperature of arterial blood retroperfused into coronary veins.

Relationship Between Myocardial Temperature and Necrosis

Interest in the use of therapeutic hypothermia for acute myocardial infarction was rejuvenated in the mid-1990s. At that time, several investigators demonstrated that there is an important relationship between myocardial temperature and the extent of tissue necrosis after coronary artery occlusion (36–38). Chien et al. found that small changes of temperature within the normothermic range significantly influenced myocardial infarct size, independent of changes in heart rate. In fact, infarct size was reduced by about 10% for each 1°C of myocardial hypothermia (36) (Fig. 1). These data highlighted the importance of controlling for myocardial temperature in experimental models of myocardial infarction, but also led to

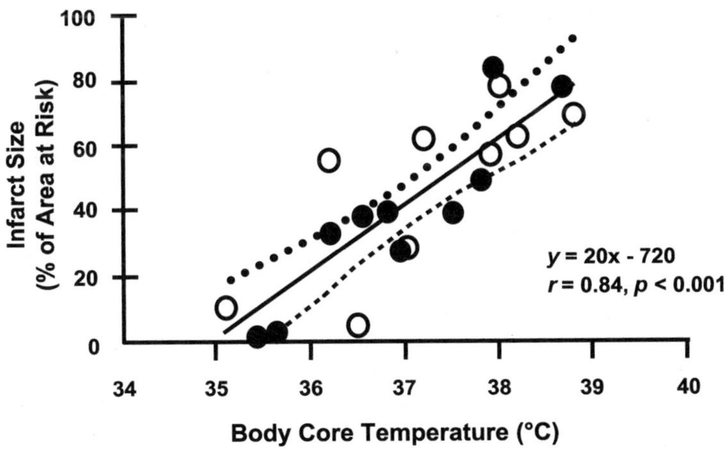

Figure 1 Relationship between body core temperature and infarct size produced by 45 min of coronary artery occlusion in 10 control swine (closed circles) and nine swine pretreated with adenosine-receptor blocker 8-phenyltheophylline (8-PT, 5mg/kg i.v.) and adenosine deaminase (ADA, 50 U/kg i.c., open circles). Relationship between temperature and infarct size was not different between the two treatment groups. Solid line represents regression line for all 19 animals. Dashed lines represent 95% confidence intervals. (From Ref. 37.)

Table 3 Experimental Studies of Mild Hypothermia in Acute Myocardial Infarction

Author	Model	Target temperature[a]	Technique	Onset of cooling	Duration of cooling	Results
Before coronary occlusion						
Hale and Kloner (39)	Rabbit	35°C (3.6°C)	TRH	20 min before occlusion	65 min	↓ Infarct size with cooling (16% vs. 46% of area at risk)
van den Doel (40)	Rat	30–31°C	Surface	Before	15–120 min	Hypothermia enhanced protective effect of ischemic preconditioning, but no benefit with prolonged occlusion
Dave et al. (41)	Rabbit	34°C (5°C)	CCP	30 min before occlusion	55 min	↓ Infarct size with cooling (18% vs. 35% of area at risk)
After coronary occlusion						
Boyer and Gerstein (29)	Dog	32°C	Surface	Not reported	Not reported	↓ Myocardial O_2 consumption and LVEDP with hypothermia

Hale et al. (42)	Rabbit	32°C (6.3°C)	TRH	10 or 25 min after occlusion	5 or 25 min	Early cooling ↓ infarct size (23% vs. 44%); however, no benefit with late cooling
Miki et al. (43)	Rabbit	32°C or 35°C	Heat exchanger	5 min before, and 10 or 20 min after	35–40 min	Better cardioprotection at 32°C then 35°C and with early cooling
Hale and Kloner (44)	Rabbit	30°C (10°C)	TRH	30 min after occlusion	90 min[b]	At 120 min, ↓ infarct size with cooling (59% vs. 72% of area at risk)
Dae et al. (45)	Pig	34°C (4°C)	Endovascular	20 min after occlusion	55 min + gradual rewarming	↓ Infarct size with hypothermia (9% vs. 45% of area at risk)
Hale et al. (46)	Rabbit	32°C	Surface	10 min before and 2 hr after reperfusion	2 hr	↓ Anatomic no-reflow and infarct size, and ↑ regional myocardial flow in risk region with hypothermia

TRH = Topical regional hypothermia; CCP = closed circuit pericardioperfusion.
[a] Mean temperature reduction from baseline shown in parentheses.
[b] Model of prolonged coronary ischemia.

further investigation into the potential therapeutic effects of mild hypothermia.

Effect of Mild Hypothermia

Several animal studies have demonstrated that reducing the temperature of the heart by even a few degrees centigrade is beneficial during regional myocardial ischemia (Table 3) (39–46). However, the cardioprotective effect of mild hypothermia appears to depend on several factors including the timing of cooling, depth of hypothermia, and duration of ischemia.

As might be expected, hypothermia provides most protection when cooling is initiated before the onset of myocardial ischemia. In a rabbit model, Hale and coworkers induced mild hypothermia using topical cooling 20 min before coronary artery occlusion (39). After 5 min of occlusion, the myocardial temperature in the risk region was reduced by 3.6°C. Cooling was associated with a profound reduction in mean infarct size (16 ± 3% vs. 46 ± 4% of the risk zone, $p < 0.0001$) and appeared to alter the relationship between the size of the risk region and extent of necrosis (Fig. 2). Similar results were found in another study using a pericardial catheter to cool the heart before ischemia (41).

Subsequent studies confirmed that mild hypothermia is also beneficial when applied after coronary occlusion, although the protective effect diminishes when cooling is started late after the onset of ischemia (42,43). In a 30-min rabbit occlusion model, Hale et al. started cooling either 10 or 25 min after occlusion (42). Early cooling reduced myocardial temperature from 38.5 ± 0.1°C to 32.2 ± 0.4°C, whereas late cooling lowered the myocardial temperature to 32.5 ± 0.8°C. Compared with the control group, early cooling resulted in a significant reduction in infarct size (23 ± 4% vs. 44 ± 4% of the risk region, $p = 0.01$); however, there was no benefit in the late cooling group (43 ± 4% vs. 44 ± 4%). Miki et al. also found that the protective effect of hypothermia was time-dependent (43). These investigators employed a novel heat exchanger between the carotid artery and jugular vein to induce hypothermia. Rabbit hearts were cooled either before coronary occlusion, or

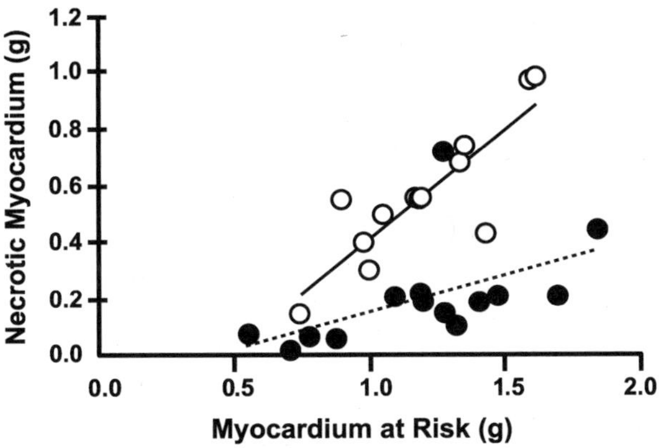

Figure 2 Effect of mild regional hypothermia before the onset of myocardial ischemia. Scatterogram of the necrotic area plotted against risk area of hearts in control (○) and topical regional hypothermia (●) groups. For any given size of the risk zone, a substantially smaller infarct developed in the hypothermia-treated hearts. (From Ref. 39.)

10 or 20 min after occlusion. Studies were performed at a target temperature of both 32°C and 35°C. In contrast to the study by Hale et al., late onset cooling was associated with a significant reduction in infarct size when the temperature was lowered to 32°C; however, protection was not observed at 35°C (Fig. 3). These data suggest that cooling needs to be initiated as soon as possible after the onset of ischemia to optimally protect the myocardium from ischemic injury.

In a more recent study, Dae et al. evaluated the effect of mild hypothermia on infarct size in human-sized pigs using an endovascular heat-exchange catheter (45). Cooling was started 20 min after occlusion of the left anterior descending coronary artery and was continued for 15 min after reperfusion. The catheter was used to lower the core body temperature to 34°C or to maintain normothermia (38°C). Although the size of the area-at-risk was similar in both hypothermic animals and normothermic controls, infarct size was significantly reduced in the hypothermic group ($9 \pm 6\%$ vs. $45 \pm 8\%$, $p < 0.0001$) (Fig. 4). Moreover, additional studies with sestamibi autoradiography

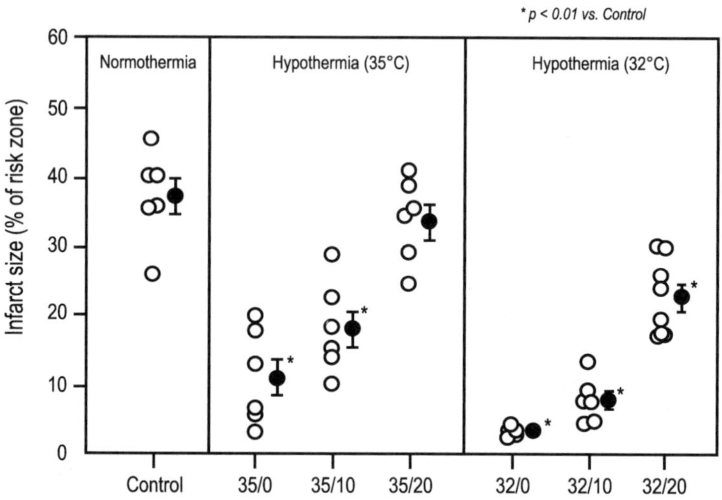

Figure 3 Effect of mild hypothermia (32°C or 35°C) on infarct size in rabbits after a 30-min coronary artery occlusion. Hypothermia was commenced either before ischemia (0), or 10 or 20 min after occlusion. Infarct size is normalized as a percent of the risk zone and is plotted for each group. Open and closed circles indicate individual experiments and group means, respectively. Note that the protection observed depends both on the temperature and the duration of cooling. (From Ref. 43.)

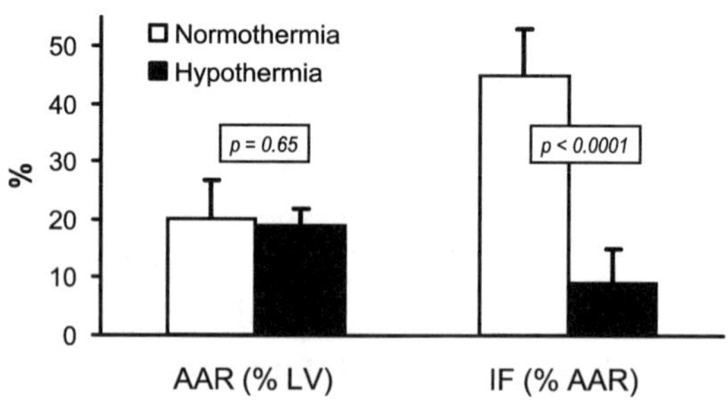

Figure 4 Infarct size in hypothermic pigs and normothermic controls after coronary occlusion and reperfusion. The size of the area-at-risk (AAR) was comparable in both groups; however, infarct size (IF) was significantly reduced in the hypothermia group. (From Ref. 45.)

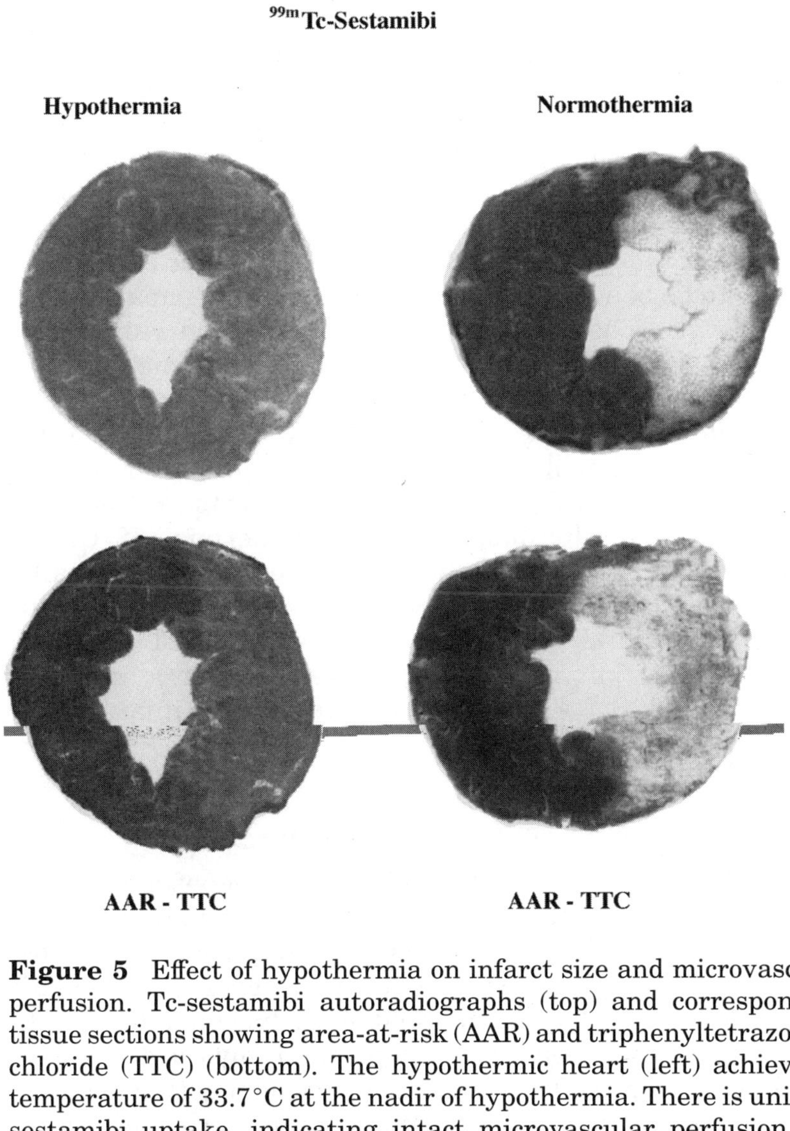

Figure 5 Effect of hypothermia on infarct size and microvascular perfusion. Tc-sestamibi autoradiographs (top) and corresponding tissue sections showing area-at-risk (AAR) and triphenyltetrazolium chloride (TTC) (bottom). The hypothermic heart (left) achieved a temperature of 33.7°C at the nadir of hypothermia. There is uniform sestamibi uptake, indicating intact microvascular perfusion and myocyte viability, and TTC positivity in the AAR. The normothermic heart (right) was maintained at a temperature of 38.2°C. There is a dense sestamibi perfusion defect that corresponds to the TTC-negative region shown at the bottom, indicating infarction. (From Ref. 45.)

demonstrated that salvaged myocardium showed normal radiotracer uptake, thus suggesting that cooling exerts a protective effect for both myocytes and the microcirculation (Fig. 5).

The optimal duration of cooling after reperfusion remains unclear, as no studies have directly compared the effect of short vs. prolonged hypothermia in the reperfusion period. Most of the aforementioned studies started rewarming soon after reperfusion. Nonetheless, prolonged cooling after reperfusion is likely to be beneficial, given that progressive impairment of myocardial flow associated with reperfusion injury may occur over several hours (47). Prolonged hypothermia may be especially important when cooling is initiated late after the onset of myocardial ischemia. Recent data from Hale et al. suggest that maintenance of hypothermia for several hours after reperfusion attenuates reperfusion injury and protects the microvasculature (46). In this model, mild hypothermia (32°C) was induced 10 min before reperfusion and continued for 2 hr after reperfusion. Hypothermia-treated animals had significantly higher myocardial flow in the risk region (1.21 ± 0.15 vs. 0.65 ± 0.11 mL/min/g, $p = 0.0048$), less anatomic no-reflow ($11 \pm 3\%$ vs. $37 \pm 3\%$, $p = 0.0001$), and smaller infarcts than normothermic controls.

Potential Mechanisms for Cardioprotection

Although it is generally believed that the beneficial effect of hypothermia is due to reducing metabolic demand in the risk region, the precise mechanisms by which cooling provides protection during myocardial ischemia–reperfusion remain poorly defined (Table 4). In isolated perfused rabbit hearts, hypothermia has been shown to preserve myocardial adenosine triphosphate (ATP) stores during ischemia, thus facilitating the maintenance of cell membrane integrity (48). More recent data suggest that cooling also reduces myocyte apoptosis in response to ischemia by altering expression of anti- or proapoptotic genes (49). Furthermore, hypothermia enhances production of heat shock proteins, which are believed to have a protective role in ischemia–reperfusion (48). However, it is likely that the cardioprotective effects of hypothermia are far

Table 4 Potential Mechanisms of Action of Hypothermia in the Heart: Supportive Evidence

Possible mechanism	Model	Results
↓ Metabolic demand in the risk region	Isolated rabbit perfused heart (48)	Preservation of ATP during ischemia reperfusion
↓ Myocyte apoptosis	Isolated rabbit perfused heart (49)	↑ Expression antiapoptotic gene (Bcl-2 homologue Bcl-x) and ↓ expression of the proapoptotic Bcl-2 homologue Bak
? Induction of heat shock proteins	Isolated rabbit perfused heart (48)	↑ Levels of inducible heat shock protein (HSP70-1) mRNA after ischemia in hypothermic hearts
? ↓ Reperfusion injury	Rabbit (46)	↓ Infarct size with cooling initiated just before reperfusion
? ↓ Free radical production	—	—
? ↓ Inflammatory response	—	—

more complex; further studies are thus required to determine whether myocardial cooling influences other biochemical and cellular processes such as free radical production or the inflammatory response following reperfusion. The protective effect of myocardial cooling appears to be independent of hypothermia-induced bradycardia, as the effect persists when the heart rate is maintained with pacing (39). One of the principal advantages of hypothermia for cell protection is that the myocardium is cooled by conduction from the blood pool and, unlike pharmacological therapies, does not require antegrade flow to the ischemic region.

Cardiac Effects of Hypothermia

Early experimental data demonstrated that hypothermia improves cardiac function, even in animals with cardiogenic shock (29). Specifically, reductions in left ventricular end-

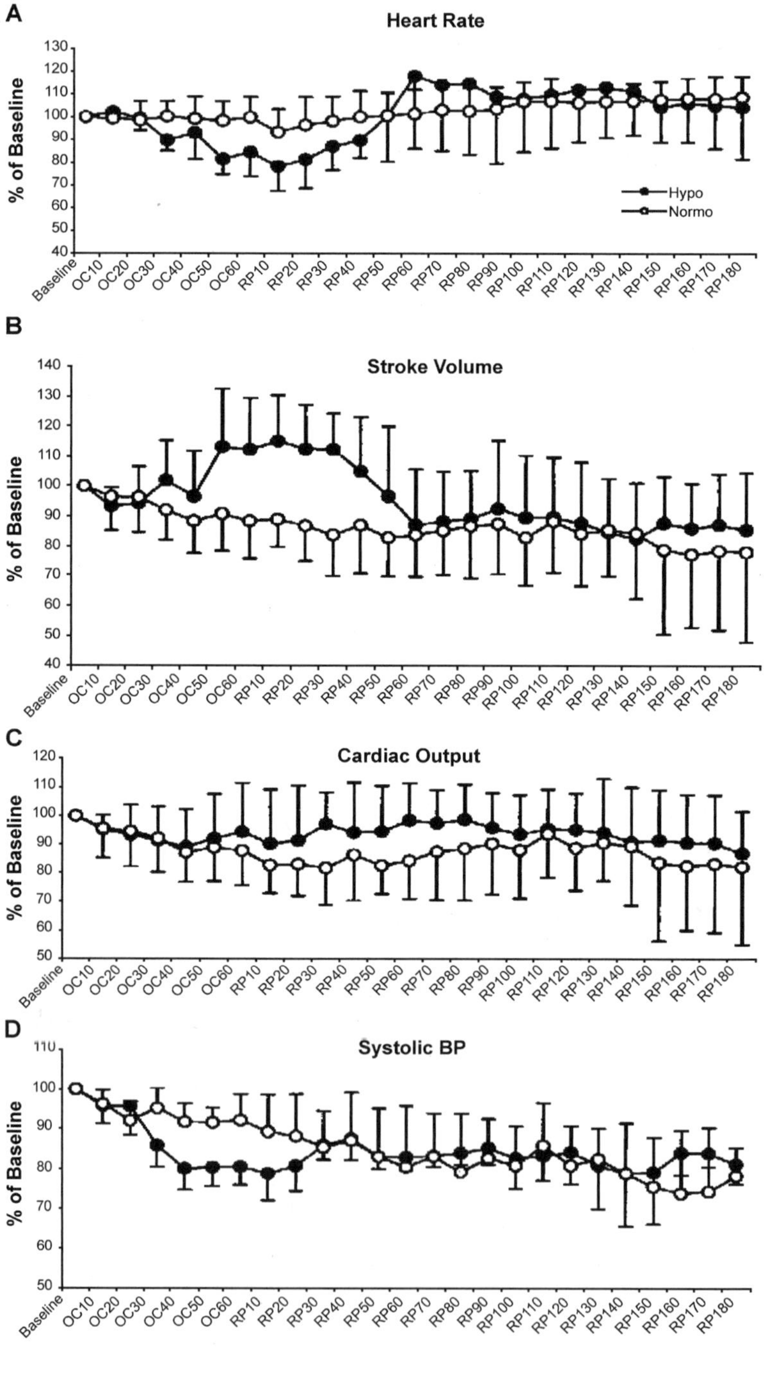
A
Heart Rate
% of Baseline
Hypo
Normo
B
Stroke Volume
% of Baseline
C
Cardiac Output
% of Baseline
D
Systolic BP
% of Baseline
Baseline
OC10
OC20
OC30
OC40
OC50
OC60
RP10
RP20
RP30
RP40
RP50
RP60
RP70
RP80
RP90
RP100
RP110
RP120
RP130
RP140
RP150
RP160
RP170
RP180

diastolic pressure (LVEDP) and heart rate were noted with cooling, while cardiac output and stroke work were unchanged (29). More recent studies have confirmed that induction of mild hypothermia in animals is well tolerated without adverse hemodynamic effects (39, 43, 45, 50). Although a small decrease in heart rate and systolic blood pressure may be observed during cooling, cardiac output is maintained as a result of an increase in stroke volume (Fig. 6) (45, 50). Mild hypothermia has been shown to improve myocardial contractility in normal hearts, without an increase in sarcoplasmic reticulum Ca^{2+} content (51,52). This effect is likely to explain the improved hemodynamic parameters observed with cooling. In contrast, other studies have shown left ventricular dysfunction following rewarming with deeper levels of hypothermia (25°C) (53). Mild hypothermia does not appear to affect coronary blood flow or flow reserve in normal animals (54,55), nor alter blood flow in the ischemic region following coronary artery occlusion (33).

Clinical Experience with Hypothermia in Myocardial Infarction

Techniques to Induce Hypothermia During Myocardial Infarction

One of the major challenges facing investigators in this field has been to develop clinically effective and practical techniques to induce therapeutic hypothermia in patients with acute myocardial infarction. Although external cooling with ice packs and cooling blankets has been used successfully in clinical studies of cardiac arrest, stroke, and brain trauma (56–62), these methods are too cumbersome and imprecise for this setting. On the other hand, methods such as extracorporeal blood cooling circuits, cardiopulmonary bypass, pericardial perfusion, and peritoneal cooling can be used to rapidly induce

---

Figure 6 Heart rate, stroke volume, cardiac output, and systolic blood pressure (BP) in hypothermic pigs (●; $n = 5$) and normothermic controls (○; $n = 5$) during coronary occlusion (OC) and reperfusion (RP). Values are expressed as a % of baseline. (From Ref. 45.)

hypothermia, but are too invasive to permit widespread application of cooling in myocardial infarction.

The introduction of catheter-based techniques to induce hypothermia has been a major advance in this field. Three endovascular cooling systems are currently under investigation in the United States for the treatment of acute myocardial infarction (Table 5). These systems utilize a heat-exchange catheter that is placed percutaneously in the inferior vena cava via the femoral vein, and a central controller that circulates cool or warm saline to alter core temperature. With these systems, mild hypothermia can be induced relatively rapidly (4–6°C/hr), and core body temperature maintained precisely at a desired target temperature.

More recently, a novel surface cooling system has been developed that also has promise in acute myocardial infarction (Arctic Sun Temperature Management System, Medivance® Inc., Louisville, CO). This system uses water-based adhesive (hydrogel) pads, which are applied to the patient's back, abdomen, and legs, to transfer heat energy by mimicking the effects of water immersion. One advantage of this system is that nursing staff can place the hydrogel pads so cooling can be initiated rapidly in the emergency room. For more information on techniques to induce hypothermia, refer to Chapter 10.

Initial Experience With Endovascular Cooling

In February 2001, we initiated a pilot study (COOL-MI pilot) to evaluate the safety and feasibility of endovascular cooling in patients with acute myocardial infarction undergoing primary angioplasty (63). Forty-two patients with anterior or large inferior infarction presenting within 6 hr of symptom onset were randomized to mechanical reperfusion with or without adjunctive mild hypothermia. Exclusion criteria included cardiogenic shock, rescue angioplasty, myocardial infarction within 1 month, Raynaud's disease, hypersensitivity to buspirone or meperidine, treatment with a monoamine oxidase inhibitor in the previous 14 days, bleeding diathesis or coagulopathy, severe hepatic or renal impairment, pregnancy, patient height <1.5 m, or the presence of an inferior vena cava filter.

Table 5 Cooling Systems Under Investigation in Acute Myocardial Infarction

Cooling system	Company	Heat exchange system	Temperature monitoring	Sheath size
Endovascular cooling				
Reprieve™ Endovascular Temperature Therapy System	Radiant Medical Inc.	Reprieve™ catheter	Naso-esophageal probe or intravenous probe (SetProbe)	10F
CoolGard® Temperature Management System	Alsius Corporation	Fortius™ catheter	Bladder catheter	12F
Celsius Control™ System	Innercool Therapies Inc.	Celsius Control™ catheter	Catheter-based thermistor	10.7 or 14F
Surface cooling				
Arctic Sun® Temperature Management System	Medivance Inc.	Hydrogel pads	Tympanic	NA

Cooling was performed using the Reprieve™ Endovascular Temperature Therapy System (Radiant Medical Inc., Redwood City, CA) (Fig. 7) and was initiated either in the emergency room or cardiac catheterization laboratory before primary angioplasty. The target core body temperature was 33°C (monitored with a naso-esophageal probe). Cooling was maintained for 3 hr after reperfusion, followed by controlled rewarming to 36.5°C. Shivering was suppressed using skin warming with a forced air blanket (Bair Hugger, Arizant Healthcare Inc., Eden Prairie, MN), oral buspirone (30–60

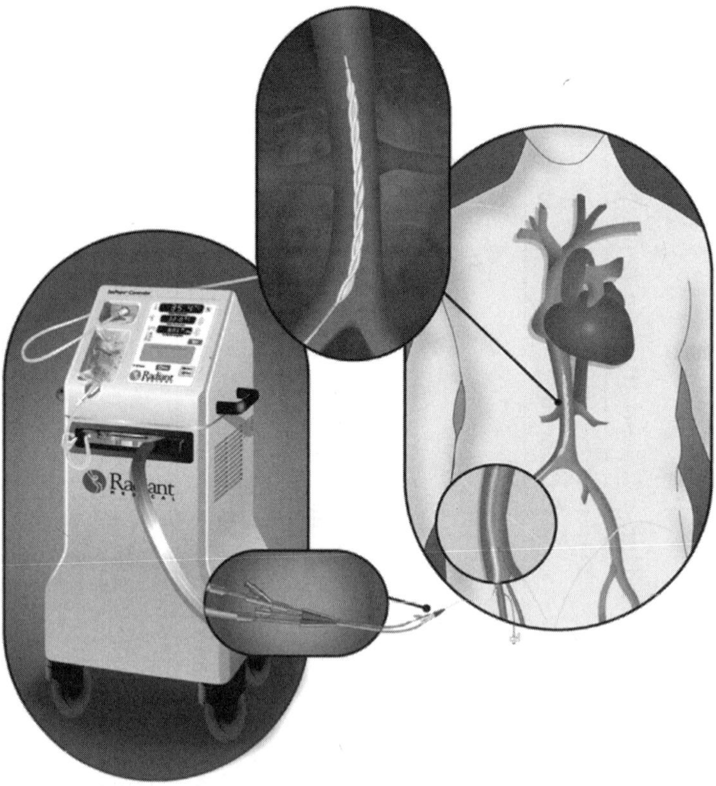

Figure 7 Diagram of the endovascular cooling system used in the COOL-MI randomized trial (Reprieve™ Endovascular Temperature Therapy System, Radiant Medical Inc., Redwood City, CA).

mg), and intravenous meperidine (75–100 mg loading dose over 15 min, followed by an intravenous meperidine infusion at 25–35 mg/hr) (64). The primary endpoint was major adverse cardiac events at 30 days.

Endovascular cooling was well tolerated, and no hemodynamic instability or increase in ventricular arrhythmia was observed in the hypothermia group. Nine patients experienced mild episodic shivering during cooling. Four of these were managed successfully with additional meperidine and surface warming; five patients required a small increase in target core temperature to between 33.5°C and 34.2°C. The mean doses of meperidine and buspirone administered were 177 ± 71 and 51 ± 17 mg, respectively. We concluded that endovascular cooling was safe and well tolerated during acute myocardial infarction and that shivering could be suppressed successfully using skin warming and pharmacological therapy.

A 20-patient feasibility study (LOWTEMP Pilot) was recently completed using the CoolGard® Temperature Management System (Alsius Corporation, Irvine, CA). This consists of a collapsible, spiral-shaped balloon catheter (Fortius™), and an external temperature control system (CoolGard®). Hypothermia was induced prior to primary percutaneous coronary intervention (PCI) to achieve a target temperature of 32–34°C for a total of 4 hr (1 hr induction, 3 hr maintenance) followed by active and passive rewarming to normothermia. Core body temperature was monitored using a thermistor mounted on a urinary bladder catheter. The CoolGard® System successfully reduced core body temperature (mean 33.7 ± 0.9°C), and there were no safety concerns, thus supporting further evaluation with this system in acute myocardial infarction (65).

Experience With Surface Cooling

In a pilot study conducted at the Montreal Heart Institute, the Arctic Sun® Temperature Management System was used to induce mild hypothermia in 11 patients with acute myocardial infarction undergoing primary angioplasty (R. Bonan, personal communication, 2003). Cooling was initiated in the emergency room and intravenous meperidine was used to suppress

Table 6 Clinical Trials of Hypothermia for Acute Myocardial Infarction

Acronym	Design	Inclusion criteria	Cooling system	Number of patients	Target temperature	Duration of cooling	Primary endpoint
Nonrandomized studies							
LOWTEMP	Registry	MI < 6 hr	CoolGard® Temperature Management System	20	32–34C	4 hr	Infarct size
NICAMI	Registry	MI < 6 hr	Arctic Sun® Temperature Management System	11	34C	3 hr	MACE
Randomized studies							
COOL-MI Pilot	Randomized, pilot study	MI < 6 hr	Reprieve™ Endovascular Temperature Therapy System	42	33C	3 hr[a]	MACE
COOL-MI	Randomized, multicenter	MI < 6 hr	Reprieve™ Temperature Therapy System	412	33C	3 hr[a]	Infarct size
ICE-IT	Randomized, multicenter	MI < 6 hr	Celsius Control™ System	Enrolling. Planned = 400	33C	6 hr	Infarct size

MACE = major adverse cardiac events.
[a] From first balloon inflation.

shivering. Results indicate that surface cooling is safe and feasible in these patients and that core body temperature can be lowered below 35°C within 60 min. A multicenter trial of hypothermia using this surface cooling system is currently being planned.

Randomized Trials of Hypothermia

Two randomized clinical trials of hypothermia for acute myocardial infarction have been undertaken in the United States: COOL-MI and ICE-IT (Table 6). The COOL-MI trial was completed in April 2003; the ICE-IT trial is currently enrolling patients. Both trials were designed to evaluate the efficacy of adjunctive hypothermia during primary angioplasty, using final infarct size as the primary study endpoint. These are the

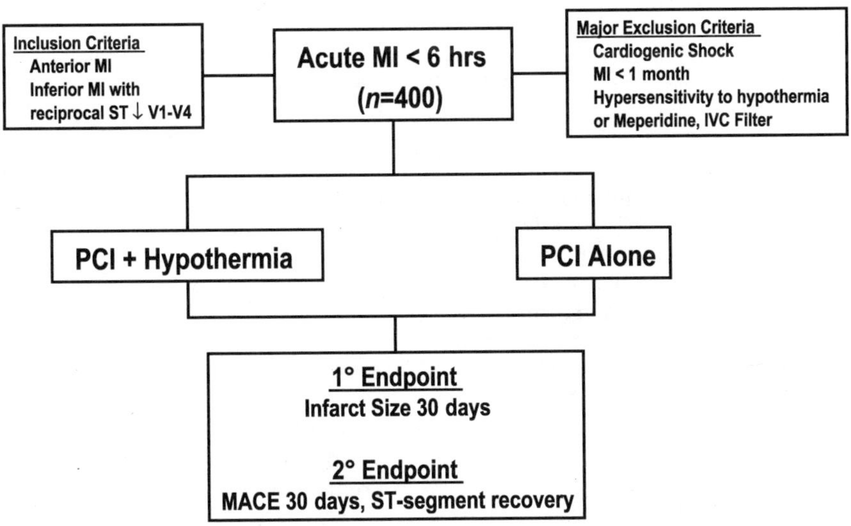

Figure 8 Design of the COOL-MI randomized clinical trial. Infarct size at 30 days was measured with ^{99m}Tc-sestamibi SPECT imaging. PCI = Primary percutaneous coronary intervention. MACE = Major adverse cardiac events (death, nonfatal reinfarction, and ischemia-driven target vessel revascularization).

first clinical trials in acute myocardial infarction to utilize infarct size as the primary efficacy endpoint of the study.

COOL-MI Trial

The COOL-MI trial enrolled 392 patients with acute myocardial infarction at 27 investigational sites from September 2001 to April 2003 (65). Patients presenting within 6 hr of symptom onset were assigned to undergo primary angioplasty with or without adjunctive hypothermia (Fig. 8). The major inclusion/exclusion criteria for the trial are shown in Table 7. Compared with the COOL-MI pilot study, the only difference in criteria was that patients with prior thrombolytic therapy were eligible for the inclusion in the randomized trial.

Table 7 Inclusion/Exclusion Criteria for the COOL-MI Randomized Clinical Trial

Inclusion criteria	Exclusion criteria
Age > 18 years	Previous MI within 1 month
Acute MI < 6 hr from symptom onset	Cardiogenic shock
	Hypersensitivity to hypothermia, including a history of Raynaud's disease
ST-segment elevation of ≥ 1 mm in two or more contiguous leads (patients with anterior or inferior infarct only; inferior infarcts must have ≥1 mm ST-segment depression in two or more contiguous precordial leads, V1 to V4)	Known hypersensitivity or contraindication to aspirin, heparin, contrast media, buspirone, meperidine
	Known history of severe hepatic or renal impairment
	Treatment with a monoamine oxidase inhibitor in the past 14 days
	Patient known or expected to be pregnant
	Patient has inferior vena cava filter in place
	Patient height < 1.5 m (4 ft. 11 in.)

Patients assigned to hypothermia were cooled using the Reprieve™ Endovascular Temperature Therapy System according to the same protocol that was used in the COOL-MI pilot trial (Figs. 9 and 10). In the hypothermia group, the investigational plan specified that cooling be initiated as early as possible before primary angioplasty was undertaken with the intent of lowering core temperature as much as possible before reperfusion. Surface skin warming, oral buspirone, and intravenous meperidine were used to prevent shivering. In the hypothermia group, core body temperature was monitored with a naso-esophageal probe or vascular probe placed in the contralateral femoral vein (SetProbe, Radiant Medical, Inc.). Cardiac catheterization was performed using conventional techniques and equipment. All patients received aspirin 325 mg before catheterization and heparin was administered during the procedure to maintain the activated clotting time >250 sec.

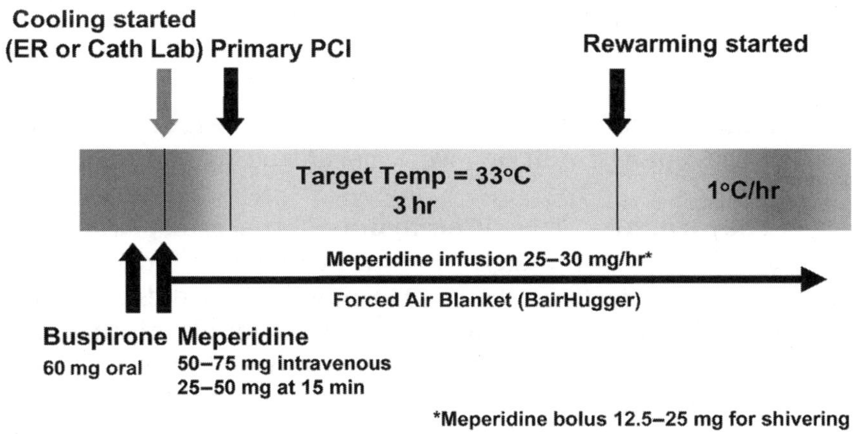

Figure 9 Diagram of the endovascular cooling and shivering suppression protocol in the COOL-MI randomized clinical trial. Cooling was initiated in the emergency room (ER) or cardiac catheterization laboratory before primary angioplasty. Surface warming, oral buspirone, and intravenous meperidine were administered to prevent shivering (see text for details). PCI = Percutaneous coronary intervention.

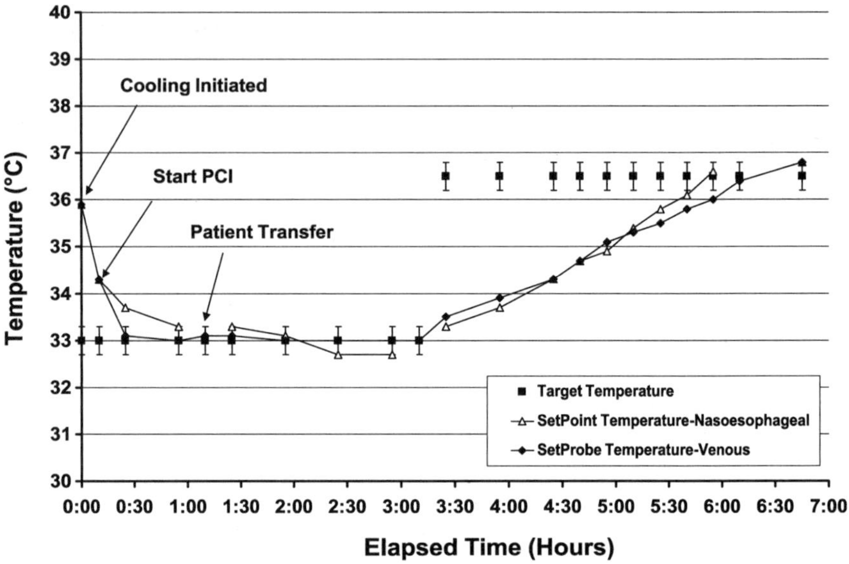

Figure 10 Core body temperature in a patient with acute myocardial infarction undergoing primary angioplasty with adjunctive endovascular cooling.

Coronary stenting, adjunctive thrombectomy, and use of glycoprotein receptor inhibitors were permitted at the operator's discretion.

The primary efficacy endpoint of the study was final infarct size at 30 ± 7 days measured using ^{99m}Tc-sestamibi SPECT imaging. The study was powered to detect a 30% difference in final infarct size between the study groups. The primary safety endpoint was the composite of major adverse cardiac events (MACE). Secondary endpoints were 1) ST-segment resolution 90 and 180 min following PCI, 2) left ventricular ejection fraction, and 3) peak creatine kinase.

Of the 392 patients, 357 underwent primary percutaneous coronary intervention. Most patients were treated with stent implantation and a glycoprotein receptor inhibitor. Approximately 40% of patients in each group had anterior wall infarction. The baseline core temperature was similar in both study groups. In the hypothermia group, the median duration of cooling before PCI was 17 min (IQR 10–27 min) and the mean temperature at the time of the first balloon inflation was 35.1 ± 0.8°C. Eighty-seven percent of patients in the hypothermia group achieved a core temperature <34°C with the cooling system; however, only 72% reached the intended target temperature of 33°C. Of those patients who reached 33°C, the median time to reach the target temperature was 68 min (IQR 43–113 min).

At 30 days the primary composite safety endpoint had occurred in 3.9% of patients in the control group and 6.2% of those in the hypothermia group ($p = 0.45$). The incidence of ventricular arrhythmia or bradycardia was similar in both groups (Table 8). The final infarct size at 30 days was 10.0%

Table 8 Clinical Events at 30 Days in the COOL-MI Randomized Trial

	Control group ($N = 180$)	Hypothermia group ($N = 177$)	P value
At 30 days			
Death	2.2	3.4	0.71
Reinfarction	1.7	0.6	0.63
Target vessel revascularization	0	2.3	0.12
Composite endpoint (MACE)	3.9	6.2	0.45
Other adverse events			
Ventricular fibrillation/tachycardia	20.0	17.5	0.64
Bradyarrhythmia	22.8	26.0	0.56
Stroke	0.6	0	0.95
Cardiogenic shock/severe hypotension	6.1	12.4	0.06
Pulmonary edema	1.7	3.4	0.49
Vascular/bleeding	13.9	18.1	0.35
Transfusion	7.8	11.3	0.34
Retroperitoneal bleed	1.1	0.6	0.95
Hematoma >6 cm	6.7	7.3	0.99
Pseudoaneurysm	0.6	1.7	0.63
AV fistula	0.6	0	0.95
Deep-vein thrombosis	0	1.7	0.24
Pulmonary embolism	1.7	0	0.24

of the left ventricle in the control group and 10.0% of the left ventricle in the hypothermia group ($p = 0.48$). However, patients with anterior infarction who had a temperature ≤35°C at reperfusion had a smaller infarct size than those patients who had a temperature >35°C (5.0% vs. 16.5%, $p = 0.007$), as well as patients in the control group (5.0% vs. 15.0%, $p = 0.03$) (Fig. 11).

Although the primary effectiveness endpoint of the trial was not met, the study provided a number of important insights regarding the use of hypothermia in acute myocardial infarction. Hypothermia was safe and well tolerated, and endovascular cooling was easily integrated into existing clinical pathways. Perhaps, the most significant observation from the study relates to the importance of cooling the heart before reperfusion. At the time the COOL-MI trial was designed we did not believe it was ethical to delay reperfusion therapy while cooling the patient, and for this reason encouraged investiga-

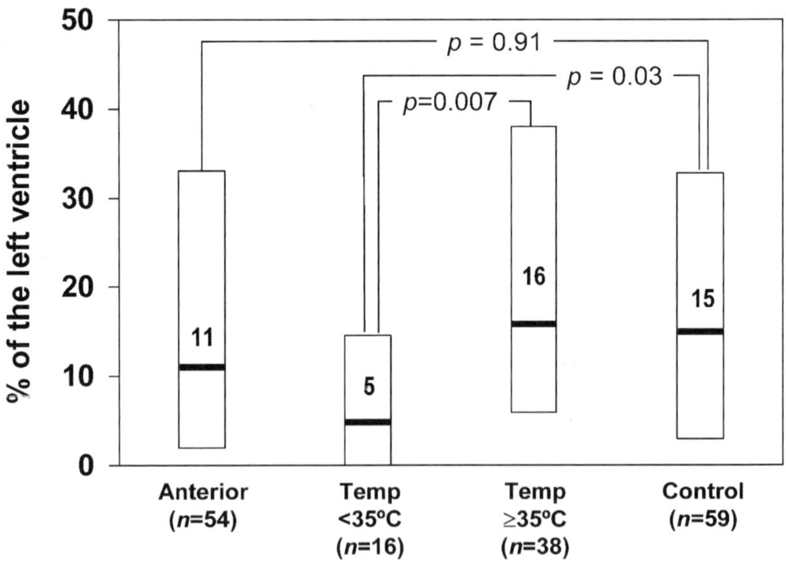

Figure 11 Final infarct size at 30 days for patients with anterior infarction assigned to hypothermia according to the core body temperature at reperfusion.

tors to proceed with intervention as soon as possible after initiation of cooling. In the trial, the median time from the onset of cooling to the first balloon inflation was only 17 min, resulting in a relatively modest 1.1°C mean reduction of core temperature at the time of reperfusion. Although 87% of patients were ultimately cooled to <34°C, the median time to achieve this temperature was 47 min, well after restoration of coronary flow. The findings of the post hoc analysis are consistent with experimental data and suggest that the heart should be cooled optimally before reperfusion to provide optimal myocyte and microvascular protection.

ICE-IT Trial

The ICE-IT randomized trial commenced in September 2002 and will enroll 400 patients with acute myocardial infarction presenting within 6 hr of symptom onset. Patients assigned to receive hypothermia are cooled with the Celsius Control™ System. The endovascular catheter (Celsius Control™ catheter) has a gold-plated flexible heat transfer element at the distal end and is available in two sizes depending on patient body size. One of the advantages of this system is that the Celsius Control™ catheter has a thermistor integrated into the shaft for temperature measurement and feedback, thus eliminating the need for bladder, esophageal, or vascular temperature probes. Compared with the COOL-MI trial, the major difference with this study is the longer duration of cooling after reperfusion (6 vs. 3 hr) (Table 6).

Table 9 Unresolved Issues Regarding Cooling in Acute Myocardial Infarction

Unresolved issues
Duration of cooling before reperfusion
Optimal myocardial temperature at reperfusion
Duration of cooling after reperfusion
Rate of rewarming
Optimal method to monitor core body temperature

CONCLUSION

Among newer therapeutic approaches in acute myocardial infarction, hypothermia has generated considerable interest as a potential cardioprotective strategy. Experimental data suggest that cooling the heart during myocardial infarction may significantly reduce infarct size and thus expand the benefit of catheter-based reperfusion. Several innovative systems have been developed to induce hypothermia in this setting. One prospective randomized trial of hypothermia for acute myocardial infarction has been completed. Although this study did not show an overall reduction in infarct size with hypothermia, results suggest that the cooling strategy needs to be refined to provide optimal myocyte protection. This will be the subject of ongoing and future clinical investigation.

Based on the results of the COOL-MI trial we believe that further investigation is required to define the optimal cooling strategy in acute myocardial infarction. In particular, future studies should focus on improving the rapidity and duration of cooling before reperfusion. To achieve this goal, one approach may be to initiate cooling earlier after presentation, but it is likely that more powerful cooling systems will also be required. Other unresolved issues include the optimal duration of cooling after reperfusion and best methods to monitor core temperature (Table 9). Additional experimental studies are also required to explore the molecular, biochemical, and cellular mechanisms that might explain the cardioprotective effects of cooling. Furthermore, there may be a role for hypothermia in cardiogenic shock to protect not only the heart but also other organs rendered ischemic by the low cardiac-output state. Finally, future clinical studies may also evaluate the role of cooling as an adjunct to pharmacological reperfusion with thrombolytic therapy.

REFERENCES

1. Reimer KA, Lowe JE, Rasmussen MM, Jennings RB. The wavefront phenomenon of ischemic cell death: 1. Myocardial

infarct size vs duration of coronary occlusion in dogs. Circulation 1977; 56:786–794.

2. White HD, Norris RM, Brown MA, Takayama M, Maslowski A, Bass NM, Ormiston JA, Whitlock T. Effect of intravenous streptokinase on left ventricular function and early survival after acute myocardial infarction. N Engl J Med 1987; 317:850–855.
3. Braunwald E. Myocardial reperfusion, limitation of infarct size, reduction of left ventricular dysfunction, and improved survival: should the paradigm be expanded. Circulation 1989; 79:441–444.
4. The GUSTO Angiographic Investigators. The effects of tissue plasminogen activator, streptokinase, or both on coronary artery patency, ventricular function, and survival after acute myocardial infarction. N Engl J Med 1993; 329:1615–1622.
5. Cerqueira MD, Maynard C, Ritchie JL, Davis KB, Kennedy JW. Long-term survival in 618 patients from the Western Washington Streptokinase in Myocardial Infarction Trials. J Am Coll Cardiol 1992; 20:1452–1459.
6. Miller TD, Christian TF, Hopfenspirger MR, Hodge DO, Gersh BJ, Gibbons RJ. Infarct size after acute myocardial infarction measured by quantitative tomographic ^{99m}Tc-sestamibi imaging predicts subsequent mortality. Circulation 1995; 92:334–341.
7. Burns RJ, Gibbons RJ, Yi Q, Roberts RS, Miller TD, Schaer GL, Anderson JL, Yusuf S. CORE Study Investigators. The relationships of left ventricular ejection fraction, end-systolic volume index and infarct size to six-month mortality after hospital discharge following myocardial infarction treated by thrombolysis. J Am Coll Cardiol 2002; 39:30–36.
8. Gersh BJ, Anderson JL. Thrombolysis and myocardial salvage. Results of clinical trials and the animal paradigm—paradoxic or predictable? Circulation 1993; 88:296–306.
9. Maroko PR, Libby P, Bloor CM, Sobel BE, Braunwald E. Factors influencing infarct size following experimental coronary occlusion. Circulation 1971; 43:67–82.
10. DeWood MA, Spores J, Notske R, Mouser LT, Burroughs R, Golden MS, Lang HT. Prevalence of total coronary occlusion

during the early hours of transmural myocardial infarction. N Engl J Med 1980; 303:897–902.

11. Ito H, Tomooka T, Sakai N, Yu H, Higashino Y, Fujii K, Masuyama T, Kitabatake A, Minamino T. Lack of myocardial perfusion immediately after successful thrombolysis. A predictor of poor recovery of left ventricular function in anterior myocardial infarction. Circulation 1992; 85:1699–1705.
12. Ito H, Maruyama A, Iwakura K, Takuchi S, Masuyama T, Hori M, Higashino Y, Fujii K, Minamino T. Clinical implications of "no-reflow" phenomenon: a predictor of complications and left ventricular remodeling in reperfused anterior wall myocardial infarction. Circulation 1996; 93:223–228.
13. Ragosta M, Camarano G, Kaul S, Powers ER, Sarembock IJ, Gimple LW. Microvascular integrity indicates myocellular viability in patients with recent myocardial infarction: new insights using myocardial contrast echocardiography. Circulation 1994; 89:2562–2569.
14. Kloner RA, Ganote CE, Jennings RB. The "no-reflow" phenomenon after temporary coronary occlusion in the dog. J Clin Invest 1974; 54:1496–1508.
15. Forman MB, Virmani R, Puett DW. Mechanisms and therapy of myocardial reperfusion injury. Circulation 1990; 81(suppl IV):IV-69–IV-78.
16. Kloner RA. Does reperfusion injury exist in humans? J Am Coll Cardiol 1993; 21:637–645.
17. Ambrosio G, Tritto I. Reperfusion injury: experimental evidence and clinical implications. Am Heart J 1999; 138:S69–S75.
18. Davies MJ. A macro and micro view of coronary vascular insult in ischemic heart disease. Circulation 1990; 82(suppl II):II-38–II-46.
19. Erbel R, Heusch G. Coronary microembolization. J Am Coll Cardiol 2000; 36:22–24.
20. Ito H, Okamura A, Iwakura K, Masuyama T, Hori M, Takiuchi S, Negoro S, Nakatsuchi Y, Taniyama Y, Higashino Y, Fujii K, Minamino T. Myocardial perfusion patterns related to thrombolysis in myocardial infarction perfusion grades after coronary angioplasty in patients with acute

anterior wall myocardial infarction. Circulation 1996; 93: 1993–1999.

21. Gerber BL, Rochitte CE, Melin JA, McVeigh ER, Bluemke DA, Wu KC, Becker LC, Lima JAC. Microvascular obstruction and left ventricular remodeling early after acute myocardial infarction. Circulation 2000; 101:2734–2741
22. Davis HC, Morse IC, Dick MM. The effect of pronestyl on experimental coronary occlusion on hypothermic dogs. Am J Surg 1957; 93:543–556
23. DeCortis A, Dalem J. Hypothermie et infarctus experimental du myocarde chez le chien. Acta Cardiol 1958; 13:299–302
24. Dimond EG, Guimpel A, Clitters RV, Cardoso S, Lin TK. Acute coronary occlusion: survival study in closed-chest dogs in controls, with hypothermia and with "lytic cocktail." J Kans Med Soc 1958; 59:249–251
25. Phibbs CM, Levy LM, MacLean LD. The influence of temperature and coronary occlusion on the ventricular fibrillation threshold. Surg Gynecol Obstet 1959; 109:216–222
26. Kuhn LA, Apter R, Weirauch H, Jacobson TE, Meltzer L. Hemodynamic and metabolic effects of skin and bloodstream cooling in experimental myocardial infarction with shock. Am J Cardiol 1963; 12:795–801
27. Kuhn LA, Weiser FM, D'Aria J, Apter R. Hemodynamic and extracorporeal circulation in experimental myocardial infarction and shock. Circ Res 1962; 10:916–924
28. Bussemaker JB, Dukta MF, Skinner DB. Hypothermia and circulatory assistance in dogs with acute myocardial infarction. J Thorac Cardiovasc Surg 1972; 64:61–65.
29. Boyer NH, Gerstein MM. Induced hypothermia in dogs with acute myocardial infarction and shock. J Thorac Cardiovasc Surg 1977; 74:286–294.
30. Abendschein DR, Tacker WA, Babbs CF. Protection of ischemic myocardium by whole-body hypothermia after coronary artery occlusion in dogs. Am Heart J 1978; 96:772–780.
31. Meerbaum S, Haendchen RV, Corday E, Povzhitkov M, Fishbein MC, Y-Rit J, Lang TW, Uchiyama T, Aosaki N,

Broffman J. Hypothermic coronary venous phased retroperfusion: a closed-chest treatment of acute regional ischemia. Circulation 1982; 65:1435–1445.

32. Haendchen RV, Corday E, Meerbaum S, Povzhitkov M, Rit J, Fishbein MC. Prevention of ischemic injury and early reperfusion derangements by hypothermic retroperfusion. J Am Coll Cardiol 1983; 1:1067–1080.

33. Voorhees WD, Abendschein DR, Tacker WA. Effect of whole-body hypothermia on myocardial blood flow and infarct salvage during coronary artery occlusion in dogs. Am Heart J 1984; 107:945–949.

34. Bergmann SR, Angelakos ET, Torres JC. Salutary effects of moderate hypothermia on the circulatory and myocardial consequences of acute coronary occlusion in dogs. Cryobiology 1985; 22:555–568.

35. Wakida Y, Haendchen RV, Kobayashi S, Nordlander R, Corday E. Percutaneous cooling of ischemic myocardium and hypothermic retroperfusion of autologous arterial blood: effects on regional myocardial temperature distribution and infarct size. J Am Coll Cardiol 1991; 18:293–300.

36. Chien GL, Wolff RA, Davis RF, van Winkle DM. "Normothermic range" temperature affects myocardial infarct size. Cardiovasc Res 1994; 28:1014–1017.

37. Duncker DJ, Klassen CL, Ishibashi Y, Herrlinger SH, Pavek TJ, Bache RJ. Effect of temperature on myocardial infarction in swine. Am J Physiol 1996; 270:H1189–H1199.

38. Schwartz LM, Verbinski SG, vander Heide RS, Reimer KA. Epicardial temperature is a major predictor of infarct size in dogs. J Mol Cell Cardiol 1997; 29:1577–1583.

39. Hale SL, Kloner RA. Myocardial temperature in acute myocardial infarction: protection with mild regional hypothermia. Am J Physiol 1997; 273:H220–H227.

40. van den Doel MA, Gho BCG, Duval SY, Schoemaker RG, Duncker DJ, Verdouw PD. Hypothermia extends the cardioprotection by ischaemic preconditioning to coronary artery occlusions of longer duration. Cardiovasc Res 1998; 37:76–81.

41. Dave RH, Hale SL, Kloner RA. Hypothermic, closed circuit

pericardioperfusion: a potential cardioprotective technique in acute regional ischemia. J Am Coll Cardiol 1998; 31:1667–1671.

42. Hale SL, Dave RH, Kloner RA. Regional hypothermia reduces myocardial necrosis even when instituted after the onset of ischemia. Basic Res Cardiol 1997; 92:351–357.
43. Miki T, Liu GS, Cohen MV, Downey JM. Mild hypothermia reduces infarct size in the beating rabbit heart: a practical intervention for acute myocardial infarction. Basic Res Cardiol 1998; 93:372–383.
44. Hale SL, Kloner RA. Myocardial temperature reduction attenuates necrosis after prolonged ischemia in rabbits. Cardiovasc Res 1998; 40:502–507.
45. Dae MW, Gao DW, Sessler DI, Chair K, Stillson CA. Effect of endovascular cooling on myocardial temperature, infarct size, and cardiac output in human-sized pigs. Am J Physiol Heart Circ Physiol 2002; 282:H1584–H1591.
46. Hale SL, Dae MW, Kloner RA. Hypothermia during reperfusion limits 'no-reflow' injury in a rabbit model of acute myocardial infarction. Cardiovasc Res 2003; 59:715–722.
47. Jeremy RW, Links JM, Becker LC. Progressive failure of coronary flow during reperfusion of myocardial infarction: documentation of the no reflow phenomenon with positron emission tomography. J Am Coll Cardiol 1990; 16:695–704.
48. Ning XH, Xu CS, Song YC, Xiao Y, Hu YJ, Lupinetti FL, Portman MA. Hypothermia preserves function and signaling for mitochondrial biogenesis during subsequent ischemia. Am J Physiol 1998; 274:H786–H793.
49. Ning XH, Chen SH, Xu CS, Li L, Yao LY, Qian K, Krueger JJ, Hyyti OM, Portman MA. Hypothermic protection of the ischemic heart via alterations in apoptotic pathways as assessed by gene array analysis. J Appl Physiol 2002; 9:2200–2207.
50. Dae MW, Gao DW, Ursell PC, Stillson CA, Sessler DI. Safety and efficacy of endovascular cooling and rewarming for induction and reversal of hypothermia in human-sized pigs. Stroke 2003; 34:734–738.
51. Weisser J, Martin J, Bisping E, Maier LS, Beyersdorf F, Hasenfuss G, Pieske B. Influence of mild hypothermia on

myocardial contractility and circulatory function. Basic Res Cardiol 2001; 96:198–205.

52. Suga H, Goto Y, Igarashi Y, Yasumura Y, Nozawa T, Futaki S, Tanaka N. Cardiac cooling increases E_{max} without affecting relation between O_2 consumption and systolic pressure–volume area in dog left ventricle. Circ Res 1988; 63:61–71.

53. Tveita T, Ytrehus K, Myhre ES, Hevroy O. Left ventricular dysfunction following rewarming from experimental hypothermia. J Appl Physiol 1998; 85:2135–2139.

54. Gerola A, Feinberg H, Katz LN. Myocardial oxygen consumption and coronary blood flow in hypothermia. Am J Physiol 1959; 196:719–725.

55. London MJ, Sybert PE, Mangano DT, Fisher DM, Bainton CR, Hickey RF. Surface-induced hypothermia: effects on coronary blood flow autoregulation and vascular reserve. J Surg Res 1988; 45:481–495.

56. Felberg RA, Kreiger DW, Chuang R, Persse DE, Burgin WS, Hickenbottom SL, Morgenstern LB, Rosales O, Grotta JC. Hypothermia after cardiac arrest. Feasibility and safety of an external cooling protocol. Circulation 2001; 104:1799–1804.

57. The Hypothermia After Cardiac Arrest Study Group. Mild therapeutic hypothermia to improve the neurologic outcome after cardiac arrest. N Engl J Med 2002; 346:549–556.

58. Bernard SA, Gray TW, Buist MD, Jones BM, Silvester W, Gutteridge G, Smith K. Treatment of comatose survivors of out-of-hospital cardiac arrest with induced hypothermia. N Engl J Med 2002; 346:557–563.

59. Schwab S, Schwarz S, Spranger M, Keller E, Bertram M, Hacke W. Moderate hypothermia in the treatment of patients with severe middle cerebral artery infarction. Stroke 1998; 29:2461–2466.

60. Krieger DW, De Georgia MA, Abou-Chebl A, Andrefsky JC, Sila CA, Katzan IL, Mayberg MR, Furlan AJ. Cooling for acute ischemic brain damage (COOL-AID). An open pilot study of induced hypothermia in acute ischemic stroke. Stroke 2001; 32:1847–1854.

61. Marion DW, Penrod LE, Kelsey SF, Obrist WD, Kochanek PM,

Palmer AM, Wisniewski SR, DeKosky ST. Treatment of traumatic brain injury with moderate hypothermia. N Engl J Med 1997; 336:540–546.

62. Clifton GL, Miller ER, Choi SC, Levin HS, McCauley S, Smith KR, Muizelaar JP, Wagner FC, Marion DW, Luerssen TG, Chesnut RM, Schwartz M. Lack of effect of induction of hypothermia after acute brain injury. N Engl J Med 2001; 344:556–563.

63. Dixon SR, Whitbourn RJ, Dae MW, Grube E, Sherman W, Schaer GL, Jenkins JS, Nguyen TT, Gibbons RJ, Kuntz RE, Baim DS, O'Neill WW. Induction of mild systemic hypothermia with endovascular cooling during primary percutaneous coronary intervention for acute myocardial infarction. J Am Coll Cardiol 2002; 40:1928–1934.

64. Mokhtarani M, Mahgoub A, Morioka N, Doufas AG, Dae M, Shaughnessy TE, Bjorksten AR, Sessler DI. Buspirone and meperidine synergistically reduce the shivering threshold. Anesth Analg 2001; 93:1233–1239.

65. Kandzari DE, Chu A, Brodie BR, Stuckey TA, Hermiller JB, Vetrovec GW, Hannan KL, Krucoff MW, Christenson RH, Gibbons RJ, Sigmon KN, Garg J, Hasselblad V, Collins K, Harrington RA, Berger PB, Chronos NA, Hochman JS, Califf RM. Feasibility of endovascular cooling as an adjunct to primary percutaneous coronary intervention (Results of the LOWTEMP Pilot Study). Am J Cardiol 2004; 93:636–639.

66. Dixon SR, Kuntz RE, Griffin JJ, Rizik DG, Carrozza JP, Rutherford BD, Seyfarth M, Thambar ST, Gibbons RJ, Popma JJ, Dae MW, O'Neill WW. Mild hypothermia during primary percutaneous coronary intervention for acute myocardial infarction: a randomized trial. 2004. Submitted for publication.

17

Hypothermia in Neurological and Cardiac Anesthesia

BRADLEY J. HINDMAN

Department of Anesthesiology,
Roy J. and Lucille A. Carver College of Medicine,
The University of Iowa, Iowa City, Iowa, U.S.A.

INTRODUCTION

Hypothermia as a neuroprotective intervention was introduced into surgical and anesthetic practice in the 1950s. In 1952, moderate systemic hypothermia (28°C, surface cooling) was first used in a cardiac procedure that employed 5.5 min of systemic circulatory arrest (1). In 1954, mild-to-moderate hypothermia (~30°C, surface cooling) was introduced to intracranial aneurysm surgery, where temporary or permanent occlusion of cerebral arteries was, and still is, sometimes necessary (2,3). The first case series using cardiopulmonary bypass (CPB) was reported in 1954 (4) and, by 1958, moderate hypothermia was routinely incorporated into CPB (5,6). By 1959, the literature was replete with descriptions of the physiologic effects of hypothermia, methods of inducing and reversing mild-to-moderate systemic hypothermia and limiting complications, and possible surgical and nonsurgical applications (7).

However, as early as the mid-1960s, serious doubt had been cast upon the protective value of mild-to-moderate hypothermia during cerebral aneurysm surgery (8–11). Consequently, except for procedures requiring deep hypothermic systemic circulatory arrest (12,13), hypothermia was not routinely used during neurological surgery during the 1970s and 1980s (14). In contrast, throughout the 1960s, 1970s, and 1980s, moderate hypothermia (27–30°C) was routinely used during cardiac surgery utilizing CPB. CPB provides systemic (and cerebral) perfusion while the heart and lungs are isolated from the circulation. Mild-to-moderate hypothermia during CPB was considered essential to limit cardiac rewarming between doses of cold (4–10°C) cardioplegia and decrease systemic oxygen requirements during CPB. As neurologic injury became increasingly recognized as a common complication of cardiac surgery (15,16), hypothermia also became increasingly regarded as a key element of "brain protection." By decreasing cerebral metabolic rate, hypothermia was thought to increase brain tolerance to low systemic pressure, flow, and oxygen content (anemia) frequently present during CPB, factors considered to contribute to much of the neurologic injury associated with cardiac surgery. Hence, in cardiac surgery, mild-to-moderate systemic hypothermia became considered a vital protective intervention for both heart and brain.

Two developments at the start of the 1990s lead to dramatic and opposing changes in use of mild-to-moderate hypothermia during neurologic and cardiac surgery. The first was a series of animal experiments demonstrating that mild hypothermia (32–34°C) conferred significant neurologic protection against a wide variety of temporary ischemic insults (17–20). On this basis, intraoperative hypothermia was reintroduced to intracranial aneurysm surgery in the early 1990s. It was postulated that mild intraoperative hypothermia (33–34°C) would decrease neurologic injury resulting from brain retraction, temporary vessel occlusion, and hypotension (21,22). Counterbalancing renewed enthusiasm for the potential neurologic benefits of mild hypothermia were studies showing that even very mild perioperative hypothermia (~35.5°C) was associated with an increased incidence of cardiovascular (23,24), bleeding (25), and infectious (26) complications in patients undergoing nonneurosurgical procedures. Although mild-to-moderate hypothermia was once again commonly used during neurosurgery, by the end of the 1990s the balance of benefit to risk remained undefined (22).

The other major development in the early 1990s was the introduction of normothermic ("warm") cardioplegia (27,28). Warm cardioplegia eliminated one of the main indications for systemic hypothermia during CPB—keeping the heart cold. There was concern that normothermic ("warm") CPB would be associated with worse neurologic outcomes compared to traditional moderately hypothermic CPB. Perhaps surprisingly, a series of randomized clinical trials indicated there was no apparent neurologic benefit to moderate hypothermia (28–30°C) during cardiac surgery and CPB. Hence, in the 1990s, after more than a 20-year hiatus, mild systemic hypothermia was reintroduced into neurologic surgery and appeared potentially beneficial (22). Paradoxically, in cardiac surgery, after 30 years of routine use, moderate hypothermia was used progressively less often because of an apparent lack of neurologic benefit.

This chapter reviews the clinical application of mild-to-moderate systemic hypothermia in the setting of neurological and cardiac surgery from the perspective of the anesthesiologist. Emphasis is placed on: (1) key physiological effects of mild-to-moderate systemic hypothermia and how these influence intraoperative management and monitoring; (2) how hypothermia influences the pharmacokinetics and pharmacodynamics of common anesthetic medications; and (3) practical elements involved in inducing and reversing hypothermia. Thereafter, the results of controlled clinical trials of mild-to-moderate hypothermia in neurologic and cardiac surgery will be reviewed.

REVIEW

Physiology of Mild-to-Moderate Perioperative Hypothermia

Direct Effect of Hypothermia on Chemical Reaction Rates

Biologic processes are mediated by chemical and enzymatic reactions. The temperature dependence of chemical reactions is described by the Arrhenius equation:

$$\text{Chemical reaction rate} = Ae^{(-E/RT)}$$

where A is a constant, E is the activation energy of the reaction, R is the gas constant, and T is temperature in Kelvin.

Most biochemical processes have activation energies that result in a 50–60% decrease in reaction rate over a 10°C decrease in temperature. When calculated on a per °C basis, hypothermia decreases biological reaction rates by about 7–9% per °C. This value is an important benchmark to use when considering the clinical effects of mild-to-moderate hypothermia. It will be observed that the physiologic effects of hypothermia are, in fact, almost always within this range.

Mild-to-Moderate Hypothermia and the Nervous System

Anesthetic Requirements

Hypothermia reduces anesthetic requirements. Animal studies demonstrate that hypothermia decreases the minimum anesthetic concentration (MAC) of volatile anesthetics (e.g., halothane, isoflurane, desflurane) in the range of 5–8% per °C (29–31). The same is true in humans. In children undergoing surface cooling prior to CPB, isoflurane MAC decreased from 1.7 ± 0.1% at 37°C to 1.2 ± 0.2% at 31°C (~5.3% per °C) (32). A different study examined the interaction between hypothermia and propofol blood concentration at which patients responded to command (CP_{50}-awake) (33). Although there was not a statistically significant difference between group mean CP_{50}-awake in normothermic (36.9°C; CP_{50} = 3.41 μg/mL) and hypothermic (34.1°C; CP_{50} = 2.65 μg/mL) patients, large interindividual differences decreased this study's power to detect the effect of hypothermia. Using group mean values, hypothermia appears to have reduced CP_{50}-awake by 8–9% per °C. This decrease is consistent with the effect of hypothermia on the MAC of volatile anesthetics. This latter study shows there is a two- to threefold variation among individuals in anesthetic requirements at a given temperature. This normal interindividual variation is much greater than the effect of hypothermia. Thus, hypothermia-mediated decreases in anesthetic requirements are small and are less than the variation expected among patients at any given temperature. Hence, clinically, it is often difficult to perceive that mild systemic hypothermia has a meaningful effect on anesthetic requirement in a given patient.

Very deep hypothermia is needed to completely eliminate the need for anesthesia. In goats, Antognini (31) observed that the abolition of purposeful responses to painful stimuli occurred at 20°C. However, motor responses to pain may be largely mediated at the spinal level and may be relatively resistant to hypothermia. Early pioneers of hypothermic anesthesia indicated that when patient temperature approaches 28–30°C, hypothermia largely negates the need for further anesthetic agent (34).

Higher Cortical Function/Amnesia

Indeed, higher cortical function appears to be quite sensitive to hypothermia. In 1940, Fay (35) reported patients cooled to 31–32°C, and who were given little to no pharmacologic sedation, were uniformly amnesic during the hypothermic period. In unanesthetized humans, Coleshaw et al. (36) reported a 70% impairment of acquisition of new memory at core temperatures of 34–35°C. The amnesic effects of mild hypothermia (37) may explain why, in the course of neurologic and cardiac surgery, relatively low levels of anesthesia are only very rarely associated with intraoperative recall.

Monitoring: Estimating Brain Temperature

Brain temperature depends on the interaction of four factors: (1) the temperature of the blood perfusing the brain (arterial blood temperature), (2) cerebral metabolism (brain heat production), (3) cerebral blood flow (heat clearance), and

(4) heat transfer to the environment through the skull (38). Under steady-state conditions, brain metabolic heat production results in brain temperatures that are slightly greater than arterial blood temperature. In humans (closed cranium), direct measurements of brain temperature show that deep brain temperature is 0.3–0.6°C greater than core temperature (i.e., esophagus or nasopharynx) (39–43).

There are also temperature gradients within the brain. Deep brain temperatures are 0.5–1.0°C warmer than temperatures in the outer cortex (42,44,45). Lower brain temperature in the outer cortex is largely a result of conductive heat loss through the skull. Nevertheless, the adult skull is a good insulator. Compared to a child's skull, the adult skull is thicker and has a smaller surface area/brain volume ratio; these properties increase its insulating effect. Accordingly, in adults, surface cooling of the closed cranium has negligible effect on average brain temperature (38,46). In contrast, in infants, surface cooling of the skull may meaningfully decrease average brain temperature (38).

In neurosurgical procedures where portions of the skull are removed, the exposed brain surface can become quite cool. Stone et al. (45) demonstrated exposed brain (the outer 1–2 cm) may be more than 3°C cooler than deep brain temperature; see Table 1. Accordingly, this author routinely maintains operating room temperature at about 20°C during open cranial procedures to decrease brain surface temperature as much as possible. In open cranial procedures, irrigation fluids can also transiently affect brain temperature. For example, Iatrou et al. (47) reported irrigation of the brain with 30°C saline decreased deep brain temperature a maximum of 1.5°C for 5 min.

Direct measurement of brain temperature is rare in clinical settings. Average brain temperature is nearly the same as arterial blood temperature because, at steady-state, deep brain temperature is usually about 0.5°C greater than arterial blood temperature and outer brain temperature is about 0.5°C less than deep brain temperature. Because of their anatomic locations, nasopharyngeal (NP) (39,48) and tympanic membrane (TYMP) (40,44,45,48) temperatures often closely approximate arterial (carotid and vertebral) blood temperature

Table 1 Superficial and Deep Brain Temperatures During Open Craniotomy

Site	Temperature (°C)
Room air	20.9 ± 1.6
T_{BRAIN}: Surface	29.8 ± 2.0
T_{BRAIN}: 0.5-cm depth	32.7 ± 1.7
T_{BRAIN}: 1-cm depth	34.3 ± 1.4
T_{BRAIN}: 2-cm depth	35.7 ± 0.9
T_{BRAIN}: 3-cm depth	35.9 ± 1.0
T_{ESO}	35.7 ± 1.0
T_{TYMP}	35.6 ± 1.1

Values are mean ± standard deviation.
T_{BRAIN} = brain temperature; T_{ESO} = esophageal temperature; T_{TYMP} = tympanic temperature.
From Ref. 45.

and, consequently, average brain temperature. However, T_{TYMP} can be affected by facial temperature, giving falsely low values when the face is cooled (40). Consequently, this author monitors T_{NP} (posterior border of the soft palate) (39) in preference to T_{TYMP} as an index of T_{BRAIN}. When properly positioned, jugular bulb (JUGB) temperature should also closely approximate steady-state global brain temperature. Because at steady state, cerebral blood flow removes heat from the brain, T_{JUGB} is usually a few tenths of a degree greater than core body temperature (49,50).

At steady state, brain arterial blood temperature equals aortic blood temperature that, in turn, is equal to deep body or "core" temperature. Hence, accurate measurement of core temperature usually provides a good estimate of global brain temperature that is accurate within a few tenths of a degree. Three sites used most often to estimate core temperature are esophagus (ESO), rectum (REC), and bladder (BLAD). T_{ESO} is highly dependent on the depth of probe placement (51). Shallow placement underestimates core temperature because the lower tracheal temperature decreases T_{ESO}. Kaufman (51) reported esophageal temperature probes placed at a depth of "best heart and breath sounds," ~28 cm, underestimated maximal T_{ESO} by ~1°C. Maximal T_{ESO} was present at a probe depth of ~38–40 cm. In humans, Whitby and Dunkin (39) observed the gradient between T_{ESO} and deep T_{BRAIN} was minimized (brain warmer by 0.3–0.5°C) when esophageal temperature probes were placed ~35 cm from the incisors. At this depth, T_{ESO} and T_{NP} gave equivalent values. At 35–40 cm, esophageal temperature probes are positioned posterior to the heart and reflect true core (cardiac, aortic) temperature. Hence, to most closely estimate T_{BRAIN}, esophageal temperature probes should be inserted to a depth of 35–40 cm in adults.

T_{REC} and T_{BLAD}, while sometimes acceptable estimates of core temperature, just as often are not. T_{REC} can be affected by depth of probe placement and by the presence of feces. T_{BLAD} depends on the rate of urine output (52). Accordingly, in the operating room, this author uses either T_{NP} or T_{ESO} as the primary estimates of global brain temperature. Other temperature sites (T_{TYMP}, T_{REC}, T_{BLAD}) are only used as backups.

The described relationships between T_{BRAIN} and temperatures at other sites do not hold when arterial blood and brain are not in thermal equilibrium, such as during arterial perfusion cooling and rewarming on CPB. Until a thermal steady state is reached, during cooling, T_{BRAIN} will necessarily be warmer than perfusate temperature and, during rewarming, the opposite will be the case (Table 2). Because of their

Table 2 Brain Temperature and Temperatures at Other Sites During Arterial Perfusion Cooling and Rewarming on Cardiopulmonary Bypass

Phase of CPB	$T_{PERFUSATE}$ (°C)	T_{BRAIN} (°C)	T_{NP} (°C)	T_{TYMP} (°C)	T_{ESO} (°C)
Midway cooling	14.9 ± 1.9	23.4 ± 2.2	24.0 ± 2.5	25.3 ± 2.9	23.1 ± 2.2
Circulatory arrest	12.7 ± 1.8	16.7 ± 1.7	17.5 ± 2.5	18.4 ± 2.8	17.3 ± 2.2
Midway rewarming	32.1 ± 1.8	27.4 ± 2.3	23.8 ± 2.6	24.7 ± 1.7	25.1 ± 2.3
End rewarming	37.5 ± 0.9	35.8 ± 1.6	35.8 ± 1.4	35.5 ± 2.1	35.7 ± 1.9

Values are mean ± standard deviation.
CPB = cardiopulmonary bypass; $T_{PERFUSATE}$ = perfusate temperature; T_{BRAIN} = brain temperature; T_{NP} = nasopharyngeal temperature; T_{TYMP} = tympanic temperature; T_{ESO} = esophageal temperature.
From Ref. 48.

anatomic locations and perfusion patterns, T_{ESO}, T_{NP}, and T_{TYMP} best approximate T_{BRAIN}. However, with rapid changes in temperature, they are far from perfect. Stone et al. (48) compared deep T_{BRAIN} (3 cm under the surface) to other temperatures during arterial perfusion cooling and rewarming in 27 patients undergoing deep hypothermic circulatory arrest for cerebral aneurysm surgery. Although mean values for T_{NP}, T_{TYMP}, and T_{ESO} closely approximated mean values for T_{BRAIN} (Table 2), within individual patients, there were substantial gradients between T_{BRAIN} and the other sites (Table 3). For example, as shown in Figure 1, at circulatory arrest T_{NP} varied from 4.7°C less than to 4.9°C greater than T_{BRAIN}; with only 9 of 27 patients (33%) having gradients between T_{BRAIN} and T_{NP} that were ≤1°C.

Monitoring: Electroencephalography and Evoked Potentials

Electroencephalography (EEG), evoked potential (EP) monitoring, or both are often used during surgery to monitor the functional integrity of the nervous system. Studies characterizing the effect of hypothermia upon EEG and EP have largely been conducted during cardiac surgery and CPB, often making it difficult to separate the effect of temperature from the

Table 3 Temperature Gradients (Absolute Values) Between Brain and Other Temperature Sites During Arterial Perfusion Cooling and Rewarming on Cardiopulmonary Bypass

	Absolute value of individual temperature gradients (°C) between T_{BRAIN} and site		
Phase of CPB	T_{NP}	T_{TYMP}	T_{ESO}
Midway cooling	2.4 ± 1.8	2.7 ± 1.9	2.5 ± 2.3
Circulatory arrest	2.1 ± 1.6	2.6 ± 1.5	1.9 ± 1.7
Midway rewarming	2.4 ± 2.2	2.6 ± 1.5	2.2 ± 1.6
End rewarming	1.2 ± 1.3	1.5 ± 1.6	1.6 ± 1.5

Values are mean ± standard deviation.
CPB = cardiopulmonary bypass; T_{NP} = nasopharyngeal temperature; T_{TYMP} = tympanic temperature; T_{ESO} = esophageal temperature.
From Ref. 48.

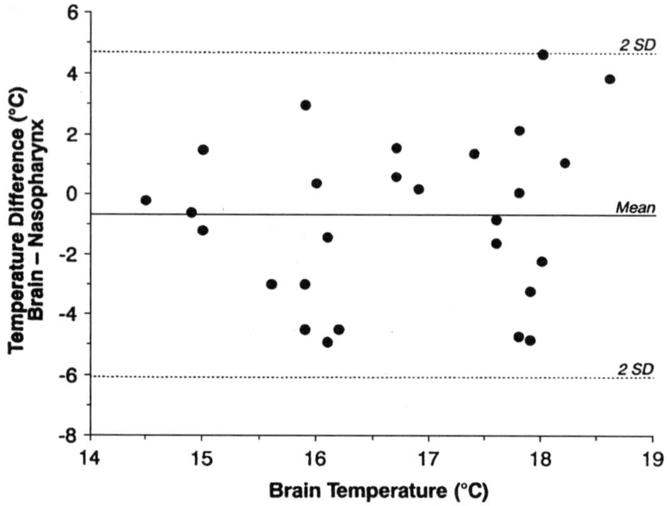

Figure 1 Individual differences between brain temperature and nasopharyngeal temperature at onset of hypothermic circulatory arrest. (From Ref. 48.)

multitude of other physiologic changes that occur with CPB (53). In general, hypothermia results in a progressive decrease in high-frequency EEG activity (~0.4–0.5 Hz per °C) (54–58) and a decrease in total EEG power (~4% per °C) (56). Because power is the square of the voltage, the decrease in voltage is about 2% per °C. Such small changes in frequency and voltage are often difficult to detect when the EEG is visually assessed. For example, in a study of 74 patients surface-cooled to 30°C, 39% had no visually detectable EEG change and 59% had only slight slowing (~3 Hz) (54). More recently, Levy et al. (58) used approximate entropy analysis to characterize the relationship between temperature and EEG. This analytic technique measures the variability of an analog signal, reflecting changes in both frequency and amplitude from the original signal. Approximate entropy was maintained at values >95% of baseline at temperatures greater than 31°C. The authors explain this indicates that only minimal EEG changes occur at temperatures greater than 31°C. With deep hypothermia, the cumulative effect of hypothermia results in the EEG becoming electrically silent ("flat") at 16–19°C (58,59). The temperature at which electrical silence occurs varies markedly among individuals. In a recent study of 109 patients undergoing hypothermic circulatory arrest, T_{NP} at onset of electrical silence ranged between 27.2 and 12.5°C (59). As discussed above, some of this variability is likely a result of inaccuracy in surrogate measures of brain temperature.

Deepening hypothermia results in progressive increases in latency and decreases in amplitude of EP signals. The effect of hypothermia upon EPs is explained by its two basic effects on neural activity: slowing of axon conduction velocity and increasing synaptic transmission delay. With hypothermia, temporal dispersion of the arriving presynaptic signal, combined with slowing of synaptic transmission results in a progressive increase in internuclear delay, i.e., latency (60). Below a certain temperature, nuclear transmission can be inhibited entirely, resulting in a total loss of signal amplitude (60–62). The late polysynaptic potentials are generally much more sensitive to hypothermia than the early mono- or bisynaptic potentials (60–63). Cortical EPs generally disappear (zero amplitude) at about 21–25°C (59,60,62). As with EEG, the majority of studies examining relationships between EP and temperature have been conducted during CPB. In CPB studies, the effect of temperature upon EP differs between the cooling and rewarming phases. With rewarming, EP signals recover at temperatures that are less than the temperatures at which the signals were lost (61–63). This discrepancy is not well understood, but may be related to inaccurate estimates of neural temperatures during perfusion cooling and rewarming (see above). This discrepancy is minimized if CPB perfusate temperature is used as the index of neural temperature (63).

Few studies have examined the effect of temperature upon EP in the absence of CPB. Recently, Lang et al. (64) reported that surface rewarming from 32 to 36°C decreased EP latencies in the range of 3–5% per °C. These values are consistent with the effect of temperature on EP latencies observed in CPB studies. In practice, extremities exposed to very cool temperatures during surface cooling may become so cold as to cause marked slowing of peripheral nerve conduction. This slowing of peripheral conduction can be misinterpreted as a sign of neural ischemia (65).

Hypothermic Acid–Base Management: Alpha-Stat and pH-Stat

Perspective

Poikilotherms and hibernators use two very different acid–base strategies under hypothermic conditions: Alpha-stat and pH-stat, respectively (defined below). Because humans are neither poikilotherms nor hibernators, nor do humans normally become systemically hypothermic, it is unclear which hypothermic acid–base strategy might be optimal for humans during mild-to-moderate hypothermia.

Chemistry and Physiology

Water spontaneously dissociates into hydrogen (H^+) and hydroxyl (OH^-) ions. Electrochemical neutrality is defined as the point where hydrogen ion concentration ($[H^+]$) equals the hydroxyl ion concentration ($[OH^-]$). When aqueous solutions are cooled, $[H^+]$ and $[OH^-]$ both decrease because of a decrease in spontaneous dissociation of water. At 37°C, the $[H^+]$ at neutrality = 1.58×10^{-7} mol/L, giving a pN = 6.80 (66). At 25°C, $[H^+] = [OH^-] = 1 \times 10^{-7}$ mol/L, giving a neutral pH (pN) = 7.00. At 17°C, the $[H^+]$ at neutrality = 0.7×10^{-7} mol/L, giving a neutral pH (pN) = 7.14. Thus, with anaerobic cooling of aqueous solutions (including blood) pN spontaneously increases, following the relationship: $\Delta pN/\Delta T \approx -0.017$ pH units/°C (67).

With some exceptions (67), poikilotherms (animals that remain active at core temperatures less than 37°C) tend to maintain intracellular pH near pN over a wide range of body temperatures. Simultaneously, they maintain extracellular pH at more alkalotic values, keeping a fairly constant intra- to extracellular pH gradient of 0.5–0.7 pH units (66). Thus, at 37°C, intracellular pH is ~6.8 and extracellular (blood) pH is ~7.4. As poikilotherms cool, both intra- and extracellular pH increase in a manner virtually identical to the anaerobic cooling of water: $\Delta pH/\Delta T \approx -0.017$ pH units/°C (68). Reeves (69) observed that the pK of the histidine imidazole group varies with temperature in a manner almost identical to that of water: $\Delta pK/\Delta T \approx -0.016$ pK units/°C. By maintaining intracellular pH near pN, poikilotherms maintain the ionization state of histidine imidazole at a constant level, despite their changing body temperature. The histidine imidazole ionization state is called alpha. Hence, the name assigned to this acid–base strategy is "alpha-stat." The alpha-stat hypothesis contends that histidine imidazole ionization state is the key determinant of both the charge state and pH-dependent function of many key enzymes and structural proteins (67). Poikilotherms, by preserving alpha (alpha-stat), maintain protein charge state, structure, and function at near normal over a wide range of body temperatures, and remain active largely independent of their temperature.

Poikilotherms keep pN and histidine ionization constant by appearing to anaerobically cool their blood. As poikilotherms cool, both intracellular and extracellular (blood) pH increase as described above. Simultaneously, because gas solubility increases with decreasing temperature, the partial pressure of carbon dioxide [$p(CO_2)$] decreases, although total blood CO_2 content does not change. Thus, poikilotherms establish what appears to be a respiratory alkalosis when blood gases are corrected to their actual in vivo temperature, "worsening" with deepening hypothermia relative to normothermic blood gas values. Alpha-stat proponents suggest that in humans, as in poikilotherms, this respiratory alkalosis is, in fact, physiologically appropriate, and results in a better preservation of intracellular electrochemical neutrality and "normal" cellular function and structure.

The other hypothermic acid–base strategy, referred to as "pH-stat," approximates that of hibernators. In contrast to poikilotherms, hibernators become inactive when hypothermic. pH-Stat management maintains arterial pH = 7.40 and $p(CO_2)$ = 40 mm Hg as measured at (or corrected to) the subject's actual in vivo temperature (i.e., blood gases are temperature-corrected); hence the name "pH-stat." As discussed above, anaerobic cooling of blood results in a spontaneous shift of pH to more alkaline values and a decrease of $p(CO_2)$. To maintain constant (temperature-corrected) values of pH and

$p(CO_2)$ during cooling, H^+ (CO_2) must be added to the blood. Thus, with pH-stat management, it is necessary to increase the total CO_2 content of blood as temperature decreases. As shown in Table 4, pH-stat management results in relative hypercarbia and acidemia compared to alpha-stat management, with the difference between strategies increasing in magnitude as temperature decreases (70).

Monitoring: Blood Gases and End-Tidal Carbon Dioxide

In hypothermic humans, alpha-stat management is achieved by maintaining arterial pH = 7.40 and $p(CO_2)$ = 40 mm Hg as measured at 37°C, regardless of the patient's actual in vivo temperature (blood gases are not temperature-corrected). If corrected to actual in vivo temperature, this approach is seen to result in a progressive respiratory alkalosis [$p(CO_2) < 40$ mm Hg, pH > 7.40]; a consequence of the spontaneous shift of pH and $p(CO_2)$ with decreasing temperature; see Table 4. Clinically, one can approximate alpha-stat management by keeping alveolar ventilation fixed at normothermic values as the patient cools. Because systemic CO_2 production decreases about 7% per °C, keeping ventilation constant as the patient cools will lead to mild hypocarbia (as measured at 37°C). This mild hypocarbia is easily corrected by small reductions in minute ventilation guided by blood gas analysis.

Clinically, pH-stat management is achieved by maintaining arterial pH = 7.40 and $p(CO_2)$ = 40 mm Hg as corrected to the patient's actual in vivo temperature (blood gases are temperature-corrected). Because of decreasing systemic CO_2 production and increasing blood CO_2 solubility, progressive decreases in minute ventilation are needed to maintain a temperature-corrected arterial $p(CO_2)$ of 40 mm Hg as patients cool.

End-tidal CO_2 monitoring is used clinically to approximate arterial $p(CO_2)$. If arterial $p(CO_2)$ is measured at 37°C (alpha-stat approach; blood gases are not temperature-corrected), one observes a progressive increase in the gradient between end-tidal CO_2 and arterial $p(CO_2)$ as patient temperature decreases. This is because $p(CO_2)$ in exhaled alveolar gas

Table 4 Alpha-Stat Versus pH-Stat Management: Values for pH and $p(CO_2)$ as a Function of Temperature

Actual in vivo temperature (°C)	Measured and reported at 37°C				Corrected to actual in vivo temperature			
	pH		$p(CO_2)$ [mm Hg]		pH		$p(CO_2)$ [mm Hg]	
	Alpha-stat	pH-stat	Alpha-stat	pH-stat	Alpha-stat	pH-stat	Alpha-stat	pH-stat
37	7.40	7.40	40	40	7.40	7.40	40	40
33	7.40	7.34	40	47	7.44	7.40	35	40
30	7.40	7.30	40	54	7.50	7.40	29	40
27	7.40	7.26	40	62	7.55	7.40	26	40
23	7.40	7.21	40	74	7.60	7.40	22	40
20	7.40	7.18	40	84	7.65	7.40	19	40
17	7.40	7.14	40	96	7.60	7.40	17	40

Corrections for temperature are from Andritsch et al. (70).

reflects actual in vivo $p(CO_2)$, which, because of increasing gas solubility, decreases as temperature decreases. On the other hand, if one corrects arterial $p(CO_2)$ to the patient's actual in vivo temperature (pH-stat approach), arterial to end-tidal gradients stay nearly constant (71,72).

Nervous System Effects

The reader is referred to Chapter 5 of this book for a complete review of the effect of hypothermia upon cerebral metabolism, blood flow, and autoregulation. In brief, however, both cerebral blood flow (CBF) and cerebral metabolic rate for oxygen ($CMRO_2$) decrease with hypothermia, ~8–9% per °C. Because the cerebral vasculature retains its responsiveness to carbon dioxide (73,74), the relative hypercarbia of pH-stat management results in greater CBF compared to alpha-stat management (75–77) and greater impairment of cerebral autoregulation compared to alpha-stat management (78,79).

Inspection of Table 4 shows pH and $p(CO_2)$ differences between alpha-stat and pH-stat management are actually quite small at temperatures greater than 33°C. Thus, with mild hypothermia (32–34°C), it is unlikely that acid–base strategy should have a significant effect on brain physiology, operative conditions, or neurologic outcome in the setting of neurologic surgery. Conceivably, the slightly greater $p(CO_2)$ associated with pH-stat management might result in slightly greater CBF (potential advantage) and very slightly greater hemoglobin P_{50} (potential advantage), but also slightly greater brain volume (potential disadvantage).

No clinical studies have been conducted that compare alpha-stat vs. pH-stat during neurosurgical procedures. There are only two animal studies comparing the effect of alpha-stat vs. pH-stat management upon neurologic outcome in the setting of mild hypothermia and temporary ischemia. Each experiment took a different approach and each came to a different conclusion. Nagai et al. (80) subjected rats to 2 hr of transient middle cerebral artery occlusion (MCAO) at 30°C under alpha-stat or pH-stat conditions. Following the ischemic interval, the brain was reperfused and animals were rewarmed. Although pH-stat management was associated with greater preischemic CBF, neither intraischemic CBF nor 24-hr infarction volumes differed between alpha-stat and pH-stat groups. In contrast, Kollmar et al. (81) subjected rats to 2 hr of normothermic MCAO followed by 5 hr of postischemic hypothermic (33°C) reperfusion. At 5 hr postischemia, pH-stat management was associated with significantly greater CBF, less infarction volume, and less brain edema. Thus, in these experiments, intraischemic acid–base management had no effect on outcome (hypothermia was equally protective with either alpha-stat and pH-stat management), whereas postischemic hypothermia appeared more beneficial with pH-stat conditions. Although these are provocative results, it may be premature to extrapolate these findings to perioperative management. Outcomes were assessed only hours after the insult in both of these animal studies. How (or if) alpha-stat vs. pH-stat management might affect long-term neurologic outcome in the setting of neurological surgery conducted with mild hypothermia is not known.

The effect of alpha-stat vs. pH-stat management in the setting of cardiac surgery favors alpha-stat. For this and other reasons (discussed in the section that follows), most anesthesiologists employ alpha-stat management during neurological surgery conducted under mild systemic hypothermia.

Cardiorespiratory Effects

Systemic Hemodynamics and Metabolism

In 1965, Michenfelder et al. (82) were among the first to quantitate the cardiorespiratory effects of systemic hypothermia in anesthetized humans. They studied four halothane-anesthetized adult neurosurgical patients surface-cooled to T_{ESO} of 30°C. More than 30 years later, Bacher et al. (83) reexamined these relationships in 13 adult neurosurgical patients anesthetized with propofol and fentanyl (Table 5). Despite 30 years, different anesthetics, and different measurement methods, the results were virtually identical. Under general anesthesia, systemic hypothermia as low as 30–32°C is generally well tolerated in healthy adults. The effects of

Table 5 Cardiorespiratory Effects of Mild Systemic Hypothermia During Neurosurgery

Variable	35.5°C	32.0°C	Effect of hypothermia
Heart rate (beats/min)	59 ± 7	55 ± 16	No change
Mean arterial pressure (mm Hg)	87 ± 9	91 ± 7	No change
Right atrial pressure (mm Hg)	7 ± 4	5 ± 5	No change
Cardiac index (L min^{-1} m^{-2})	2.4 ± 0.3	2.4 ± 0.5	No change
Systemic vascular resistance index (dyne sec cm^{-5} m^{-2})	2806 ± 547	2929 ± 397	No change
Systemic oxygen delivery (mL min^{-1} m^{-2})	350 ± 50	360 ± 50	No change
Systemic oxygen consumption (mL min^{-1} m^{-2})	100 ± 13	77 ± 11	Decrease 23±13%; 7% per °C
Systemic oxygen extraction (%)	29 ± 5	22 ± 3	Decrease
Systemic carbon dioxide production (mL min^{-1} m^{-2})	75 ± 7	57 ± 7	Decrease 24 ± 9%; 7% per °C
Respiratory quotient	0.77 ± 0.15	0.75 ± 0.11	No change
Plasma lactate (mmol/L)	1.4 ± 0.7	1.1 ± 0.8	No change

Values are mean ± standard deviation.
From Ref. 83.

hypothermia on systemic arterial pressure, cardiac output, and vascular resistance are usually minor (82,83). Most notable is the decrease in systemic oxygen consumption and CO_2 production, each decreasing about 7% per °C (82,83). This decrease in systemic metabolism is exactly what might be expected from the effect of hypothermia on chemical and enzymatic reaction rates.

Because systemic oxygen delivery was maintained while systemic oxygen consumption decreased, systemic oxygen extraction decreased. Neither the respiratory quotient nor the plasma lactate changed. This suggests that the decrease in systemic oxygen extraction was probably not the result of impaired oxygen off-loading from hemoglobin caused by an increase in hemoglobin oxygen affinity (P_{50}) [P_{50}(37°C) = 26.8 mm Hg; P_{50}(32°C) = 19.0 mm Hg] (84), but simply because systemic oxygen consumption decreased more than systemic oxygen delivery.

Some investigators have noted that hypothermia increases systemic lactate concentration. Stayer et al. (85) surface-cooled neonates to 31 ± 0.6°C prior to CPB. Although systemic arterial pressure was maintained during cooling, there was an increase in serum lactate from 1.7 ± 0.6 to 3.5 ± 1.6 mEq/L. There was no increase in pyruvate, plasma-free fatty acids, acetoacetate, or beta-hydroxybutyrate with cooling. Whether lactate accumulated as a result of anaerobic metabolism in hypoperfused tissue beds or on the basis of hypothermia-related reduced hepatic lactate clearance could not be determined in this study. This author has occasionally observed adult patients who exhibit an otherwise unexplained mild-to-moderate metabolic acidosis during rewarming. It may be that, in some instances, surface cooling causes sufficient peripheral vasoconstriction as to produce peripheral anaerobic metabolism. So long as vasoconstriction is maintained, metabolic acids are constrained to the periphery. With peripheral rewarming and reperfusion, metabolic acids may enter the systemic circulation (see Chapter 7 for further discussion of the physiology of rewarming).

Monitoring: Cardiac Rate and Rhythm

The studies of Michenfelder et al. (82) and Bacher et al. (83) observed little change in heart rate although, in the experience of this author, bradycardia is common at temperatures below 34°C. Mild-to-moderate hypothermia is known to have significant effects on cardiac automaticity and conduction. As temperature decreases, sinus bradycardia, ectopic atrial pacemakers, as well as PR-, QRS-, QT-, and QT_c-prolongation occur (86–90). Although there is marked interindividual variability, heart rate decreases by about 10% per °C, PR interval increases about 4–6% per °C, and QRS and QT intervals increase about 5–7% per °C (87,89,90). The classic electrographic manifestation of hypothermia, the dome or hump elevation in the terminal portion of the QRS complex (the J wave; also called the Osborn wave) is rare above 32°C, but is common at lesser temperatures and increases in size as hypothermia becomes more profound (91). Below ~30°C, atrial fibrillation becomes progressively more likely (86–90,92), and below ~28°C, ventricular arrhythmias and ventricular fibrillation are frequent (90).

The pioneers of systemic hypothermia were of the opinion that, in the absence of CPB, 30°C was the approximate safe lower thermal limit (10,93). At lesser temperatures, arrhythmias and/or hemodynamic instability often resulted in cardiac arrest. These pioneers emphasized the need to "hyperventilate" patients to reduce ventricular irritability (34). In the 1980s, animal (94) and clinical (95) studies showed that hypothermic acid–base strategy affects ventricular fibrillation thresholds. The relatively hypocarbic alpha-stat strategy (see Table 4 and Hypothermic Acid–Base Management: Alpha-Stat and pH-Stat Section) decreases the propensity toward hypothermic ventricular fibrillation (94,95). Also, in dogs, surface-cooled to 30°C, alpha-stat management results in lesser systemic vascular resistance and greater cardiac index than pH-stat management (96). The pioneers thus appear to have been correct regarding hypothermic ventilatory management: relative hyperventilation (i.e., alpha-stat management) appears to slightly better preserve systemic cardiovascular function and decreases the risk of serious arrhythmias.

Left Ventricular Function

Using echocardiography, Kuwagata et al. (97) assessed left ventricular (LV) performance in seven adults cooled to ~34°C as part of a head trauma management strategy. Mean arterial pressure, end diastolic dimension, and stroke volume index were not affected by temperature. Between 36 and 34°C, cardiac index decreased ~15% (2.6–2.2 L min^{-1} m^{-2}) as the result of a 12% decrease in heart rate (83–69 beats/min). LV performance indices depending on temporal factors (ejection time, rates of systolic contraction and diastolic relaxation) were significantly affected (slowed) by hypothermia. In contrast, indices depending on spatial factors such as fractional shortening and stroke volume index were not affected. Under hypothermia, the decreased rate of LV contraction was compensated for by a prolonged ejection time (i.e., slower heart rate) resulting in relatively constant fractional shortening and stroke volume. In this study, there did not appear to be compensatory mechanisms for the decreased rate of diastolic relaxation, although LV filling remained adequate. Lewis et al. (98) made similar conclusions in a study of paced human hearts between 31 and 37°C. These investigators found that, under hypothermic conditions, LV contractility increased as heart rate decreased. With hypothermia, a slow heart rate compensates for the slower rate of LV contraction, allowing time for complete LV contraction to take place. Thus, hypothermia-induced bradycardia is beneficial because it preserves net LV performance. Therefore, in the operating room, this author does not attempt to reverse bradycardia during mild-to-moderate systemic hypothermia.

Sympathetic Nervous System Responses and the Heart

In patients with known, or at high risk of, coronary artery disease, perioperative hypothermia is associated with a two- to ninefold increase in the incidence of postoperative cardiovascular complications (23,24). The mechanism underlying this increase is not established, but may be related to sympathetic nervous system responses to hypothermia. In the absence of anesthesia, a 1°C decrease in core temperature is sufficient to provoke marked increases in systemic concentrations of epinephrine and norepinephrine with accompanying increases in heart rate, blood pressure, and cardiac output (99). These responses may be sufficient to provoke myocardial ischemia in patients with coronary disease (24). Under general anesthesia, sympathetic responses to hypothermia appear to be largely prevented (100). It is only with emergence from anesthesia that catecholamines are seen to increase (100,101).

Recently, in adults undergoing intracranial aneurysm surgery anesthetized with isoflurane (1.2%) and nitrous oxide, Chi et al. (102) reported a very different pattern of catecholamine responses. Patients assigned to hypothermia during surgery (34.2 ± 0.2°C) had significantly lower systemic concentrations of epinephrine and norepinephrine during surgery and at extubation than patients maintained normothermic (36.9 ± 0.3°C). Hypothermic patients also had lesser increases in plasma antidiuretic hormone (ADH) and adrenocorticotrophic hormone (ACTH) at these same intervals. It is not obvious why these patients' responses to hypothermia appear to differ so greatly from other studies. Nevertheless, it suggests that the catecholamine responses to hypothermia may be attenuated under certain circumstances, such as when residual anesthetic concentrations remain high, which is often the case with neurosurgical patients.

Pharmacokinetics and Pharmacodynamics

Anesthetics and Paralytics

Most medications are cleared by enzymatic processes taking place within the liver and/or kidney. Because hypothermia decreases enzymatic reaction rates 7–9% per °C, one would expect the duration of effect of most drugs would increase at least this much. To the extent that hypothermia may also decrease hepatic and renal blood flow (103), drug duration may increase even more.

Remifentanil and Atracurium: As expected, agents cleared exclusively by chemical and/or enzymatic processes (i.e., independent of hepatic and renal blood flow) appear to be least affected by hypothermia. For example, spontaneous recovery of muscle paralysis induced by atracurium (T_{25-75} recovery) slows from 20 ± 4 min at 37°C to 23 ± 5 min at 34°C; ~4.6% per °C. (103). Similarly, hypothermia decreases remifentanil clearance 4.7% to 6.4% per °C (104,105).

Propofol, rocuronium, and vecuronium: Agents undergoing hepatic and renal clearance are more greatly affected by hypothermia. At a fixed infusion rate (~80 μg/kg/min), blood propofol concentrations were ~28% greater at 34°C than at 37°C (103). This indicates steady-state propofol clearance decreased ~9% per °C. Beaufort et al. (106) reported rocuronium clearance decreased ~9% per °C. Caldwell et al. (107) reported hypothermia decreased vecuronium clearance 11% per °C. These investigators also noted that hypothermia decreased the rate constant for drug equilibration between plasma and effect site (muscle) by 0.02 $\text{min}^{-1}/°\text{C}$. Thus, hypothermia delays the equilibration of vecuronium between the bloodstream and the neuromuscular junction, probably the result of a decrease in muscle blood flow during hypothermia. Slowed rates of equilibration delay both the onset (108) and the resolution of drug effect. The net result of slowed drug clearance and delayed blood–muscle equilibration is a twofold increase in duration of action of vecuronium between 37 and 34°C (107) (Figure 2).

Hypothermia may also slightly increase the sensitivity of the neuromuscular junction to muscle relaxants, but the effect is small. Heier et al. (108) reported the ED_{95} of vecuronium at 36.8 and 34.3°C was 272 ± 92 and 236 ± 80 ng/mL, respectively, which was not statistically significant. However, inspection of their data (Figure 3) reveals a key point. The difference among individuals in ED_{95} at the same temperature (~threefold variation) is much greater than the ED_{95} differ-

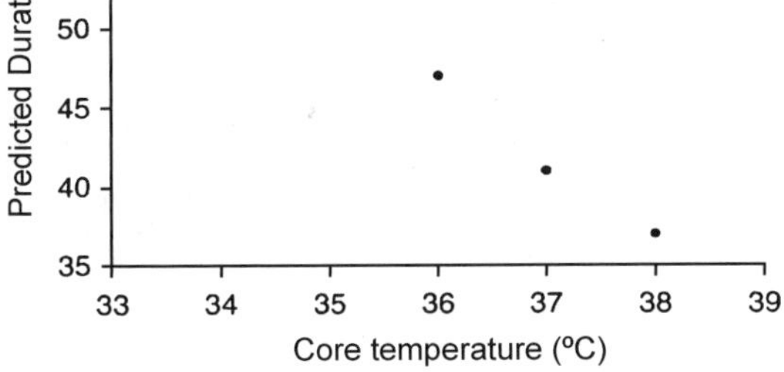

Figure 2 Pharmacokinetic/pharmacodynamic model of the effect of hypothermia to increase the duration of action of a 0.1 mg/kg dose of vecuronium. Duration of action is the time from drug injection to 25% recovery of baseline twitch tension. (From Ref. 107.)

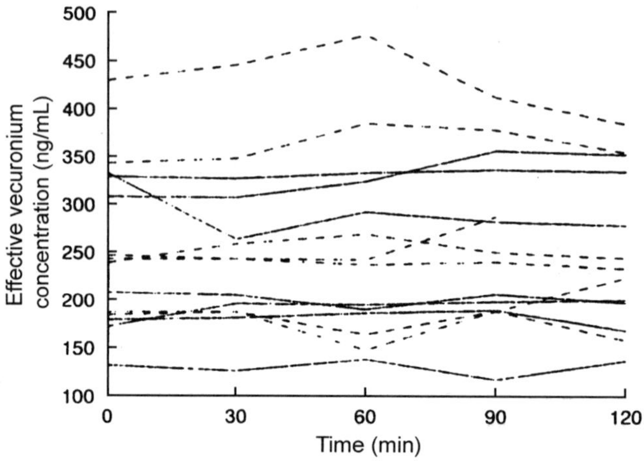

Figure 3 Effect of hypothermia upon vecuronium concentration required to produce a 95% depression of baseline twitch tension under normothermic (dashed lines) and hypothermic (solid lines) conditions. (From Ref. 108.)

ence caused by hypothermia within individuals. Anesthesiologists compensate for the large variation among patients in drug kinetics and effects by adjusting drug dose to a monitored effect. The small changes in net drug effect that result from mild-to-moderate hypothermia are considerably less than normal (normothermic) interindividual variation and, in practice, cannot be distinguished from it.

Neostigmine: Heier et al. (108) reported hypothermia (34.3°C) did not change the clearance, maximum reversing effect, or duration of action of neostigmine. Hence, mild systemic hypothermia does not have any meaningful impact upon the pharmacologic reversal of neuromuscular blocking agents.

Monitoring: Neuromuscular Blockade

In a cold operating room, exposed extremities often become cool, and they become very cool when they are exposed to surface cooling methods. Peripheral tissue temperatures can be much lower (10°C) than core temperature, particularly in superficial structures such as the ulnar nerve and adductor pollicis. Below a threshold temperature of about 35 °C, decreasing tissue (muscle) temperature results in a progressive decrease in twitch response, ~16% per °C (109–111). When tissue temperature approaches 25 °C, there is no twitch response at all (111). Hence, cold extremities can exaggerate the effect of neuromuscular blocking agents, resulting in an overestimate of the true degree of neuromuscular blockade. One may think the patient is pharmacologically paralyzed when they are not. It is thus prudent to measure neuromuscular transmission in an area that is kept nearly normothermic during systemic hypothermia.

Other Physiologic Effects

Renal/Electrolyte

Hypothermia typically results in a "cold diuresis" due in part to inhibition of renal tubular reabsorption of solutes and water. In a study of head injury patients cooled to 31.8 ± 0.8 °C, urine output increased from 219 ± 70 to 485 ± 209 mL/hr during the cooling period, returning to baseline with establishment of stable hypothermia (112). During cooling, urinary excretion of magnesium, phosphate, and potassium increased. Despite attempts to keep up with urinary electrolyte losses, cooling resulted in significantly decreased serum concentrations of magnesium, phosphate, calcium, and potassium. During surgery, depletion of intravascular volume may contribute to hemodynamic instability, and electrolyte disturbances may predispose patients to arrhythmias.

Hyperglycemia

Hypothermia can result in hyperglycemia, due in part to inhibition of insulin secretion and/or insulin receptor function. (113). In a recent study of patients experiencing cardiac arrest, patients assigned to hypothermia (33 °C) had significantly greater serum glucose than normothermic patients; ~16 vs. 11 mmol/L, respectively (114). In our pilot study of intraoperative hypothermia (33.5 °C) vs. normothermia in cerebral aneurysm surgery (22), hypothermic patients had slightly greater intraoperative blood glucose values compared to normothermic patients; 8 ± 2 vs. 7 ± 2 mmol/L, respectively (Hindman, unpublished observations, 2003). Thus while moderate hypothermia increases plasma glucose concentrations, the increase is modest and can easily be managed.

Pancreatitis

Pancreatitis of varying severity is a long recognized complication of accidental hypothermia (115). Studies of mild sustained hypothermia (32–34°C for 24–72 hr) in the treatment of patients with head injury (116,117) and severe stroke (118,119) report that 15–40% of patients have biochemical evidence of pancreatic injury (e.g., elevated systemic amylase or lipase). In almost all instances, these abnormalities resolve with rewarming without apparent adverse effect. This author is not aware of any reports or instances of pancreatitis associated with short-term intraoperative hypothermia for neurological surgery.

Surface Cooling and Rewarming in the Operating Room

Perspective

Hypothermia can be induced and reversed by either surface or central (e.g., perfusion) techniques. With surface cooling, cooling efforts are directed toward the peripheral thermal compartment, the skin and subcutaneous tissue of the arms, legs, abdomen, and thorax. Cool venous blood from these tissues returns to the central circulation, decreasing central venous, arterial, and brain temperatures in turn. Rewarming occurs in reverse. Depending on its relative size, the peripheral compartment acts as a thermal buffer, slowing and minimizing changes in core temperature caused by changes in body surface temperature. As a result, most surface cooling techniques are relatively slow, achieving maximum cooling rates of 1–1.5°C/hr (71,83).

Until recently, the only central cooling technique was that of CPB, where cooled oxygenated blood (perfusate) is directly introduced into the arterial circulation. With this technique, the brain and body can be perfused with very cold blood and hypothermia can be induced very quickly (e.g., T_{BRAIN} from 37 to 17°C in 20 min or less, ~1.0°C/min). Very recently, new percutaneous vascular cooling catheters have been described. These devices are placed in the central venous circulation, cooling the blood that comes into contact with them (120–124). Maximal cooling rates with these catheters approach 4–6 °C/hr (~0.07–0.10°C/min) (121–123).

Contraindications

There are a few conditions that are considered to be contraindications to the induction of systemic hypothermia; these include (1) cold-reactive proteins (e.g., cold agglutins or cryoglobulinemia), (2) Raynaud's phenomena, (3) hypokalemic periodic paralysis, and (4) homozygote sickle cell disease.

Whether or not patients with sickle-trait (heterozygotes) may be safely surface-cooled remains unclear. Almost all articles relating to sickle trait and hypothermia describe patients undergoing arterial perfusion cooling (24–32°C) with CPB (125–129). Clinically, all patients did well and were free of obvious systemic complications. The coldest patient had a systemic temperature nadir of 20°C, and there was no clinical sign of sickling (125). Nevertheless, one report where investigators serially examined blood for sickle formation observed that all the cells that could sickle did so (at least transiently) during a postoperative period of residual hypothermia, peripheral vasoconstriction, and shivering (126). Indeed, the literature stresses peripheral vasoconstriction, tissue and hemoglobin desaturation, and vascular stasis act synergistically to result in sickle hemoglobin polymerization. When mild-to-moderate hypothermia (core 30–32°C) is induced by surface cooling, peripheral temperatures (arms/legs) may easily approach 20°C. This degree of hypothermia, coexisting with peripheral vasoconstriction and reduced peripheral perfusion, may result in tissue that is relatively hypoxic, potentially causing desaturation and subsequent polymerization of the sickle hemoglobin. Some might thus consider sickle trait to be at least a relative contraindication to surface cooling.

Overview of Thermoregulation during General Anesthesia

Thermoregulation during general anesthesia has been recently reviewed (130). In conscious humans at standard room temperature, the peripheral thermal compartment is normally 3–4 °C cooler than the thermal core. This temperature gradient is established and controlled by central nervous system (CNS) thermoregulatory control mechanisms that maintain tonic vasoconstriction in cutaneous blood vessels. This peripheral vasoconstriction tends to constrain metabolic heat to the thermal core. Anesthetics inhibit this tonic CNS-mediated vasoconstriction. In addition, many anesthetics also have direct vasodilator properties. With induction of anesthesia, peripheral vasodilation results in a rapid redistribution of heat from the warmer core to the cooler periphery. This initial redistribution of heat typically decreases core temperature 1–2 °C over the first hour of anesthesia.

Following this initial redistribution, core temperature continues to decrease unless preventive measures are taken. This second phase of core temperature reduction occurs because, in the presence of anesthetic-induced peripheral vasodilation, cutaneous heat loss exceeds metabolic heat production. Finally, when patients become sufficiently hypothermic, usually at core temperatures of ~33–35 °C, CNS-mediated thermoregulatory vasoconstriction is reestablished. With restoration of thermoregulatory cutaneous vasoconstriction, core cooling slows, the combined result of decreased cutaneous heat loss (minor) and constraint of metabolic heat to the thermal core (major). Surface cooling methods modify one or more of these processes to increase core and/or whole body heat loss.

Heat Redistribution

The initial redistribution of heat from the warmer core to the cooler periphery can be increased by acute coadministration of an additional vasodilator. Vassilieff et al. (131) reported 10 mg of sublingual nifedipine given just before anesthetic induction resulted in a slightly greater decrease in core temperature in the first hour of surgery compared with controls; -2.0 ± 0.2 vs.

−1.7 ± 0.2°C, respectively. Conversely, vasoconstrictors decrease redistribution hypothermia. Ikeda et al. (132) reported patients receiving phenylephrine (0.5 μg/kg/min) had less reduction in core temperature than controls; −0.5 ± 0.2 vs. −1.2 ± 0.4°C, respectively ($P < 0.001$). Hence, in theory, selecting an anesthetic with relatively greater peripheral vasodilating properties and limiting vasoconstrictor administration as much as possible, the rate of initial (redistribution) cooling should be maximized. Further facilitation of core cooling depends on increasing cutaneous heat loss and inhibiting the reestablishment of thermoregulatory vasoconstriction.

Cutaneous Heat Loss

Plattner et al. (133) compared the effectiveness of intraoperative cooling methods. As shown in Table 6, methods that increased cutaneous heat loss were the most effective. Circulating water mattresses and forced-air cooling blankets are the two methods currently used most often in the operating room. They are roughly equally effective. These methods increase clearance of heat from the peripheral thermal compartment by both conduction and convection. Cool venous blood returning from the periphery reduces core temperature. To speed up core cooling, peripheral tissues are usually cooled to temperatures much less than the desired core temperature. This is an

Table 6 Efficacy of Intraoperative Cooling Methods

Method	Core cooling rate
Bladder lavage 300 mL iced Ringer's every 10 min	0.8 ± 0.3°C/hr
Circulating water mattress 5°C, anterior and posterior body surface	1.6 ± 1.1°C/hr
Forced air (convection) 10°C, anterior body surface only	1.7 ± 0.5°C/hr
Ice water immersion (~0°C)	9.7 ± 4.4°C/hr

Values are mean ± standard deviation.
Adapted from Ref. 133.

important point and will be discussed again when discussing the phenomenon of "afterdrop." Because dependent surfaces are compressed by body weight and are less well perfused, heat transfer largely occurs via the nondependent surface, i.e., the anterior surface of a supine patient.

Water immersion is extremely effective, but is generally considered so inconvenient that it is now rarely used. However, very recently, new technologies that approximate immersion physiology have begun to enter clinical practice (134).

Cooling methods that increase cutaneous heat loss depend on surface area. The greater the surface area participating in heat exchange, the more effective surface cooling will be. Skin exposed to cooling methods should thus be maximized, ensuring all available nondependent surfaces are covered by the forced-air cover (or water mattress). To maximize convective heat exchange, no clothing or sheets should be permitted between the blanket and skin. It is also helpful to ensure that full flow to the forced-air blanket is maintained by preventing external compression of the forced air blanket by straps used to secure the patient to the table.

Thermoregulatory Vasoconstriction

The effectiveness of surface cooling methods is diminished by the reestablishment of thermoregulatory vasoconstriction that, depending on a number of factors (see below), typically occurs at core temperatures in the range of 33–35°C. Vasoconstriction reduces blood flow to the peripheral tissues, reducing the amount of cool venous blood returning to the core. However, the main effect of restored thermoregulatory vasoconstriction is constraint of metabolic heat to the thermal core, which limits further cooling of the core. This phenomenon was characterized by Kurz et al. (135) in a group of 26 neurosurgical patients undergoing forced-air surface cooling. In roughly half of the patients, thermoregulatory vasoconstriction returned at a core temperature of 34.5°C, whereas in the other half, vasoconstriction occurred at lesser core temperatures. Table 7 shows that the early reappearance of thermoregulatory vasoconstriction significantly increased times required to

Table 7 Effect of Thermoregulatory Vasoconstriction Upon Rate of Surface Cooling

	Patients who vasocontricted	Patients who did not vasoconstrict
Time to cool to 34°C (hr)	2.3 ± 0.6	1.7 ± 0.4
Time to cool to 33°C (hr)	3.4 ± 0.6	2.6 ± 0.6[a]
Time to cool to 32°C (hr)	4.8 ± 0.8	3.6 ± 0.7[a]

Values are mean ± standard deviation, n = 13/group.
[a] $P < 0.01$ between groups.
From Ref. 135.

reach desired levels of hypothermia. In this report, there were no obvious physiologic or morphologic differences between patients who vasoconstricted at 34.5°C and those who did not.

A number of factors have been identified as affecting thermoregulatory vasoconstriction thresholds. Age affects the vasoconstriction threshold. Under isoflurane/nitrous oxide anesthesia, Kurz et al. (136) observed younger patients (30–50 years) had greater (warmer) vasoconstriction thresholds than older patients (60–80 years), 35.1 ± 0.2 vs. 33.9 ± 0.6°C, respectively. Gender also affects thermoregulatory thresholds. Women vasoconstrict at 0.3–0.4°C greater core temperature than men (137). Skin temperature also affects vasoconstriction thresholds. Each 1.0°C decrease in mean skin surface temperature increases the vasoconstriction threshold by about 0.25°C (138). Hence, surface cooling is to some extent self-limiting because as mean skin temperature decreases, the vasoconstriction threshold tends to increase. Thermoregulatory vasoconstriction is effective and restricts development of further hypothermia.

With the exception of midazolam (139), literally all anesthetics, sedatives, and opioids that have been studied have been found to markedly decrease the thermoregulatory vasoconstriction threshold, including propofol (140), alfentanil (141), dexmedetomidine (142), and meperidine (143)—all in a dose-dependent manner. As shown in Figure 4, increasing isoflurane concentration decreases the vasoconstriction

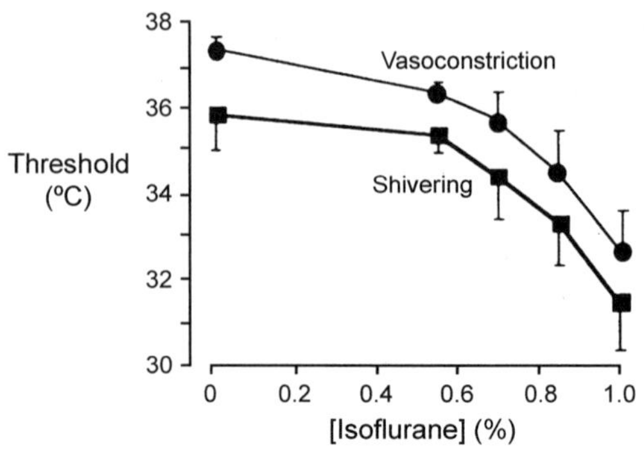

Figure 4 Nonlinear effect of isoflurane concentration on the thermoregulatory vasoconstriction and shivering thresholds. Results are mean ± standard deviation. (From Ref. 144.)

threshold (144). However, the effect is not linear. With both isoflurane (144) and desflurane (145), there is only a minor decrease of the vasoconstriction threshold at concentrations less than 0.5 MAC. The substitution of nitrous oxide for isoflurane appears to increase the vasoconstriction threshold (146).

In theory, maintaining a relatively high concentration of volatile anesthetic (or "deep" level of anesthesia) should promote surface cooling by decreasing the hypothermic vasoconstriction threshold. In practice, however, this is difficult to do. Anesthetic requirements decrease as patients cool. Attempting to maintain anesthetic concentrations at normothermic values usually results in unacceptable hypotension. Because of additive interactions among anesthetics and sedatives, substituting one agent for another is not likely to avoid the hypotensive effect of relatively deep anesthesia. Administration of vasoconstrictors (e.g., phenylephrine) to correct hypotension may slow core cooling (see above). When used to achieve surgical anesthesia, most anesthetics (isoflurane (144,146), desflurane (145), propofol (140), fentanyl/nitrous oxide (147)) appear to be roughly equivalent in terms of decreasing the hypothermic vasoconstriction threshold to somewhere in the range of 33–35°C. Hence, the decrease in the vasoconstriction threshold appears to be mostly related to the generalized CNS (central thermoregulatory) depression that results from anesthesia. Likewise, differences among anesthetics in direct peripheral vascular effects do not appear sufficiently great as to have a meaningful impact on surface cooling. For example, a recent study of adult neurosurgical patients anesthetized with either sevoflurane/nitrous oxide or propofol/nitrous oxide observed no differences in peripheral vasoconstriction or in the rates of surface cooling or rewarming (148). Thus, currently, choice of general anesthetic agents does not appear to meaningfully affect an individual patient's hypothermic vasoconstriction threshold and/or rate of cooling.

Probably through a combination of effects, intravenous amrinone administration has been shown to increase the rate of surface cooling and rewarming by 30–40% (149). The vasodilating properties of amrinone likely promote acute redistribution hypothermia. Forearm minus fingertip temperature gradients were significantly less in patients receiving amrinone as compared to controls. This suggests amrinone may also inhibit thermoregulatory vasoconstriction, preventing or delaying the constraint of metabolic heat to the core. (Such inhibition is almost certainly a direct vascular- rather than CNS-mediated process.) Cardiac index tended to be greater in patients receiving amrinone. Hence, amrinone may result in a relatively greater proportion of cardiac output being directed toward the peripheral compartment, thereby promoting heat exchange between the peripheral and core thermal compartments.

Afterdrop

As discussed above, to speed surface cooling, the skin surface and peripheral compartment are almost always cooled to temperatures much less than the desired target core hypothermic value. For example, forced-air devices are often set to achieve skin surface temperatures of 10 °C, and water mattresses are commonly set to achieve temperatures in the range of 4–10 °C. Because peripheral vasoconstriction limits peripheral perfusion, there is a considerable time delay between temperature change in the peripheral compartment and the resulting change in core temperature. As a result of these two factors, even when active surface cooling is stopped, core temperature usually continues to decrease by 0.5–1.0°C over the next 30–60 min (133). This phenomenon is called "afterdrop." To minimize afterdrop, this author stops active surface cooling when core temperatures decrease to within ~0.5°C of the target value, and often starts to warm peripheral tissues with forced-air temperatures approximating the final desired core temperature (e.g., 32–33°C during neurosurgery). These steps decrease the likelihood that core temperature will decrease much below target levels and helps speed rewarming as well.

Body Morphology

In addition to vasoconstriction, the other major factor influencing the effectiveness of surface cooling is body morphology (150). Metabolic heat production is roughly proportional to body weight (Wt), whereas heat loss is proportional to cutaneous surface area (SA) (130). As the Wt/SA ratio increases, there is an increase in the amount of heat that must be lost per unit SA to maintain core normothermia. To do this, there is a reduction in the level of tonic vasoconstriction to the periphery, increasing cutaneous blood flow and cutaneous heat loss. Hence, as the Wt/SA ratio increases, (1) there is less tonic peripheral vasoconstriction, (2) peripheral tissues become increasingly warm, and (3) as a result, there is a smaller tonic thermal gradient between the core and periphery (150). Because of their smaller tonic core-to-peripheral thermal gradient, with induction of anesthesia, patients with a greater Wt/SA ratio have a lesser initial decrease in core temperature due to redistribution. Kurz et al. (150) demonstrated that the amount of redistribution hypothermia is, in fact, inversely proportional to the Wt/SA ratio. In the second phase of cooling, prior to the return of thermoregulatory vasoconstriction, cutaneous heat loss exceeds metabolic production. However, a greater Wt/SA ratio tends to slow the decrease in core temperature because the greater metabolic heat generation can more readily keep up with cutaneous heat loss (150). Finally, although SA increases as Wt increases, SA does not increase proportionately. In particular, when an increase in Wt/SA ratio is on the basis of a larger peripheral compartment (e.g., obesity), the SA available for heat transfer per unit weight of peripheral tissue also decreases. Thus, the greater the weight of the peripheral thermal compartment relative to the weight of the core, the less efficient cutaneous heat transfer becomes. In this way, an increasing Wt/SA ratio buffers the core against changes in cutaneous temperature, slowing the rate of core cooling.

A large Wt/SA ratio may decrease the rate of core cooling so greatly that it can be impossible to achieve desired levels of core hypothermia with surface cooling within a reasonable time frame. In a pilot trial of mild hypothermia during cerebral aneurysm surgery, our group reported that 7 of 57 (12%) assigned to hypothermia could not be cooled to within 1°C of target temperature (target $T_{\mathrm{ESO}} = 33.5\,^{\circ}\mathrm{C}$) by time of aneurysm clipping (22). Four of these seven patients were obese, with body mass indices (BMIs) exceeding 35 kg/m^2. Failure to reach target temperature in 10–20% of neurosurgical patients has been reported by others (151). This is a substantial limitation of existing methods of surface cooling.

Surface cooling by water immersion is much more rapid than forced-air cooling (Table 6), but this method has largely fallen out of favor and will still be relatively less efficient in obese patients. The only way to circumvent the problem of slow surface cooling in obese patients may be to employ endovascular (central venous) cooling catheters (123).

Cold Intravenous Fluids

In cases where surface cooling is insufficiently rapid, core temperature can be temporarily decreased by the intravenous administration of cold fluid. Baumgarder et al. (152) reported 5 mL/kg of ice-cold 5% albumin decreased core temperature by $0.6 \pm 0.1\,^{\circ}\mathrm{C}$ when given over 5 min and $0.4 \pm 0.1\,^{\circ}\mathrm{C}$ when given over 30 min. The decrease in core temperature was greater than expected if the cold albumin had been distributed evenly throughout total body volume. Essentially, the “cold” appeared to be constrained to the core. This same phenomenon was also observed by Rajeck et al. (153). In this later study, 40 mL/kg of 4°C normal saline was given over 30 min. Core temperature decreased 2.5 ± 0.4°C. This decrease was 0.8°C greater than expected if the change in body heat content were distributed in proportion to body mass. In both studies, core temperature returned toward baseline values within 20–30 min.

Rewarming

Conceptually, surface rewarming should be just the opposite of surface cooling but, practically, it is not. Because of the risk of burn injury (see below), one cannot greatly overheat the skin and subcutaneous tissue of the peripheral compartment to speed warming. Hence, one cannot create as great a thermal gradient between periphery and core during rewarming as is possible during cooling. As the core temperature increases, CNS-mediated thermoregulatory peripheral vasoconstriction is withdrawn. Paradoxically, this can result in a decrease in core temperature (another "afterdrop") as metabolic heat is no longer constrained to the core, once again being redistributed to the (still) cooler periphery. The threshold core temperature needed to result in the withdrawal of peripheral vasoconstriction is greater than core temperature needed to trigger its onset. Ozaki et al. (154) observed that, during cooling, peripheral thermoregulatory vasoconstriction was induced at a core temperature of 35.2 ± 0.6°C. In contrast, during rewarming, a core temperature of 36.2 ± 0.5°C was needed for its withdrawal ($P < 0.01$). Collectively, these factors create a considerable delay (often 45–60 min) between the onset of surface rewarming and any detectable increase in core temperature and a slower rate of warming than cooling. Also, if the peripheral compartment is relatively large (greater Wt/SA ratio) there is greater absolute peripheral thermal deficit that must be repaid before the temperature of the peripheral compartment can be increased.

In neurosurgical patients, both Baker et al. (21) and Szmuk et al. (155) observed that rewarming rate was inversely related to surface area. This is a paradoxical finding. Greater surface area would be expected to increase heat transfer and rewarming rate, not decrease it. The probable explanation for this apparent paradox is that a greater SA was, in fact, associated with a greater Wt/SA ratio. A reexamination of the data of Szmuk et al. (155) supports this contention (see Table 8 and Figure 5). Hence, with surface techniques, an increasing Wt/SA ratio is associated with both slower cooling and slower rewarming.

Active warming and humidification of ventilatory gases is an ineffective method of warming hypothermic patients (156,157). This is because respiratory heat exchange is so small relative to cutaneous heat exchange. Active airway heating and humidification thus has no benefit relative to passive heat-and-moisture exchanging filters. And even these should be used only to provide respiratory humidity because they have no important influence on core temperature.

One aspect of surface rewarming deserving special attention is the risk of burn injury. Burns result when heat input exceeds heat dissipation to the point that tissue temperatures exceed that of viability (~45°C) (130). There are numerous

Table 8 Morphometric and Temperature Characteristics during Surface Cooling and Rewarming in Adults and Children

	Body weight category			
	<15 kg (n = 11)	16–30 kg (n = 11)	31–90 kg (n = 11)	>90 kg (n = 11)
Age (years)	1 ± 1	5 ± 2	26 ± 19	44 ± 12
Weight (kg)	10 ± 5	21 ± 4	61 ± 22	109 ± 15
Surface area (m^2)	0.4 ± 0.2	0.8 ± 0.1	1.6 ± 0.4	2.3 ± 0.2
Weight/surface area ratio (kg/m^2)[a]	22.7 ± 3.6	26.3 ± 2.8	37.0 ± 2.8	45.5 ± 0.6
Cooling rate (°C/hr)	1.7 ± 0.2	1.6 ± 0.4	1.2 ± 0.6	0.7 ± 0.1
Rewarming rate (°C/hr)	1.8 ± 0.5	1.3 ± 0.2	0.9 ± 0.3	0.6 ± 0.1

Values are mean ± standard deviation.
[a] Calculated as the inverse of the surface area/weight ratio reported by the authors.
From Ref. 155.

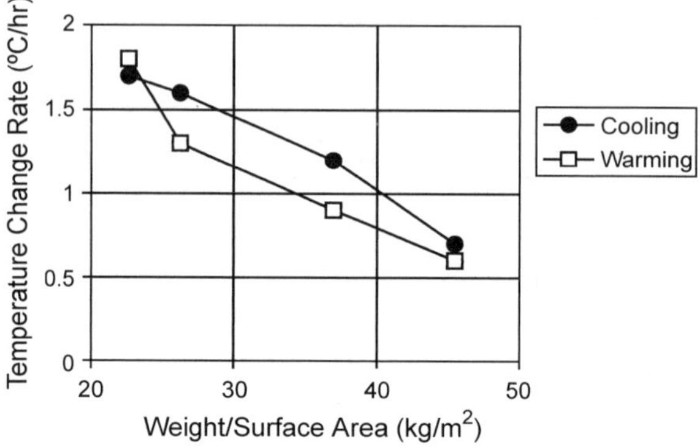

Figure 5 Relationship between weight to surface area ratio and rates of cooling and rewarming in adults and children. Data are from Table 8. (From Ref. 155.)

reports of burns from the use of water-filled heating blankets and mattresses (158–161). Usually, burns resulting from water blankets and mattresses occur in tissues that are compressed and/or poorly perfused such that applied heat could not be readily dissipated. Warming device malfunction is rarely responsible. However, perhaps surprisingly, in a 1994 American Society of Anesthesiologists closed claims analysis of intraoperative burn injury (before the common use of forced-air devices), warming blankets were not the most common cause of burns (160). The most common cause of burns (80%) was associated with the use of warm (hot) intravenous fluid bags or water filled bottles placed directly on the skin. This type of burn injury continues to be reported (162). Because surface warming is dependent on surface area, placing a hot bag or bottle on a small area of skin cannot be expected to meaningfully increase body temperature, but is dangerous. This practice should therefore be avoided.

Forced-air devices have largely supplanted water blankets/mattresses for both cooling and warming. Although considered to be an improvement over water-driven devices, there have been reports of burns associated with the use of forced-air rewarming (163–166). These burns appear to be associated with limited air clearance from the exposed areas, such that a superheated microenvironment was created. Similarly, burns resulted when the specifically designed forced-air blanket was not used; practitioners simply placing the warm air delivery hose under standard fabric blankets. The temperature of the air leaving the hose of the forced-air rewarming device is greater than the displayed target skin temperature. In addition to distributing the heat, the forced-air blanket cools the delivered air by ~2–5°C. If the specifically designed forced-air blanket is not used, it is possible for dangerously warm air to be applied to a small surface area. With the use of any warming method, heating should not be applied to tissues with compromised perfusion.

Postoperative Hypothermia and Shivering

Because rewarming is so slow, it is often difficult to completely rewarm patients by the completion of surgery (49). In adult neurosurgical patients cooled to 34.3 ± 0.4°C, Baker et al. (21) reported intraoperative surface rewarming took place at a rate of 0.7 ± 0.6°C/hr. Mean temperature upon ICU admission was 35.8 ± 1.0°C, with 7 of 12 (58%) patients shivering.

In neurosurgical patients, postoperative shivering is undesirable because it may result in hypertension (167) and increased intracranial pressure. Ideally, one would inhibit shivering while avoiding sedation. This can sometimes be achieved by increasing mean skin temperature by surface warming. Warmer skin temperatures will decrease the hypothalamic shivering threshold ~0.25°C for each 1°C increase in mean skin temperature (138). Hence, active surface warming may be sufficient to inhibit postoperative shivering in patients who are only slightly hypothermic or who have substantial residual anesthetic concentrations. For example, a mean skin temperature of 37°C decreases the shivering threshold to about 35.3 ± 0.8°C in males, with perhaps a slightly greater shivering threshold (~36.0°C) in women (137,138). There are several reports indicating selective warming of the face (168,169) and/or hands (170) inhibits shivering. Despite a report to the contrary, isolated face and/or hand warming is only marginally effective in eliminating shivering because of the small skin surface area that is exposed.

If surface warming fails to stop shivering, pharmacologic suppression is the next step (171). Almost all agents demonstrated to significantly decrease shivering thresholds have sedative properties, including propofol (140), alfentanil (141), dexmedetomidine (142), and meperidine (143). In postoperative patients, this author's first choice for an antishivering medication is usually meperidine (0.1–1.0 mg/kg), largely because (1) it is so effective and (2) many patients also require postoperative analgesia. Meperidine is the most commonly used antishivering agent in the United States. However, either propofol (140) or dexmedetomidine (142) infusions can suppress shivering while the patient is being rewarmed, with a rapid resolution of sedative effect with discontinuation of the drug. Other agents reported to have antishivering properties include clonidine (1.5 μg/kg) (167,172), physostigmine (0.04 mg/kg) (172), methylphenidate (10,173), and buspirone (174). Clonidine is the most commonly used antishivering agent in Europe.

Clinical Trials of Mild-to-Moderate Hypothermia in Neurosurgery

To date, there has been only a single randomized trial of mild systemic hypothermia in neurosurgery (22). Five centers studied 114 patients undergoing cerebral aneurysm clipping, with (n = 52) and without (n = 62) acute aneurysmal subarachnoid hemorrhage (SAH). Patients were randomized to either systemic hypothermia (forced-air surface cooling, target T_{ESO} at time of clip application was 33.5°C) vs. normothermia (target T_{ESO} = 36.5°C). After clip application, hypothermic patients were warmed as rapidly as possible with warmed forced air, warmed intravenous fluids, and warmed airway gases. Neurological status and secondary outcomes were assessed by individuals who were not aware of intraoperative temperatures.

At the time of clip application, patients assigned to hypothermia were significantly cooler (33.9 ± 0.9°C; median = 33.7°C) than those assigned to normothermia (36.5 ± 0.6°C; median = 36.6°C). Ninety-five percent (54/57) of patients assigned to normothermia were within 1.0°C of the target temperature of 36.5°C, whereas only 88% (50/57) of the patients assigned to hypothermia were within 1.0°C of target (i.e., ≤34.5°C). As discussed above, four of the seven patients assigned to hypothermia who could not be cooled to within 1.0°C of target temperature were obese, with BMIs exceeding 35 kg/m^2. Temperature groups did not differ with respect to (1) use of induced hypotension, (2) use or duration of temporary clipping, (3) use of supplemental pharmacologic cerebral protection (e.g., thiopental), or (4) intraoperative blood loss.

Despite intraoperative rewarming efforts, patients assigned to hypothermia arrived to the postoperative care area cooler (35.4 ± 1.1°C; median = 35.7°C) than patients who had been maintained normothermic throughout surgery (36.6 ± 0.8°C; median = 36.6°C). Consistent with the results reported by Baker et al. (21), our intraoperative rewarming rate was also 0.7 ± 0.5°C/hr. In the recovery area, 60% (34/57) of hypothermic group patients required continued forced-air rewarming as compared to 9% (5/57) of patients assigned to normothermia. Likewise, a greater percentage of patients assigned to hypothermia required mechanical ventilation as compared to normothermic patients, 42% (24/57) vs. 28% (10/56), respectively ($P < 0.06$). However, by 2 hr after arrival to the recovery area, the percentage of intubated patients in the two temperature groups did not differ (18%).

Neurologic outcome results are summarized in Table 9. In patients with acute SAH ($n = 52$), at 24 and 72 hr after surgery, a smaller percentage of patients assigned to hypothermia had increases in National Institute of Health Stroke Scale (NIHSS) score ≥4 points (neurologic deterioration) than patients assigned to normothermia (21% vs. 37–41%, respectively). The incidence of delayed ischemic neurologic deficit (DIND, also called vasospasm) did not differ between temperature groups (50–60%). Nevertheless, a smaller percentage of patients assigned to hypothermia were considered to have a resultant neurologic deficit at discharge as compared to patients in the normothermic group (33% vs. 56%, respectively). In addition, patients with acute SAH assigned to intra-

Table 9 Neurologic Outcomes in Cerebral Aneurysm Surgery Patients Managed With and Without Intraoperative Hypothermia

	Subarachnoid hemorrhage ($n = 52$)		No subarachnoid hemorrhage ($n = 62$)	
Outcome	Hypothermia	Normothermia	Hypothermia	Normothermia
In hospital death	1/24 = 4%	2/28 = 7%	2/33 = 6%	0/29 = 0%
≥4 increase in NIHSS				
At 24 hr	5/24 = 21%	10/27 = 37%[a]	7/33 = 21%	5/29 = 17%
At 72 hr	5/24 = 21%	11/27 = 41%[a]	6/31 = 19%[b]	6/27 = 22%[c]
DIND	12/24 = 50%	16/27 = 59%[a]	Not applicable	Not applicable
Resultant deficit	4/24 = 33%	9/27 = 56%		
Discharge destination				
Home	18/24 = 75%	16/28 = 57%	25/31 = 81%	23/29 = 79%
Rehabilitation	5/24 = 21%	10/28 = 36%	4/31 = 13%	6/29 = 21%
Glasgow outcome score at 3–6 months				
Good	17/24 = 71%	16/28 = 57%	23/30 = 77%[d]	22/29 = 76%
Moderate	3/24 = 13%	6/28 = 21%	4/30 = 13%	3/29 = 10%
Severe	2/24 = 8%	3/28 = 11%	1/30 = 3%	4/29 = 14%
Dead	2/24 = 8%	3/28 = 11%	2/30 = 7%	0/29 = 0%

NIHSS = National Institutes of Health Stroke Scale. DIND = Delayed ischemic neurologic deficit (vasospasm).
[a] Excludes one patient who died on postoperative day 1.
[b] Data from 31 of 33 patients.
[c] Data from 27 of 29 patients.
[d] Data from 30 of 33 patients.
Adapted from Ref. 22.

operative hypothermia had a greater frequency of discharge to home than those assigned to normothermia (75% vs. 57%, respectively). At 3–6 months follow-up, patients with acute SAH who had been assigned to intraoperative hypothermia had a numerically greater incidence of good outcome than those assigned to normothermia (71% vs. 57%, respectively). All deaths were on a neurologic basis. Separately, none of these apparent outcome differences achieved statistical significance. Nevertheless, each of these differences suggested that, in patients with SAH, intraoperative hypothermia was associated with an early and sustained neurologic benefit.

Notably, and perhaps surprisingly, no such benefit was apparent in patients without SAH. Accordingly, we hypothesized that the apparent neurologic benefit of intraoperative hypothermia in patients with SAH might be related to a decrease in additional (secondary) intraoperative brain injury (retractors, temporary clips) occurring in patients who were only days out from a primary neurologic injury (their SAH). The patients without acute SAH had no primary injury predisposing them to additional secondary (intraoperative) injury. A decrease in intraoperative brain injury might also increase the brain's tolerance to any subsequent insults, such as vasospasm. We noted that although the incidence of DIND was equivalent between the temperature groups, SAH patients who had been assigned to intraoperative hypothermia appeared to better tolerate DIND, having a lesser incidence of resulting neurologic deficits. As before, patients without SAH had no such delayed (tertiary) insult to tolerate. Support for this possible mechanism of intraoperative hypothermic protection in SAH patients was subsequently reported by Karibe et al. (175). In patients undergoing clipping of ruptured internal carotid or middle cerebral artery aneurysms, patients randomized to intraoperative hypothermia (n = 12, T_{REC} = 33.5°C) had greater cerebral blood flow in the ipsilateral frontal ($P < 0.01$) and frontoparietal cortex 4 days after surgery compared to those who had been normothermic during surgery. Although not significant at postoperative days 7 or 14, the trend toward greater CBF was still present in patients assigned to intraoperative hypothermia. This study suggests that, in patients with SAH, intraoperative hypothermia somehow results in better postoperative cerebral perfusion characteristics. Better postoperative perfusion may increase the brain's tolerance to subsequent insults.

Adverse events are summarized in Table 10. In nonneurosurgical patients, prior studies indicated perioperative hypothermia was associated with increased intraoperative blood loss (25), delayed emergence from anesthesia (176), increased postoperative cardiac morbidity (23,24), and increased rates of wound infection (26). In our study, intraoperative hypothermia did not appear to be associated with greater intraoperative blood loss. As noted earlier, because many patients assigned to hypothermia were not completely rewarmed by the end of surgery, this group more frequently required a brief period of postoperative intubation and rewarming. However, by 2 hr after surgery, all hypothermic patients were restored to normothermia and the fraction of patients that remained intubated did not differ between groups. Postoperative cardiovascular complications were relatively rare. There were no perioperative myocardial infarctions and no deaths were on a cardiovascular basis. Patients presenting with aneurysmal SAH are relatively young (median age ~50 years) and have a low incidence (3–5%) of preexisting coronary artery disease (177). Therefore, the threat of cardiovascular complications appears to be small relative to the neurologic threats posed by aneurysmal SAH itself. Likewise, we found no indication that hypothermia was associated with increased rates of infection (e.g., pneumonia) although, in this pilot trial, our surveillance of infectious complications did not include surgical wound infection or meningitis.

Although inconclusive, our pilot study suggested mild intraoperative hypothermia may improve the neurologic outcome of patients undergoing surgery to clip an acutely ruptured intracranial aneurysm. Mild intraoperative hypothermia did not appear to carry increased risk of bleeding, infectious, or cardiovascular complications, but this pilot study was simply too small to have sufficient statistical power to make definitive conclusions. The only apparent disadvantage associated with intraoperative hypothermia was the

Table 10 Adverse Events in Cerebral Aneurysm Surgery Patients Managed With and Without Intraoperative Hypothermia

	Subarachnoid hemorrhage (n = 52)		No subarachnoid hemorrhage (n = 62)	
Adverse event	Hypothermia[a]	Normothermia[a]	Hypothermia	Normothermia
Median intraoperative blood loss (mL)	325	400	325	250
Intubated				
At arrival to recovery	11/24 = 46%	8/28 = 29%	13/33 = 39%	8/29 = 28%
At 2 h in recovery	6/24 = 25%	6/28 = 21%	4/32 = 13%[b]	4/28 = 14%[c]
At 24 h after surgery	0/24 = 0%	3/27 = 11%	3/33 = 9%	2/29 = 7%
Postoperative reintubation (any cause)	4/24 = 17%	4/28 = 15%	1/33 = 3%	1/29 = 3%
Cardiovascular				
Myocardial ischemia	2/24 = 8%	1/28 = 4%	2/33 = 6%	2/29 = 7%
Congestive failure	1/24 = 4%	0/28 = 0%	0/33 = 0%	0/29 = 0%
Respiratory				
Pneumonia	1/24 = 4%	3/28 = 11%	0/33 = 0%	0/29 = 0%
Respiratory failure	3/24 = 13%	1/28 = 4%	1/33 = 3%	1/29 = 3%
Any major complication	12/24 = 50%	22/28 = 79%	6/33 = 19%	7/29 = 24%
Intensive care				
At 24 h after surgery	12/24 = 50%	22/28 = 79%	20/33 = 61%	10/29 = 34%
At 72 h after surgery	11/24 = 46%	14/27 = 52%	5/33 = 15%	4/29 = 14%
Median interval from surgery to live discharge (days)	17	16	4	5

[a] One patient in this group died on postoperative day 1. Rates based on n = 27 for all events after 24 hr.
[b] Data from 32 of 33 patients.
[c] Data from 28 of 29 patients.
Adapted from Ref. 22.

frequent occurrence of mild postoperative hypothermia and the associated need for brief postoperative warming and intubation. In theory, delays in detection of acute postoperative neurologic deficits following neurosurgery could delay implementation of critical therapeutic interventions. Although this was not observed in this pilot trial (with a total of 57 hypothermic patients), our larger follow-up trial [Intraoperative Hypothermia for Aneurysm Surgery Trial, Part 2 (IHAST2), 1001 patients] will have much greater power to address this and other potential risks associated with mild intraoperative hypothermia.

Mild-to-Moderate Hypothermia for Cardiac Surgery

Basics of Arterial Perfusion Cooling and Rewarming

Perspective

Currently, arterial perfusion-based methods of cooling and warming are exclusively used during cardiac surgery and CPB. The CPB pump delivers oxygenated blood (perfusate) directly into the central arterial system via the ascending aorta or, occasionally, the femoral artery. Venous cannulas in the right atrium and/or vena cavae divert blood that would normally enter the right ventricle into the venous reservoir of the CPB circuit. The perfusionist determines the temperature of the water that flows through the heat-exchanger component of the CPB oxygenator. Because the heat exchanger water temperature can be made very cold (10°C) or very warm (41°C), perfusate temperature can be rapidly changed. Because brain temperature depends most greatly on the temperature of the blood perfusing it (38), brain temperature can be very rapidly changed with arterial perfusion.

Cooling

The rate of change of brain temperature varies directly with the magnitude of temperature gradient between the perfusate and brain. Greater gradients (colder perfusate) increase the rate of cooling proportionately (38). During arterial perfusion cooling, a perfusate-to-brain temperature gradient exceeding 10°C is generally avoided. As blood temperature decreases, both blood oxygen solubility and hemoglobin oxygen affinity (P_{50}) increase, i.e., blood becomes more oxygen-avid (84). In theory, with a large perfusate-to-brain temperature gradient, oxygen transfer between cold (oxygen-avid) blood and warm (less oxygen-avid) brain could be limited, resulting in brain tissue hypoxia. Therefore, during cooling, perfusate temperatures are usually adjusted to avoid perfusate-to-brain gradients greater than 10°C. However, even with this limitation, brain cooling during CPB takes place very rapidly. Average brain temperature can be reduced from 37 to 27°C over the course of 12–15 min, or less (38,48). Thus, arterial perfusion cooling can easily achieve an average brain cooling rate of ~1°C/min, which is 40- to 60-fold greater than that accomplished by conventional surface cooling methods (1–1.5°C/hr).

Because cooling rates also depend on blood flow, there is considerable heterogeneity among body regions in rates of cooling during CPB (130). Because of relatively lesser blood flow, the peripheral thermal compartment cools considerably less rapidly than the central (high flow) compartment.

Rewarming

A common practice, now largely abandoned, was to maximize the rate of rewarming on CPB by increasing arterial perfusate temperature to supraphysiologic values, e.g., 40–41°C (178). This practice was associated with jugular venous desaturation, very rapid rates of brain rewarming and, sometimes, overt cerebral hyperthermia (178). Each of these elements could have an adverse effect upon the brain, as discussed below.

Clinical Trials of Mild-to-Moderate Hypothermia in Cardiac Surgery

Alpha-Stat Vs. pH-Stat

Under hypothermic conditions, two different acid–base strategies can be used, alpha-stat or pH-stat. As discussed previously, pH-stat management results in a relative acidemia and hypercarbia compared to alpha-stat, and results in greater CBF. At issue was whether the greater CBF of pH-stat management resulted in better cerebral perfusion and neurologic outcome compared to alpha-stat, or increased delivery of cerebral emboli and worse neurologic outcome compared to alpha-stat.

Five randomized clinical trials have examined the impact of alpha-stat vs. pH-stat on neurologic outcomes (Table 11). The first study to address this question was that of Bashein et al. (179), in which 86 adults were randomized to alpha-stat or pH-stat management during CPB (30°C). Short-term (8 days) and long-term (7 months) neurocognitive status were not affected by choice of acid–base management. Three subsequent studies indicated that there was a modest benefit with alpha-stat management. Stephan et al. (75) randomized 65 adults to alpha-stat or pH-stat management during CPB (26°C). During CPB, pH-stat patients had greater CBF, but $CMRO_2$ did not differ between groups. Postoperative neurologic deficits 7 days after surgery were more common in pH-stat patients (10/35 = 29%) as compared with alpha-stat patients (2/30 = 7%), $P = 0.04$. In a similar study, Patel et al.

Table 11 Clinical Trials of Alpha-Stat Versus pH-Stat Management in Adult Cardiac Surgery Using Cardiopulmonary Bypass

Author, year; (ref.)	*n*	Neurologic outcome result: alpha-stat versus pH-stat
Bashein, 1990; (179)	86	Cognitive at 8 days and 7 months: no difference
Stephan, 1992; (75)	65	Neurologic at 7 days: alpha-stat better
Murkin, 1995; (180)	316	Neurologic and cognitive at 7 days and 2 months: no difference CPB duration >90 min, cognitive at 2 months: alpha-stat better
Patel, 1996; (77)	70	Cognitive at 6 weeks: alpha-stat better
Engelhardt, 1996; (181)	45	Neurologic, cognitive, and electrophysiological at 7 days: no difference

(77) randomized 70 adults to alpha-stat or pH-stat management during CPB (28°C). During CPB, pH-stat patients had greater CBF and lesser $CMRO_2$ (~25% decrease) compared to alpha-stat patients. Six weeks after surgery, neurocognitive abnormalities were more common in pH-stat patients (17/35 = 49%) as compared with alpha-stat patients (7/35 = 20%; $P = 0.02$). Murkin et al. (180) randomized 316 adults to alpha-stat or pH-stat management during CPB (26–28°C). Overall, there was no difference in acute or chronic neurologic outcomes between the groups. However, in patients undergoing CPB for 90 min or more, those managed with alpha-stat had a lesser incidence of neurocognitive abnormalities at 2 months postoperatively (17/62 = 27%) than those managed with pH-stat (28/63 = 44%; $P = 0.05$). Finally, Engelhardt et al. (181) randomized 45 adults to alpha-stat or pH-stat management during CPB (29°C). In the first week after surgery, there were no differences between groups in level of consciousness, neurologic abnormalities, neurocognitive scores, or auditory evoked potentials.

Thus, there is no neurologic disadvantage, but perhaps a slight advantage, to alpha-stat management during moderately hypothermic (26–30°C) CPB. Although pH-stat management results in greater CBF than alpha-stat management, this greater CBF is not associated with greater $CMRO_2$. If anything, $CMRO_2$ may actually be slightly less under pH-stat conditions (77). Thus, the lesser CBF and P_{50} of alpha-stat management do not appear to significantly limit cerebral oxygen availability (76,84). Why alpha-stat results in slightly better neurologic outcome during moderately hypothermic CPB is not truly known. It has been postulated that the lesser CBF associated with alpha-stat management may decrease the number of cerebral emboli entering the cerebral circulation during CPB. The neurologic benefits of alpha-stat management are not overwhelming and may, as shown by Murkin et al., only become detectable with longer CPB durations.

"Warm" Vs. "Cold" Cardiopulmonary Bypass

In the early 1990s, normothermic ("warm") cardioplegia and CPB were reintroduced into cardiac surgery (27,28). At the same time, animal experiments were demonstrating the rather dramatic neuroprotective value of mild hypothermia. There was widespread concern that normothermic CPB would result in worse neurologic outcomes compared to traditional moderately hypothermic CPB. This concern resulted in seven separate randomized clinical trials addressing this issue (Table 12).

Three studies reported no difference in neurologic or neurocognitive outcomes between "normothermic" and hypo-

Table 12 Randomized Trials of Hypothermic Versus Normothermic Cardiopulmonary Bypass and Neurologic Outcome

Author, year; (ref.)	*n*	Groups	Neurologic outcome result: effect of temperature
The Warm Heart Investigators, 1994; (182)	1,732	25–30°C; 33–37°C	Stroke by discharge: no difference
McLean, 1994; (183)[a]	155	28°C; 34°C	Cognitive at 5 days and 3 months: no difference
Martin, 1994; (184)	1,001	28°C; 36°C	Neurologic by discharge: cold better
Mora, 1996; (185)[b]	138	28°C; 36°C	Neurologic at 7 days: cold better Cognitive at 7 days and 6 weeks: no difference
Regragui, 1996; (186)	70	28°C; 32°C; 36°C	Cognitive at 6 weeks: cold (32°) better
Engelman, 1996; (187)	130	23–28°C; 32–33°C; 35–36°C	Neurologic outcome at 1 month: no difference
Plourde, 1997; (188)	54	29°C; 36°C	Cognitive at 7 days: no difference
Grimm, 2000; (189)	144	32°C; 37°C	Cognitive and electrophysiological at 4 months: no difference
Grigore, 2001; (190)	300	28°C; 36°C	Neurologic at discharge: no difference Cognitive at 6 weeks: no difference

[a] Patients reported in this study were a subset of those reported by The Warm Heart Investigators (182).

[b] Patients reported in this study were a subgroup of those reported by Martin et al. (184).

thermic (28°C) CPB (182,183,188). Because, in these three studies, most "normothermic" patients were actually modestly hypothermic (~34.5°C), it is possible that these "normothermic" patients may actually have had some hypothermic protection, decreasing outcome differences between groups. In contrast, three other studies reported worse neurologic outcomes with "normothermic" CPB (184–186). However, in these three studies, active warming during CPB probably resulted in "normothermic" patients with brain temperatures that were actually slightly hyperthermic throughout CPB (185). Even mild hyperthermia (just 1–2°C above normal) markedly increases injury following a neurologic insult (191–193). Thus, "normothermic" patients in these later three studies could have had some hyperthermic worsening of neurologic injury. Engelman et al. (187) largely avoided these limitations by randomizing 130 patients to core temperatures of 23–28°C ("cold") vs. 32–33°C ("tepid") vs. 35–36°C ("warm") during CPB, and avoiding hyperthermia during rewarming. This study found no difference in neurologic outcomes among the three temperature groups. Likewise, subsequent studies that have been careful to avoid or limit hyperthermia during the rewarming phase of CPB have not observed any neurologic benefit with hypothermic CPB. Grigore et al. (190) randomized 300 adults to either hypothermic (28–30°C) or normothermic (35.5–36.5°C) CPB. During normothermic CPB, perfusate inflow temperature was maintained at 36°C, and patients were rewarmed to a T_{NP} = 37°C with a maximum perfusate temperature of 38°C. During hypothermic CPB, perfusate temperature was maintained at 28°C and patients were rewarmed to a T_{NP} = 37°C with a maximal difference between perfusate and T_{NP} of 4–6°C, and a maximum perfusate temperature of 38°C. The incidence of adverse neurologic events occurring by time of discharge was equivalent between groups (~14%). Likewise, the incidence of new cognitive deficits 6 weeks after surgery was also equivalent between groups (~39%).

Because moderate hypothermia during CPB does not confer clear-cut neurologic or neurocognitive benefit, it would seem most neurologic insults occurring in adult cardiac surgery patients are of a type not greatly affected by hypothermia (e.g., permanent emboli), or principally occur during normothermic periods of cardiac surgery (e.g., aortic cannulation, aortic cross-clamp removal, emergence from CPB, or postoperatively). Alternatively, the neurologic benefits afforded by hypothermic CPB might be negated by some adverse effect or feature unique to CPB. Accordingly, considerable attention has been given to the rewarming phase of CPB.

Rewarming Issues

Jugular Venous Desaturation

Jugular bulb blood is usually representative of mixed cerebral venous blood (194). As such, jugular bulb oxyhemoglobin saturation provides a rough index of the relationship between global brain oxygen delivery and consumption. A normal (normothermic) jugular venous saturation is about 60%. During moderately hypothermic CPB (alpha-stat), jugular venous saturation is usually about 75% (195–199). There have been numerous reports describing decreases in jugular venous saturation during CPB rewarming, with jugular venous saturations less than 50% occurring in 15–30% of patients (196–202). In some studies, the degree of jugular desaturation appears to be related to rewarming rate, with more rapid rewarming leading to greater desaturation (198,202,203). At issue was whether marked jugular venous desaturation and rapid rewarming during CPB were adversely affecting the brain, negating the neuroprotection expected from moderately hypothermic CPB.

A series of studies from Duke University assessed the relationship between jugular venous desaturation and postoperative neurocognitive outcome. Their first report found no association (200). Two subsequent reports, each derived from the same patient population, that indicated that greater jugular venous desaturation at completion of rewarming (specifically, greater arterio–venous oxygen content difference) was associated with a greater incidence of acute postoperative cognitive deficits (201,204). Notably, patients who exhibited marked jugular venous desaturation at completion of rewarming tended to have lesser CBF, greater $CMRO_2$, and greater brain oxygen extraction before the start of rewarming (201). This suggested that patients who desaturated the most during rewarming differed from the rest of the study population before rewarming was initiated. Perhaps this preexisting difference was responsible for their greater postoperative cognitive impairment, not the jugular venous desaturation per se.

This hypothesis was supported by Goto et al. (205). These investigators observed that patients with greater abnormalities on preoperative brain magnetic resonance imaging (MRI) had greater degrees of jugular venous desaturation during CPB rewarming. Thus, patients with preexisting neurologic injury, even if subclinical, may have limited cerebral perfusion reserves. Both conditions may predispose patients to new postoperative neurocognitive deficits.

The final report from the Duke group on this topic indicated that jugular venous desaturation had only a minor independent effect on early postoperative neurocognitive outcome when baseline neurocognitive status, educational level, and age were considered (206). More recently, Robson et al. (207), who also adjusted for baseline cognitive status, reported averaged jugular venous saturation values during CPB and in the early postoperative phase had no association with cognitive status 3 months after surgery. Therefore, it appears that when baseline cognitive status is taken into consideration, jugular saturation (desaturation) has, at most, only a very small short-term impact on cognitive status, but no effect on long-term outcome. Jugular venous desaturation during the rewarming phase of CPB appears to largely be a marker of preexisting cerebrovascular abnormalities.

Rewarming Rate and Hyperthermia

An obvious difference between the animal (non-CPB) experiments that observed marked protective efficacy with mild-to-moderate hypothermia and clinical CPB studies that did not was the rate of rewarming. Rewarming during clinical CPB was, and remains, much faster than achieved in non-CPB animal studies. Brain rewarming rates in the range of 0.5–1.5°C/min were, and still are, common during cardiac surgery

(202,206). To achieve such rapid rewarming, it was common practice to increase arterial perfusate temperature to 40°C or even warmer (178). A number of studies indicate brain temperatures of 38–39°C frequently occurred because of this aggressive rewarming or inaccurate temperature monitoring (178,203,206,208). Rapid rewarming rates and transient cerebral hyperthermia are interrelated phenomena, and either one or both could have an adverse effect on the brain.

Rapid Rewarming: Observations suggest that rapid rewarming is poorly tolerated by the brain. In a rabbit CPB model, rapid brain rewarming (0.8–1.0°C/min) was associated with a transient uncoupling of flow and metabolism (209). Specifically, CBF did not increase sufficiently to match increases in $CMRO_2$, resulting in moderate cerebral venous desaturation. This apparent uncoupling was not present at slower rewarming rates (0.3°C/min). Subsequently, in a gerbil model of transient forebrain ischemia (5 min at normothermia, followed by 2 hr of postischemic reperfusion at 24°C), animals that were rapidly rewarmed (0.43°C/min) had lesser CBF and greater extracellular glutamate and lactate concentrate at the end of rewarming compared to animals slowly rewarmed (0.1–0.2°C/min) (210). Also, at 7 days after ischemia, rapidly rewarmed animals had greater hippocampal injury than slowly rewarmed animals. The mechanistic basis of these observations is unknown. However, two in vitro studies—one using rat microvessels (211) and one using human middle cerebral arteries (212)—have observed rapid rewarming results in transient hypercontractile vascular responses. Such vascular responses might have an adverse effect on postischemic reperfusion and could explain our observation of impaired flow–metabolism coupling. This would also be consistent with the observations of some investigators that the degree of jugular venous desaturation occurring during CPB rewarming varies with rewarming rate.

There have been few studies that have formally assessed the effect of rewarming rate on cognitive outcome. Newman et al. (206) observed that with increasing age, greater rewarming rates had a borderline association with poorer cognitive performance. More recently, Grigore et al. (213) compared cognitive outcomes between patients who were warmed rapidly (4–6°C difference between T_{NP} and CPB perfusate temperature) vs. those rewarmed slowly (2°C difference between T_{NP} and perfusate temperature). Maximum rewarming rates were 0.56°C/min in the rapid rewarming group vs. 0.49°C/min in the slow rewarming group ($P = 0.03$). Maximum T_{NP} was 38.2°C in the rapid group vs. 37.8°C in the slow group ($P = 0.01$). Despite these rather minor differences between groups, multivariable linear regression analysis indicated patients in the slow rewarming group had significantly less decrease of cognitive performance 6 weeks after surgery compared to patients who were rapidly rewarmed ($P = 0.047$). However, the effect of rewarming rate was not robust. When cognitive deficits were considered as a dichotomous outcome (one standard deviation decrease in one or more factors) in a model controlling for age, education, and baseline cognitive performance, rewarming rate did not predict the presence of postoperative cognitive deficits ($P = 0.11$). It remains possible, though, that this result represents a type II statistical error and that the difference would be statistically significant with a larger sample size.

A different approach to this issue was taken in a study of patients undergoing moderately hypothermic (32°C) CPB (214). Patients were randomized to partial (T_{NP} = 34°C) vs. complete (T_{NP} = 37°C) rewarming prior to separation from CPB. Patients in the partial rewarming group underwent additional postoperative surface warming and returned to normothermia approximately 2 hr later than the other group. Hence, the partial rewarming group was, in fact, a slow rewarming group. At 10 days after surgery, cognitive impairment was less common in the partial (slow) rewarming group (45/94 = 48%) vs. the complete (rapid) rewarming group (62/100 = 62%; $P = 0.048$). At 3 months after surgery, cognitive outcome was slightly better in the partial (slow) rewarming group. These two clinical studies are suggestive but not definitive. Nevertheless, given the collective observations regarding the potentially unfavorable effect of rapid rewarming, it may be prudent to restrict CPB rewarming rates ≤0.4°C/min.

Hyperthermia: There is considerable laboratory (191–193) and clinical evidence (215–218) that hyperthermia has an independent adverse effect upon the acutely injured brain. At issue is whether rewarming-induced cerebral hyperthermia could exacerbate neurologic injuries, negating the benefits of hypothermic CPB. Reexamining the data from the McLean et al. study, Buss et al. (208) reported that 44% of patients were rewarmed to nasopharyngeal temperatures ≥38°C. Nevertheless, neuropsychologic outcome did not appear significantly worse in these patients compared to those rewarmed to lesser temperature. The authors suggested the duration of cerebral hyperthermia during rewarming may not be sufficient to adversely affect outcome. Whether transient hyperthermic overshoot during rewarming from hypothermic CPB has adverse neurologic effects is unclear. On the other hand, postoperative fever is very common following CPB and is of a much greater duration (219–221). Using multivariable linear regression (controlling for age, baseline cognitive function, education, and CPB temperature group assignment), Grocott et al. (221) reported that greater values of maximum postoperative temperature were associated with greater degrees of cognitive dysfunction 6 weeks after cardiac surgery.

FUTURE DIRECTIONS

As we progress into the first decade of the 21st century, the balance of risk vs. benefit associated with mild-to-moderate hypothermia during surgery and anesthesia remains undefined. Hypothermia is certainly not a panacea. Like any other therapeutic intervention, for every potential benefit there is also potential risk.

Cardiac Surgery

In the setting of adult cardiac surgery and CPB, mild-to-moderate hypothermia does not appear to confer any clear-cut neurologic benefit. One can only conclude that the insults that lead to stroke and cognitive impairment with cardiac surgery are of a type not meaningfully affected by intraoperative hypothermia. Animal studies indicate mild-to-moderate hypothermia has very limited protective efficacy in the setting of permanent focal cerebral ischemia (20,222,223). Thus, if an aortic atherosclerotic plaque is embolized to the brain (a permanent occlusion), intraoperative hypothermia may not have any appreciable effect on neurologic outcome. Another factor that may decrease the apparent efficacy of intraoperative hypothermia in the setting of cardiac surgery may relate to the fact that 50% of perioperative strokes have their onset well into the postoperative period (224). Intraoperative brain temperature is less likely to affect neurologic outcome when neurologic insults have their onset days later. Finally, there are indications that some of the potential benefits of mild-to-moderate hypothermia during cardiac surgery and CPB may be negated by rapid rewarming (213) and intraoperative or postoperative hyperthermia (221). Hence, future investigations may focus more on postoperative temperature management and fever control and less on intraoperative hypothermia per se.

A rapidly increasing fraction of coronary revascularization procedures are performed without CPB, the so called "off-pump" procedures (225,226). In these procedures, coronary revascularization takes place on the spontaneously beating heart. Off-pump procedures utilize temporary coronary artery occlusion while distal anastomoses are created. Accordingly, patients experience one or more periods of regional myocardial ischemia. These periods of myocardial ischemia may result in systemic hypotension and myocardial ischemia and infarction. A recent animal study showed mild systemic hypothermia (34°C) significantly decreases infarct size following transient coronary occlusion (121). Likewise, Dixon et al. (122) reported that, in patients undergoing emergent percutaneous coronary revascularization, mild systemic hypothermia (34°C for 3–4 h in the reperfusion phase) appeared to decrease infarct size.

Both of these studies used a percutaneous cooling catheter placed in the inferior vena cava to rapidly induce mild systemic hypothermia. Although invasive compared to cooling blankets and forced-air devices, the great advantage of percutaneous cooling catheters is their rapidity of cooling. Systemic hypothermia in the range of 33–34°C can be achieved within 1 hr as opposed to 3–4 hr with surface cooling techniques. Therefore, in an attempt to limit myocardial injury from periods of temporary myocardial ischemia, it is possible "off-pump" coronary revascularization might be performed in patients cooled to 33–34°C. To the extent that neurologic injury associated with these procedures might be caused by transient periods of hypotension or low cardiac output, mild systemic hypothermia also has the potential to improve neurologic outcome.

Neurosurgery

It remains unknown whether mild-to-moderate hypothermia confers any meaningful neurologic benefit in the setting of neurological surgery. A large prospective randomized clinical trial of mild systemic hypothermia (33.0°C) vs. normothermia (36.5°C) during cerebral aneurysm surgery completed enrollment in April 2003 (1001 patients). This trial, the Intraoperative Hypothermia for Aneurysm Surgery Trial, Part 2 (IHAST2), was powered to detect an absolute increase of 10% in the rate of good neurologic outcome (Glasgow Outcome Scale) 3 months after surgery (e.g., 75% good outcome vs. 65% good outcome). Secondary outcome measures included other functional measures (Rankin, Barthel's scale), as well as a host of intermediate measures such as duration of hospitalization, need for rehabilitative care, and various medical complications (neurological, cardiovascular, bleeding, infection, etc.). Many of the neurologic insults occurring during cerebral aneurysm surgery are temporary in nature, e.g., hypotension, brain retraction, temporary vessel occlusion. It is these types of insults for which hypothermia is most consistently effective in laboratory settings. As discussed above, the pilot work (22,175) suggests that mild intraoperative systemic hypothermia is likely to improve neurologic outcome in the setting of cerebral aneurysm surgery. However, until the results of IHAST2 are published (late 2004), the risks and benefits remain speculative.

Aneurysm surgery per se may become far less common with the increasing use of endovascular methods for the treatment of cerebral aneurysms and arteriovenous malformations. In patients with ruptured aneurysms, a recent randomized trial indicated short-term outcomes may be slightly better with endovascular treatment (cooling) as compared to traditional surgical clipping (227). Nevertheless, if IHAST2 confirms the safety and efficacy of mild systemic hypothermia during aneurysm surgery, the next logical question will be the extent to which mild-to-moderate hypothermia confers protection during other forms of CNS intervention—neurosurgical, endovascular, or otherwise. Of course, even if the outcome of IHAST2 is positive, there is no guarantee that hypothermia will meaningfully improve outcome with every type of neurologic intervention because the mechanisms of injury and determinants of outcome vary from condition to condition.

Present and Future

Outside of the operating room, studies of the efficacy of mild-to-moderate hypothermia as a neuro-resuscitative intervention have had mixed results. Two randomized trials conducted in head trauma patients did not observe any apparent benefit with mild systemic hypothermia (32–34°C for 48–96 hr) as compared to normothermia (117,228). In contrast, two other randomized trials in cardiac arrest patients observed an apparent neurologic benefit with mild hypothermia (33°C for 12–24 hr) (114,229). It is clear that the neurologic benefits of mild-to-moderate hypothermia can be overwhelmed by other determinants of outcome such as (1) differences in nature of the neurologic insult (trauma, focal ischemia, global ischemia, subarachnoid hemorrhage, inflammation, vasospasm), (2) differences in the application of hypothermia (temperature and duration, rates of cooling and rewarming), (3) differences among patient populations (age, coexisting disease and injury), and (4) differences in the management of hypothermia-related side effects (fluids, vasopressors, electrolytes, infection). In the prevention and treatment of neurologic injury, we stand on the threshold of either another in a long series of disappointments (230) or a meaningful new advance. Hopefully, therapeutic hypothermia in the neurocritical care setting represents that long-sought advance.

REFERENCES

1. Lewis FJ, Taufic M. Closure of atrial septal defects with the aid of hypothermia; experimental accomplishments and the report of one successful case. Surgery 1953; 33:52–59.
2. Botterell EH, Lougheed WM, Scott JW, Vandewater SL. Hypothermia and interruption of carotid, or carotid and vertebral circulation, in the surgical management of intracranial aneurysms. J Neurosurg 1956; 13:1–42.
3. Pool JL. The development of modern intracranial aneurysm surgery. Neurosurgery 1977; 1:233–237.
4. Gibbon JH. Application of a mechanical heart and lung apparatus to cardiac surgery. Minn Med 1954; 37:171–180.
5. Sealy WC, Brown IW Jr, Young WG Jr. A report on the use of both extracorporeal circulation and hypothermia for open heart surgery. Ann Surg 1958; 147:603–613.
6. Swan H, Paton B. The combined use of hypothermia and extracorporeal circulation in cardiac surgery. J Cardiovasc Surg 1960; 1:169–175.
7. Little DM. Hypothermia. Anesthesiology 1959; 20:842–877.
8. Hale DE, Collis JS Jr, King MH. Intracranial aneurysmal surgery with and without hypothermia. Surgery 1962; 52:338–341.
9. Hamby WB. Intracranial surgery for aneurysm: effect of hypothermia upon survival. J Neurosurg 1963; 20:41–45.
10. Michenfelder JD, Terry HR Jr. Current practices and trends in neuroanesthesia. Clin Neurosurg 1965; 13:252–264.
11. Paul RL, Arnold JG. Operative factors influencing mortality in intracranial aneurysm surgery: analysis of 186 consecutive cases. J Neurosurg 1970; 32:289–294.
12. Michenfelder JD, Kirklin JW, Uihlein A, Svien HJ, MacCarty CS. Clinical experience with a closed-chest method of producing profound hypothermia and total circulatory arrest in neurosurgery. Ann Surg 1964; 159:125–131.
13. Young WL, Lawton MT, Gupta DK, Hashimoto T. Anesthetic management of deep hypothermic circulatory arrest for

cerebral aneurysm clipping. Anesthesiology 2002; 96:497–503.

14. McDowal DG. The current usage of hypothermia in British neurosurgery. Br J Anaesth 1971; 43:1084–1087.
15. Ehrenhaft JL, Claman MA, Layton JM, Zimmerman GR. Cerebral complications of open-heart Surgery: further observations. J Thorac Cardiovasc Surg 1961; 42:514–526.
16. Arrowsmith JE, Grocott HP, Reves JG, Newman MF. Central nervous system complications of cardiac surgery. Br J Anaesth 2000; 84:378–393.
17. Busto R, Dietrich WD, Globus MYT, Valdes I, Scheinberg P, Ginsberg MD. Small differences in intraischemic brain temperature critically determine the extent of ischemic neuronal injury. J Cereb Blood Flow Metab 1987; 7:729–738.
18. Minamisawa H, Nordstrom C-H, Smith M-L, Siesjö BK. The influence of mild body and brain hypothermia on ischemic brain damage. J Cereb Blood Flow Metab 1990; 10:365–374.
19. Clifton GL, Jiang JY, Lyeth BG, Jenkins LW, Hamm RJ, Hayes RL. Marked protection by moderate hypothermia after experimental traumatic brain injury. J Cereb Blood Flow Metab 1991; 11:114–121.
20. Ridenour TR, Warner DS, Todd MM, McAllister AC. Mild hypothermia reduces infarct size resulting from temporary but not permanent focal ischemia in rats. Stroke 1992; 23:733–738.
21. Baker KZ, Young WL, Stone JG, Kader A, Baker CJ, Solomon RA. Deliberate mild intraoperative hypothermia for craniotomy. Anesthesiology 1994; 81:361–367.
22. Hindman BJ, Todd MM, Gelb AW, Loftus CM, Craen RA, Schubert A, Mahla ME, Torner JC. Mild hypothermia as a protective therapy during intracranial aneurysm surgery: a randomized prospective pilot trial. Neurosurgery 1999; 44:23–33.
23. Frank SM, Beattie C, Christopherson R, Norris EJ, Perler BA, Williams GM, Gottlieb SO. Unintentional hypothermia is

associated with postoperative myocardial ischemia. Anesthesiology 1993; 78:468–476.

24. Frank SM, Fleisher LA, Breslow MJ, Higgins MS, Olson KR, Kelly S, Beattie C. Perioperative maintenance of normothermia reduces the incidence of morbid cardiac events. A randomized clinical trial. JAMA 1997; 277:1127–1134.
25. Schmied H, Kurz A, Sessler DI, Kozek S, Reiter A. Mild hypothermia increases blood loss and transfusion requirements during total hip arthroplasty. Lancet 1996; 347:289–292.
26. Kurz A, Sessler DI, Lenhardt R. Perioperative normothermia to reduce the incidence of surgical-wound infection and shorten hospitalization. N Engl J Med 1996; 334:1209–1215.
27. Lichtenstein SV, Ashe KA, El Dalati H, Cusimano RJ, Panos A, Slutsky AS. Warm heart surgery. J Thorac Cardiovasc Surg 1991; 101:269–274.
28. Christakis GT, Koch JP, Deenar KA, Fremes SE, Sinclair L, Chen E, Salerno TA, Goldman BS, Lichtenstein SV. A randomized study of the systemic effects of warm heart surgery. Ann Thorac Surg 1992; 54:449–457.
29. Vitez TS, White PF, Eger EI II. Effects of hypothermia on halothane MAC and isoflurane MAC in the rat. Anesthesiology 1974; 41:80–81.
30. Eger EI II, Johnson BH. MAC of I-653 in rats, including a test of the effect of body temperature and anesthetic duration. Anesth Analg 1987; 66:974.
31. Antognini JF. Hypothermia eliminates isoflurane requirements at 20°C. Anesthesiology 1993; 78:1152–1156.
32. Liu M, Hu X, Liu J. The effect of hypothermia on isoflurane MAC in children. Anesthesiology 2001; 94:429–432.
33. Leslie K, Bjorksten AR, Ugoni A, Mitchell P. Mild core hypothermia and anesthetic requirement for loss of responsiveness during propofol anesthesia for craniotomy. Anesth Analg 2002; 94:1298–1303.
34. Virtue RW. Hypothermic Anesthesia. Springfield, IL: Charles C Thomas, 1955.

35. Fay T. Observations on prolonged human refrigeration. NY State J Med 1940; 40:1351–1354.

36. Coleshaw SRK, Van Someren RNM, Wolff AH, Davis HM, Keatinge WR. Impaired memory registration and speed of reasoning caused by low body temperature. J Appl Physiol (Respirat Environ Exercise Physiol) 1983; 55:27–31.

37. Castellani JW, Young AJ, Sawka MN, Backus VL, Canete JJ. Amnesia during cold water immersion: a case report. Wilderness Environ Med 1998; 9:153–155.

38. Dexter F, Hindman BJ. Computer simulation of brain cooling during cardiopulmonary bypass. Ann Thorac Surg 1994; 57:1171–1179.

39. Whitby JD, Dunkin LJ. Cerebral, oesophageal and nasopharyngeal temperatures. Br J Anaesth 1971; 43:673–676.

40. Shiraki K, Sagawa S, Tajima F, Yokota A, Hashimoto M, Brengelmann GL. Independence of brain and tympanic temperatures in unanesthetized human. J Appl Physiol 1988; 65:482–486.

41. Mellergård P, Nordstrom CH. Intracerebral temperature in neurosurgical patients. Neurosurgery 1991; 28:709–713.

42. Mellergård P. Intracerebral temperature in neurosurgical patients. Intracerebral temperature gradients and relationships to consciousness level. Surg Neurol 1995; 43:91–95.

43. Henker RA, Brown SD, Marion DW. Comparison of brain temperature with bladder and rectal temperatures in adults with severe head injury. Neurosurgery 1998; 42:1071–1075.

44. Mariak Z, Lewko J, £uczaj J, Polocki B, White MD. The relationship between directly measured human cerebral and tympanic temperatures during changes in brain temperatures. Eur J Appl Physiol 1994; 69:545–549.

45. Stone JG, Goodman RR, Baker KZ, Baker CJ, Solomon RA. Direct intraoperative measurement of human brain temperature. Neurosurgery 1997; 41:20–24.

46. Mellergård P. Changes in human intracerebral temperature in response to different methods of brain cooling. Neurosurgery 1992; 31:667–671.

47. Iatrou CC, Domaingue CM, Thomas RD, Nye DH. The effect of selective brain cooling on intracerebral temperature during craniotomy. Anaesth Intens Care 2002; 30:167–170.

48. Stone JG, Young WL, Smith CR, Solomon RA, Wald A, Ostapkovich N, Shrebnick DB. Do standard monitoring sites reflect true brain temperature when profound hypothermia is rapidly induced and reversed? Anesthesiology 1995; 82:344–351.

49. Crowder CM, Tempelhoff R, Theard A, Cheng MA, Todorov A, Dacey RG. Jugular bulb temperature: comparison with brain surface and core temperatures in neurosurgical patients during mild hypothermia. J Neurosurg 1996; 85:98–103.

50. Clausen T, Rieger A, Roth S, Soukup J, Furka I, Lindner J, Telgmaa L, Hennig C, Radke J, Menzel M. Cerebrovenous blood temperature-influence of cerebral perfusion pressure changes and hyperventilation: evaluation in a porcine study and in man. J Neurosurg Anesth 2000; 12:2–9.

51. Kaufman RD. Relationship between esophageal temperature gradient and heart and lung sounds heard by esophageal stethoscope. Anesth Analg 1987; 66:1046–1048.

52. Horrow JC, Rosenberg H. Does urinary temperature reflect core temperature during cardiac surgery? Anesthesiology 1988; 69:986–989.

53. Bashein G, Nessly ML, Bledsoe SW, Townes BD, Davis KB, Coppel DB, Hornbein TF. Electroencephalography during surgery with cardiopulmonary bypass and hypothermia. Anesthesiology 1992; 76:878–891.

54. Pearcy WC, Virtue RW. The electroencephalogram in hypothermia with circulatory arrest. Anesthesiology 1959; 20:341–347.

55. Russ W, Kling D, Sauerwein G, Hempelmann G. Spectral analysis of the EEG during hypothermic cardiopulmonary bypass. Acta Anaesthesiol Scand 1987; 31:111–116.

56. Levy WJ. Quantitative analysis of EEG changes during hypothermia. Anesthesiology 1984; 60:291–297.

57. Doi M, Gajraj RJ, Mantzaridis H, Kenny GNC. Effects of

cardiopulmonary bypass and hypothermia on electroencephalographic variables. Anaesthesia 1997; 52:1048–1055.

58. Levy WJ, Pantin E, Mehta S, McGarvey M. Hypothermia and the approximate entropy of the electroencephalogram. Anesthesiology 2003; 98:53–57.

59. Stecker MM, Cheung AT, Pochettino A, Kent GP, Patterson T, Weiss SJ, Bavaria JE. Deep hypothermic circulatory arrest: I. Effects of cooling on electroencephalogram and evoked potentials. Ann Thorac Surg 2001; 7:14–21.

60. Markand ON, Warren C, Mallik GS, King RD, Brown JW, Mahomed Y. Effects of hypothermia on short latency somatosensory evoked potentials in humans. Electroencephalogr Clin Neurophysiol 1990; 77:416–424.

61. Markand ON, Warren C, Mallik GS, Williams CJ. Temperature-dependent hysteresis in somatosensory and auditory evoked potentials. Electroencephalogr Clin Neurophysiol 1990; 77:425–435.

62. Markand ON, Warren CH, Moorthy SS, Stoelting RK, King RD. Monitoring of multimodality evoked potentials during open heart surgery under hypothermia. Electroencephalogr Clin Neurophysiol 1984; 59:432–440.

63. Russ W, Sticher J, Scheld H, Hempelmann G. Effects of hypothermia on somatosensory evoked responses in man. Br J Anaesth 1987; 59:1484–1491.

64. Lang M, Welte M, Syben R, Hansen D. Effects of hypothermia on median nerve somatosensory evoked potentials during spontaneous circulation. J Neurosurg Anesth 2002; 14:141–145.

65. Reynolds PC, Antoine JA, Bettencourt J, Starck TW. Regional hypothermia affects somatosensory evoked potentials. Anesth Analg 1991; 73:653–656.

66. Rahn H, Reeves RB, Howell BJ. Hydrogen ion regulation, temperature, and evolution. Am Rev Respir Dis 1975; 112: 165–172.

67. Nattie EE. The alpha-stat hypothesis in respiratory control and acid–base balance. J Appl Physiol 1990; 69:1201–1207.

68. Malan A, Wilson TL, Reeves RB. Intracellular pH in cold-blooded vertebrates as a function of body temperature. Respir Physiol 1976; 28:29–47.

69. Reeves RB. An imidazole alphastat hypothesis for vertebrate acid–base regulation: tissue carbon dioxide content and body temperature in bullfrogs. Respir Physiol 1972; 14:219–236.

70. Andritsch RF, Muravchick S, Gold MI. Temperature correction of arterial blood–gas parameters: a comparative review of methodology. Anesthesiology 1981; 55:311–316.

71. Sitzwohl C, Kettner SC, Reinprecht A, Dietrich W, Klimscha W, Fridrich P, Sladen RN, Illievich UM. The arterial to end-tidal carbon dioxide gradient increases with uncorrected but not with temperature-corrected $PaCO_2$ determination during mild to moderate hypothermia. Anesth Analg 1998; 86:1131–1136.

72. Hansen D, Syben R, Vargas O, Spies C, Welte M. The alveolar–arterial difference in oxygen tension increases with temperature-corrected determination during moderate hypothermia. Anesth Analg 1999; 88:538–541.

73. Prough DS, Stump DA, Roy RC, Gravlee GP, Williams T, Mills SA, Hinshelwood L, Howard G. Response of cerebral blood flow to changes in carbon dioxide tension during hypothermic cardiopulmonary bypass. Anesthesiology 1986; 64:576–581.

74. Hindman BJ, Funatsu N, Harrington J, Cutkomp J, Dexter F, Todd MM, Tinker JH. Cerebral blood flow response to $PaCO_2$ during hypothermic cardiopulmonary bypass in rabbits. Anesthesiology 1991; 75:662–668.

75. Stephan H, Weyland A, Kazmaier S, Henze T, Menck S, Sonntag H. Acid–base management during hypothermic cardiopulmonary bypass does not affect cerebral metabolism but does affect blood flow and neurological outcome. Br J Anaesth 1992; 69:51–57.

76. Hindman BJ, Dexter F, Cutkomp J, Smith T, Tinker JH. Hypothermic acid–base management does not affect cerebral metabolic rate for oxygen ($CMRO_2$) at 27°C. A study during cardiopulmonary bypass in rabbits. Anesthesiology 1993; 79:580–587.

77. Patel RL, Turtle MR, Chambers DJ, James DN, Newman S, Venn GE. Alpha-stat acid–base regulation during cardiopulmonary bypass improves neuropsychologic outcome in patients undergoing coronary artery bypass grafting. J Thorac Cardiovasc Surg 1996; 111:1267–1279.

78. Murkin JM, Farrar JK, Tweed A, McKenzie FN, Guiraudon G. Cerebral autoregulation and flow/metabolism coupling during cardiopulmonary bypass: the influence of $PaCO_2$. Anesth Analg 1987; 66:825–832.

79. Verhaegen M, Todd MM, Hindman BJ, Warner DS. Cerebral autoregulation during moderate hypothermia. Stroke 1993; 24:407–414.

80. Nagai S, Irikura K, Maruyama S, Miyasaka Y. The significance of hypothermic acid–base management induced before ischemia in a rat model of transient middle cerebral artery occlusion. Neurol Res 1999; 21:204–208.

81. Kollmar R, Frietsch T, Georgiadis D, Schäbitz W-R, Waschke KF, Kuschinsky W, Schwab S. Early effects of acid–base management during hypothermia on cerebral infarct volume, edema, and cerebral blood flow in acute focal cerebral ischemia in rats. Anesthesiology 2002; 97:868–874.

82. Michenfelder JD, Uihlein A, Daw EF, Theye RA. Moderate hypothermia in man: haemodynamic and metabolic effects. Br J Anaesth 1965; 37:738–745.

83. Bacher A, Illievich UM, Fitzgerald R, Ihra G, Spiss CK. Changes in oxygenation variables during progressive hypothermia in anesthetized patients. J Neurosurg Anesth 1997; 9:205–210.

84. Dexter F, Hindman BJ. Theoretical analysis of cerebral venous blood hemoglobin oxygen saturation as an index of cerebral oxygenation during hypothermic cardiopulmonary bypass. A counterproposal to the "luxury perfusion" hypothesis. Anesthesiology 1995; 83:405–412.

85. Stayer SA, Steven JM, Nicolson SC, Jobes DR, Stanley C, Baumgart S. The metabolic effects of surface cooling neonates prior to cardiac surgery. Anesth Analg 1994; 79:834–839.

86. Gunton RW, Scott JW, Lougheed WM, Botterell EH. Changes

in cardiac rhythm and in the form of the electrocardiogram resulting from induced hypothermia in man. Am Heart J 1956; 52:419–429.

87. Hicks CE, McCord MC, Blount SG Jr. Electrocardiographic changes during hypothermia and circulatory occlusion. Circulation 1956; 13:21–28.

88. Fleming PR, Muir FH. Electrocardiographic changes in induced hypothermia in man. Br Heart J 1957; 19:59–66.

89. Emslie-Smith D, Sladden GE, Stirling GR. The significance of changes in the electrocardiogram in hypothermia. Br Heart J 1959; 21:343–351.

90. Schwab RH, Lewis DW, Killough JH, Templeton JY III. Electrocardiographic changes occurring in rapidly induced deep hypothermia. Am J Med Sci 1964; 248:290–303.

91. Vassallo SU, Delaney KA, Hoffman RS, Slater W, Goldfrank LR. A prospective evaluation of the electrocardiographic manifestations of hypothermia. Acad Emerg Med 1999; 6: 1121–1126.

92. Okada M. The cardiac rhythm in accidental hypothermia. Electrocardiology 1984; 17:123–128.

93. Swan H. Clinical hypothermia: a lady with a past and some promise for the future. Surgery 1973; 73:736–758.

94. Swain JA, White FN, Peters RM. The effect of pH on the hypothermic ventricular fibrillation threshold. J Thorac Cardiovasc Surg 1984; 87:445–451.

95. Kroncke GM, Nichols RD, Mendenhall JT, Myerowitz PD, Starling JR. Ectothermic philosophy of acid–base balance of prevent fibrillation during hypothermia. Arch Surg 1986; 121:303–304.

96. Ohmura A, Wong KC, Westenskow DR, Shaw CL. Effects of hypocarbia and normocarbia on cardiovascular dynamics and regional circulation in the hypothermic dog. Anesthesiology 1979; 50:293–298.

97. Kuwagata Y, Oda J, Ninomiya N, Shiozaki T, Shimazu T, Sugimoto H. Changes in left ventricular performance in patients with severe head injury during and after mild

hypothermia. J Trauma Inj Infect Crit Care 1999; 47:666–672.

98. Lewis ME, Al-Khalidi A-H, Townend JN, Coote J, Bonser RS. The effects of hypothermia on human left ventricular contractile function during cardiac surgery. J Am Coll Cardiol 2002; 39:102–108.
99. Frank SM, Cattaneo CG, Wieneke-Brady MB, El-Rahmany H, Gupta N, Lima JAC, Goldstein DS. Threshold for adrenomedullary activation and increased cardiac work during mild core hypothermia. Clin Sci 2002; 102:119–125.
100. Breslow MJ, Parker SD, Frank SM, Norris EJ, Yates H, Raff H, Rock P, Christopherson R, Brosenfeld BA, Beattie C. Determinants of catecholamine and cortisol responses to lower extremity revascularization. Anesthesiology 1993; 79:1202–1209.
101. Frank SM, Higgins MS, Breslow MJ, Fleisher LA, Gorman RB, Sitzmann JV, Raff H, Beattie C. The catecholamine, cortisol, and hemodynamic responses to mild perioperative hypothermia. Anesthesiology 1995; 82:83–93.
102. Chi OZ, Choi YK, Lee DI, Kim YS, Lee I. Intraoperative mild hypothermia does not increase the plasma concentration of stress hormones during neurosurgery. Can J Anaesth 2001; 48:815–818.
103. Leslie K, Sessler DI, Bjorksten AR, Moayeri A. Mild hypothermia alters propofol pharmacokinetics and increases the duration of action of atracurium. Anesth Analg 1995; 80:1007–1014.
104. Russell D, Royston D, Rees PH, Gupta SK, Kenny GN. Effect of temperature and cardiopulmonary bypass on the pharmacokinetics of remifentanil. Br J Anaesth 1997; 79:456–459.
105. Michelsen LG, Holford NH, Lu W, Hoke JF, Hug CC, Bailey JM. The pharmacokinetics of remifentanil in patients undergoing coronary artery bypass grafting with cardiopulmonary bypass. Anesth Analg 2001; 93:1100–1105.
106. Beaufort AM, Wierda JMKH, Belopavlovic M, Nederveen PJ, Kleef UW, Agoston S. The influence of hypothermia (surface cooling) on the time–course of action and on the pharmaco-

kinetics of rocuronium in humans. Eur J Anaesth 1995; 12(suppl 11):95–106.

107. Caldwell JE, Heier T, Wright PMC, Lin S, McCarthy G, Szenohradszky J, Sharma ML, Hing JP, Schroeder M, Sessler DI. Temperature-dependent pharmacokinetics and pharmacodynamics of vecuronium. Anesthesiology 2000; 92:84–93.

108. Heier T, Clough D, Wright PM, Sharma ML, Sessler DI, Caldwell JE. The influence of mild hypothermia on the pharmacokinetics and time course of action of neostigmine in anesthetized volunteers. Anesthesiology 2002; 97:90–95.

109. Heier T, Caldwell JE, Sessler DI, Kitts JB, Miller RD. The relationship between adductor pollicis twitch tension and core, skin, and muscle temperature during nitrous oxide-isoflurane anesthesia in humans. Anesthesiology 1989; 71:381–384.

110. Heier T, Caldwell JE, Sessler DI, Miller RD. The effect of local surface and central cooling on adductor pollicis twitch tension during nitrous oxide/isoflurane and nitrous oxide/fentanyl anesthesia in humans. Anesthesiology 1990; 72:807–811.

111. Young ML, Hanson CW 3rd, Bloom MJ, Savino JS, Muravchick S. Localized hypothermia influences assessment of recovery from vecuronium neuromuscular blockade. Can J Anaesth 1994; 41:1172–1177.

112. Polderman KH, Peerdeman SM, Girbes ARJ. Hypophosphatemia and hypomagnesemia induced by cooling in patients with severe head injury. J Neurosurg 2001; 94:697–705.

113. Curry DL, Curry KP. Hypothermia and insulin secretion. Endocrinology 1970; 87:750–755.

114. Bernard SA, Gray TW, Buist MD, Jones BM, Silvester W, Gutteridge G, Smith K. Treatment of comatose survivors of out-of-hospital cardiac arrest with induced hypothermia. N Eng J Med 2002; 346:557–563.

115. Coniam SW. Accidental hypothermia. Anaesthesia 1979; 34:250–256.

116. Metz C, Holzschuh M, Bein T, Woertgen C, Frey A, Frey I, Taeger K, Brawanski A. Moderate hypothermia in patients with severe head injury: cerebral and extracerebral effects. J Neurosurg 1996; 85:533–541.

117. Shiozaki T, Hayakata T, Taneda M, Nakajima Y, Hashiguchi N, Fujimi S, Nakamori Y, Tanaka H, Shimazu T, Sugimoto H. A multicenter prospective randomized controlled trial of the efficacy of mild hypothermia for severely head injured patients with low intracranial pressure. J Neurosurg 2001; 94:50–54.

118. Schwab S, Schwarz S, Spranger M, Keller E, Bertram M, Hacke W. Moderate hypothermia in the treatment of patients with severe middle cerebral artery infarction. Stroke 1998; 29:2461–2466.

119. Steiner T, Friede T, Aschoff A, Schellinger PD, Schwab S, Hacke W. Effect and feasibility of controlled rewarming after moderate hypothermia in stroke patients with malignant infarction of the middle cerebral artery. Stroke 2001; 32:2833–2835.

120. Georgiadis D, Schwarz S, Kollmar R, Schwab S. Endovascular cooling for moderate hypothermia in patients with acute stroke. First results of a novel approach. Stroke 2001; 32:2550–2553.

121. Dae MW, Gao DW, Sessler DI, Chair K, Stillson CA. Effect of endovascular cooling on myocardial temperature, infarct size, and cardiac output in human-sized pigs. Am J Physiol (Heart Circ Physiol) 2002; 282:H1584–H1591.

122. Dixon SR, Whitbourn RJ, Dae MW, Grube E, Sherman W, Schaer GL, Jenkins S, Baim DS, Gibbons RJ, Kuntz RE, Popma JJ, Nguyen TT, O'Neill WW. Induction of mild systemic hypothermia with endovascular cooling during primary percutaneous coronary intervention for acute myocardial infarction. J Am Coll Cardiol 2002; 40:1928–1934.

123. Doufas AG, Akça O, Barry A, Petrusca DA, Suleman M-I, Morioka N, Guarnaschelli JJ, Sessler DI. Initial experience with a novel heat-exchanging catheter in neurosurgical patients. Anesth Analg 2002; 95:1752–1756.

124. Schmutzhard E, Engelhardt K, Beer R, Brössner G, Pfausler B, Spiss H, Unterberger I, Kampfl A. Safety and efficacy of a novel intravascular cooling device to control body temperature in neurologic intensive care patients: a prospective pilot study. Crit Care Med 2002; 30:2481–2488.

125. Somanathan S. Anaesthesia and hypothermia in sickle cell disease. Anaesthesia 1976; 31:113.

126. Heiner M, Teasdale SJ, David T, Scott AA, Glynn MFX. Aorta-coronary bypass in a patient with sickle cell trait. Can Anaesth Soc J 1979; 26:428–434.

127. Fox MA, Abbott TR. Hypothermic cardiopulmonary bypass in a patient with sickle-cell trait. Anaesthesia 1984; 39:1121–1123.

128. Baxter MRN, Bevan JC, Esseltine DW, Bernstein M. The management of two pediatric patients with sickle cell trait and sickle cell disease during cardiopulmonary bypass. J Cardiothorac Anesth 1989; 3:477–480.

129. Ohashi Y, Akamatsu T, Hirata T, Uchida O, Kuro M. Cardiac surgery using cardiopulmonary bypass in a patient with sickle-cell trait. Jpn J Anesth 1996; 45:1269–1271.

130. Sessler DI. Perioperative heat balance. Anesthesiology 2000; 92:578–596.

131. Vassilieff N, Rosencher N, Sessler DI, Conseiller C, Lienhart A. Nifedipine and intraoperative core body temperature in humans. Anesthesiology 1994; 80:123–128.

132. Ikeda T, Ozaki M, Sessler DI, Kazama T, Ikeda K, Sato S. Intraoperative phenylephrine infusion decreases the magnitude of redistribution hypothermia. Anesth Analg 1999; 89:462–465.

133. Plattner O, Kurz A, Sessler DI, Ikeda T, Christensen R, Marder D, Clough D. Efficacy of intraoperative cooling methods. Anesthesiology 1997; 87:1089–1095.

134. Stanley TO, Grocott HP, Phillips-Bute B, Mathew JP, Landolfo KP, Newman MF. Preliminary evaluation of the arctic sun temperature-controlling system during off-pump coronary artery bypass surgery. Ann Thorac Surg 2003; 75:1140–1144.

135. Kurz A, Sessler DI, Birnbauer F, Illievich UM, Spiss CK. Thermoregulatory vasoconstriction impairs active core cooling. Anesthesiology 1995; 82:870–876.

136. Kurz A, Plattner O, Sessler DI, Huemer G, Redl G, Lackner

F. The threshold for thermoregulatory vasoconstriction during nitrous oxide/isoflurane anesthesia is lower in elderly than in young patients. Anesthesiology 1993; 79:465–469.

137. Lopez M, Sessler DI, Walter K, Emerick T, Ozaki M. Rate and gender dependence of the sweating, vasoconstriction, and shivering thresholds in humans. Anesthesiology 1994; 80:780–788.

138. Cheng C, Matsukawa T, Sessler DI, Ozaki M, Kurz A, Merrifield B, Lin H, Olofsson P. Increasing mean skin temperature linearly reduces the core-temperature thresholds for vasoconstriction and shivering in humans. Anesthesiology 1995; 82:1160–1168.

139. Kurz A, Sessler DI, Annadata R, Dechert M, Christensen R, Bjorksten AR. Midazolam minimally impairs thermoregularoy control. Anal Analg 1995; 8:393–398.

140. Matsukawa T, Kurz A, Sessler DI, Bjorksten AR, Merrifield B, Cheng C. Propofol linearly reduces the vasoconstriction and shivering thresholds. Anesthesiology 1995; 82:1169–1180.

141. Kurz A, Go JC, Sessler DI, Kaer K, Larson MD, Bjorksten AR. Alfentanil slightly increases the sweating threshold and markedly reduces the vasoconstriction and shivering thresholds. Anesthesiology 1995; 83:293–299.

142. Talke P, Tayefeh F, Sessler DI, Jeffrey R, Noursalehi M, Richardson C. Dexmedetomidine does not alter the sweating threshold, but comparably and linearly decreases the vasoconstriction and shivering thresholds. Anesthesiology 1997; 87:835–841.

143. Kurz A, Ikeda T, Sessler DI, Larson MD, Bjorksten AR, Dechert M, Christensen R. Meperidine decreases the shivering threshold twice as much as the vasoconstriction threshold. Anesthesiology 1997; 86:1046–1054.

144. Xiong J, Kurz A, Sessler DI, Plattner O, Christensen R, Dechert M, Ikeda T. Isoflurane produces marked and nonlinear decreases in the vasoconstriction and shivering thresholds. Anesthesiology 1996; 85:240–245.

145. Annadata R, Sessler DI, Tayefeh F, Kurz A, Dechert M. Desflurane slightly increases the sweating threshold but

produces marked, nonlinear decreases in the vasoconstriction and shivering thresholds. Anesthesiology 1995; 83:1205–1211.

146. Goto T, Matsukawa T, Sessler DI, Uezono S, Ishiguro Y, Ozaki M, Morita S. Thermoregulatory thresholds for vasoconstriction in patients anesthetized with various 1-minimum alveolar concentration combinations of xenon, nitrous oxide, and isoflurane. Anesthesiology 1999; 91:626–632.

147. Sessler DI, Olofsson CI, Rubinstein EH. The thermoregulatory threshold in humans during nitrous oxide-fentanyl anesthesia. Anesthesiology 1988; 69:357–364.

148. Iwata T, Inoue S, Kawaguchi M, Takahashi M, Sakamoto T, Kitaguchi K, Furuya H, Sakaki T. Comparison of the effects of sevoflurane and propofol on cooling and rewarming during deliberate mild hypothermia for neurosurgery. Br J Anaesth 2003; 90:32–38.

149. Inoue S, Kawaguchi M, Sakamoto T, Kitaguchi K, Furuya H, Sakaki T. High-dose amrinone is required to accelerate rewarming from deliberate mild intraoperative hypothermia for neurosurgical procedures. Anesthesiology 2001; 97:116–123.

150. Kurz A, Sessler DI, Narzt E, Lenhardt R, Lackner F. Morphometric influences on intraoperative core temperature changes. Anesth Analg 1995; 80:562–567.

151. Théard MA, Tempelhoff R, Crowder CM, Cheng MA, Todorov A, Dacey RG Jr. Convection versus conduction cooling for induction of mild hypothermia during neurovascular procedures in adults. J Neurosurg Anesth 1997; 9:250–255.

152. Baumgardner JE, Baranov D, Smith DS, Zager EL. The effectiveness of rapidly infused intravenous fluids for inducing moderate hypothermia in neurosurgical patients. Anesth Analg 1999; 89:163–169.

153. Rajek A, Greif R, Sessler DI, Baumgardner J, Laciny S, Bastanmehr H. Core cooling by central venous infusion of ice-cold (4°C and 20°C) fluid. Isolation of core and peripheral thermal compartments. Anesthesiology 2000; 93:629–637.

154. Ozaki M, Sessler DI, McGuire J, Blanchard D, Schroeder M, Moayeri A. The direction dependence of thermoregulatory

vasoconstriction during isoflurane/epidural anesthesia in humans. Anesth Analg 1993; 77:811–816.

155. Szmuk P, Rabb MF, Baumgartner JE, Berry JM, Sessler AM, Sessler DI. Body morphology and the speed of cutaneous rewarming. Anesthesiology 2001; 95:18–21.

156. Hynson JM, Sessler DI. Intraoperative warming therapies: a comparison of three devices. J Clin Anesth 1992; 4:194–199.

157. Goheen MSL, Ducharme MB, Kenny GP, Johnston CE, Frim J, Bristow GK, Giesbrecht GG. Efficacy of forced-air and inhalation rewarming by using a human model for severe hypothermia. J Appl Physiol 1997; 83:1635–1640.

158. Crino MH, Nagel EL. Thermal burns caused by warming blankets in the operating room. Anesthesiology 1968; 29:149–150.

159. Sadove RC, Furgasen TG. Major thermal burn as a result of intraoperative heating blanket use. J Burn Care Rehabil 1992; 13:443–445.

160. Cheney FW, Posner KL, Caplan RA, Gild WM. Burns for warming devices in anesthesia. A closed claims analysis. Anesthesiology 1994; 80:806–810.

161. Acikel C, Kale B, Celikoz B. Major thermal burn due to intraoperative heating blanket malfunction. Burns 2002; 28:283–284.

162. Rosenfield LK, Pitlyk PJ. Intraoperative burns secondary to warming IV bags: a warning. Anesthesiology 1999; 90:616–618.

163. Anonymous. Augustine Medical Bair Hugger patient warming systems models 200 and 250. Health Devices 1990; 19:373.

164. Anonymous. Hazard Report: misusing forced-air hyperthermia units can burn patients. Health Devices 1999; 28:229–230.

165. Azzam FJ, Krock JL. Thermal burns in two infants associated with a forced air warming system. Anesth Analg 1995; 81: 654.

166. Truell KD, Bakerman PR, Teodori MF, Maze A. Third degree burns due to intraoperative use of a Bair Hugger warming device. Ann Thorac Surg 2000; 69:1933–1934.

167. Rosa G, Pinto G, Orsi P, De Blasi RA, Conti G, Sanitá R, La Rosa I, Gasperetto A. Control of post anaesthetic shivering with nefopam hydrochloride in mildly hypothermic patients after neurosurgery. Acta Anaesthesiol Scand 1995; 39:90–95.

168. Mekjavic IB, Eiken O. Inhibition of shivering in man by thermal stimulation of the facial area. Acta Physiol Scand 1985; 125:633–637.

169. Iaizzo PA, Jeon YM, Sigg DC. Facial warming increases the threshold for shivering. J Neurosurg Anesth 1999; 11:231–239.

170. Sweney MT, Sigg DC, Tahvildari S, Iaizzo PA. Shiver suppression using focal hand warming in unanesthetized normal subjects. Anesthesiology 2001; 95:1089–1095.

171. De Witte J, Sessler DI. Perioperative shivering. Anesthesiology 2002; 96:467–484.

172. Horn E-P, Standl T, Sessler DI, von Knobelsdorff G, Büchs C, Schulte am Esch J. Physostigmine prevents postanesthetic shivering as does meperidine or clonidine. Anesthesiology 1998; 88:108–113.

173. Dodson ME, Fryer JM. Postoperative effects of methylphenidate. Br J Anaesth 1980; 52:1265–1270.

174. Mokhtarani M, Mahgoub AN, Morioka N, Doufas AG, Dae M, Shaughnessy TE, Bjorksten AR, Sessler DI. Buspirone and meperidine synergistically reduce the shivering threshold. Anesth Analg 2001; 93:1233–1239.

175. Karibe H, Sato K, Shimizu H, Tominaga T, Koshu K, Yoshimoto T. Intraoperative mild hypothermia ameliorates postoperative cerebral blood flow impairment in patients with aneurysmal subarachnoid hemorrhage. Neurosurgery 2000; 47:594–599.

176. Lenhardt R, Marker E, Goll V, Tschernich H, Kurz A, Sessler DI, Narzt E, Lackner F. Mild intraoperative hypothermia prolongs postanesthesia recovery. Anesthesiology 1997; 87:1318–1323.

177. Kassell NF, Torner JC, Haley EC, Jane JA, Adams JP, Kongable GL. The international cooperative study on the timing of aneurysm surgery. Part 1: Overall management results. J Neurosurg 1990; 73:18–36.

178. Nathan HJ, Lavallee G. The management of temperature during hypothermic cardiopulmonary bypass: I—Canadian survey. Can J Anaesth 1995; 42:669–671.

179. Bashein G, Townes BD, Nessly ML, Bledsoe SW, Hornbein TF, Davis KB, Goldstein DE, Coppel DB. A randomized study of carbon dioxide management during hypothermic cardiopulmonary bypass. Anesthesiology 1990; 72:7–15.

180. Murkin JM, Martzke JS, Buchan AM, Bentley C, Wong CJ. A randomized study of the influence of perfusion technique and pH management strategy in 316 patients undergoing coronary artery bypass surgery. II. Neurologic and cognitive outcomes. J Thorac Cardiovasc Surg 1995; 110:349–362.

181. Engelhardt W, Dierks T, Pause M, Hartung E. Early cerebral functional outcome after coronary artery bypass surgery using different acid–base management during hypothermic cardiopulmonary bypass. Acta Anaesthesiol Scand 1996; 40:457–465.

182. The Warm Heart Investigators. Randomised trial of normothermic versus hypothermic coronary bypass surgery. Lancet 1994; 343:559–563.

183. McLean RF, Wong BI, Naylor CD, Snow WG, Harrington EM, Gawel M, Fremes SE. Cardiopulmonary bypass, temperature, and central nervous system dysfunction. Circulation 1994; 90:II-250–II-255. Part 2.

184. Martin TD, Craver JM, Gott JP, Weintraub WS, Ramsay J, Mora CT, Guyton RA. Prospective, randomized trial of retrograde warm blood cardioplegia: myocardial benefit and neurologic threat. Ann Thorac Surg 1994; 57:298–304.

185. Mora CT, Henson MB, Weintraub WS, Murkin JM, Martin TD, Craver JM, Gott JP, Guyton RA. The effect of temperature management during cardiopulmonary bypass on neurologic and neuropsychologic outcomes in patients undergoing coronary revascularization. J Thorac Cardiovasc Surg 1996; 112:514–522.

186. Regragui I, Birdi I, Izzat MB, Black AMS, Lopatatzidis A, Day CJE, Gardner F, Bryan AJ, Angelini GD. The effects of cardiopulmonary bypass temperature on neuropsychologic outcome after coronary artery operations: a prospective ran-

domized trial. J Thorac Cardiovasc Surg 1996; 112:1036–1045.

187. Engelman RM, Pleet AB, Rousou JA, Flack JE, Deaton DW, Gregory CA, Pekow PS. What is the best perfusion temperature for coronary revascularization? J Thorac Cardiovasc Surg 1996; 112:1622–1633.

188. Plourde G, Leduc AS, Morin JE, De Varennes B, Latter D, Symes J, Robbins R, Fosset N, Couture L, Ptito A. Temperature during cardiopulmonary bypass for coronary artery operations does not influence postoperative cognitive function: a prospective, randomized trial. J Thorac Cardiovasc Surg 1997; 114:123–128.

189. Grimm M, Czerny M, Baumer H, Kilo J, Madl C, Kramer L, Rajek A, Wolner E. Normothermic cardiopulmonary bypass is beneficial for cognitive brain function after coronary artery bypass grafting—a prospective randomized trial. Eur J Cardiothorac Surg 2000; 18:270–275.

190. Grigore AM, Mathew J, Grocott HP, Reves JG, Blumenthal JA, White WD, Smith PK, Jones RH, Kirchner JL, Mark DB, Newman MF. A prospective randomized trial of normothemic versus hypothermic cardiopulmonary bypass on cognitive function after coronary artery bypass graft surgery. Anesthesiology 2001; 95:1110–1119.

191. Minamisawa H, Smith M-L, Siesjö BK. The effect of mild hyperthermia and hypothermia on brain damage following 5, 10, and 15 minutes of forebrain ischemia. Ann Neurol 1990; 28:26–33.

192. Dietrich WD, Busto R, Valdes I, Loor Y. Effects of normothermic versus mild hyperthermic forebrain ischemia in rats. Stroke 1990; 21:1318–1325.

193. Dietrich WD, Alonso O, Halley M, Busto R. Delayed posttraumatic brain hyperthermia worsens outcome after fluid percussion brain injury: a light and electron microscopic study in rats. Neurosurgery 1996; 38:533–541.

194. Stocchetti N, Paparella A, Bridelli F, Bacchi M, Piazza P, Zuccoli P. Cerebral venous oxygen saturation studied with bilateral samples in the internal jugular veins. Neurosurgery 1994; 34:38–44.

195. Croughwell N, Smith LR, Quill T, Newman M, Greeley W, Kern F, Lu J, Reves JG. The effect of temperature on cerebral metabolism and blood flow in adults during cardiopulmonary bypass. J Thorac Cardiovasc Surg 1992; 103:549–554.

196. Cook DJ, Oliver WC, Orszulak TA, Daly RC. A prospective, randomized comparison of cerebral venous oxygen saturation during normothermic and hypothermic cardiopulmonary bypass. J Thorac Cardiovasc Surg 1994; 107:1020–1029.

197. Endoh H, Shimoji K. Changes in blood flow velocity in the middle cerebral artery during nonpulsatile hypothermic cardiopulmonary bypass. Stroke 1994; 25:403–407.

198. Nakajima T, Kuro M, Hayaski Y, Kitaguchi K, Uchida O, Takaki O. Clinical evaluation of cerebral oxygen balance during cardiopulmonary bypass: on-line continuous monitoring of jugular venous oxyhemoglobin saturation. Anesth Analg 1992; 74:630–635.

199. Kiziltan HT, Baltali M, Bilen A, Seydaoglu G, Incesoz M, Tasdelen A, Aslamaci S. Comparison of alpha-stat and pH-stat cardiopulmonary bypass in relation to jugular venous oxygen saturation and cerebral glucose–oxygen utilization. Anesth Analg 2003; 96:644–650.

200. Croughwell ND, Frasco P, Blumenthal JA, Leone BJ, White WD, Reves JG. Warming during cardiopulmonary bypass is associated with jugular bulb desaturation. Ann Thorac Surg 1992; 53:827–832.

201. Croughwell ND, Newman MF, Blumenthal JA, White WD, Lewis JB, Frasco PE, Smith LR, Thyrum EA, Hurwitz BJ, Leone BJ, Schell RM, Reves JG. Jugular bulb saturation and cognitive dysfunction after cardiopulmonary bypass. Ann Thorac Surg 1994; 58:1702–1708.

202. van der Linden J, Ekroth R, Lincoln C, Pugsley W, Scallan M, Tyden H. Is cerebral blood flow/metabolic mismatch during rewarming a risk factor after profound hypothermic procedures in small children? Eur J Cardio-thorac Surg 1989; 3:209–215.

203. Cook DJ, Orszulak TA, Daly RC, Buda DA. Cerebral hyperthermia during cardiopulmonary bypass in adults. J Thorac Cardiovasc Surg 1996; 111:268–269.

204. Newman MF, Croughwell ND, Blumenthal JA, White WD, Lewis JB, Smith LR, Frasco P, Towner EA, Schell RM, Hurwitz BJ, Reves JG. Effect of aging on cerebral autoregulation during cardiopulmonary bypass. Association with postoperative cognitive dysfunction. Circulation 1994; 90:II-243–II-249. Part 2.

205. Goto T, Yoshitake A, Baba T, Shibata Y, Sakata R, Uozumi H. Cerebral ischemic disorders and cerebral oxygen balance during cardiopulmonary bypass surgery: preoperative evaluation using magnetic resonance imaging and angiography. Anesth Analg 1997; 84:5–11.

206. Newman MF, Kramer D, Croughwell ND, Sanderson I, Blumenthal JA, White WD, Smith LR, Towner EA, Reves JG. Differential age effects of mean arterial pressure and rewarming on cognitive dysfunction after cardiac surgery. Anesth Analg 1995; 81:236–242.

207. Robson MJA, Alston RP, Deary IJ, Andrews PJD, Souter MJ, Yates S. Cognition after coronary artery surgery is not related to postoperative jugular bulb oxyhemoglobin desaturation. Anesth Analg 2000; 91:1317–1326.

208. Buss MI, McLean RF, Wong BI, Fremes SE, Naylor CD, Harrington EM, Snow WG, Gawel M. Cardiopulmonary bypass, rewarming, and central nervous system dysfunction. Ann Thorac Surg 1996; 61:1423–1427.

209. Enomoto S, Hindman BJ, Dexter F, Smith T, Cutkomp J. Rapid rewarming causes an increase in the cerebral metabolic rate for oxygen that is temporarily unmatched by cerebral blood flow: a study during cardiopulmonary bypass in rabbits. Anesthesiology 1996; 84:1392–1400.

210. Nakamura T, Miyamoto O, Yamagami S-I, Hayashida Y, Itano T, Nagao S. Influence of rewarming conditions after hypothermia in gerbils with transient forebrain ischemia. J Neurosurg 1999; 91:114–120.

211. Ogura K, Takayasu M, Dacey RG. Effects of hypothermia and hyperthermia on the reactivity of rat intracerebral arterioles in vitro. J Neurosurg 1991; 75:433–439.

212. Sagher O, Huang D-L, Webb RC. Induction of hypercontractility in human arteries by rewarming following hypothermia:

a possible role for tyrosine kinase. J Neurosurg 1997; 87:431–435.

213. Grigore AM, Grocott HP, Mathew JP, Phillips-Bute B, Stanley TO, Butler A, Landolfo KP, Reves JG, Blumenthal JA, Newman MF. Rewarming rate affects neurocognitive dysfunction after cardiac surgery. Anesth Analg 2002; 94:4–10.

214. Nathan HJ, Wells GA, Munson JL, Wozny D. Neuroprotective effect of mild hypothermia in patients undergoing coronary artery surgery with cardiopulmonary bypass. A randomized trial. Circulation 2001; 104(suppl I):I-85–91.

215. Azzimondi G, Bassein L, Nonino F, Fiorani L, Vignatelli L, Re G, D'Alessandro R. Fever in acute stroke worsens prognosis. A prospective study. Stroke 1995; 26:2040–2043.

216. Reith J, Jørgensen HS, Pedersen PM, Nakayama H, Raaschou HO, Jeppesen LL, Olsen TS. Body temperature in acute stroke: relation to stroke severity, infarct size, mortality, and outcome. Lancet 1996; 347:422–425.

217. Kammersgaard LP, Jørgensen HS, Rungby JA, Reith J, Nakayama H, Weber UJ, Houth J, Olsen TS. Admission body temperature predicts long-term mortality after acute stroke. The Copenhagen stroke study. Stroke 2002; 33:1759–1762.

218. Wang Y, Lim LL-Y, Levi C, Heller RF, Fisher J. Influence of admission body temperature on stroke mortality. Stroke 2000; 31:404–409.

219. Bissonnette B, Holtby MH, Davis AJ, Pua H, Gilder FJ, Black M. Cerebral hyperthermia in children after cardiopulmonary bypass. Anesthesiology 2000; 93:611–618.

220. Thong WY, Strickler AG, Li S, Stewart EE, Collier CL, Vaughn WK, Nussmeier NA. Hyperthermia in the forty-eight hours after cardiopulmonary bypass. Anesth Analg 2002; 95:1489–1495.

221. Grocott HP, Mackensen GB, Grigore AM, Mathew J, Reves JG, Phillips-Bute B, Smith PK, Newman MF. Postoperative hyperthermia is associated with cognitive dysfunction after coronary artery bypass graft surgery. Stroke 2002; 33:537–541.

222. Kader A, Brisman MH, Maraire N, Huh JT, Solomon RA. The

effect of mild hypothermia on permanent focal ischemia in the rat. Neurosurgery 1992; 31:1056–1061.

223. Morikawa E, Ginsberg MD, Dietrich WD, Duncan RC, Kraydieh S, Globus MYT, Busto R. The significance of brain temperature in focal cerebral ischemia: histopathological consequences of middle cerebral artery occlusion in the rat. J Cereb Blood Flow Metab 1992; 12:380–389.

224. Hogue CW Jr, Murphy SF, Schechtman KB, Dávila-Román VG. Risk factors for early or delayed stroke after cardiac surgery. Circulation 1999; 100:642–647.

225. Nierich AP, Diephuis J, Jansen EWL, van Dijk D, Lahpor JR, Borst C, Knape JTA. Embracing the heart: perioperative management of patients undergoing off-pump coronary artery bypass grafting using the octopus tissue stabilizer. J Cardiothorac Vasc Anesth 1999; 13:123–129.

226. Mack M, Bachand D, Acuff T, Edgerton J, Prince S, Dewey T, Magee M. Improved outcomes in coronary artery bypass grafting with beating heart techniques. J Thorac Cardiovasc Surg 2002; 124:598–607.

227. International Subarachnoid Aneurysm Trial (ISAT) Collaborative Group. International Subarachnoid Aneurysm Trial (ISAT) of neurosurgical clipping versus endovascular coiling in 2143 patients with ruptured intracranial aneurysms: a randomised trial. Lancet 2002; 360:1267–1274.

228. Clifton GL, Miller ER, Choi SC, Levin HS, McCauley S, Smith KR, Muizelaar JP, Wagner FC, Marion DW, Luerssen TG, Chesnut RM, Schwartz M. Lack of effect of induction of hypothermia after acute brain injury. N Engl J Med 2001; 344:556–563.

229. The Hypothermia after Cardiac Arrest Study Group. Mild therapeutic hypothermia to improve the neurologic outcome after cardiac arrest. N Engl J Med 2002; 346:549–556.

230. Gladstone DJ, Black SE, Hakim AM. Toward wisdom from failure. Lessons from neuroprotective stroke trials and new therapeutic directions. Stroke 2002; 33:2123–2136.

Appendix

Columbia University Medical Center

Hypothypothermia Protocol
(Target Temperature 33°C)

INDICATIONS:
A. Hypoxic-ischemic brain injury after cardiac arrest
B. Elevated intracranial pressure
C. Large hemispheric ischemic stroke
D. Severe traumatic brain injury

1. **Admit to ICU**
2. **Diagnosis:** ______________
3. **Condition:** Critical
4. **Allergies:** ______________
5. **Activity:** Bedrest with the head of bed at 30 degrees
6. **Diet:** NPO for 48 hours
7. **Vitals:** q 15 minutes for one hour, then q 1 hour, including assessments for shivering

8. **Nursing:**
   a. Place Foley catheter with thermistor (YSI 400 series) and connect to cooling device
   b. Palpate masseter and pectoralis muscles q 1 h to assess for shivering

9. **Labs:** Basic Metabolic Panel, Complete Blood Count, PT/PTT, Ionized Calcium, Arterial Blood Gas, Lactate, Troponin I, Creatine Kinase, and Amylase at admission, 12 hours, 24 hours and 48 hours.

10. **Arterial line** for BP monitoring

11. **Initiate cooling device** (specify device________) set to **AUTOMATIC mode** to maintain patient temperature at **33° Celsius** for 24 hours after patient reaches target temperature. *Mark time that patient attained T = 33°C on nursing flow sheet.*

12. **IV fluids:** Normal saline at 1 mL/kg/hr:_________ mL/hr

13. **Ventilator Settings:** cool air to 30° Celsius, Assist Control rate_______, TV_______, FiO_2_______%, PEEP_______cm H_2O

14. **Medications:**
   a. Fentanyl 4 mg/250 mL 0.9% saline IV (starting at 25–50 mcg/kg/min), titrate to quiet motionless state and/or to prevent shivering.
   b. Meperidine 50–100 mg IV q 1 hour PRN shivering
   c. Vecuronium 0.1 mg/kg IVP q 1 hour for shivering refractory to meperidine PRN
   d. Norepinephrine 4 mg/250NS IV, titrate to maintain MAP / CPP (circle one) > ____ mm Hg
   e. Pantoprazole 40 mg IVSS qd
   f. Regular human insulin (100 U/100 mL) titrate to maintain blood glucose between 100–125 mg/dl.
   g. Enoxaparin 30 mg SC q12 hours
   h. Potassium 10 mEq/100 mL normal saline ×4 runs for K^+ ≤3.4 mEq/L

15. **Controlled Rewarming:** 24 hours after attaining temperature <33°C, begin controlled rewarming to target temperature of 37°C over 12 hours. *Set maximal device water temperature to 34°C, the rewarming target temperature to 37°C, then set the warming rate to 0.3°C per hour.* Keep the cooling device on to maintain body temperature at 37°C for 24 hours after the target temperature of 37°C is attained.

16. **Call MD for:**
    a. Uncontrolled shivering
    b. HR <50 or >110 BPM
    c. SBP <80 mmHg or >180 mmHg
    d. If cooling device water temperature drops below 8°C after target temperature has been attained (to indicate febrile response).

Index